Focus on
PHARMACOLOGY

ESSENTIALS FOR HEALTH PROFESSIONALS

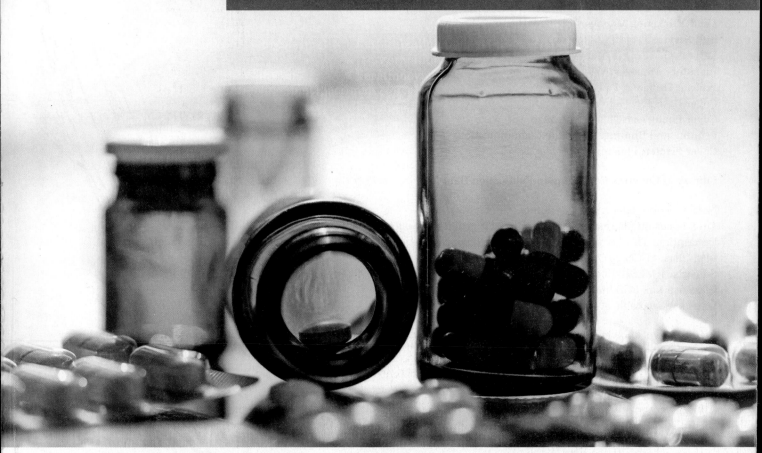

Jahangir **Moini**, MD, MPH

Professor of Science and Health, Eastern Florida State College

 Pearson

330 Hudson Street, NY NY 10013

Vice President, Health Science and TED: Julie Levin Alexander
Director of Portfolio Management: Marlene McHugh Pratt
Portfolio Manager: Derril Trakalo
Development Editor: Joan Gill
Portfolio Management Assistant: Emily Edling
Vice President, Content Production and Digital Studio: Paul DeLuca
Managing Producer, Health Science: Melissa Bashe
Content Producer: Faye Gemmellaro
Project Monitor: Meghan DeMaio
Operations Specialist: Mary Ann Gloriande
Creative Director: Blair Brown
Creative Digital Lead: Mary Siener
Vice President, Product Marketing: David Gesell
Field Marketing Manager: Brittany Hammond
Full-Service Project Management and Composition: SPi Global
Full-Service Project Manager: Benjamin Gilbert
Inventory Manager: Vatche Demirdjian
Interior Designer: Pam Verros
Cover Designer: Pam Verros
Cover Photo: Getty Images/zozzzzo
Printing and Binding: Lake Side Communications
Cover Printer: Phoenix Color

Library of Congress Cataloging-in-Publication Data

Names: Moini, Jahangir, 1942- author.
Title: Focus on pharmacology : essentials for health professionals / Jahangir Moini.
Description: Third edition. | Upper Saddle River, New Jersey : Pearson Education, 2017. | Includes Index
Identifiers: LCCN 2017000583 | ISBN 9780134525044
Subjects: | MESH: Pharmacological Phenomena | Drug Therapy | Pharmacokinetics | Allied Health Personnel
Classification: LCC RM300 | NLM QV 4 | DDC 615/.1--dc23
LC record available at https://lccn.loc.gov/2017000583

1 17

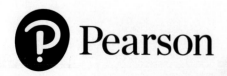

ISBN 13: 978-0-13-452504-4
ISBN 10:   0-13-452504-3

Dedication

This book is dedicated to the memory of my Mother, to my wife Hengameh, my daughters Mahkameh and Morvarid, and to my granddaughters, Laila Jade and Anabelle Jasmine Mabry.

Brief Contents

Preface

The Third Edition of *Focus on Pharmacology: Essentials for Health Professionals* has been updated with the latest drug information available. It is accompanied by a new Student Workbook, which contains many different types of review questions, including multiple-choice, fill-in-the-blank, true/false, and some labeling exercises. There are seven new chapters in this edition:

* Chapter 2—Pharmacodynamics
* Chapter 3—Pharmacokinetics
* Chapter 4—Drug Toxicity and Pharmacogenomics
* Chapter 13—Dietary Supplements and Alternative Therapies
* Chapter 17—Antiviral Agents
* Chapter 19—Antiprotozoal Agents
* Chapter 29—Drugs Used to Treat Hyperlipidemia and Related Conditions

Other key changes and updates:

* Chapter 1 was divided into four chapters (1—Introduction to Pharmacology, 2—Pharmacodynamics, 3—Pharmacokinetics, and 4—Drug Toxicity and Pharmacogenomics).
* Basic Mathematics was renamed Principles of Math in Medicine.
* Nutritional Aspects of Pharmacology and Herbal Substances was divided and expanded to become Chapter 12—Nutritional Aspects of Pharmacology, and Chapter 13—Dietary Supplements and Alternative Therapies.
* Substance Abuse was renamed and expanded as Chapter 15—Substance Abuse and Misuse
* Antibacterial and Antiviral Agents was divided into two chapters: Chapter 16—Antibacterial Agents and Chapter 17—Antiviral Agents.
* Second-edition chapter on Antifungal, Antimalarial, and Antiprotozoal Agents was divided into two chapters: Chapter 18—Antifungal Agents, and Chapter 19—Antiprotozoal Agents.

There also have been changes to the appendices:

* Appendix A—The Top 200 Drugs by prescription
* The previous Appendix D (Immunization Schedules) was removed because it is now in the body of the book

Pharmacology is often a challenging subject for allied health students. To the rescue comes this text uniquely designed to use a *focused* approach to learning pharmacology. Introductory chapters lay the groundwork for learning this subject by explaining the history of pharmacology, discussing the legal and ethical principles involved, illustrating drug administration techniques, reviewing math, explaining drug calculations, and a discussion of medication errors and their prevention. Additionally, substance abuse is focused on in detail. The chapters that follow focus on drugs specific to body systems, pharmacotherapy of certain age groups (pediatrics and geriatrics), pharmacology for pregnant women, and broad drug categories such as antibiotics.

Structured Presentation of Pharmacologic Principles

Each drug chapter focuses on drugs used to treat a certain body system and its associated disorders. The chapters open with a concise review of anatomy and physiology, providing a foundation for understanding the actions, effects, and uses of each drug. These pharmacologic principles are succinctly explained by using clearly identifiable headings in question format that help focus students' attention on the most important points about a drug class or an individual drug:

✳ How do they work?

✳ How are they used?

✳ What are the adverse effects?

✳ What are the contraindications and interactions?

✳ What are the most important points patients should know?

Sometimes these question headings focus on a class of drugs, for example, beta-adrenergic blockers. Other times, the question headings focus on a *prototype* (representative) drug—that is, the drug that was either the first developed in the class or is the most widely used drug in its class. Whichever approach is taken in the chapter, the five-question headings are used so students can easily focus on the key "need-to-know" drug information.

Focus On

Chloroquine

Chloroquine is one of the most commonly used drugs for prophylaxis and the treatment of acute malarial attacks that are caused by *P. vivax, Plasmodium malariae, Plasmodium ovale,* and susceptible strains of *P. falciparum.*

How does it work?

Chloroquine is a protozoacidal drug. The agent destroys *Plasmodia* organisms by interfering with their metabolism or inhibiting normal replication of the **protozoan.**

How is it used?

Chloroquine is used for the control of acute attacks of *P. vivax* malaria and for suppression against all plasmodia except chloroquine-resistant *P. falciparum.* The drug is neither a prophylactic nor a radical curative agent in *P. vivax* malaria. In regions where *P. falciparum* is generally sensitive to chloroquine, it is markedly effective in terminating acute attacks of nonresistant *P. falciparum* malaria and usually brings about a complete cure in this type of malaria. Chloroquine is the drug of choice for the oral treatment of all malaria except that caused by resistant *P. falciparum.*

What are the adverse effects?

Adverse effects include pigmentation of the skin and nail beds, pruritus, fatigue, toxic psychosis, and ototoxicity.

Chloroquine may also cause clouding of the corneas of the eyes and retinopathy.

What are the contraindications and interactions?

Chloroquine is contraindicated in patients with liver disease, hypersensitivity to 4-aminoquinolines, psoriasis, porphyria, and renal disease. This drug should also not be used by children or by pregnant or lactating women. Certain antacids and laxatives decrease chloroquine absorption, and chloroquine may interfere with the response to the rabies vaccine.

What are the important points patients should know?

Advise patients to promptly report visual or hearing disturbances, muscle weakness, loss of balance, and symptoms of blood dyscrasia, which include fever, sore mouth or throat, unexplained fatigue, easy bruising, or bleeding. Instruct them to wear dark glasses in sunlight and bright light because of photophobia, to reduce the risk of ocular damage, and to avoid driving or other potentially hazardous activities until a reaction to the drug is known. Inform patients that this drug may cause rusty yellow or brown discoloration of the urine.

. . . .

Doxycycline

Doxycycline is also known as *doxycycline calcium oral suspension* (syrup), *doxycycline hyclate* (capsules or film-coated tablets), and *doxycycline monohydrate* (for oral suspension). It is active against many different types of bacteria as well as parasites.

How does it work?

Doxycycline inhibits bacterial protein synthesis by binding to ribosomal subunits and is bacteriostatic against a broad range of Gram-positive and Gram-negative bacteria.

How is it used?

Doxycycline should be used only to treat or prevent infections that are proven or strongly suspected to be caused by bacteria, in order to reduce development of drug-resistant bacteria and maintain effectiveness of this and other antibacterial drugs. This drug is primarily indicated for Rickettsial infections such as Rocky Mountain spotted fever and typhus fever and for chlamydia. Doxycycline is used for the prevention of malaria.

Teach-and-Test Approach

Learning small amounts of information and testing themselves on what they've just learned is a proven way for students to retain new information. This text includes a large number of exercises, implemented in three ways: (1) *Practical Scenarios* (two per chapter) with critical thinking questions; (2) within-chapter *Apply Your Knowledge* questions; and (3) end-of-unit *Checkpoint Reviews*. This approach makes learning about pharmacology an engaging, interactive process. The Teach-and-Test approach truly differentiates the text from others and has been positively received by educators.

PRACTICAL SCENARIO

Each chapter concludes with two short scenarios involving fictional patients with real-life problems concerning medications. A list of two or three questions follows. These scenarios relate to the knowledge that students have gained from reading each chapter. After completing each chapter, individual students can write short answers to the questions, or the class as a whole can discuss the answers.

PRACTICAL SCENARIO 2

A 75-year-old man was taking several different medications for hypertension, hyperplasia of the prostate, and rheumatoid arthritis. Four of his medications were to be taken before bed, and three were to be taken in the morning. One night, he recalled that he had forgotten to take one of his medications. He got out of bed, went into his kitchen, and avoided turning on the light so as not to disturb his son-in-law, who was sleeping in the adjacent family room. In the darkness, he inadvertently took one of the medications he had already taken earlier. After 2 hours, he woke up to go to the bathroom and felt chest pain and dizziness, which caused him to collapse, awakening his wife.

Monkey Business Images/Shutterstock

Critical Thinking Questions

1. Which of his medications would cause lower blood pressure, chest pain, and dizziness?
2. What are the disadvantages of taking several drugs at the same time?

APPLY YOUR KNOWLEDGE

The second implementation of the "teach-and-test" approach includes exercises that are strategically placed *within* the chapters (rather than at the end). These exercise sections, called *Apply Your Knowledge*, appear after each component of the chapter content, including anatomy and physiology, and the individual pathophysiology/pharmacology sections.

The exercise sections include a variety of exercises in which students need to recall and apply the content they just learned. Exercise types include fill-in-the blank, labeling, matching, and multiple-choice, as well as more pharmacology-specific exercises such as dosage calculations and drug name exercises (sound-alike and look-alike and generic-to- brand). The goal in these sections is to provide the student with an immediate review of all vital content. All drugs and drug classes mentioned in the content are "tested" in these exercise sections.

✸ Apply Your **Knowledge 39.1**

The following questions focus on what you have just learned about pediatric pharmacokinetics. See Appendix F for answers.

CRITICAL THINKING

1. What physiologic processes may influence pharmacokinetics in children?
2. What are the definitions of the terms *neonate, infant,* and *toddler*?
3. What is the cause of kernicterus?
4. What is the result of lower metabolic activities in neonates?
5. Compare the GFR of newborns to older children and adults.

CHECKPOINT REVIEWS

The third component of our teach-and-test approach is unit "tests" called *Checkpoint Reviews*. These review questions reflect the format on most certifying and licensing exams, and include multiple-choice and essay questions. Answers to the Apply Your Knowledge and Checkpoint Reviews are found at the end of the book in Appendix E.

Checkpoint Review 1

Select the best answer for the following questions.

1. The half-life is the major determinant of which of the following?
   a. The adverse effects of a drug after a single dose
   b. The interaction with another single dose
   c. The duration of elimination of a drug after administration of multiple doses
   d. The duration of action of a drug after a single dose

2. *Hypersensitivity* is often used synonymously with which of the following terms?
   a. Immunogen
   b. Allergy
   c. Antigen
   d. Allergen

3. Which of the following agencies oversees controlled substances and prosecutes individuals who illegally distribute them?
   a. HIPAA
   b. FDA
   c. DEA
   d. CDC

4. Which of the following federal laws offers a 7-year monopoly on drug sales and tax breaks to induce drug companies to undertake development and manufacturing of drugs used for rare diseases that affect small numbers of people in the United States?
   a. Orphan Drug Act of 1983
   b. Prescription Drug Marketing Act of 1987
   c. Durham–Humphrey Amendment of 1951
   d. Comprehensive Drug Abuse Prevention and Control Act of 1970

5. Which of the following phases of drug approval evaluates toxicology data?
   a. Phase I
   b. Phase II
   c. Phase III
   d. Phase IV

6. The angle of insertion for intradermal injections is which of the following degrees?
   a. 30
   b. 90
   c. 15
   d. 45

7. Which of the following is the route of administration of a drug that is placed between the gums and the cheek?
   a. Buccal
   b. Topical
   c. Sublingual
   d. Transdermal

8. Which of the following is a drug that was withdrawn after postmarketing surveillance?
   a. Penbutolol
   b. Atenolol
   c. Furosemide
   d. Celecoxib

9. The proprietary drug name is also called the:
   a. Chemical name
   b. Generic name
   c. Trade name
   d. None of the above

10. The study of drugs derived from herbal and other natural sources is called:
    a. Pharmacodynamics
    b. Pharmacotherapy
    c. Pharmacognosy
    d. Pharmacology

11. Which of the following drugs carries a black box warning?
    a. Rifampin
    b. Rofecoxib
    c. Valdecoxib
    d. Celecoxib

12. Herbal products and dietary supplements are controlled by the
    a. Center for Disease Control and Prevention
    b. Center for Biologics Evaluation and Research
    c. Center for Food Safety and Applied Nutrition
    d. Center for Drug Evaluation and Research

13. Which of the following can determine the dose-effect relationship?
    a. Pharmacodynamics
    b. Pharmacokinetics
    c. Both A and B
    d. Pharmacology

Drug Dosing Information

Each drug chapter includes tables of all drugs discussed in the chapter, arranged by drug classes and formatted to include generic and trade names, adult dosing, and route of administration.

Table 17-1 ■ Examples of Effective Antiviral Agents

GENERIC NAME	TRADE NAME	AVERAGE ADULT DOSAGE	ROUTE OF ADMINISTRATION
acyclovir	Zovirax	IV: 5–15 mg/kg q8h for 7–21 days; PO: 20–400 mg (800 mg max) 4–5 times/d for 5–14 days; Topical: 5% cream 5 times/d for 4 days	IV, PO, topical
amantadine	Symmetrel	Two 100 mg tablets/d or 4 teaspoons of syrup/d; may be split into 1 tablet bid or 2 teaspoons of syrup bid	PO (tablets and syrup)
didanosine	Videx, Videx EC	EC Capsules: 400 mg once/d (or 250 mg once/d with tenofovir); Oral solution: 200 mg bid	PO (enteric-coated capsules or oral solution) (take 30 minutes before meals or 2 hours after)
ganciclovir	Cytovene, Vitrasert, Zirgan	IV infusion: 5 mg/kg over 1 hour q12h for 14–21 days; Oral: 1000 mg tid with food; Ocular implant: inserted surgically and replaced q5–8m; Ocular 0.15% gel: 1 drop in affected eye 5 times/d prn, followed by 1 drop tid for 7 days	IV, PO, ocular implant, ocular gel
ribavirin	Virazole	20 mg/mL as starting solution in SPAG-2 unit with continuous aerosol administration for 12–18 hours/d for 3–7 days (this concentration = 190 micrograms/liter of air)	Inhalation (powder for solution)
zanamivir	Relenza	10 mg, provided in 2 inhalations using Diskhaler	Inhalation (powder for PO inhalation)
zidovudine	Retrovir	200 mg tid or 300 mg bid	PO

IV, intravenous; PO, oral; bid, twice a day; tid, three times a day.

Special Populations and Important Drug-Related Points

* **Focus Points:** These marginal features highlight significant or difficult concepts in pharmacology.
* **Focus on Pediatrics** and **Focus on Geriatrics:** Each of these boxes highlights pediatric or geriatric information specific to pharmacology.
* **Focus on Natural Products:** This boxed feature highlights drug interactions related to complementary and alternative medicines. Herbs, supplements, and foods are included in these boxes.

Focus Point

Mechanism of Action of HIV Medications

It is important to understand how specific drugs used against HIV listed above. The drug called maraviroc affects Step 1, blocking H receptor. The drug called enfuvirtide blocks the fusion process of S drugs inhibit the reverse transcriptase enzyme's effects in Step 3. T integrase enzyme and its effects in Step 5. Several drugs target HIV protease and its effects in Step 10.

During all stages of HIV infection, the virus replicates very quickly, but particularly during the initial stage. This is because the amount of CD4 cells is still very large, and th response against the virus. Therefore, plasma levels of HIV can initia Patients often experience acute retroviral syndrome as a result. In the decline sharply but eventually level off to between 1,000 and 100,0 seems, since the HIV plasma half-life is 6 hours, meaning that one- every 6 hours. Therefore, to remain a relatively steady level when infe between 1 and 10 billion virions per day. Even so, the patient is usually asymptomatic for approximately 10 years. After this period, advanced signs and symptoms appear.

HIV mutates very quickly due to errors in reverse transcriptase. U incorporated into HIV DNA with each replication. Therefore, HIV can even though it was previously in a drug-sensitive form. The chance o related to the total viral load. There is more chance of at least one viri amounts of total virions. Therefore, patients are treated with combina

Focus Point

Medical Errors During the Prescribing Process

The three most common forms of prescribing errors include dosing errors, prescribing medications to which the patient has had an allergic response, and errors involving the prescribing of inappropriate dosage forms.

Focus Point

Heparin Injections

For subcutaneous heparin injections, make sure that 0.1 to 0.2 mL of air is in the syringe to prevent heparin leakage into tissue, thus avoiding localized hemorrhaging.

Focus on Geriatrics

Medications May Stain Teeth and Dentures

Advise elderly patients who have dentures to remove them before taking certain medications. Some oral liquid drugs, such as liquid iron or iodides, may stain the teeth.

Focus on Natural Products

Lobelia Dangers

Lobelia is found in dietary supplements that are marketed for use by children and infants as well as pregnant women. Lobelia may be very dangerous to use because it contains alkaloids with pharmacologic actions that are similar to nicotine. It can cause autonomic nervous system depression or stimulation, bronchial dilation, increased respiratory rate, respiratory depression, sweating, rapid heart rate, hypotension, and even coma or death.

Each chapter includes:

* Chapter Objectives
* Key Terms with pronunciations
* Chapter Capsule: A review of each chapter objective with bulleted summaries of the key information for each objective

The focused teach-and-test approach of this textbook provides allied health students with the perfect blend of concise content and an enjoyable—even fun—learning process. Pharmacology and fun have never been joined in the same sentence—until now!

Acknowledgments

This textbook is the culmination of the efforts of many people, including my students of many years who inspired me to write it. Thank you to Julie Levin Alexander, Marlene Pratt, Derril Trakalo, and Faye Gemellaro—all of whom believed in this project from the start—and those dedicated professionals on the editorial team who helped produce this book. Melissa Bashe (Managing Content Producer) has been invaluable in helping me with the media. Joan Gill (Developmental Editor) was vital in coordinating all the steps needed to create this edition from the initial book. Many thanks to the team at SPi Global for their inspired design and excellent production process.

My special thanks go to Greg Vadimsky, who has been my personal editorial assistant from the first edition through the completion of this third edition. He also assisted me in completing the *Instructor's Manual*, student website, and PowerPoint presentations.

About the Author

Jahangir Moini, MD, MPH, was Assistant Professor at Tehran University School of Medicine for 9 years, teaching medical and allied health students. The author was also Professor (for 24 years) and Director (for 15 years) of allied health programs at Everest University. He was Brevard County Epidemiologist and Biological Scientist for 18 years. Dr. Moini was also Physician Liaison for the American Association of Medical Assistants (AAMA) in Florida and an Advisory Member of NACCAS. He is now Professor of Science and Health at Eastern Florida State College, and a member of their book selection and nursing student selection committees.

Dr. Moini is actively involved in teaching and helping students prepare for service in various health professions. He has been a published author of 20 allied health books since 1999.

Courtesy of the author

Contributors/Reviewers

CONTRIBUTORS

Karen Bills, PharmD, CPH
HealthFirst, Palm Bay Hospital
Palm Bay, Florida

Jeffrey R. Mabry, DMD
Melbourne, Florida

Mahkameh Moini, DMD
Melbourne, Florida

Stephanie K. Mullen, RN, MSN, CPNP
Private Practice
Cleveland, Ohio

Norman Tomaka, CRPh, LHCRM
HealthFirst Pharmacist Consultant
Melbourne, Florida

THANK YOU TO OUR REVIEWERS

Reviewers of the Third Edition

Peter F. Andrus, MD
Clinical Instructor
Albany Medical College
Albany, New York

Carole Berube, MA, MSN, BSN, RN
Bristol Community College
Fall River, Massachusetts

Sara K. Daniel, MS, CHES, RHIA
Arkansas Tech University
Russellville, Arkansas

Pilar Perez-Jackson, CPhT, RPhT
Sanford Brown Institute
Iselin, New Jersey

Paula D. Silver, PharmD
ECPI University
Newport News, Virginia

Reviewers of the Second Edition

Elenora Alvarado
Nashville State Community College
Nashville, Tennessee

Sonya Burns, CMA (AAMA), BBA
Augusta Technical College
Waynesboro, Georgia

Sue Coleman
National College
Lynchburg, Virginia

Chanta Hall
Mountain View College
Dallas, Texas

Barbara Jareo, RN, BSN, CCM, CEN
Davenport University
Saginaw, Michigan

Patricia Sell, RMA(AMT), RN, AAS, BS, MSEd
National College
Princeton, West Virginia

Paula Silver, PharmD
Medical Careers Institute
Newport News, Virginia

Phaedra Spartan, RMA, BS
Vatterott College
Springfield, Missouri

Cindy Thompson
Davenport University
Saginaw, Michigan

Christy Tinnin, RN
Vatterott College
Fairview Heights, Illinois

Cynthia Watkins, RN, BSN
Lorain County Community College
Elyria, Ohio

Stephanie Weller
Carrington College California
Stockton, California

Reviewers of the First Edition

Patricia J. Allee, RN
Blinn College
Brenham, Texas

Kristen Anderson, RN, BSN
Southwest Wisconsin Technical College
Fennimore, Wisconsin

Deborah Bedford, CMA
North Seattle Community College
Seattle, Washington

Susan Boggs, RN, CNOR
Piedmont Technical College
Greenwood, South Carolina

Vince Druash, CMA, BS
Medical Careers Institute
Virginia Beach, Virginia

Judy Ehninger, MA
Lehigh Carbon Community College
Schnecksville, Pennsylvania

Rosemary Fischer, RN, BSN, MS
Alfred State College (retired)
Alfred, New York

Steve Forshier, RT(R), MEd
Pima Medical Institute
Mesa, Arizona

Nancy D. Glass, RN, PhD
Austin Community College
Austin, Texas

Robyn Gohsman, RMA, CMAS, AAS
Medical Careers Institute
Newport News, Virginia

Henry Gomez, MD
ASA Institute
Brooklyn, New York

Jeanette Goodwin, CMA, BSN
Southeast Community College
Lincoln, Nebraska

Corrine C. Harmon, RN, MS, EdD, AOCN
Clemson University
Clemson, South Carolina

Elizabeth Hoffman, MAEd, CMA, CPT, (ASPT)
Baker College of Clinton Township
Clinton Township, Michigan

Robin Kern, RN, BSN
Moultrie Technical College
Moultrie, Georgia

Len Lichtblau, PhD
University of Minnesota School of Nursing
Edina, Minnesota

Douglas Lytle, PhD, MBA
Widener University
Pottstown, Pennsylvania

David Martinez, RHE, BA
International Business College
El Paso, Texas

Nancy Matyunas, PharmD
Jefferson Community & Technical College
Louisville, Kentucky

Gayle Mazzocco, RN, CMA, BSN
Oakland Community College
Waterford, Michigan

Carol McMahon, RN, BSN, MEd
Capital Community College
Simsbury, Connecticut

Michele G. Miller, MEd, CMA, COMT
Lakeland Community College
Kirtland, Ohio

Lisa Nagle, BSed, CMA
Augusta Technical College
Augusta, Georgia

Eva Ruth Oltman, CMA, CPC, EMT, LMR, MA
Kentucky Community & Technical College System
Prospect, Kentucky

Christopher Owens, PharmD, BCPS
Idaho State University
Pocatello, Idaho

Steve Peterson, CPhT, MEd
Apollo College
Scottsdale, Arizona

Diane Premeau, RHIA, CHP, MBA
Chabot College
Fremont, California

Myra Resnick, RN
Southwestern College
Florence, Kentucky

Jackie Smith, RN, CPhT
National College of Business and Technology
Pounding Mill, Virginia

Karen Snipe, CPhT, MAEd
Trident Technical College
Charleston, South Carolina

Pat Stroupe, RN, MSN
Waukesha County Technical College
Pewaukee, Wisconsin

Joe Tinervia, CPhT, MBA
Community Care College
Tulsa, Oklahoma

Robert Tralongo, RRT-NPS, MBA
Molloy College
Rockville Centre, New York

Jana Tucker, CMA, LPRT
Salt Lake Community College
Salt Lake City, Utah

Gail Tuohig, RN, PhD
St. Mark's Hospital
Salt Lake City, Utah

Lori Warren, RN, CPC, CCP, CLNC, MA
Spencerian College
Louisville, Kentucky

Tonia Webster, RN, CMA
Southwest Wisconsin Technical College
Platteville, Wisconsin

Mary Ann Woods, RN, CMA, MS, PhD
Fresno City College
Fresno, California

Judith Wulff, RN, BSN
D.G. Erwin Technical Center
Tampa, Florida

MEDIA REVIEWERS

Reviewers of the Third Edition Media

Peter F. Andrus, MD
Albany Medical College,
Albany, New York

Carole Berube, MA, MSN, BSN, RN
Bristol Community College
Fall River, Massachusetts

Sara K. Daniel, MS, CHES, RHIA
Arkansas Tech University
Russellville, Arkansas

Pilar Perez-Jackson, CPhT, RPhT
Sanford Brown Institute
Iselin, New Jersey

Paula D. Silver, PharmD.
ECPI University: College of Health Science
Newport News, Virginia

Reviewers of the Second Edition Media

Sonya Burns, CMA (AAMA), BBA
Augusta Technical College
Waynesboro, Georgia

Barbara Jareo, RN, BSN, CCM, CEN
Davenport University
Saginaw, Michigan

Patricia Sell, RMA(AMT), RN, AAS, BS, MSEd
National College
Princeton, West Virginia

Paula Silver, PharmD.
Medical Careers Institute
Newport News, Virginia

Phaedra Spartan, RMA, BS
Vatterott College
Springfield, Missouri

Cindy Thompson
Davenport University
Saginaw, Michigan

Christy Tinnin, RN
Vatterott College
Fairview Heights, Illinois

Cynthia Watkins, RN, BSN
Lorain County Community College
Elyria, Ohio

Reviewers of the First Edition Media

Joyce B. Benedetti, RN, MS, JD, CMA-AC
Allan Hancock College
Santa Maria, California

Peggy Bush, PhD, RPh
Durham Technical Community College
Durham, North Carolina

Carol Buttz
Dakota County Technical College
Rosemount, Minnesota

Jennifer Chang, BS, MS
College of Marin
Kentfield, California

June A. Griffith, PharmD, CGP
Florida Community College
Jacksonville, Florida

Lynda Harkins, PhD
Texas State University–San Marcos
San Marcos, Texas

Anne P. LaVance, BS, CPhT
Delgado Community College
New Orleans, Louisiana

Vivian C. Lilly, PhD, MBA, RN
North Harris College
Houston, Texas

Patricia McLane, RHIA, MA
Schoolcraft College
Garden City, Michigan

Michele G. Miller, MEd, CMA, COMT
Lakeland Community College
Kirtland, Ohio

Lisa Nagle, BSed, CMA
Augusta Technical College
Augusta, Georgia

Geraldine Twomey, MEd, RRT, RN
North Shore Community College
Danvers, Massachusetts

Contents

Unit 5   Special Populations   670

UNIT 1

General Principles

" To administer a drug safely, one must know its usual dose, frequency, route of administration, indications, contraindications, significant adverse reactions, and major drug interactions. "

Chapter 1

Introduction to Pharmacology

Chapter Objectives

After completing this chapter, you should be able to:

1. Compare and define pharmacognosy and pharmacotherapeutics.

2. Define *drugs* and *CAM therapies*.

3. Compare prescription drugs with over-the-counter drugs.

4. Explain biologic agents and give four examples.

5. Describe the role of the Food and Drug Administration.

6. Explain drug approval.

7. Describe the longest stage of drug approval.

8. Define *postmarketing surveillance*.

Key Terms

biologics (p. 5)
black box warning (p. 8)
complementary and alternative medicine (CAM) therapies (p. 5)

dose (p. 5)
drug (p. 5)
medication (p. 5)
NDA review (p. 8)

pharmacognosy (p. 5)
pharmacology (p. 5)
pharmacotherapeutics (p. 5)
prescription (p. 5)

Introduction

Pharmacology is the study of drugs, including their action and effects in living body systems. Clinical pharmacology is the study of drugs in humans. It is involved with all aspects of the interaction between drugs and patients. The term *drug* is defined as "any substance or product that is used or intended to be used to modify or improve a physiologic or pathologic condition." The terms *medication* and *medicine* refer to drugs mixed in a formulation with other ingredients to improve the stability, taste, or physical form to allow appropriate administration of the active drug.

Pharmacology deals with all the types of drugs used in society today (legal, illegal, prescription, and over-the-counter [OTC] medications). To administer a drug safely, one must know its usual **dose**, frequency, route of administration, indications, contraindications, significant adverse reactions, and major drug interactions. Knowledge of the patient's medication allergies, weight, and liver and kidney functions is also essential.

Pharmacognosy is the study of drugs derived from herbal and other natural sources. By studying the compositions of natural substances and how the body reacts to them, one gains better knowledge for developing purified versions. **Pharmacotherapeutics** is the study of how drugs may be best used in the treatment of illnesses and which drug is most or least appropriate to use for a specific disease. In this chapter, I consider classifications of prescription and over-the-counter drugs, the role of the FDA, and drug approval.

Classification of Drugs

Therapeutic agents may be classified as drugs (medications), biologics, or complementary and alternative medicine (CAM) therapies.

✳ A **drug** is any agent that produces biologic responses within the body. When a drug response is desired, it is referred to as *therapeutic*. When the response is undesired, it is referred to as *adverse*. Once a drug has been administered to a patient, it is referred to as a **medication**, yet both drugs and medications are thought of as components of normal physiological activities. Drugs differ from other products such as cosmetics, foods, and household chemicals, such as toothpaste, shampoo, and others.

✳ **Biologics** are agents produced inside animal cells from the actions of microorganisms, or by the entire body itself. They are natural substances, whereas most drugs used today are synthesized in laboratories. Biologics treat many different conditions or illnesses, and include hormones, vaccines, interferons, monoclonal antibodies, and natural blood products.

✳ **Complementary and alternative medicine (CAM) therapies** use herbs, plant extracts, dietary supplements, vitamins, and minerals. Additionally, therapies such as acupuncture, massage, hypnosis, and biofeedback are also considered CAM therapies.

✳ Apply Your Knowledge 1.1

The following questions focus on what you have just learned about drug classifications.

CRITICAL THINKING

1. Describe biologic drugs.
2. Define *complementary* and *alternative medicine therapies*.
3. What is the definition of a *medication*?

PRESCRIPTION DRUGS

Prescription agents are legal drugs that can only be dispensed using a prescription from an authorized health practitioner. A **prescription** is an order, usually written, for medications or other therapies to be supplied to a specific individual patient. They are based on examinations and diagnoses of patients by physicians, nurse practitioners, and other health practitioners. Prescriptions contain dosage information that is designed to provide the most accurate treatment for the diagnosed condition. Another advantage of using prescription agents is that, should there be any interactions with other drugs, supplements, or foods, the health care practitioner is able to ascertain the safe use of what is being prescribed for the patient. Sometimes, usage of a prescription medication over many years, with little or no safety concerns resulting, means that the medication may later become available over the counter (OTC).

OVER-THE-COUNTER DRUGS

Over-the-counter agents are those that do not require a prescription from a health care provider. For the majority of OTC drugs, the patient is able to treat him- or herself safely as long as the dosage instructions are followed. However, misuse of OTC drugs can result in serious adverse effects, in the same way that misuse of prescription drugs can. Comparing the two types of agents, OTC drugs are preferred by patients since they are easily obtained, do not require an appointment with a health care provider, and are usually of lower cost. The difficulty when using OTC drugs is correctly deciding which specific drug is correct for the patient's own condition. Also, there are interactions between various OTC drugs with prescription medications, other OTC drugs being taken, herbal supplements, and even foods. Patients may not be aware of these potential interactions. Certain OTC drugs impair the ability to function normally, drive a car, or operate machinery, and the patient may be unaware. Also, some OTC drugs are simply not potent enough to successfully treat a condition, and the patient may be harmed if the disease progresses because of insufficient treatment.

✺ Apply Your Knowledge 1.2

The following questions focus on what you have just learned about prescription and OTC drugs.

CRITICAL THINKING

1. Define the term *prescription*.
2. How may a prescription drug eventually become an OTC drug?
3. Why are OTC drugs preferred by patients?

The Food and Drug Administration

The Food and Drug Administration (FDA) is part of the United States Department of Health and Human Services. The determination of the correct use of prescription and OTC agents is controlled by the branch of the FDA known as the Center for Drug Evaluation and Research (CDER). This administration focuses on the use of safe and effective drugs, and keeping unsafe or ineffective drugs from being marketed. They also improve the health of citizens by publishing easily understandable drug information to ensure safety and efficacy. Before a drug can be marketed, all pharmaceutical laboratories must receive approval by the FDA.

Biologics are controlled by another branch of the FDA called the Center for Biologics Evaluation and Research (CBER). In 1986, the Childhood Vaccine Act authorized the FDA to collect information about patients receiving vaccines, to recall biologic products, and to enact civil penalties when guidelines about biologics were not followed.

Herbal products and dietary supplements are controlled by yet another FDA branch known as the Center for Food Safety and Applied Nutrition (CFSAN). They are also regulated by the Dietary Supplement Health and Education Act of 1994. However, herbal and dietary supplements can still be marketed without FDA approval. After being marketed, their package inserts and other information are monitored by the FDA. CAM therapies are controlled by the National Center for Complementary and Alternative Medicine (NCCAM). This agency studies the usefulness and safety of these therapies in improving health care.

Drug Approval

The FDA reviews therapeutic drugs and biologics in four phases: preclinical investigation, clinical investigation, review of the New Drug Application (NDA), and postmarketing surveillance. Figure 1-1 ■ shows the drug development process.

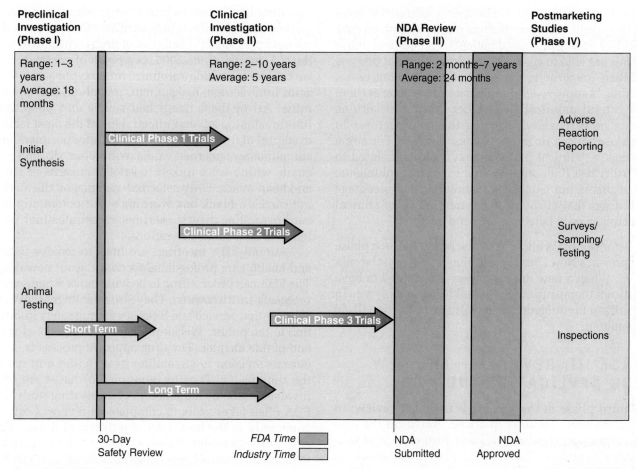

Preclinical Investigation (Phase I)	Clinical Investigation (Phase II)	NDA Review (Phase III)	Postmarketing Studies (Phase IV)
Range: 1–3 years Average: 18 months	Range: 2–10 years Average: 5 years	Range: 2 months–7 years Average: 24 months	

Initial Synthesis

Clinical Phase 1 Trials

Clinical Phase 2 Trials

Animal Testing

Short Term

Clinical Phase 3 Trials

Long Term

Adverse Reaction Reporting

Surveys/ Sampling/ Testing

Inspections

30-Day Safety Review

FDA Time
Industry Time

NDA Submitted

NDA Approved

Figure 1-1 ■ The drug development process.

Source: Adams, Michael Patrick; Holland, Leland; Urban, Carol, *Pharmacology for Nurses: A Pathophysiologic Approach, 4th Ed.,* ©2014. Reprinted and Electronically reproduced by permission of Pearson Education, Inc., New York, NY

PHASE I: PRECLINICAL INVESTIGATION

Preclinical investigation, the first stage of new drug testing, involves extensive research on human and microbial cells in a laboratory. Also, cultured cells and animal studies are used to determine dosages, effectiveness, and adverse effects. This phase is always inconclusive since results may be insufficient or excessive in comparison to how human subjects will actually react to a new product. The FDA Critical Path Initiative of 2007 was implemented to better utilize bioinformation for safety, effectiveness, and manufacturability of new drug products. It improved the areas of bioinformatics, imaging, genomics (the study of DNA sequencing), and proteomics (the study of proteins). Preclinical investigation usually takes between 1 and 3 years, on average 18 months, to complete, with animal pharmacology and toxicology data being obtained.

PHASE II: CLINICAL INVESTIGATION

Clinical investigation is the second phase of new drug testing, and also the longest, occurring over 2 to 10 years, 5 years being the average. It is subdivided into three different clinical phase trials:

✳ **Clinical phase 1 trials** occur over several months. Dosages and adverse effects are assessed on approximately 20–100 human volunteers initially, who have the disease or condition that the drug is being tested to treat. Manufacturers most often start developing their trade name for the new drug during this phase. Doses are often subtherapeutic, but ascending (increasing) doses are used. This determines whether the drug is safe so that it can be checked for effectiveness. The percentage of drugs that move on to the next phase of clinical testing is 70%.

✳ **Clinical phase 2 trials** occur over several months to 2 years and use between several dozen and 300 volunteers that have the disease or condition that the drug is being tested to treat. The investigators come from a variety of medical specialty areas. Together, they assess the new drug's effectiveness, harmful effects upon other medical conditions, unsafe drug interactions, or differences in effects upon certain types of patients. The drug is assumed not to have a therapeutic effect until further testing occurs. The percentage of drugs that move on to the next phase of clinical testing is only 33%.

✳ **Clinical phase 3 trials** occur over 1 to 4 years, and test the drug on several hundred to approximately 3,000 volunteers with the disease or condition for which the drug is being tested. The drug is assumed to have a therapeutic effect during this phase. Responses vary widely among the tested patients, and clinical phase trials are able to speed up the drug approval process if there are no serious adverse effects. In some cases, a drug is approved for immediate use as long as there is careful monitoring. In other cases, precautions may be discovered, causing the manufacturer to make changes in the new drug product. For some drugs, a "clinical phase 4" may be implemented to further test it amongst several thousand volunteers, but this is not extremely common. The percentage of drugs that move on to the next phase of clinical testing is only between 25% and 30%.

Before a drug is allowed to proceed to the next phase of approval, a New Drug Application (NDA) must be submitted. When a new drug has been determined to have significant therapeutic benefits and be reasonably safe in humans, an Investigational New Drug Application (IND) is submitted.

PHASE III: REVIEW OF THE NEW DRUG APPLICATION (NDA)

The third phase of the process is the **NDA review**, in which the trade name is finalized. Based on the preclinical testing, clinical trials and further animal testing may continue. Though the FDA must make its initial NDA review within 6 months, the overall time period for this phase may be from 2 months to 7 years. If approved, the process continues. If rejected, concerns must be addressed by the manufacturer and then the process resumes. For a new drug, it usually takes about 24 months for the full NDA review.

PHASE IV: POSTMARKETING SURVEILLANCE

Postmarketing surveillance is the final phase of the new drug approval process, and begins after completion of clinical trials and the NDA review. By the time a new drug has reached a much larger population via the market, adverse effects may manifest that were not discovered previously. Examples of drugs withdrawn from the U.S. market since 2005, as a result of postmarketing surveillance, include aprotinin, propoxyphene, gatifloxacin, lumiracoxib, ozogamicin, pergolide, and sibutramine. All of these drugs had severe and potentially life-threatening adverse effects. One of the most famous examples of drugs being withdrawn after postmarketing surveillance concerned valdecoxib, celecoxib, and rofecoxib, which were linked to safety concerns of stroke and heart attack. Only celecoxib remains on the market, but carries a **black box warning** about potentially fatal cardiovascular disease, serious gastrointestinal problems, and bleeding ulcerations.

Annual FDA meetings are held to receive patient and health care professional feedback about new drugs. The FDA can order a drug to be withdrawn when serious problems are discovered. They also offer their MedWatch subscription service and a variety of drug safety information to the public. Websites for the FDA are listed at the end of this chapter. The drug approval process is under current revision to streamline its activities and reduce the time factor. Tens of thousands of pages are often involved in the documentation of a new drug study. The FDA often takes years to complete its review. Costs are commonly in the hundreds of millions of dollars for a single drug to be developed. Regardless, the FDA strives to make sure that all new drugs are safe for use. The Prescription Drug User Fee Act was established on a 5-year trial basis in 1992, requiring manufacturers to provide yearly product user fees. This income allowed the FDA to expand, restructure, and become more efficient in drug approval activities. It also greatly increased the amount of approved drugs and reduced review times significantly. The Prescription Drug User Fee Act was then authorized as part of the FDA Modernization Act, further expanding the FDA. The FDA Amendments Act then allocated additional funding for new drug reviews, and the FDA Food Safety Modernization Act increased recalls on tainted products and improved the ability to detect illnesses and outbreaks occurring from food products.

✳ Apply Your **Knowledge** 1.3 ▬▬▬▬▬▬

The following questions focus on what you have just learned about the drug approval process.

CRITICAL THINKING

1. Why must therapeutic drugs be approved by the Food and Drug Administration (FDA)?

2. What are the four stages of drug approval?

3. Describe clinical stage trials.

4. List the three most famous examples of drugs being withdrawn after postmarketing surveillance.

PRACTICAL SCENARIO 1

A 52-year-old female was suffering from constipation for 4 days, and bought an OTC drug for this condition. Also, her sister advised her to take the herbal supplement *Cascara sagrada*.

Auremar/Shutterstock

Critical Thinking Questions

1. What are the indications of *Cascara sagrada*?
2. If this patient took the drug and the supplement together, what may be the effects?

PRACTICAL SCENARIO 2

A patient went to the pharmacy for a refill of a medication. The pharmacy technician told him that he must obtain a new prescription because no refills were allowed. The pharmacy technician said she would contact the patient's physician for this.

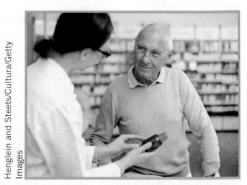

Henglein and Steets/Cultura/Getty Images

Critical Thinking Questions

1. What is the definition of a *prescription*?
2. What is the difference between a prescription drug and an OTC drug?

Chapter Capsule

This section repeats the objectives from the beginning of the chapter and then provides a summary of the most important concepts for that objective. Use this section as a quick review and to check your knowledge.

Objective 1: Compare and define *pharmacognosy* and *pharmacotherapeutics*.

- Pharmacognosy is the study of drugs derived from herbal and other natural sources. By studying the compositions of natural substances and how the body reacts to them, one gains better knowledge for developing purified versions.

- Pharmacotherapeutics is the study of how drugs may be best used in the treatment of illnesses and which drug is most or least appropriate to use for a specific disease.

Objective 2: Define *drugs* and *CAM therapies*.

- A drug is any agent that produces biologic responses within the body. When a drug response is desired, it is referred to as *therapeutic*. When the response is undesired, it is referred to as *adverse*. Once a drug has been administered to a patient, it is referred to as a *medication*, yet both drugs and medications are thought of as components of normal physiological activities. Drugs differ from other products such as cosmetics, foods, and household chemicals, such as toothpaste, shampoo, and others.

- Complementary and alternative medicine (CAM) therapies use herbs, plant extracts, dietary supplements, vitamins, and minerals. Additionally, therapies such as acupuncture, massage, hypnosis, and biofeedback are also considered CAM therapies.

Objective 3: Compare prescription drugs with over-the-counter drugs.

- Prescription agents are legal drugs that can only be dispensed using a prescription from an authorized health practitioner. A prescription is an order, usually written, for medications or other therapies to be supplied to a specific individual patient. Prescriptions contain dosage information that is designed to provide the most accurate treatment for the diagnosed condition.

- Over-the-counter agents are those that do not require a prescription from a health care provider. For the majority of OTC drugs, the patient is able to treat him- or herself safely as long as the dosage instructions are followed. Comparing the two types of agents, OTC drugs are preferred by patients since they are easily obtained, do not require an appointment with a health care provider, and are usually of lower cost.

Objective 4: Explain biologic agents and give four examples.

- Biologics are agents produced inside animal cells from the actions of microorganisms, or by the entire body itself. They are natural substances, whereas most drugs used today are synthesized in laboratories. Biologics treat many different conditions or illnesses.

- Examples of biologic agents include hormones, vaccines, interferons, monoclonal antibodies, and natural blood products.

Objective 5: Describe the role of the Food and Drug Administration.

- The determination of the correct use of prescription and OTC agents is controlled by the branch of the FDA known as the Center for Drug Evaluation and Research (CDER). This administration focuses on the use of safe and effective drugs and keeping unsafe or ineffective drugs from being marketed. They also improve the health of citizens by publishing easily understandable drug information to ensure safety and efficacy. Before a drug can be marketed, all pharmaceutical laboratories must receive approval by the FDA.

- The FDA also controls or monitors biologics, vaccines, herbal products, dietary supplements, and CAM therapies.

Objective 6: Explain drug approval.

- The FDA reviews therapeutic drugs and biologics in four phases: preclinical investigation, clinical investigation (with three subphases), review of the New Drug Application (NDA), and postmarketing surveillance.

- Preclinical investigation, the first stage of new drug testing, involves extensive research on human and microbial cells in a laboratory. Also, cultured cells and animal studies are used to determine dosages, effectiveness, and adverse effects. This phase is always inconclusive since results may be insufficient or excessive in comparison to how human subjects will actually react to a new product.

- Clinical investigation is the second phase of new drug testing, and is divided into three different *clinical phase trials (1, 2, and 3)*. In clinical phase 1 trials, dosages and adverse effects are assessed on approximately 20–100 human volunteers initially, and between several dozen and 300 volunteers in clinical phase 2 trials. Patients who have the disease being studied are selected to receive the new medication. Clinical phase 3 trials test the drug on several hundred to approximately 3,000 volunteers. Before a drug is allowed to proceed to the next phase of approval, a New Drug Application (NDA) must be submitted. When a new drug has been determined to have significant therapeutic benefits and be reasonably safe in humans, an *Investigational New Drug Application (IND)* is submitted.

- The third phase of the process is the NDA review, in which the trade name is finalized. Based on the preclinical testing, clinical phase 3 trials and further animal testing may continue. Though the FDA must make its initial NDA review within 6 months, the overall time period for this phase may be from 2 months to 7 years. If approved, the process continues. If rejected, concerns must be addressed by the manufacturer and then the process resumes. For a new drug, it usually takes about 24 months for the full NDA review.

- Postmarketing surveillance is the final phase of the new drug approval process, and begins after completion of clinical trials and the NDA review. By the time a new drug has reached a much larger population via the market, adverse effects may manifest that were not discovered previously. Annual FDA meetings are held to receive patient and health care professional feedback about new drugs. The FDA can order a drug to be withdrawn when serious problems are discovered. The FDA often takes years to complete its review.

Objective 7: Describe the longest stage of drug approval.

- Phase II (clinical investigation) is the most time-consuming of all, occurring over 2 to 10 years, with 5 years being the average. It has three substages, all of varying lengths.

Objective 8: Define *postmarketing surveillance*.

- Postmarketing surveillance involves monitoring of additional adverse effects and other results of the use of a particular drug. This often takes many years. It begins after clinical trials and the NDA review have been completed. Postmarketing surveillance may result in a drug being changed by the manufacturer or withdrawn from the market.

 ## Internet Sites of Interest

- The FDA's free e-mail subscription service concerning alerts about withdrawn drugs and other medical products: **www.fda.gov/safety/MedWatch**
- The FDA's Drug Safety Communications, Podcasts, and Newsletters: **www.fda .gov/drugs/drugsafety/PostmarketDrugSafetyInformationForPatientsAndProviders/ default.htm**
- An encyclopedia of medical and pharmacology terms, health news, and information on disorders: **www.sciencedaily.com/terms/pharmacology.htm**
- The FDA provides new drug approvals, prescription and OTC drug information, and drug safety and side effect information: **www.fda.gov/drugs/default.htm**
- Medscape Pharmacists contains a wealth of information about drugs, natural therapies, FDA drug warnings, and even continuing education programs for health professionals: **www.medscape.com/pharmacists**

Chapter 2

Pharmacodynamics

Chapter Objectives

After completing this chapter, you should be able to:

1. Define the term *pharmacodynamics*.
2. Identify what is represented by the frequency distribution curve.
3. Explain the dose–effect relationship.
4. Discuss how the therapeutic index of a drug is calculated.
5. Describe the affinity of a drug.
6. Identify various types of second-messenger events.
7. Briefly explain the four primary drug-receptor families.
8. Explain the equation used to calculate drug-receptor interactions.
9. Differentiate between agonists and antagonists.
10. Explain competitive and noncompetitive antagonists.

Key Terms

adverse effects (p. 13)
affinity (p. 15)
agonist (p. 17)
agonist-antagonists (p. 18)
antagonist (p. 18)
dose–effect relationship (p. 13)

frequency distribution curve (p. 13)
maximal efficacy (p. 13)
median effective dose (p. 13)
median lethal dose (p. 15)
median toxicity dose (p. 15)
pharmacodynamics (p. 13)

receptor (p. 15)
second messenger (p. 15)
target molecules (p. 17)
therapeutic (p. 13)
therapeutic index (TI) (p. 14)

Introduction

When a drug enters the body systems, many alterations and interferences with cell function may occur. It is important to understand that a specific drug may cause widely different and often unpredictable responses in different patients. Prescribers must choose the optimal dose of a medication for the individual patient while avoiding as many adverse effects as possible. In this chapter, I consider pharmacodynamics, the dose–effect relationship, the frequency distribution curve, the therapeutic index, drug safety, cellular receptors, drug action, types of drug receptors, drug-receptor interactions, agonists, and antagonists.

Pharmacodynamics

The **pharmacodynamics** process describes all matters concerned with the pharmacologic actions of a drug—whether they are determinants of **therapeutic** effects or **adverse effects**. It describes how a medication causes changes in the body. Pharmacodynamics studies the biochemical as well as the physiologic effects of drugs, along with the molecular mechanisms used to produce these effects. Knowledge of pharmacodynamics in regard to drug actions is essential so that medications can be safely prescribed, used with effectiveness, and evaluated for patient responses. The health care professionals of today must be able to predict whether a specific medication will produce significant benefits when administered.

DOSE–EFFECT RELATIONSHIP

A basic understanding of the factors that control drug concentration at the site of action is important for the optimal use of drugs. There should be knowledge of dose–effect relationships, drug-receptor interactions, and therapeutic indexes.

Blood is the most commonly sampled fluid used to characterize the pharmacologic actions of drugs. The drugs must dissolve before being absorbed. Then, they are able to pass through the small intestine and enter the blood circulation. Some of these drugs are absorbed and metabolized before reaching the site of action. The factors that may influence the onset, duration, and intensity of drug effects include absorption, metabolism, reabsorption, excretion, site of action, and observed response. Usually, there are correlations between pharmacokinetics and pharmacodynamics that demonstrate the relationship between drug dose and blood or other biological fluid concentrations.

Pharmacokinetics and pharmacodynamics can determine the **dose–effect relationship** (also called *dose–response relationship*), which is the relationship between the dose of a drug (or other agent) that produces therapeutic effects and the potency of the effects on an individual person (Figure 2-1 ■). A graph is used to illustrate the relationship: The maximum response for each drug (%) is plotted along the y-axis and the dose along the x-axis, increasing from left to right. The resulting plotted relationship is a characteristic curve, as the figure shows. The body's response to a drug (or toxic agent) increases as its overall exposure to the substance increases; for example, in the case of toxic agents, a small dose of carbon monoxide may cause drowsiness, but a large dose can be fatal. In the figure, drug A's curve is to the left of drug B's curve, which indicates that drug A has a higher potency. This means that a smaller dose of drug A will produce the same effect as a larger dose of drug B. The amount of drug required to cause an effect is referred to as its *relative potency*. Note that potency is rarely important overall. Drug A reaches a maximum response of 100% at the same dose as drug B, which reaches a maximum response of about 60%. Therefore, drug A's efficacy (or effectiveness) is greater than that of drug B. The largest effect that a drug can produce is also known as its **maximal efficacy**. It is important to understand that a drug's potency does not indicate anything about its maximal efficacy.

FREQUENCY DISTRIBUTION CURVE

The number of patients that respond to a drug's action at different doses is shown in the **frequency distribution curve** (see Figure 2-2 ■). It represents the number of patients that respond to the actions of a drug at different doses. A few patients are shown to have responded to a medication at very low doses, whereas increasing numbers of patients responded as the dosage was increased. Note that at the top of the curve, the **median effective dose**

Focus Point

Blood Drug Testing

Approximately 68% of all adults who are illegal drug users are employed full or part time. Preemployment workplace drug testing usually requires that applicants give urine samples, but also may require blood, saliva, sweat, or hair. Blood drug tests measure the actual amount of drugs in the blood at the time of the test.

A

Figure 2-1 ■ The dose–effect relationship, showing (**A**) drug potency and (**B**) drug efficacy (or effectiveness).

B

✳ Apply Your **Knowledge 2.1**

The following questions focus on what you have just learned about pharmacodynamics and the dose–effect relationship.

CRITICAL THINKING

1. Explain what pharmacodynamics describes.
2. Identify the factors that may influence drug effects.
3. Explain the dose–effect relationship.

or ED_{50} is shown, which is the amount of medication needed to produce a specific response in 50% of patients. It is important to understand that the frequency distribution curve does not indicate the magnitude of drug response, but does indicate if a measurable response occurred in the test group of patients.

THERAPEUTIC INDEX AND DRUG SAFETY

The **therapeutic index (TI)** of a drug is used to predict whether a certain dosage is safe for a specific patient. Like the median effective dose, frequency distribution curves are also used to determine the

Figure 2-2 ■ The frequency distribution curve of a drug.
Source: Adams, Michael Patrick; Holland, Leland; Urban, Carol, Pharmacology for Nurses: *A Pathophysiologic Approach, 4th Ed.,* ©2014. Reprinted and Electronically reproduced by permission of Pearson Education, Inc., New York, NY

$$\text{Drug X : TI} = \frac{LD_{50}}{ED_{50}} = \frac{40}{10} = 4$$

A

$$\text{Drug Z : TI} = \frac{LD_{50}}{ED_{50}} = \frac{20}{10} = 2$$

B

Figure 2-3 ■ The therapeutic indexes for two drugs.
Source: Adams, Michael Patrick; Holland, Leland; Urban, Carol, Pharmacology for Nurses: *A Pathophysiologic Approach, 4th Ed.,* ©2014. Reprinted and Electronically reproduced by permission of Pearson Education, Inc., New York, NY

median lethal dose or LD_{50} of a drug during preclinical trials. The LD_{50} represents the dose of a medication that is lethal in 50% of a group of test animals. The median effective and median lethal doses are then compared to understand the drug's safety by determining its average effective and average lethal doses. The therapeutic index is then calculated using the following formula:

$$\frac{\text{Median lethal dose (LD}_{50})}{\text{Median effective dose (ED}_{50})} = \text{Therapeutic index}$$

A larger therapeutic index means that the difference between the two doses is larger. Also, the higher the value of the therapeutic index, the safer the medication is to use. Figures 2-3A ■ and 2-3B show the therapeutic indexes for two drugs.

It is important to understand that the median lethal dose cannot be tested in humans, and therefore, the **median toxicity dose** or TD_{50} is used. It is the dose that produces a given toxicity in 50% of patients, and can be determined from animal testing data or because of adverse effects occurring during patient clinical trials.

CELLULAR RECEPTORS AND DRUG ACTION

Drugs produce their effects by altering the function of the cells and tissues of the body or of organisms such as bacteria. Each drug has a specific **affinity** (attractive force) for a target receptor. The cell recipient is known as a **receptor**—usually a specific protein—situated in cell membranes on cell surfaces. *Intracellular receptors* are located within the cellular cytoplasm. Some drugs act on intracellular receptors; these include corticosteroids, which act on cytoplasmic steroid receptors, and thyroid hormone. A term called *receptor theory* is used to explain how most drugs produce their effects in the body. Most drug receptors are proteins, though they can be any type of macromolecule. These receptors consist of protein subunits that surround a central channel. Additional protein segments attach to the plasma membrane. The channels are opened by voltage changes or chemicals (see Figure 2-4 ■).

Once bound to a receptor, a drug may trigger **second-messenger** events inside cells. Examples include release of intracellular calcium, activation of enzymes and specific G proteins, and conversion of adenosine triphosphate (ATP) to cyclic adenosine monophosphate (cyclic AMP). Inhibition or stimulation of cellular activities cause a drug's actions to occur. Certain receptors are not bound to plasma membranes, such as DNA or cytoplasmic enzymes. Some medications interact with these to regulate metabolism or cellular replication, as well as in the inhibition of protein synthesis. The agents that bind these intracellular components include hormones, steroid medications, retinoids, and vitamin D.

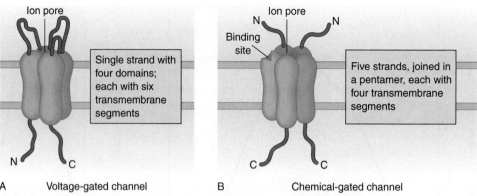

Figure 2-4 ■ Drug action through channels, via voltage changes or chemicals.

Source: Adams, Michael Patrick; Holland, Leland; Urban, Carol, Pharmacology for Nurses: *A Pathophysiologic Approach, 4th Ed.,* ©2014. Reprinted and Electronically reproduced by permission of Pearson Education, Inc., New York, NY

There are two basic receptor types, known as alpha and beta these also have subtypes known as α_1, α_2, β_1, and β_2. Medications may affect only alpha or beta receptor types, or only certain specific subtypes. Other medications act independently of cellular receptors by either changing cellular membrane permeability, by changing how cellular pumps work, or by depressing membrane excitability. These actions are called *nonspecific cellular responses.* Agents that work via these responses include general anesthetics, osmotic diuretics, and ethyl alcohol.

Types of Drug Receptors

The human body has many different receptors, but they can all be classified under four primary receptor families (see Figure 2-5 ■). The specific region of a receptor where the binding of drugs and endogenous regulatory molecules occurs is known as a *ligand-binding domain.*

The four primary drug-receptor families are:

✳ **Enzymes embedded in cell membranes** The ligand-binding domain is the specific region of the receptor where drug binding occurs, as well as the binding of endogenous regulatory molecules. With the enzymes embedded in cell membranes, the domain is located on the cell surface; the catalytic sites of the enzymes are inside. Binding of agonist drugs or endogenous regulatory molecules causes activation of the enzymes, increasing catalytic activities. Responses follow within a few seconds. Example: insulin, an endogenous ligand that acts through these enzymes.

✳ **Ligand-gated ion channels** The receptors span the cell membrane, regulating ions flowing in and out of cells. Each channel is specific for a certain ion. The ligand-binding domain is on the cell surface, and the channels open when an agonist drug or endogenous ligand binds the receptor. The ion's

Figure 2-5 ■ The four primary drug-receptor families.

✳ Apply Your Knowledge 2.2

The following questions focus on what you have just learned about the therapeutic index, cellular receptors, and drug action.

CRITICAL THINKING

1. Describe the structure of proteins that act as drug receptors.
2. Identify agents that work via nonspecific cellular responses.
3. Explain which drug-receptor family has actions that occur within milliseconds, and which has actions that occur over hours to days.

concentration gradient determines direction of flow across the membrane. Responses are very fast, within milliseconds in most cases. Examples: acetylcholine, gamma-aminobutyric acid (GABA).

✳ **G protein–coupled receptor systems** These involve three factors: the receptor itself, a G protein, and an effector such as an enzyme or ion channel. These systems bind agonist drugs or endogenous ligands, which then activates a G protein, and then the effector. Responses are fast. The ligand-binding domain may be on the cell surface or in a pocket-like structure accessed from the cell surface. Examples: Norepinephrine, histamine, serotonin, and many peptide hormones, which use these systems.

✳ **Transcription factors** These factors are located on DNA in the cell nucleus and regulate protein synthesis. Their responses are delayed. Activation stimulates transcription of messenger RNA molecules, which stimulate protein synthesis. Actions occur over hours to days. Transcription factors are activated only by ligands that cross the cell membrane because they have high lipid solubility. Examples: Thyroid hormone and all steroid hormones such as testosterone and progesterone, which use transcription factors for their actions.

DRUG-RECEPTOR INTERACTIONS

Drugs are chemicals that produce their effects by interacting with other chemicals, which are known as receptors inside the body. A receptor is a macromolecule inside a cell to which a drug binds. In the body, the term *receptor* is mostly used in reference to regulatory molecules such as neurotransmitters and hormones.

Enzymes, ribosomes, and other macromolecules are referred to as **target molecules** rather than true receptors.

Drug-receptor interactions are explained in the following equation:

$$D + R \Leftrightarrow D\text{–}R \text{ Complex} \longrightarrow \text{Response}$$

Receptors are considered either "on" or "off." When "on," they are referred to as being "activated." Physiologically, they are activated by endogenous compounds, or by drugs that either mimic or block actions of these compounds. For example, the effects of norepinephrine upon the heart involves the following things to occur:

✳ If increased cardiac output is needed by the body, autonomic neurons to the heart fire more quickly, which increases release of norepinephrine

✳ This neurotransmitter binds to cardiac receptors

✳ The rate and force of cardiac contractions increase, which increases cardiac output

✳ Once demand is no longer required, the process reverses itself, and the cardiac output is returned to resting levels

It is important to understand that in this example, the same cardiac receptors can also be receptors for drugs. Binding of drugs to these receptors can imitate actions of endogenous norepinephrine to increase cardiac output. Alternately, drugs can block the action of endogenous norepinephrine, preventing the heart from being stimulated by autonomic neurons.

Agonists, Agonist-Antagonists, and Antagonists

An **agonist** is a drug that binds to a receptor and produces a stimulatory response that is similar to what an endogenous substance (such as a hormone) would

Focus Point

Target Molecules and Drug Design

Biological targets, or target molecules, are used for the development of new medications. Drug design involves the design of molecules that are complementary to the shapes and electrical charges of target molecules, so that they will interact and bind to them.

have done if it were bound to the receptor. For example, adrenaline is an agonist at beta (β)-adrenoceptors. When adrenaline binds to β-adrenoceptors in the heart, the heart rate increases. Agonist drugs have affinity, which allows them to bind to receptors, as well as high intrinsic activity, which allows them to activate the functions of receptors. Examples of drugs that function as agonists include dobutamine, insulin, and norethindrone. Agonists may produce a greater maximal response than that of an endogenous chemical.

Agonists that produce weaker or less effective responses than endogenous chemicals are referred to as **agonist-antagonists** or *partial agonists*. They have only slight intrinsic activity. An example drug is pentazocine, which has much lower pain-relieving actions than a full agonist such as meperidine. Agonist-antagonists have the ability to act as both agonists and antagonists. An example is when pentazocine acts as an agonist when it is administered alone, but when it antagonizes the effects of meperidine when administered concurrently. In this case, it occupies the opioid receptors to prevent them from being activated by meperidine. The pentazocine in this example acts as an agonist to provide moderate pain relief while also acting as an antagonist to block the higher pain-relieving actions of meperidine.

An **antagonist** is a drug or another agent that blocks or antagonizes the effects of another substance or function. Therefore, antagonists are often used when treating overdoses of other drugs. Antagonists often compete with agonists for their receptor binding sites. For example, in most cases, antibacterial therapy involves the use of a single drug, but combining two antibiotics may actually decrease each drug's effects. If incorrect combinations are prescribed, the use of multiple antibiotics may also increase the potential to promote resistance.

Antagonists have almost no effects upon receptor function on their own. If no agonist is present, the administered antagonist will have no observable effect.

However, not all antagonists are associated with receptors, with *functional antagonists* inhibiting agonists by changing their pharmacokinetics, and not by competing for receptors. They may slow drug absorption and speed up drug excretion by affecting metabolism. Antagonist interactions with agonists are the basis of drug–drug and drug–food interactions. Examples of drugs used as antagonists include antihistamines and naloxone.

The majority of antagonists are classified as *competitive antagonists*. Also referred to as *surmountable antagonists*, they bind reversibly to receptors, producing receptor blockade because they compete with agonists for receptor binding. When an agonist and a competitive antagonist have equal affinity for a receptor, the receptor will be occupied by which of the two agents is present in the highest concentration. The result can be "surmounted" (overcome) if the concentration gradient changes so that the opposite agent reaches a higher concentration.

There are also *noncompetitive antagonists*. Also referred to as *insurmountable antagonists*, they bind irreversibly to receptors. Their effect is equivalent to reducing the total amount of receptors that are available to be activated by an agonist. Therefore, noncompetitive antagonists reduce the *maximal response* that an agonist can trigger. The effects of an agonist may be blocked completely if there is a high enough concentration of antagonist present. Noncompetitive antagonists cannot be overcome regardless of how high the concentration of an agonist. Therefore, noncompetitive antagonists are rarely used as therapeutic agents. Their effects are not permanent, however, since cells break down older receptors and synthesize new ones.

Focus Point

Antidotes

Antagonists commonly used as antidotes include acetylcysteine (for acetaminophen overdose), activated charcoal (for many poisons), digibind (for digoxin overdose), naloxone (for various narcotics overdoses), and penicillamine (for various metal ion poisonings).

❋ Apply Your Knowledge 2.3

The following questions focus on what you have just learned about drug-receptor interactions, agonists, and antagonists.

CRITICAL THINKING

1. Describe what physiologically activates drug receptors.
2. Identify what allows agonists to bind to receptors.
3. Describe the actions of *functional antagonists*

PRACTICAL SCENARIO 1

A 75-year-old man was admitted to the hospital after suffering from confusion, nausea, dizziness, and sleepiness. He had a history of type 2 diabetes mellitus, hypertension, aortic valve stenosis, and atrial fibrillation. His drug history included tolbutamide, pravastatin, bumetanide, bisoprolol, warfarin, and digoxin. Tests revealed that he did not have a systemic infection, but did have decreased renal function, and that his digoxin levels were very high.

Critical Thinking Questions

1. What is the likelihood that this patient was experiencing digoxin toxicity?
2. What health conditions may contribute to digoxin toxicity?
3. Are there other drugs that could be used instead of digoxin for patients who are at risk of digoxin toxicity?

PRACTICAL SCENARIO 2

A 47-year-old female cancer patient underwent insulin potentiation chemotherapy, which is a safe approach to treating aggressive forms of cancer. Since cancer cells have up to 20 times more insulin receptors than normal cells, insulin is able to open channels in cancer cell walls and allow nutrients to enter. The administration of insulin triggers cancer cells to open their membranes in order to obtain the glucose they require. When a chemotherapy drug is then administered, followed quickly by glucose, the cancer cells take in almost the entire dose of the chemotherapy drug, which poisons and kills them. Because of this insulin potentiation, only about one-tenth the amount of standard chemotherapy is needed.

Critical Thinking Questions

1. Why do normal, healthy cells not experience any significant toxic reactions to the chemotherapy drug administered by this method?
2. What are the signs and symptoms of overdose of insulin?

Chapter Capsule

This section repeats the objectives from the beginning of the chapter and then provides a summary of the most important concepts for that objective. Use this section as a quick review and to check your knowledge.

Objective 1: Define the term *pharmacodynamics.*

- Pharmacodynamics is concerned with the pharmacologic actions of a drug, including both therapeutic effects and adverse effects.
- It describes how a medication causes changes in the body.

Objective 2: Identify what is represented by the frequency distribution curve.

- A frequency distribution curve represents the number of patients that respond to the actions of a drug at different doses. A few patients are shown to have responded to a medication at very low doses, whereas increasing numbers of patients responded as the dosage was increased. The median effective dose is shown at the top of the curve. It is important to understand that the frequency distribution curve does not indicate the magnitude of drug response, but does indicate if a measurable response occurred in the test group of patients.

Objective 3: Explain the dose–effect relationship.

- The dose–effect (or dose–response) relationship is the relationship between the dose of a drug or other agent that produces therapeutic effects and the potency of these effects.

Objective 4: Discuss how the therapeutic index of a drug is calculated.

- The therapeutic index of a drug is used to predict whether a certain dosage is safe for a specific patient.
- It is calculated by dividing the median lethal dose (LD_{50}) by the median effective dose (ED_{50}).

Objective 5: Describe the affinity of a drug.

- A drug's affinity is its attractive force for a target receptor. The cell recipient is known as a receptor—usually a specific protein—situated either in cell membranes on cell surfaces or within the cellular cytoplasm. However, some drugs act on intracellular receptors; these include corticosteroids, which act on cytoplasmic steroid receptors.

Objective 6: Identify various types of second-messenger events.

- Once bound to a receptor, a drug may trigger second-messenger events inside cells. Examples include release of intracellular calcium, activation of enzymes and specific G proteins, and conversion of adenosine triphosphate (ATP) to cyclic adenosine monophosphate (cyclic AMP).

Objective 7: Briefly explain the four primary drug-receptor families.

- Enzymes are embedded in cell membranes. The ligand-binding domain is where drug and endogenous regulatory molecule binding occurs. It is on the cell surface, and catalytic sites of the enzymes are inside. Example: insulin
- Ligand-gated ion channels are receptors that span the cell membrane, regulating ions flowing in and out, with ion-specific channels. Channels open when an agonist drug or endogenous ligand binds the receptor. Direction of flow is determined by the ion's concentration gradient. Examples: acetylcholine, GABA
- G protein-coupled receptor systems involve a receptor, a G protein, and an effector. Agonist drugs or endogenous ligands are bound. Examples: norepinephrine, histamine, serotonin, peptide hormones
- Transcription factors are located on DNA in the nucleus. They regulate protein synthesis with delayed responses. Activation requires highly lipid-soluble cell membrane ligands. Examples: thyroid hormone, all steroid hormones

Objective 8: Explain the equation used to calculate drug-receptor interactions.

- Drug-receptor interactions are calculated by the equation:

$$D + R \Leftrightarrow D-R \text{ Complex} \longrightarrow \text{Response}$$

Objective 9: Differentiate between agonists and antagonists.

- An agonist is a drug that binds to a receptor and produces a stimulatory response that is similar to what an endogenous substance (such as a hormone) would have done if it were bound to the receptor. Agonist drugs have affinity, which allows them to bind to receptors, as well as high intrinsic activity, which allows them to activate the functions of receptors.

- An antagonist is a drug or another agent that blocks or antagonizes the effects of another substance or function. Antagonists often compete with agonists for their receptor binding sites. Antagonists have almost no effects upon receptor function on their own.

Objective 10: Explain competitive and noncompetitive antagonists.

- Most antagonists are classified as *competitive (surmountable) antagonists*. They bind reversibly to receptors, producing receptor blockade because they compete with agonists for receptor binding. The receptor will be occupied by which of the two agents is present in the highest concentration. The result can be "surmounted" (overcome) if the concentration gradient changes so that the opposite agent reaches a higher concentration.

- There are also *noncompetitive (insurmountable) antagonists*. They bind irreversibly to receptors, effectively reducing the total amount of receptors that are available to be activated by an agonist. They reduce the *maximal response* that an agonist can trigger, and may completely block agonist effects if there is a high enough concentration of antagonist present. Noncompetitive antagonists cannot be overcome regardless of agonist concentrations, so they are rarely used therapeutically. Effects are not permanent, however, since receptors are replaced.

 ## Internet Sites of Interest

- Overview of pharmacodynamics: **www.merckmanuals.com/professional/clinical-pharmacology/pharmacodynamics/overview-of-pharmacodynamics**
- Therapeutic index: **http://pharmacologycorner.com/therapeutic-index/**
- Functions of cell surface receptors: **www.ncbi.nlm.nih.gov/books/NBK9866/**
- Agonists and antagonists: **http://wings.buffalo.edu/aru/Agonists&Antagonists.html**
- Mechanism of drug actions: **http://howmed.net/pharmacology/mechanism-of-drug-action-drug-receptor-interactions/**
- Variation in drug responses: **www.phgfoundation.org/tutorials/pharmacogenomics/2.html**

Chapter 3

Pharmacokinetics

Chapter Objectives

After completing this chapter, you should be able to:

1. Identify the four primary processes of pharmacokinetics.
2. Explain the primary ways that drugs cross cell membranes.
3. Discuss the main site variables that affect drug absorption.
4. Discuss how drugs are distributed throughout the body.
5. Explain the metabolism of drugs and its applications to drug therapy.
6. Identify major processes by which drugs are excreted.
7. Explain the four main stages of biotransformation.
8. Explain the applications of a drug's plasma half-life to pharmacotherapy.
9. Explain how a drug reaches and maintains its therapeutic range in the plasma.
10. Differentiate between loading and maintenance doses.

Key Terms

absorption (p. 25)
bioavailability (p. 25)
biotransformation (p. 23)
blood–brain barrier (p. 27)
cytochrome P450 (p. 28)
dissolution (p. 25)
distribution (p. 27)
enzyme induction (p. 28)
excretion (p. 31)
first-pass effect (p. 25)
glucuronidation (p. 28)
half-life (p. 32)
hydrophilic (p. 28)
lipophilic (p. 24)

loading dose (p. 34)
maintenance dose (p. 34)
metabolic acidosis (p. 29)
metabolic alkalosis (p. 29)
metabolic tolerance (p. 31)
metabolism (p. 28)
microsomal enzymes (p. 29)
minimum effective concentration (p. 33)
peak concentration (p. 33)
P-glycoprotein (p. 24)
pharmacodynamic tolerance (p. 30)
pharmacokinetics (p. 23)
pH partitioning (p. 25)
placebo (p. 30)

plasma albumin (p. 27)
plateau (p. 34)
polar molecules (p. 24)
respiratory acidosis (p. 29)
respiratory alkalosis (p. 29)
side effects (p. 29)
tachyphylaxis (p. 31)
therapeutic range (p. 33)
thermodynamics (p. 25)
tolerance (p. 30)
toxic concentration (p. 33)
trough concentration (p. 33)

Introduction

The term **pharmacokinetics** is derived from two Greek words: *pharmakon* ("drug or poison") and *kinesis* ("motion"). Pharmacokinetics is the study of drug movement throughout the body. Pharmacokinetics is a core subject in pharmacology. It assists health care professionals in understanding the mechanism of action and adverse effects of drugs. There are four principle pharmacokinetic processes: absorption, distribution, **biotransformation** (metabolism), and excretion (Figure 3-1 ■). The combination of drug metabolism and excretion is also known as *elimination*. Absorption, distribution, metabolism, and excretion are related to drug concentrations, drug metabolites, and mechanisms of action. In this chapter, I consider movement of drug plasma membranes, drug absorption, drug distribution, drug metabolism, and special considerations of drug metabolism.

Movement of Drugs Across Plasma Membranes

In order for drugs to move throughout the body, they must cross plasma membranes. These membranes consist of two layers of molecules called *phospholipids*, which are fats that contain one atom of phosphate. Phospholipids have a round "head," which contains the phosphate, and two "tails," which are long-chain hydrocarbons. Other substances embedded in the membrane include cholesterol, carbohydrates, and proteins.

Drugs may cross plasma membranes by two primary processes: diffusion (passive transport) and active transport. Lipid-soluble drugs and small molecules that are nonionized pass through plasma membranes by simple diffusion, and easily reach the target cells (see Figure 3-2 ■). Simple diffusion involves movement of molecules from

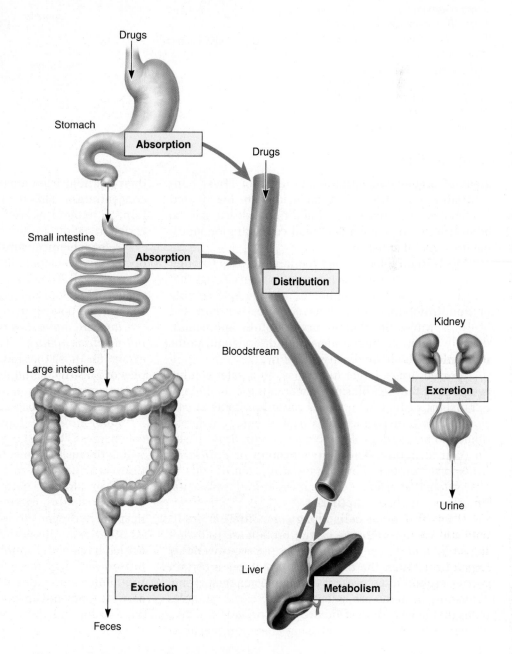

Figure 3-1 ■ The four processes of pharmacokinetics (i.e., movement) are absorption, distribution, metabolism, and excretion.

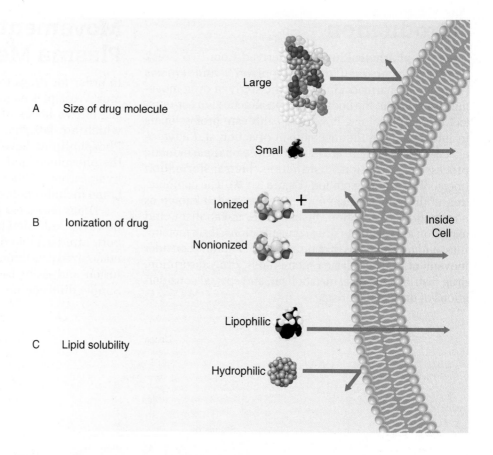

A — Size of drug molecule

B — Ionization of drug

C — Lipid solubility

Large

Small

Ionized +

Nonionized

Lipophilic

Hydrophilic

Inside Cell

Figure 3-2 ■ Passage of drugs across plasma membranes: (**A**) small drugs, (**B**) non-ionized drugs, and (**C**) lipophilic drugs are more likely to cross membranes.

Source: Urban, Carol, Pharmacology: Connection to Nursing Practice, 2nd Ed., ©2013. Reprinted and Electronically reproduced by permission of Pearson Education, Inc., New York, NY.

areas of higher concentration to areas of lower concentration. Over time, drug molecules are inactivated (metabolized) by tissues, and additional doses may be administered to create a continual concentration gradient, from blood to tissue.

Most drug molecules are too large to pass through pores or channels and lack transport systems. Drugs that directly penetrate the membranes must be lipid soluble or **lipophilic** since membranes are mostly composed of lipids. Molecules that are not lipophilic and cannot directly penetrate membranes include ions and **polar molecules**, which are discussed below.

Ionized drugs, larger molecules, and water-soluble agents pass through plasma membranes via the help of a transport system, which uses certain proteins as carriers. Some transport systems require energy whereas others do not, and are selective for certain drugs based on their structure. The **P-glycoprotein** or *multidrug transporter protein* moves many drugs out of cells. It is a system that is active in the liver, kidneys, placenta, intestines, and brain capillaries.

Drugs that enter cells along concentration gradients and use a membrane carrier protein are undergoing *facilitated diffusion*, which does not require energy expenditure from the cells. It only requires a certain carrier protein to be present on the plasma membrane. Transport proteins are selective, only carrying molecules that have certain structures. The process of *active transport* involves drugs crossing membranes against

their gradient from areas of low concentration to high concentration. This requires the cell, and a carrier protein, to expend energy. Carrier proteins assisting in active transport are sometimes called *pumps.*

A few chemical substances are able to pass through open pores or channels in the plasma membrane, but these are very small. Therefore, only substances with a molecular weight of less than 200 can pass through. Examples include sodium and potassium ions, alcohol, urea, and water.

Ions are molecules that have a positive or negative *net electrical charge*. They cannot cross membranes, except for those that have very small molecules. Examples of ions that cannot cross membranes include *quaternary ammonium compounds* such as tubocurarine and weak acids or bases.

Polar molecules have unevenly distributed electrical charges. The best example is the water molecule, in which the negative electrons remain closer, most of the time, near the oxygen atom in comparison to the two hydrogen atoms. Therefore, the area near the oxygen atom is usually negatively charged, whereas the area near the hydrogen atoms is usually positively charged. Another example is the drug kanamycin. Polar molecules have equal numbers of protons and electrons, but no net electrical charge that is positive or negative. Polar molecules dissolve in *polar solvents* such as water, but not in *nonpolar solvents* such as oil. A good example is how sugar will dissolve in water but not oil.

✱ Apply Your Knowledge 3.1

The following questions focus on what you have just learned about pharmacokinetics.

CRITICAL THINKING

1. What are the four stages of pharmacokinetics?
2. What determines a drug's ability to cross a membrane?
3. How do ions differ electrically from polar molecules?

Drug Absorption

The process of drug movement into the systemic circulation is **absorption**. Absorption depends on the drug's ability to cross cell membranes and resist extensive breakdown by the stomach, intestines, and liver. Presystemic metabolism occurs when enzymes in the gastrointestinal (GI) tract begin to break down the drug before it is absorbed. Presystemic metabolism affects the amount of drug that reaches the systemic circulation intact and the speed at which this happens—a concept termed **bioavailability**.

Bioavailability depends on pharmaceutical factors (such as the rate at which a tablet or capsule dissolves or the use of binding products in formulating the medication) and variable factors that affect GI absorption (such as food in the stomach, other drugs taken concurrently, intestinal motility, or certain disease states). Lipid-soluble drugs (e.g., diazepam and phenytoin) and weak acids (such as acetylsalicylic acid and penicillin V) may be absorbed directly from the stomach. Weak bases (e.g., morphine and atropine) are not normally absorbed from the site. The small intestine is the primary site of absorption because of the very large surface area across which drugs may diffuse. Acids (such as ibuprofen and warfarin) are normally absorbed more extensively in the intestines than in the stomach even though the intestines have a higher pH.

FACTORS THAT AFFECT THE RATE OF DRUG ABSORPTION

A drug's physical and chemical properties influence how quickly it is absorbed. Also, the anatomic and physiologic qualities of the absorption site play a role. In the GI tract, many factors influence the rate of drug absorption, including:

1. **Acidity of the stomach** Aspirin and other drugs that have an acidic pH are easily absorbed in the stomach's acidic environment. The small intestine, which has an alkaline environment, more readily absorbs alkaline medications. The pH of the stomach tends to be changed by milk products and antacids. Some drugs are not absorbed properly as a result. For this reason, infants who are consuming milk or formula may need to be given certain medications on an empty stomach. A factor known as **pH partitioning** influences absorption, such as when it is sped up by differences between plasma pH and the pH at the site of drug administration. This means that the drug's molecules are more likely to be ionized in the plasma.

2. **Physiochemical properties** The rate of a drug's absorption may be greatly affected by the rate at which the drug is made available to the biologic fluid at the administration site. Some of the factors that affect a drug's rate of **dissolution** (the process of dissolving) from a solid form include intrinsic physiochemical properties, such as solubility and **thermodynamics**. A drug must dissolve before it can be absorbed, so its rate of dissolution aids in determining its rate of absorption. Therefore, drugs that are formulated for rapid dissolution take effect faster than those formulated for slower dissolution.

3. **Presence of food in the stomach or intestine** The rate and extent of drug absorption may be greatly influenced by the presence of food. Whereas an empty stomach increases the rate of absorption of some medications, food in the stomach decreases the absorption rate. However, if a medication causes irritation to the stomach, the patient should eat food with the medication; the food serves as a buffer to decrease irritation.

4. **Routes of administration** Orally administered drugs are usually absorbed in the stomach and the small intestine. From the small intestine, drugs are absorbed and immediately move to the liver for metabolism, involving various enzymes, to reach the systemic circulation. This process is called the **first-pass effect** (see Figure 3-3 ■). After the drug is in the liver, it is partly metabolized before being sent to where systemic effects occur. As a result, medications that are metabolized too quickly in the liver should not be given orally. Dopamine (generic), and lidocaine (Xylocaine) are some examples of drugs that exhibit first-pass metabolism. To determine the suitability of a drug for each patient, it is crucial that the route of administration be correctly chosen. Depending on the degree of first-pass elimination

Figure 3-3 ■ The first-pass effect.

and the formulation of some drugs, oral administration is feasible for some drugs and not for others. Drugs that are directly injected into the bloodstream bypass the process of absorption and are distributed throughout the body. The time before the drug becomes effective for these injections is typically short compared with other types of injections. Also, drugs may be injected deeply into skeletal muscle. The vascularity of the muscle site and the lipid solubility of the drug determine the rate of absorption. Because the subcutaneous region is less vascular than the muscle tissues, subcutaneous injections are absorbed less rapidly. Transdermal injections (tuberculin test), transdermal patches, and otic or ophthalmic administration are other routes. Topical drugs may be absorbed through several layers of skin for a local effect. Transdermal nitroglycerin (Nitrostat) is absorbed rapidly and provides sustained blood levels after application to the skin in the form of either an ointment or a transdermal patch. Some drugs, such as fentanyl patches (Duragesic), also provide certain systemic effects, such as pain relief. Drugs administered in low concentrations tend to be less rapidly absorbed than those administered in high concentrations.

5. **Lipid solubility** Generally, drugs with high lipid solubility are absorbed more quickly than those with low lipid solubility. Those with high lipid solubility also readily cross membranes separating them from the blood.

6. **Blood flow** Drug absorption is faster from sites with high blood flow. This is because the blood that contains the newly absorbed drug is replaced quickly by blood that is drug-free. A large gradient between drug concentrations outside the blood and in the blood exists. Therefore, absorption is faster with greater concentration gradients.

7. **Surface area** The rate of absorption is mostly determined by the amount of surface area available. Larger surface areas mean faster absorption. This is why orally administered drugs are more commonly absorbed from the small intestine, which has a larger surface area, than from the stomach.

✳ Apply Your Knowledge 3.2

The following questions focus on what you have just learned about drug absorption.

CRITICAL THINKING

1. Explain bioavailability, and upon what it depends.
2. List the factors that affect the rate of drug absorption.
3. Which routes of administration protect drugs from chemical decomposition that may occur in the stomach or liver?

Drug Distribution

The movement of pharmacologic drugs throughout the body after they are absorbed is known as **distribution**. Drugs may interact with components in the blood, and can be chemically or physically altered prior to reaching their targets. Many drugs are bound to circulating proteins, usually albumin, and lipoproteins or glycoproteins. Only the fraction of drugs that is not bound to protein can bind to cellular receptors, pass across tissue membranes, and gain access to cellular enzymes, thus being distributed to body tissue. Changes in protein binding can therefore sometimes cause changes in drug distribution. The initial rate of distribution of a drug depends heavily on the blood flow to various organs. Lipid-soluble drugs enter the central nervous system (CNS) rapidly. Because of the **blood–brain barrier**, certain drugs are poorly distributed to the CNS because they pass through the barrier.

There are three major influencing factors related to drug distribution: blood flow to the body tissues, how drugs are able to exit the vascular system, and how drugs are able to enter body cells. After administration, a drug is carried in the blood to body tissues and organs, with the flow rate influencing the speed at which the drug is delivered. Low regional blood flow affects drug therapy in two specific conditions: tumors and abscesses. When a tumor is solid, there is a limited blood supply, with the lowest amount of blood flow in the tumor's core. High drug levels, therefore, cannot reach the deeper parts of a tumor. Therefore, solid tumors are highly resistant to drug therapy. Pus-filled pockets of infection, or *abscesses*, lack internal blood vessels. Therefore, antibiotics cannot reach the bacteria they contain and, instead, surgical drainage is required initially.

Once a drug reaches a tissue or organ, it then leaves the vascular system. This step is required for the drug to reach its target cells, and so the drug can be metabolized and excreted. In the vascular system, drugs leave the blood at the capillary beds. They usually pass directly through the capillary walls via pores. This does not impede movement into the interstitial space. The tight junctions between the cells that compose most capillary walls in the CNS are referred to as the *blood–brain barrier*. Drugs are prevented from passing through this tight barrier. Instead, a drug must be able to pass through the capillary wall cells themselves. This can only occur when a drug is lipid soluble or has a transport system. Another factor is P-glycoprotein, which is the transporter that pumps many drugs out of cells. In the CNS, P-glycoprotein pumps drugs back to the blood and helps to stop them from entering the brain. While the blood–brain barrier protects the brain from many toxic substances, it can also keep helpful antibiotics from treating CNS infections. The barrier is not fully developed in newborns, making them more susceptible to drug effects and CNS toxicities.

During pregnancy, the placenta is able to transfer drugs from the mother to the fetus. The substances most likely to pass through the placenta are those that are lipid soluble and nonionized. These agents are linked to birth defects, drug dependency, and respiratory depression.

Drugs can also bind to **plasma albumin** and other body proteins. Albumin remains in the bloodstream because of its size and lack of a transport system. Only some drug molecules are bound, at any given time, to albumin. This is related to the strength of attraction between the drug and albumin. An example of a drug that is highly bound to albumin is warfarin. An example of a drug that is only slightly bound to album is gentamicin. Drugs that are highly bound to albumin cannot leave the bloodstream, meaning they cannot reach their sites of action, metabolism, or excretion. Protein binding is also a source of drug interactions, since one drug can displace another for a protein such as albumin. Competition can increase drug responses and cause toxicity.

Nearly all drugs must enter cells in order to be metabolized and excreted, and some drugs must enter cells in order to reach their sites of action. Lipid solubility and the existence of a transport system also influence this situation. Many drugs bind with receptors on cell membrane surfaces in order to become effective, and do not need to cross cell membranes.

✱ Apply Your Knowledge 3.3 ▬▬▬▬

The following questions focus on what you have just learned about drug distribution.

CRITICAL THINKING

1. On what does the initial rate of drug distribution heavily depend?
2. How do tumors or abscesses affect drug distribution?
3. Explain the blood–brain barrier in relation to drug distribution.

Drug Metabolism

Most drug **metabolism**, also referred to as *biotransformation*, occurs in the liver through the same biochemical pathways and reactions that affect nutrients, vitamins, and minerals. The majority of metabolism in the liver occurs through the *hepatic microsomal enzyme system* or *P450 system*. Its key component is **cytochrome P450**, which is actually a group of 12 enzyme families.

Drug metabolism may cause six therapeutically significant outcomes:

✱ Faster drug excretion via the kidneys occurs by converting lipid-soluble drugs into more water-soluble (**hydrophilic**) forms, speeding up excretion of many drugs; methods of conversion include the structural addition of a hydroxyl group or by **glucuronidation**

✱ Inactivation of drugs in which an active form of a drug is converted to its inactive form

✱ More therapeutic action in which the drug's effectiveness is increased

✱ "Prodrug" activation in which an inactive form of a drug is administered, which is then converted to an active form, or *prodrug*

✱ More toxicity by converting a relatively safe compound into a toxic form

✱ Less toxicity by converting a drug into its inactive form

Focus Point

Drug Metabolism

In infants, drug metabolism is limited until about 1 year of age. Until the liver is mature, extreme care must be taken to prevent injury caused by drug administration.

Certain drugs cause the liver to increase rates of metabolism, often by synthesizing drug-metabolizing enzymes, which is called **enzyme induction**. In this situation, the drug can increase the rate of its own metabolism, requiring increased dosages. Induction of drug-metabolizing enzymes can also speed up metabolism of concurrent drugs, requiring increased dosages as well.

The *first-pass effect* is an important mechanism that influences drug action and metabolism. When oral drugs are absorbed from the GI tract, they move to the liver through the hepatic portal vein. Metabolism accomplishes the conversion of molecules as well as biodegration of foreign substances. Substances absorbed across the intestinal wall enter blood vessels. This is known as *hepatic portal circulation*, a process that carries blood directly to the liver (see Figure 3-3). If the liver has a high metabolic capacity, the drug is totally inactivated on its first pass, and no therapeutic effects occur.

A drug may be given parenterally in order to avoid the first-pass effect. The liver is temporarily bypassed, and the drug reaches therapeutic levels in the systemic blood. An example is nitroglycerin, which may avoid the first-pass effect via sublingual administration, since this method allows it to be absorbed directly into the systemic circulation. The drug moves to its sites of action prior to being exposed to liver enzymes.

Enzymes act on most drugs in the body and convert drugs to end-products called *metabolites* during metabolism. Biotransformation is the process of conversion of drugs via enzymatic actions. Biotransformation may be divided into four main stages:

1. **Oxidation**—combination with oxygen

2. **Reduction**—a reaction with a substance that involves the gaining of electrons

3. **Hydrolysis**—the cleaving of a compound into simpler compounds with the uptake of the hydrogen and hydroxide parts of a water molecule

4. **Conjugation**—the combination of substances with glucuronic or sulfuric acid, terminating biologic activity and making them ready for excretion

All these activities occur primarily in the liver via **microsomal enzymes**, with cytochrome P450 playing an essential role in drug metabolism. Toxic drug action can be influenced by drug metabolism, interactions, activation, toxicity, and **adverse effects**. **Side effects** are usually less serious than adverse effects, are predictable, and may occur even at therapeutic doses.

Another important factor to consider is *enterohepatic recirculation*, in which a drug is moved from the liver, through the bile duct, to the duodenum. It is then moved in the portal blood back to the liver. However, this only occurs with drugs that have gone through glucuronidation. The process of enterohepatic recirculation means that susceptible drugs can stay in the body for a much longer time than other drugs. Fortunately, not all glucuronidated drugs experience this recycling, and are excreted intact in the feces.

SPECIAL CONSIDERATIONS OF DRUG METABOLISM

Many factors may influence drug response and should be considered prior to drug administration. These factors include age; body weight; gender; race; diurnal body rhythms; acid–base, fluid, and electrolyte balance; diseases; genetics; immunology; psychology; environment; tolerance; drug excretion, clearance, accumulation, and interactions; diet; and failure to follow medication regimens.

Age

Drug effects may vary in patients according to their different metabolic rates. Age often affects metabolic rates. Drug dosages may need to be adjusted in children or elderly patients by using specific conversion formulas. In infants, increased sensitivity to medications is because of organ immaturity. In older adults, it is often due to organ degeneration, but may also be caused by multiple drug therapies, more than one disease or condition being present, and the severity of these diseases or conditions. Commonly, older adults have reduced absorption and distribution, changes in biotransformation, and less effective excretion. As a result, many medications are packaged with recommended doses for elderly patients. Regardless of whether the patient is a child or an older adult, there should be close monitoring of drug effects. The rule of thumb with pediatric and geriatric individuals is "start low and go slow!"

Body Weight

Body weight is an important factor for drug action. In general, this is based on an average 150-pound adult. The same dosage of medication can have varied effects in patients whose weights differ. Some medication doses must be adjusted based on body weight and body surface area, especially in children. This is because the percentage of body fat is calculated when body surface area is assessed. The percentage of body fat is a significant factor concerning drug distribution. The calculation of correct dosage of drugs based on body weight is discussed in Chapter 10.

Gender

Male and female patients respond to drugs differently. Drugs administered intramuscularly are absorbed faster by men than by women. Such drugs remain in women's tissues longer than in men's tissues because women have a higher body fat-to-muscle ratio. Other factors include higher cerebral blood flow in males. Examples of differences between males and females in relation to drug response include the increased effects of certain opioid analgesics in women and increased mortality in women when treated with digoxin or quinidine. Today, more drug trials focusing on females are being conducted in order to better understand these many differences in drug response. Another important factor is that women must be questioned about the possibility of pregnancy since the use of drugs in pregnant women is generally not recommended unless benefits outweigh risks to the fetus.

Race

In regard to a person's race, drug responses are most influenced by genetic variations and psychosocial factors. An example of an agent that has proven effectiveness in African Americans is the combination of the vasodilators called isosorbide dinitrate and hydralazine. This combination drug has reduced 1-year mortality among African Americans, yet has not yet been tested with significant results in any other racial group. The racial component in drug response is still largely unproven, but is constantly being explored for potentially important significances related to drug development.

Diurnal Body Rhythms

Diurnal, or circadian, rhythms can affect the intensity of a person's response to a drug. For example, at night, the circadian clock sets the stage for sleep. By administering sleep-inducing medications at night, the drug actions may be more pronounced. In contrast, administering corticosteroids during the day is meant to mimic the circadian variations in endogenous cortisol.

Acid–Base, Fluid, and Electrolyte Balances

Acid–base, fluid, and electrolyte balances also play a part in drug effects, both in how the drug affects the body and how the body reacts. If desired effects are not achieved, a review of these balances should be made in conjunction with the timing of the drug administration. Changes in acid–base balance can affect drug absorption, distribution, metabolism, and excretion. The four main types of disorders involved are **respiratory acidosis**, **respiratory alkalosis**, **metabolic acidosis**, and **metabolic alkalosis**. Altered electrolyte status, most commonly of the electrolytes potassium, sodium, calcium, and magnesium, can result in many disruptions of cellular processes. These disruptions most often affect muscular and nervous tissue. However, electrolyte disturbances do not cause widespread effects in drug response. The most significant example of altered drug response due to electrolyte imbalance is with digoxin. When potassium levels are lower than normal, digoxin toxicity may occur, causing potentially fatal dysrhythmias.

Diseases

Because the liver is the major site of detoxification and the kidneys are the major sites of elimination of chemical substances, a person with liver or kidney disease may respond differently to medications than does a healthy individual. Since the liver is the major site of drug metabolism, liver disease may result in drugs accumulating in the body. Kidney disease often reduces drug excretion, meaning that drugs may accumulate in the body, reaching toxic levels.

Genetics

In some people, genetic background affects therapeutic or adverse effects of certain drugs. This is basically due to genes that code for enzymes that metabolize drugs and for drug targets. Today, genetic testing is regularly performed for specific drugs, including maraviroc, trastuzumab, warfarin, and carbamazepine. It is believed that in the future, genetic testing will be conducted for specific individuals on a regular basis to determine the most effective and safest drugs and dosages required.

In most cases, genetic variants alter drug responses by increasing or decreasing drug metabolism. Most commonly, the drug is ineffective or becomes toxic. When the therapeutic index is low, genetic variants play a more serious part in drug responses. Examples of drugs affected by gene variants include:

✳ Tamoxifen—gene variants of cytochrome P450-2D6 (CYP2D6)

✳ Clopidogrel—gene variants of CYP2C19

✳ Isoniazid—in Caucasians, 52% metabolize this drug slowly whereas 48% metabolize it quickly

✳ Codeine conversion into morphine—in Caucasians, about 7% have a form of CYP2D6 that cannot convert codeine into morphine for pain relief

✳ Warfarin—gene variants that code for CYP2C9 can increase risk of bleeding

✳ Thiopurine methyltransferase—gene variants can reduce activity of this agent, delaying metabolic inactivation of the cancer drugs thioguanine and mercaptopurine

✳ Fluorouracil—approximately 1% of Americans produce a type of dihydropyrimidine dehydrogenase that cannot adequately metabolize fluorouracil

Gene variants can also change the structure of normal cell receptors and other drug targets, such as those for beta$_1$-adrenergics and warfarin. Gene variants that affect cancer cell and virus drug targets have effects related to trastuzumab, cetuximab, and maraviroc. Gene variants that can increase risks of severe hypersensitivity to immunomodulators involve the drugs carbamazepine and abacavir.

Immunology

Drug allergies may result in development of antibodies once the patient is exposed to its proteins. When another exposure occurs, a serious allergic reaction can develop. Mild reactions include skin rashes; severe reactions can include anaphylaxis, shock, and even death.

Psychology

A patient's response to a drug that is related to psychological factors, and not the actual properties of the drug, is called the *placebo effect*. A **placebo** is a drug preparation that lacks any intrinsic pharmacologic activity. Its effects occur because of the patient's psychologic reaction to the "drug." Placebos are most often used as control preparations in clinical drug trials. The placebo effect is usually perceived to be positive, but this is not always true. Responses to a placebo may promote recovery when the patient believes the placebo will be effective, but if the patient believes it to be harmful or ineffective, the outcome may be negative or neutral. Today, after much research, it is believed that the placebo effect is much less significant than was previously thought.

Environment

Even a person's surrounding environment can affect drug therapy. Sedatives are shown to work more effectively when the patient is put into a quiet environment that lacks excessive stimulation. Another environmental influence is temperature. Antihypertensives may have increased effectiveness in hotter climates since natural vasodilation occurs with increased temperature. The combined effects of an antihypertensive with the already-present vasodilation may result in results that are for more than desired.

Tolerance

When a patient has a decreased response to a drug because of repeated drug administration, **tolerance** has developed. Higher doses are then needed to produce effects that were previously achieved with lower doses. The three categories of tolerance are pharmacodynamic tolerance, metabolic tolerance, and tachyphylaxis.

Pharmacodynamic tolerance is related to long-term administration of a drug, when increased drug levels are needed to achieve the desired effects. The minimum effective concentration of the drug is excessively high. This type of tolerance results from the receptors adapting to the drug over time, and takes several days to occur. Cross-tolerance may also occur, in which tolerance develops to drugs that are within the same class, and not only to the specific drug that was originally being used when tolerance developed.

Metabolic tolerance results from increased drug metabolism, when the drug causes the liver to synthesize drug-metabolizing enzymes. This increases drug metabolism and results in the dosage having to be increased to maintain therapeutic levels. Metabolic tolerance does not affect the minimum effective concentration of the drug, and also takes several days to occur.

Tachyphylaxis is a reduction in response to a drug caused by repeated doses over a short period of time. This develops much more quickly than pharmacodynamic or metabolic tolerance, and is not as common. An example of a drug for which tachyphylaxis may develop is nitroglycerin.

✳ Apply Your Knowledge 3.4

The following questions focus on what you have just learned about drug metabolism.

CRITICAL THINKING

1. Describe hepatic portal circulation.
2. Explain the four main stages of biotransformation.
3. Where are the microsomal enzymes found and what are their roles?
4. What is meant by the side effects of a drug?
5. Explain the phrase "start low and go slow."
6. Why may drugs remain in women's tissues longer than in men's tissues?
7. Which type of drug tolerance is a reduction in response to a drug caused by repeated doses over a short period of time?

Drug Excretion

Drug **excretion** is the last stage of pharmacokinetics that removes drugs from the body via the kidneys. The kidneys remove waste and harmful agents in the blood circulation. Because most drugs are excreted by the kidneys, diseases of the kidneys can significantly prolong the duration of drug action. Drugs that affect the kidneys and the processes the kidneys use to remove substances from the body are discussed in Chapter 31.

The steps used in renal excretion include:

✳ **Glomerular filtration** Occurs at the glomerulus of the kidney tubule. Drugs are forced through pores of capillary walls, then into the tubular urine. However, blood cells and large molecules such as proteins cannot undergo this process due to their size; therefore, drugs bound to albumin remain in the blood.

✳ **Passive tubular reabsorption** Since lipid-soluble drug concentrations in the blood are lower than those in the tubule, this concentration gradient moves drugs out of the tubule and back into the blood. In contrast, non-lipid-soluble drugs remain in the urine for excretion. Conversion of lipid-soluble drugs into more polar forms reduces passive reabsorption and speeds up excretion of these drugs.

✳ **Active tubular secretion** Pumps drugs from the blood to the tubular urine. One type of pump is used for organic acids and another for organic bases. Tubule cells also contain P-glycoprotein, which is able to pump many different drugs into the urine. They have a relatively high capacity, playing an important role in excretion of certain compounds.

Renal drug excretion is modified by pH-dependent ionization and by competition for active tubular transport, which has an age-related component in newborns. In pH-dependent ionization, since ions are not lipid-soluble, drugs ionized at tubular urine pH will stay in the tubule and be excreted. Therefore, manipulation of urinary pH results in decreased passive reabsorption and increased excretion. Regarding competition for active tubular transport, if two drugs are administered concurrently that both use the same transport system, excretion of each drug is delayed by the other's presence.

Other routes of drug elimination include:

✳ **Lungs**—important for the elimination of alcohol and anesthetic gases

✳ **Breast milk**—important for the elimination of aspirin, barbiturates, and other drugs

✳ **Sweat, tears, urine, and feces**—elimination that may be alarming if the patient is not expecting the orange-red discoloration caused by phenazopyridine or rifampicin

✳ **Bile**—leading to the recirculation of compounds, such as chloramphenicol (its inactive metabolites are reactivated by hydrolysis in the gut), morphine, rifampicin, tetracycline, and digitoxin

✳ **Saliva**—sometimes used in monitoring drug concentrations in body fluids

To aid in the proper excretion of drugs, the patient should follow these guidelines:

✳ Take medications as ordered.

✳ Cough and breathe deeply after general anesthesia to help eliminate anesthetics more quickly.

✳ Chew gum or suck on hard candy to decrease the unpleasant effects of drugs that are eliminated through saliva.

✳ Increase intake of fluids because this will increase the filtration of urine and increase blood volume, thereby assisting in proper excretion.

✳ Maintain proper diet and amount of physical activity because both of these speed drug excretion.

✳ Keep skin clean to help avoid irritation from drugs that are eliminated through the sweat glands.

✳ Discuss use of all medications, including OTC drugs, with your physician to avoid possible risks to the fetus if you are pregnant.

Drug Clearance

Drug clearance is the pharmacokinetic measurement of plasma volume that is completely cleared of a drug per unit of time. Total body clearance is equal to renal, hepatic, and lung clearance combined. The clearance of a drug is calculated by dividing its rate of elimination by its plasma concentration, usually in mL per minute. Most drugs experience clearance at a relatively constant rate over a large range of plasma concentrations. For different drugs, the amounts of clearance range from small percentages of blood flow to a maximum of total blood flow to the organs of elimination. Therefore, in every patient, drug clearance is based on the drug administered, blood flow, and the healthiness of the organs of elimination. Clearance is, therefore, equivalent to the extraction capability multiplied by the rate that the drug is delivered to these organs.

Blood flow to the organs of elimination limits rates of drug clearance. Total clearance of a drug is directly affected by the amount of blood flow to the organs of elimination. The rate of drug clearance can also be significantly affected by cardiac disease, as well as drugs that alter blood flow. Also, for some drugs, clearance is not constant.

DRUG PLASMA HALF-LIFE

A drug's plasma **half-life** ($t\frac{1}{2}$) is defined as the time taken for the blood or plasma concentration of the drug to decrease from full to one-half (50%) after the last dose is taken. The half-life is the major determinant of the duration of drug action, and the half-life of each drug may be different. The longer the half-life of the drug, the longer the drug remains in the body. A drug with a short half-life of 2 or 3 hours must be administered more often than one with a longer half-life of 12 hours. This is because a shorter half-life means the drug leaves the body more quickly.

No matter how much drug was administered, the half-life still means *how long it takes for 50% to leave the*

✳ Apply Your **Knowledge 3.5**

The following questions focus on what you have just learned about drug excretion.

CRITICAL THINKING

1. List the main route of drug excretion and the factors that may change it.

2. List and briefly explain the three steps of renal excretion.

3. Which alternate route is important for excretion of alcohol and anesthetic gases?

4. Explain drug clearance and how it is calculated.

5. Briefly explain a drug's "half-life."

Focus on Geriatrics

Drug Elimination in Elderly Patients

Older adults with chronic active hepatitis, cirrhosis of the liver, or drug-induced hepatitis can have markedly affected drug elimination. Consequently, some drugs, such as diazepam, may cause coma in patients with severe liver damage when given in ordinary doses.

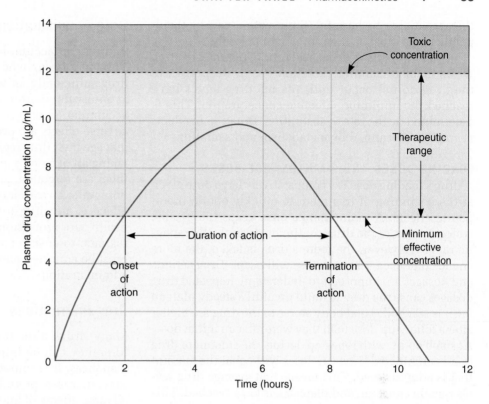

Figure 3-4 ▪ The therapeutic range of a drug.

body. However, the more the drug is present in the body, the larger the amount that is lost during one half-life. Remember that a drug's half-life determines how much time must pass between each dose. Drugs with a shorter half-life have shorter dosing intervals, and vice versa.

DRUG PLASMA CONCENTRATION AND THERAPEUTIC RESPONSE

Generally, the concentration of a drug in the plasma is directly related to the amount of time the drug will exert its effects. Drug plasma concentrations are regularly monitored in order to control a patient's responses to a drug. These concentrations can be adjusted by changing dosage size, timing, or both. It is important to remember that drug responses are related to concentrations at the sites of action. There is a direct correlation between therapeutic and toxic responses compared to how much drug is present in the plasma. Therefore, plasma concentrations are able to predict therapeutic as well as toxic responses.

The **minimum effective concentration** is the plasma drug level below which therapeutic effects do not occur. A beneficial drug must have concentrations that meet or exceed the minimum effective concentration. The **toxic concentration** is the plasma level at which toxic effects begin to occur. Toxicity happens when plasma drug levels become too high. Therefore, doses are kept small enough to avoid reaching the toxic concentration. The **peak concentration** is the highest level at which a drug is present in the body, whereas the **trough concentration** is the lowest level at which a drug is present in the body.

The **therapeutic range** of a drug is between the minimum effective concentration and the toxic concentration (see Figure 3-4 ▪). The goal of drug dosing is to keep plasma drug levels within the therapeutic range. Drugs with a narrow therapeutic range are more dangerous to use. An example of a drug with a narrow therapeutic range is lithium; an example of a drug with a large therapeutic range is acetaminophen. Though all drugs have

✳ Apply Your Knowledge 3.6

The following questions focus on what you have just learned about drug plasma concentration and therapeutic response.

CRITICAL THINKING

1. At which site in the body can drug concentrations predict drug responses?
2. Which drugs are more dangerous to use in regard to their type of therapeutic range and why?
3. Give an example of a drug with a narrow therapeutic range and one with a large therapeutic range.

the potential to be harmful, those with a narrow therapeutic range must be monitored more closely.

Drug levels rise during absorption, but then decline while metabolism and excretion occur. Responses to the drug do not occur until plasma drug levels have reached the minimum effective concentration. This is determined by the rate of absorption. Duration of effects is greatly determined by metabolism and excretion.

LOADING DOSES AND MAINTENANCE DOSES

A drug's **loading dose** is a comparatively large dose given at the beginning of treatment to quickly obtain therapeutic effects. A **maintenance dose** keeps the plasma concentration of the drug continuously in the therapeutic range. However, the more a drug is taken, the more chance that drug accumulation will occur. Drug actions and dosages are important to understand. Repeated drug dosages cause the drug to build up until a steady **plateau** level is reached. Total body stores of the drug are higher after a follow-up dose than they were after an initial dose. At some point, with repeated dosing, the amount of drug that is eliminated between doses will equal the amount that is administered. This means that average drug levels remain constant, and plateau has been reached. This is true because the actual amount of drug that is lost between doses increases each day. Although 50% of the total amount of the drug in the body is still lost every day, the amount in grams or milligrams gets continually larger as total body stores increase day after day.

If a drug is taken repeatedly in the same dose, plateau is reached in about four half-lives. Therefore, for a drug that has a half-life of 1 day, plateau would be reached in 4 full days after beginning treatment (see Figure 3-5 ■). When the dosage stays the same, the time needed to reach plateau does not depend on dosage size.

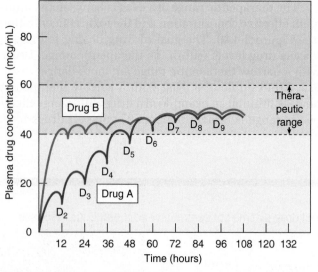

Figure 3-5 ■ A drug's plateau level.

Source: Adams, Michael Patrick; Holland, Leland; Urban, Carol, Pharmacology for Nurses: *A Pathophysiologic Approach, 4th Ed.,* ©2014. Reprinted and Electronically reproduced by permission of Pearson Education, Inc., New York, NY

Drug Accumulation

A drug can accumulate in the body in several ways. This may occur when the body cannot eliminate the drug sufficiently, or when it is taken in multiple doses at intervals shorter than recommended. When drug accumulation occurs, toxic levels can be reached, and adverse effects are prevalent. Many individuals do not manage their drug regimens correctly. Examples include taking all of a day's medications at once so that none of them are forgotten, and the taking of a drug in double doses after an earlier dose was missed. If serious adverse effects to any drug are occurring, the physician or other health care professional must review the patient's drug regimen to ensure correct administration. The patient must be educated about the importance of correct drug administration.

Drug Interactions

Many drugs alter the effects of other drugs. Therefore, they can be important in relation to varied drug responses. It is important to understand that one drug may increase or reduce the therapeutic as well as adverse effects of another drug. Also, the combination of two drugs may result in unique responses that differ widely from the effects of either drug used individually. Drug interactions may occur due to direct chemical or physical interactions; alterations in absorption, distribution, metabolism, or renal excretion; and interactions involving P-glycoprotein. Other interactions between drugs occur due to those using the same receptor, interactions from actions at separate sites, and because of combined toxicity.

Diet

Since diet affects overall health, it can also affect drug responses. In general, a person in good general health experiences better therapeutic drug responses. In a person who is clinically considered to be in starvation, protein binding of drugs is reduced, and responses are intensified. However, only a few nutrients directly affect drug responses. The best example involves the monoamine oxidase inhibitors (MAOIs), used for depression, which may cause serious malignant hypertension. This condition can be triggered by foods containing tyramine, so patients taking MAOIs must avoid foods such as yeast products, ripe cheeses, beef liver, and Chianti wine.

Failure to Follow Medication Regimens

When any medication is not administered exactly as prescribed or otherwise required, variances in drug response often occur. Common examples are when a patient forgets to take a medication per the correct schedule or when a hospitalized patient is the victim of a medication administration error. Regarding self-medication, related factors include lack of money to pay for needed medications, attitudes toward drugs, psychological problems, cognitive problems, visual problems, and even reduced manual dexterity, such as in elderly patients. Also, medication errors occur, which involve patients, physicians, nurses, pharmacists, and pharmacy technicians.

❋ Apply Your Knowledge 3.7

The following questions focus on what you have just learned about the types of drug doses.

CRITICAL THINKING

1. How is a drug's plateau reached?
2. In what ways can a drug accumulate in the body?
3. What are the reasons that drug interactions can occur?

PRACTICAL SCENARIO 1

A 73-year-old man with a 25-year history of alcoholism was prescribed the sedative phenobarbital by his family physician after he reported anxiety and trouble sleeping. The patient was also taking the anticoagulant warfarin (Coumadin) that had been prescribed by his cardiologist. Warfarin is a drug that is metabolized more rapidly when given with phenobarbital. This patient was later brought into the emergency room with a possible hemorrhagic stroke.

Michal Heron/Pearson Education/PH College

Critical Thinking Questions

1. How might the patient's age be related to the drug toxicity?
2. How could the family physician have helped prevent this emergency?

PRACTICAL SCENARIO 2

A female patient with diabetes and chronic glomerulonephritis has developed a urinary tract infection. Her physician must aggressively prescribe antibiotics.

Thinkstock/Stockbyte/Getty Images

Critical Thinking Questions

1. What is the main route of elimination for antibiotics?
2. What considerations should the physician take regarding dosage for this patient?
3. What complications could this patient have in relation to medication dosages?

Chapter Capsule

This section repeats the objectives from the beginning of the chapter and then provides a summary of the most important concepts for that objective. Use this section as a quick review and to check your knowledge.

Objective 1: Identify the four primary processes of pharmacokinetics.

- Absorption—the process of drug movement into the systemic circulation
- Distribution—the passage of a drug or agent through blood or lymph to various body sites
- Metabolism (biotransformation)—the utilization of a drug by the body via (mostly) liver enzymes
- Excretion—the removal of a drug from the body, via (mostly) the kidneys

Objective 2: Explain the primary ways that drugs cross cell membranes.

- To move throughout the body, drugs must cross membranes in order to enter the blood, then cross others to move from the vascular system, eventually reaching their sites of action. Additional membranes are crossed in order for drugs to be metabolized and excreted. Therefore, the three primary ways in which drugs cross cell membranes are by directly penetrating the cell membrane (most common method), by using a transport system, or by passing through pores or channels.

Objective 3: Discuss the main site variables that affect drug absorption.

- Drug absorption depends on the drug's ability to cross cell membranes and resist extensive breakdown by the stomach, liver, and intestines.

Objective 4: Discuss how drugs are distributed throughout the body.

- Many drugs are bound to circulating proteins, including albumin, globulins, lipoproteins, or glycoproteins
- The initial rate of drug distribution depends heavily on blood flow to various organs
- Lipid-soluble drugs enter the central nervous system rapidly
- The three major related factors are blood flow to body tissues, how drugs can exit the vascular system, and how drugs can enter body cells
- Once reaching target cells, the drug can be metabolized and excreted

Objective 5: Explain the metabolism of drugs and its applications to drug therapy.

- Most drug metabolism (biotransformation) occurs in the liver through the same biochemical pathways and reactions that affect nutrients, vitamins, and minerals
- The majority of metabolism in the liver occurs through the hepatic microsomal enzyme (P450) system
- The first-pass effect influences drug action and metabolism via the hepatic portal circulation, which carries blood directly to the liver
- A drug may be given parenterally to avoid the first-pass effect
- Other drugs that have undergone glucuronidation are transported via the enterohepatic recirculation system—from the liver, through the bile duct, to the duodenum, then back to the liver

■ Drug therapy involves consideration of the following aspects of drug metabolism: age, weight, gender, race, diurnal body rhythms, acid–base balance, fluid balance, electrolyte balance, diseases, genetics, immunology, psychology, environment, and tolerance

Objective 6: Identify major processes by which drugs are excreted.

■ Most drugs are excreted by the kidneys, via glomerular filtration, passive tubular reabsorption, and active tubular secretion

■ Other routes include the lungs, breast milk, sweat, tears, urine, feces, bile, and saliva

Objective 7: Explain the four main stages of biotransformation.

■ Oxidation—combination with oxygen

■ Reduction—a reaction with a substance that involves the gaining of electrons

■ Hydrolysis—the cleaving of a compound into simpler compounds with the uptake of the hydrogen and hydroxide parts of a water molecule

■ Conjugation—the combination of substances with glucuronic or sulfuric acid, terminating biologic activity and making them ready for excretion

Objective 8: Explain the applications of a drug's plasma half-life to pharmacotherapy.

■ A drug's plasma half-life is the time taken for the blood or plasma concentration to decrease from full to one-half (50%) after the last dose is taken; this is the major determinant of duration of drug action

■ The more a drug is present in the body, the larger the amount that is lost during one half-life

■ Half-life determines how much time must pass between each dose; drugs with a shorter half-life have shorter dosing intervals, and vice versa

Objective 9: Explain how a drug reaches and maintains its therapeutic range in the plasma.

■ The minimum effective concentration is the plasma drug level below which therapeutic effects do not occur—a beneficial drug must have concentrations that meet or exceed the minimum effective concentration, but do not reach the toxic concentration; doses are kept small enough to avoid reaching this level

■ Drug levels rise during absorption, but then decline while metabolism and excretion occur

■ Responses to the drug do not occur until plasma drug levels have reached the minimum effective concentration, as determined by the rate of absorption

■ Duration of effects is greatly determined by metabolism and excretion

Objective 10: Differentiate between loading and maintenance doses.

■ A drug's loading dose is a comparatively large dose given at the beginning of treatment to quickly obtain therapeutic effects

■ A maintenance dose keeps the plasma concentration of the drug continuously in the therapeutic range; however, the more the drug is taken, the more chance that drug accumulation will occur

Internet Sites of Interest

- Review of pharmacokinetic concepts: **www.rxkinetics.com/pktutorial/1_1.html**
- Drug absorption: **www.merckmanuals.com/professional/clinical-pharmacology/pharmacokinetics/drug-absorption**
- Drug distribution: **http://howmed.net/pharmacology/distribution-of-drugs/**
- Drug metabolism: **www.sigmaaldrich.com/technical-documents/articles/biofiles/phase-i-drug-metabolism.html**
- Drug excretion: **www.forcon.ca/learning/excretion.html**
- Drug plasma concentration: **http://learnpkpd.com/2011/02/19/blood-or-plasma-which-should-you-assay-for-drug-concentration/**
- Drug actions and dosages: **http://ndri.com/article/factors_modifying_the_dose_and_actions_of_drugs-396.html**

Chapter 4

Drug Toxicity and Pharmacogenomics

Chapter Objectives

After completing this chapter, you should be able to:

1. Differentiate between the terms *toxicity* and *overdose*.
2. Define *adverse drug reaction* and give examples.
3. Differentiate between toxic effects and side effects.
4. Describe what type of medicine has evolved from both pharmacogenomics and the understanding of polymorphisms.
5. Explain genome medicine.
6. Explain the functions of plasma membrane transporters.
7. Describe idiosyncratic drug reactions.
8. Compare teratogenic and carcinogenic effects of drugs.
9. Differentiate between hypersensitivity and autoimmune reactions.
10. Describe types of hypersensitivity reactions.

Key Terms

abstinence syndrome (p. 43)
alanine aminotransferase (ALT) (p. 45)
anaphylactic shock (p. 43)
antidote (p. 40)
apoptosis (p. 40)
aspartate aminotransferase (AST) (p. 45)
autoimmunity (p. 42)
comorbidities (p. 40)
cyclic GMP (cGMP) (p. 47)
drug targets (p. 41)
embryo (p. 43)

genome (p. 41)
genome medicine (p. 41)
hapten (p. 45)
hypersensitivity (p. 42)
idiosyncratic (p. 40)
jaundice (p. 45)
necrosis (p. 40)
overdose (p. 40)
pathogens (p. 42)
peptidoglycan (p. 42)
pharmacogenomics (p. 41)

poison (p. 40)
polymorphisms (p. 41)
prophylaxis (p. 41)
red man syndrome (p. 46)
side effects (p. 40)
Stevens-Johnson syndrome (p. 42)
toxic effects (p. 40)
toxicity (p. 40)
xenobiotics (p. 42)

Introduction

Drug toxicity describes the accumulation of an excessive amount of medication in the bloodstream. Effects of the medication are more intense at toxic levels, and adverse effects may be severe. Toxicity may occur when a dose is too high, or from the inability of the liver or kidneys to remove the drug from the bloodstream. It can occur when a commonly prescribed medication accumulates in the bloodstream. *Pharmacogenomics* studies genetic variations that influence individual responses to drugs. By understanding whether a patient carries a genetic variation, drug therapy can be individualized, the effect of drugs increased, and the chance for adverse effects reduced. Pharmacogenomics combines biochemistry and other traditional pharmaceutical sciences with understanding about common human genome DNA variations. In this chapter, I cover toxicity, adverse effects, adverse drug reactions, drug targets, idiosyncratic drug reactions, physical dependence, teratogenic effects, carcinogenic effects, hepatotoxic effects, hypersensitivity reactions, and drug–drug interactions.

Drug Toxicity

Toxicity is the state of being noxious and refers to a drug's ability to poison the body by excessive dosing. Examples include severe hypoglycemia from an overdose of insulin and coma from an overdose of morphine. There may be an **antidote** for some drug toxicities. Consequences of toxicity are either called *adverse drug reactions*, **toxic effects**, or **side effects**. Side effects are peripheral or secondary effects caused by drugs and other agents. Some side effects develop soon after drug use begins, whereas others may not appear until a drug has been taken for weeks or months. Side effects are generally predictable, and their intensity is dose dependent.

Factors that determine drug toxicity include the patient's age, preexisting conditions, and genetics, as well as the drug dosage and drugs being used concurrently. Very young or very old patients often are more susceptible to toxicities because of altered pharmacokinetics or drug-metabolizing enzymes. Examples of health conditions that often result in toxicity include liver or kidney disease and the presence of allergies. Another factor is drug interactions with other drugs, herbal supplements, and even foods.

It is important to remember that toxicity occurs when cellular defenses become overwhelmed. Repeated damage can eventually harm the function of affected organs. Two different outcomes occur, based on the severity of the damage. **Apoptosis** is programmed cell death, and allows cells to self-destruct using activation of specific proteins. This is helpful when the process kills damaged cells but does not harm surrounding tissue. In cancer cells, apoptosis is often inhibited. The second outcome is **necrosis**, the death of cells and tissues, often in a localized area, in which apoptosis cannot occur because toxicity is exceedingly severe. Instead, the contents of the cells are digested by enzymes, proteins change their structure, and membranes are disrupted. Necrotic cells can damage nearby normal cells when they attract inflammatory cells. This occurs when apoptosis occurs with only slight inflammation and disruption of adjacent tissues.

Adverse Effects

An adverse effect is a harmful or abnormal result of any substance, including medications. When an adverse effect occurs from drug binding to the intended receptor, but becomes altered, it is referred to as "on target." The factors that may alter drug binding include incorrect dosages, altered pharmacokinetics, or administration into incorrect tissues. These factors are also called *class effects*. However, when drug binding for an incorrect target or receptor results in an adverse effect, it is called "off target." Adverse effects can also be mediated by the immune system, and **idiosyncratic** responses can occur because of unknown mechanisms of action. Idiosyncratic responses are unpredictable reactions to a drug, and occur rarely.

Sometimes, through medication errors or poor judgment, or as a result of attempted suicide, a patient may receive a drug **overdose**, a toxic dose of the drug that causes harm. This can be dangerous because any drug can act like a **poison** if taken in too large a dose. A drug's adverse effects are based on its *margin of safety* between the effective dose and the toxic dose. An overdose is usually linked to a drug with a large margin of safety, whereas adverse effects can occur from therapeutic doses when the margin of safety is small or nonexistent. The margin of safety applies to all drugs, prescription or nonprescription. Other factors related to margin of safety include genetic characteristics, polymorphisms or enzymes, **comorbidities**, and reduced organ function. Comorbidities consist of disorders or diseases that are present, in addition to a primary disorder or disease. They can also be effects caused by additional disorders or diseases.

Focus Point

Drug Overdoses

Every day, approximately 46 Americans die from an overdose of prescription pain medications, while many others become addicted to them. Most fatal drug overdoses are related to prescription medications, not illegal drugs. Of these, more than 74% are accidental.

ADVERSE DRUG REACTIONS

An *adverse drug reaction (ADR)* has been defined as any response to a drug that is noxious, unintended, and occurs at doses normally used in humans for the **prophylaxis**, diagnosis, or therapy of disease. Adverse drug reactions may range in intensity from mildly annoying to life-threatening.

Adverse drug reactions occur in patients of all ages and can be fatal. According to the Food and Drug Administration (FDA), they are the fourth major cause of death, especially among elderly patients. More than 770,000 adverse drug events occur annually in hospitals, often because of unclear or missing drug information. In specific groups of patients, allergies, idiosyncrasies, and intolerance may occur. During new drug application studies, all adverse events must be reported, regardless of their severity. Additionally, once the drug reaches the market, adverse events of all types must still be reported. The FDA requires serious or unexpected events to be reported within 15 days of occurrence.

Unfortunately, little attention has been given to the incidence of ADRs in neonates, infants, children, and adolescents. Before release of a new drug, few studies are undertaken in children because of issues including ethics, responsibility, cost, and regulations. This often leads prescribers to estimate dosage and hence increases the risk of ADRs in children. Today, ADRs are a significant issue in elderly and pediatric patients.

✳ Apply Your Knowledge 4.1

The following questions focus on what you have just learned about drug toxicity and adverse effects.

CRITICAL THINKING

1. Explain the difference between apoptosis and necrosis.
2. Define *toxicity*, *side effects*, and *adverse effects*.
3. Explain how adverse drug reactions are addressed during new drug development.

Pharmacogenomics

Pharmacogenomics, formerly known as *pharmacogenetics*, is the study of genetic factors that influence variations in drug responses. More than one genetic variant may play a part in varied drug responses. The field of pharmacogenomics arose from severe adverse reactions occurring in patients who were later discovered to have drug-metabolizing enzymes with **genome** variations. A genome consists of all the hereditary information of an individual organism. Since the sequencing of the human genome, this field has grown quickly. Changes in genomes are referred to as **polymorphisms**. They also occur in genes that encode cytokines, human leukocyte antigen (HLA) loci, transporters, and other proteins. Polymorphisms help to predict variations in therapeutic as well as adverse drug responses. There is an estimated 11 million different single-nucleotide polymorphisms in humans, to which individual responses to a drug are often linked. Susceptibility to specific diseases is also related to common DNA variations. Therefore, pharmacogenomics is highly focused on genes that encode metabolic enzymes that alter drug activity, as well as defects in structural proteins that increase susceptibility to disease.

Genome medicine, or *personalized medicine*, has therefore evolved, which uses genetic information to choose drugs and doses for individual patients. Guidelines have been established by the Clinical Pharmacogenetics Implementation Consortium (CPIC). As a result, drugs are now being prescribed more effectively. An example of *genome replication*, in relation to viruses, requires specific triphosphates: ribonucleoside triphosphates for RNA viruses or deoxyribonucleoside triphosphates for DNA viruses. The triphosphates are incorporated into new viral genomes either by a viral or a cellular polymerase. Understanding this process has allowed scientists to develop new antivirals that are safer and more effective than those previously available. This is because differences between viral kinases and polymerases exist, which are unique compared to the kinases and polymerases of normal body cells. Therefore, genome medicine has developed drugs, in this example, that are able to target two different steps in the viral replication pathway.

DRUG TARGETS

Drug targets are any components inside the body to which drugs or other agents bind. They are also influenced by genetic variations. Also called *biological targets*, they are often proteins within the body that may be modified by drugs, altering their activities. In most cases, common drug targets are either proteins or nucleic acids. More than 50% of drug targets are G protein–coupled receptors. The remaining 50% of

Focus Point

Benefits of Pharmacogenomics

Pharmacogenomics allows individualized drug therapy that is based on genetic variations related to drug effects and adverse effects. Advances include more powerful medicines, the choice of initial drugs that are better and safer, and higher accuracy in the determination of drug dosages.

✳ Apply Your Knowledge 4.2

The following questions focus on what you have just learned about pharmacogenomics.

CRITICAL THINKING

1. Define *pharmacogenomics* and explain how it began.
2. Explain what polymorphisms are and how they are used.
3. Identify how genome medicine may be successful in treating viral conditions.

drug targets are enzymes, ion channels, nuclear hormone receptors, structural proteins, and nucleic acids.

An important consideration concerns the presence of specific drug targets in **pathogens** or cancer cells, which are often not present in normal cells. Pathogens are defined as infectious microorganisms. For example, the bacterial **peptidoglycan** cell wall is a drug target for certain antibacterial drugs. These drugs interrupt peptidoglycan synthesis, and cell lysis results from abnormal cell wall synthesis. For example, penicillins are able to harm these drug targets while causing little toxicity to normal cells. Similarly, antifungals often target fungal cell walls. The term *peptidoglycan* is also referred to as *murein*. It is a polymer that is made of sugars and amino acids, forming a mesh-like layer outside bacterial plasma membranes, as well as the cell wall.

In addition, *plasma membrane transporters* mediate selective uptake and removal of endogenous compounds and **xenobiotics**, which include many drug products. Transporters work with drug-metabolizing enzymes to a great degree. They help to determine the plasma and tissue concentrations of drugs as well as their metabolites. When transporters have genetic variations, drugs may have widely differing effects, including toxicities. The term xenobiotic is defined as a chemical inside an organism that is not normally produced or even expected to be present.

There are also pharmacodynamic genes linked to drug receptors and drug targets. In fact, a polymorphism in human leukocyte antigen positions is related to predisposed drug toxicity. Severe **hypersensitivity** reactions occur to certain drugs, manifested as **Stevens-Johnson syndrome**, liver damage, and toxic epidermal necrosis. The term *hypersensitivity* refers to undesirable reactions produced by a normal immune system,

including allergies and **autoimmunity**. Stevens-Johnson syndrome is a life-threatening skin condition, in which cell death causes separation of the epidermis from the dermis. The drugs most often linked to hypersensitivity reactions include nonsteroidal anti-inflammatory drugs (NSAIDs), antibiotics, antiepileptic agents, methotrexate, steroids, and sulfonamides. Other related drugs include abacavir, linked to skin hypersensitivities, and flucloxacillin, linked to liver damage. Hypersensitivity reactions differ through various races of people, as do their genetic makeups. Genetic testing is an important asset in preventing gene-linked hypersensitivities to medications.

The interferon lambda-3 enzyme is encoded by the *IFNL3* gene. They are linked to hepatitis C infection, and in patients with the favorable genotype, have resulted in about double the success rate in curing the condition with proper treatment. This involves pegylated interferon with ribavirin, with or without a protease inhibitor also being used.

IDIOSYNCRATIC DRUG REACTIONS

When a patient experiences a unique, strange, or unpredicted reaction to a drug, it is termed an *idiosyncratic drug reaction* or, simply, an *idiosyncratic reaction*. Idiosyncratic reactions may be caused by underlying enzyme deficiencies resulting from genetic or hormonal variations. For example, carisoprodol (Soma®) may cause such idiosyncratic reactions as transient quadriplegia, dizziness, or temporary loss of vision. It is believed that with continuing study, idiosyncratic drug reactions may be reduced by documenting varied patient responses to different drugs, related to genetic and other mechanisms of action.

✳ Apply Your Knowledge 4.3

The following questions focus on what you have just learned about drug targets.

CRITICAL THINKING

1. List various types of unique drug targets.
2. Explain the effects of plasma membrane transporters.
3. Identify the features of Stevens-Johnson syndrome, and drugs linked to hypersensitivity reactions.

An idiosyncratic, sudden, and severe allergic reaction that may be life-threatening is termed **anaphylactic shock**. It can cause a sharp loss of blood pressure, urticaria (lesions known as *hives* or *wheals*), paralysis of the diaphragm, and swelling of the oropharynx; the end result may be cardiac collapse. Anaphylactic shock, a true medical emergency, occurs so swiftly and with such severity that controlled clinical studies of treatment have never been possible. Prevention is, of course, most important. A history of previous allergic reactions to drugs, vaccines, serum, or blood transfusions must be obtained from anyone about to undergo treatment to prevent or at least be prepared for the slightest hazard of this kind. Patients who are predisposed to allergic reactions should wear an alerting bracelet or necklace (e.g., Medic Alert). Epinephrine (adrenaline) is frequently injected to combat anaphylactic shock but must be administered soon after shock begins.

Drug allergy is an abnormal response characterized by:

✳ Occurrence in a small number of individuals

✳ Previous exposure to either the same or a chemically related drug

✳ Rapid development of an allergic reaction after re-exposure

✳ Production of clinical manifestations of an allergic reaction

Physical Dependence

Long-term use of drugs such as alcohol, amphetamines, barbiturates, and opioids results in *physical dependence*. When this occurs, the body adapts to the drug in a way that will cause **abstinence syndrome** if the drug is discontinued. Each drug's abstinence syndrome is unique. Physical dependence is most commonly related to narcotics, which include prescribed opioids as well as illegal drugs such as heroin. Many other drugs produce physical dependence, however, including amphetamines, barbiturates, and ethanol. Some drugs cause a specific type of physical dependence even though their effects are outside of the central nervous system. Withdrawal reactions from various drugs can be extremely harmful to the body. Therefore, patients must be cautioned against abruptly discontinuing any medication until they consult their health care provider.

Teratogenic Effects

A *teratogen* is any substance or illness that is able to cause harm to an **embryo**. Examples of teratogens include alcohol, cigarette smoke, various medications (such as Accutane, antibiotics, and antidepressants), illegal drugs (such as cocaine and heroin), some vaccines, certain viral infections, radiation such as x-rays, some occupational chemicals, and maternal autoimmune disorders. A *teratogenic effect* is a drug-induced birth defect.

Carcinogenic Effects

A drug's *carcinogenic effect* is its ability to cause cancer. Only a few therapeutic agents can cause cancer, but some of these include agents actually used to treat the disease. It is very difficult to determine a substance's carcinogenic effects because cancer may not appear until 20 or more years after initial exposure to the substance. Therefore, preclinical and clinical trials usually do not detect carcinogenic effects. Many new drugs are released to the public without full understanding of potential cancer-causing effects. An example is the drug diethylstilbestrol, a synthetic hormone with estrogen-like effects. Previously used to prevent spontaneous abortion in women who had high-risk pregnancies, it was later discovered that exposure to the drug *in utero* resulted in vaginal and uterine cancers.

Hepatotoxic Effects

Hepatotoxic drugs are those that cause destruction of the liver. These drugs are the leading cause of acute liver failure, which can be fatal very quickly. Most drugs are withdrawn from the United States drug market because of their hepatotoxic effects. There are more than 50 drugs known to be hepatotoxic, examples of which are listed in Table 4-1 ■. Since the liver is the

Table 4-1 ■ **Drugs That Are Toxic to the Liver**

DRUG CLASSIFICATION	EXAMPLES
Statins and Other Lipid-Lowering Drugs	atorvastatin (Lipitor)
	fenofibrate (Tricor)
	fluvastatin (Lescol)
	gemfibrozil (Lopid)
	lovastatin (Mevacor)
	niacin (Niaspan)
	pravastatin (Pravachol)
	simvastatin (Zocor)
Oral Antidiabetic Drugs	acarbose (Precose)
	pioglitazone (Actos)
	rosiglitazone (Avandia)
Antiseizure Drugs	carbamazepine (Tegretol)
	felbamate (Felbatol)
	valproic acid (Depakene)
Antifungal Drugs	itraconazole (Sporanox)
	ketoconazole (Nizoral)
	terbinafine (Lamisil)
Antituberculosis Drugs	isoniazid (generic)
	pyrazinamide (generic)
	rifampin (Rifadin)
Immunosuppressants	azathioprine (Imuran)
	methotrexate (Rheumatrex)
Antiretroviral Drugs	nevirapine (Viramune)
	ritonavir (Norvir)
Miscellaneous Drugs	acetaminophen (Tylenol), when taken with alcohol
	amiodarone (Cordarone)
	diclofenac (Voltaren)
	duloxetine (Cymbalta)
	halothane (Fluothane)
	leflunomide (Arava)
	methyldopa (Aldomet)
	nefazodone (Serzone)
	nitrofurantoin (Macrodantin)
	tacrine (Cognex)
	tamoxifen (Nolvadex)
	zileuton (Zyflo)

primary site of drug metabolism, many drugs are converted to toxic products that harm liver cells. Combinations of hepatotoxic drugs with other drugs, including alcohol, can cause severe liver injury. A good example of this situation is the combination of acetaminophen (Tylenol) with alcohol. Any patient taking a hepatotoxic drug must undergo liver function tests, which assess blood levels of the enzymes **aspartate aminotransferase**

(AST) and **alanine aminotransferase (ALT)**. Since life-threatening liver damage can develop so quickly, early detection of elevations in these enzymes is essential. Patients must also be informed about the signs of liver damage, which include yellowing of the skin and eyes that is known as **jaundice**, light-colored stools, dark urine, nausea and vomiting, abdominal discomfort, malaise, and loss of appetite.

Focus Point

Organ-Specific Toxicity

Besides the liver, many drugs are toxic to specific organs, including:

- Kidneys—amphotericin B
- Heart—doxorubicin
- Lungs—amiodarone
- Ear—gentamicin

✳ Apply Your Knowledge 4.4

The following questions focus on what you have just learned about idiosyncratic drug reactions as well as various types of drug effects.

CRITICAL THINKING

1. Describe the signs of anaphylactic shock.
2. Explain why it is difficult to assess a substance's carcinogenic effects.
3. Identify the signs of hepatotoxicity.

Hypersensitivity Reaction

The term *hypersensitivity* is often used synonymously with *allergy*. Hypersensitivity reactions are therefore also referred to as *allergic responses*. The two primary ways that drugs can cause damage are via hypersensitivity reactions and autoimmune reactions. Hypersensitivity reactions require a presensitized (immune) state of the host, and may be damaging, uncomfortable, or even fatal. Autoimmune reactions arise from abnormal immune responses against substances and tissues normally present in the body.

Regarding hypersensitivity, the diagnosis of a drug allergy is often difficult to establish because no reliable laboratory tests can identify the relevant drug, and in some cases, the symptoms can imitate infectious disease symptoms. A health care practitioner must clarify whether the patient is experiencing a true allergic reaction or drug intolerance. For example, administration of

penicillin by injection may cause a severe allergic reaction, which may be life-threatening. Conversely, when a patient takes penicillin orally, allergy to the substance may cause nausea and vomiting to an intolerable degree. Allergic reactions to drugs generally follow the Type I–IV classification as listed in Table 4-2 ■.

Type I is immediate hypersensitivity or anaphylaxis responses that result from production of IgE after being exposed to an antigen. This may be a foreign or endogenous protein that is modified by a **hapten** and becomes immunogenic. An example is when fragments of penicillin act as haptens to activate the immune system. Recurrent exposure to the antigen cause degranulation of mast cells and the release of histamine, leukotrienes, or other inflammatory mediators. A hapten is a small molecule that can cause an immune response only when it is attached to a large carrier, such as a protein. Type I reactions develop in the skin as *wheal-and-flare reactions*, which are irregular patches of raised skin

Table 4-2 ■ **Allergic Drug Reactions**

TYPE	EXAMPLES OF DRUGS OR CLASSES OF DRUGS	CAUSES
I. Immediate hypersensitivity (anaphylaxis)	Penicillins, streptomycin, local anesthetics, neuromuscular-blocking drugs, radiologic contrast media	Production of IgE after exposure to antigen, which may be a foreign protein or an endogenous protein modified by a hapten, to become immunogenic
II. Antibody dependent, cytotoxic	Quinine, quinidine, rifampicin, metronidazole	Drug binds to (usually) red blood cells and is recognized by the antibody (primarily, IgG)
III. Immune complex–mediated	Anticonvulsants, antibiotics, hydralazine, diuretics	Antibodies, usually IgG or IgM, are formed against soluble antigens; antigen–antibody complexes are then deposited in tissues
IV. Cell-mediated or delayed hypersensitivity	Local anesthetic creams, antihistamine creams	Activation of T_H1 and cytotoxic T cells

surrounded by redness. The upper respiratory tract develops hay fever symptoms such as rhinitis and conjunctivitis; the lower respiratory tract develops asthmatic bronchoconstriction.

Type II is antibody-dependent cytotoxic hypersensitivity responses that result from a drug binding to cells, mostly red blood cells, which is recognized by IgG or other antibodies. Cell lysis is triggered through complement fixation, cytolysis by cytotoxic T cells, or phagocytosis by macrophages. These are rare responses to certain drugs such as quinidine or penicillin.

Type III is immune complex–mediated hypersensitivity responses that require the formation of antibodies—usually IgG or IgM—to be formed against soluble antigens. Complexes of antigens and antibodies are then deposited in tissues, primarily the joints, kidneys, and lung vascular endothelium. Damage is then caused by *serum sickness*, which involves inflammation due to activation of complement and leukocytes inside the tissues. Examples of Type III hypersensitivity causative agents include bupropion, cefaclor, and antivenins.

Type IV is delayed-type hypersensitivity responses that are caused by activation of cytotoxic T cells and T_H1 cells. As a hapten binds to host proteins, there is usually contact dermatitis. This often occurs after subsequent exposures, not the first exposure to the causative agent. Langerhans cells are activated and migrate to local lymph nodes. T cells are then activated and return to the skin, causing an immune response. Examples of Type IV responses include reactions to latex and poison ivy. There is also a severe situation that happens when there is repeated exposure to a foreign agent. A severe immune response known as a *cytokine storm* occurs, resulting in fever, hypotension, and possible organ failure.

When the immune system attacks its own cells, *autoimmunity* occurs. Drugs that may trigger autoimmunity include hydralazine, isoniazid, methyldopa, and procainamide. **Red man syndrome** is a rare condition caused by certain drugs such as vancomycin, amphotericin B, ciprofloxacin, rifampicin, and teicoplanin. The condition involves degranulation of the mast cells, but this occurs independently of preformed complement or IgE. Usually, wheals and urticaria of the skin develop on the neck, arms, and upper trunk. The syndrome usually subsides after the drug's infusion rate is reduced or discontinued.

Other drug-related reactions include skin rashes referred to as *erythema multiforme*. Severe skin rashes such as Stevens-Johnson syndrome and epidermal necrolysis have occurred from barbiturates, antiepileptics, sulfonamides, NSAIDs, and other drugs. Injury to the immune system is known as *immunotoxicity*, and may be related to drug therapy or even an intended outcome of certain drug therapies. An example of the latter situation would be the use of cytotoxic agents used to kill specific neoplastic cells. Immune system targeting is indicated when a disease is worsened by the normal immune responses. However, this type of therapy is rigidly controlled due to the possibility of other negative results, including dangerous infections.

When the body is not able to metabolize and excrete one dose of a drug completely before the next dose is given, a cumulative effect occurs. With repeated doses, the drug starts to collect in the blood and body tissues, resulting in cumulative toxicity. Cumulative toxicity may occur rapidly, such as with ethyl alcohol, or slowly over time, such as with lead poisoning.

The combined action of two or more agents that produce an effect greater than that which would have been expected from the two agents acting separately is called *synergism*. Some drug interactions exhibit synergism, which, depending on the circumstances, may be beneficial or harmful; for example, the combination of the antibacterial drug trimethoprim with sulfamethoxazole (Bactrim, Septa) is more effective for treating infections than either drug acting alone. However, the combination of aspirin and the anticoagulant warfarin (Coumadin) can act synergistically to reduce blood clotting to the extent of spontaneous hemorrhage if doses are not carefully monitored.

An interaction between two drugs that causes an effect greater than that which would have been expected from the additive properties of the drugs involved is called *potentiation*. For example, alcohol potentiates the sedating effects of the tranquilizer diazepam (Valium) when the two drugs are ingested at the same time.

Drug–Drug Interactions

Drug–drug interactions have become more common with growing populations, longer lifespans, and polypharmacy. Drug–drug interactions may have pharmacokinetic as well as pharmacodynamic implications. A pharmacokinetic drug–drug interaction occurs when a drug alters another drug's absorption, distribution, metabolism, or excretion. This changes the concentration of active drug within the body. If two drugs are metabolized by the same P450 enzyme, there may be competitive or irreversible inhibition of the enzyme, affecting drug concentrations. The opposite effect also occurs. Certain drugs may affect the transport of other drugs in and out of body tissues. Pharmacokinetic interactions may be desired, such as when one drug is given with another that increases its beneficial actions. Some drugs may displace others by utilizing the same proteins, increasing the bioavailability of the other drug to tissues.

Regarding pharmacodynamics, drug–drug interactions occur when a drug changes how tissues respond, or do not respond, to another drug. These interactions may be toxic when the two drugs activate complementary pathways, increasing effects of both. A major example would be the use of nitroglycerin, for angina pectoris, along with sildenafil, which is used for erectile dysfunction. This combination excessively increases **cyclic GMP (cGMP)** to high levels that can result in severe hypotension. Cyclic GMP is an abbreviation for cyclic guanosine monophosphate, a cyclic nucleotide that acts as a second messenger. It is derived from guanosine triphosphate (GTP).

Drugs may also interact with herbs, herbal supplements, foods, and beverages. This is because many herbal products contain biologically active compounds that have not been thoroughly studied. Therefore, physicians must always ask patients about all possible nondrug substances that they consume when prescribing medications that may interact. An example of an herbal supplement that interacts with NSAIDs is gingko biloba. Since both of these agents inhibit platelet aggregation, concurrent use may increase risk of bleeding.

Focus Point

Allergy History

Ask all patients if they have a history of allergies, such as hay fever, rashes, or asthma, or have had unusual reactions to any drugs taken orally or by injection in the past.

✳ Apply Your **Knowledge 4.5**

The following questions focus on what you have just learned about hypersensitivity reaction and drug–drug interactions.

CRITICAL THINKING

1. Explain why it may be difficult to diagnose a drug allergy.
2. Give examples of drugs linked to Type I and Type II hypersensitivity reactions.
3. Differentiate between cumulative effect and synergism.
4. Describe what happens if two drugs are metabolized by the same P450 enzyme.

PRACTICAL SCENARIO 1

Renee, a medical assistant, works in a walk-in clinic. A child is brought in to be treated for strep throat, and the physician orders a penicillin intramuscular (IM) injection. Renee asks the child's mother if the child has any allergies to antibiotics, and the mother says he does not. Renee administers the IM injection. Ten minutes later, the child experiences anaphylactic shock. The pediatrician begins to treat the condition.

Courtesy of the author

Critical Thinking Questions

1. What was the reason that the patient had anaphylactic shock?
2. Explain the signs and symptoms of anaphylactic shock.
3. What did Renee do wrong?

PRACTICAL SCENARIO 2

A 59-year-old man came to the emergency department because of nausea and vomiting, a slight fever, abdominal tenderness, and jaundice. Upon examination, he admitted drinking as many as 12 servings of alcohol per week, which he had done for the past 10 years. Because of a recent injury to his knee, he had been taking up to eight 500 mg tablets of acetaminophen every day for the past 2 weeks. Tests revealed elevated liver enzymes, bilirubin, serum glucose, and blood acetaminophen concentrations.

Oktay Ortakcioglu/E+/Getty Images

Critical Thinking Questions

1. What is the likely outcome of the combination of regular alcohol intake with acetaminophen?
2. What is the maximum daily dose of acetaminophen for an average adult?
3. How prevalent is acetaminophen overdose in relation to acute liver failure?

Chapter Capsule

This section repeats the objectives from the beginning of the chapter and then provides a summary of the most important concepts for that objective. Use this section as a quick review and to check your knowledge.

Objective 1: Differentiate between the terms *toxicity* and *overdose*.

■ Toxicity is the state of being noxious and refers to a drug's ability to poison the body. There may be an antidote that has the opposite effect and can reverse toxic symptoms.

■ An overdose is a toxic dose of a drug that causes harm. It may occur through medication errors or poor judgment or as a result of attempted suicide. Any drug can act like a poison if taken in too large a dose.

Objective 2: Define *adverse drug reaction* and give examples.

- An adverse drug reaction is any response to a drug that is noxious, unintended, and occurs at doses normally used in humans for the prophylaxis, diagnosis, or therapy of disease.

- Examples include severe nausea, vomiting, and diarrhea.

Objective 3: Differentiate between toxic effects and side effects.

- Toxic effects are those produced by an intensification of drug effects that would normally produce a therapeutic response.

- Side effects are peripheral or secondary effects caused by drugs and other agents, which may or may not be considered "adverse."

Objective 4: Describe what type of medicine has evolved from both pharmacogenomics and the understanding of polymorphisms.

- Genome medicine or personalized medicine has evolved from pharmacogenomics and the understanding of polymorphisms. It uses genetic information to choose drugs and doses for individual patients. Drugs are now being prescribed more effectively.

Objective 5: Explain genome medicine.

- Genome medicine is also called *personalized medicine*. It uses genetic information to choose drugs and doses for individual patients.

Objective 6: Explain the functions of plasma membrane transporters.

- Plasma membrane transporters mediate selective uptake and remove (efflux) endogenous compounds and xenobiotics, including many drug products. They work with drug-metabolizing enzymes to a great degree and help to determine the plasma and tissue concentrations of drugs as well as their metabolites.

Objective 7: Describe idiosyncratic drug reactions.

- When a patient experiences a unique, strange, or unpredicted reaction to a drug, it is termed an *idiosyncratic drug reaction* (or *idiosyncratic reaction*). They may be caused by underlying enzyme deficiencies resulting from genetic or hormonal variation. Anaphylactic shock is an idiosyncratic, sudden, and severe allergic reaction that may be life-threatening.

Objective 8: Compare teratogenic and carcinogenic effects of drugs.

- A teratogen is any substance or illness that is able to cause harm to an embryo and is also described as a drug-induced birth defect.

- A drug's carcinogenic effect is its ability to cause cancer. It is very difficult to determine this since cancer may not appear until 20 or more years after initial exposure to the substance. Preclinical and clinical trials usually do not detect carcinogenic effects.

Objective 9: Differentiate between hypersensitivity and autoimmune reactions.

- The term *hypersensitivity* is often used synonymously with *allergy*. *Hypersensitivity reactions* are therefore also referred to as *allergic responses*. The two primary ways that drugs can cause damage are via hypersensitivity reactions and *autoimmune reactions*. Hypersensitivity reactions require a presensitized (immune) state of the host and may be damaging, uncomfortable, or even fatal. Autoimmune reactions arise from abnormal immune responses against substances and tissues normally present in the body.

Objective 10: Describe types of hypersensitivity reactions.

- *Type I* is immediate hypersensitivity or *anaphylaxis* responses due to production of IgE after exposure to an antigen. Recurrent exposure causes mast cell degranulation, and release of histamine, leukotrienes, or other inflammatory mediators. *Wheal-and-flare reactions* occur on the skin, hay fever symptoms include rhinitis and conjunctivitis, and asthmatic bronchoconstriction develops.

- *Type II* is antibody-dependent cytotoxic hypersensitivity responses that result from a drug binding to cells, mostly red blood cells, which is recognized by IgG or other antibodies. Cell lysis is triggered through complement fixation, cytolysis by cytotoxic T cells, or phagocytosis by macrophages. These are rare responses to certain drugs such as quinidine or penicillin.

- *Type III* is immune complex–mediated hypersensitivity responses requiring formation of antibodies—usually IgG or IgM—against soluble antigens. Complexes are then deposited in joints, kidneys, and lung vascular endothelium. Damage caused by *serum sickness* involves inflammation from activation of complement and leukocytes in tissues. Examples of causative agents include bupropion, cefaclor, and antivenins.

- *Type IV* is delayed-type hypersensitivity responses due to activation of cytotoxic T cells and T_H1 cells. There is usually contact dermatitis after re-exposure. Langerhans cells are activated, migrating to local lymph nodes. Activated T cells return to the skin, causing an immune response; examples are reactions to latex and poison ivy. A severe situation may be *cytokine storm*, with fever, hypotension, and possible organ failure.

 Internet Sites of Interest

- Drug overdose: **www.emedicinehealth.com/drug_overdose/page6_em.htm**
- Adverse drug reactions: **www.fda.gov/Drugs/DevelopmentApprovalProcess/ DevelopmentResources/DrugInteractionsLabeling/ucm110632.htm**
- Pharmacogenomics: **https://www.ama-assn.org/content/selected-topics-genetics-and-personalized-medicine**
- Genome variations: **www.genomenewsnetwork.org/resources/whats_a_genome/ Chp1_1_1.shtml**
- Drug-metabolizing enzymes: **http://tools.thermofisher.com/downloads/ o-12758dmeguide_intro.pdf**
- Genetic polymorphisms of drug targets: **http://pharmrev.aspetjournals.org/ content/63/2/437.full#title6**
- Plasma membrane transporters: **http://themedicalbiochemistrypage.org/ membranes.php**
- Idiosyncratic drug reactions: **www.ncbi.nlm.nih.gov/pmc/articles/PMC3639727/**
- Hypersensitivity: **http://beltina.org/health-dictionary/hypersensitivity-reaction-types-symptoms-treatment-allergy.html**

Chapter 5

Law and Ethics of Medications

Chapter Objectives

After completing this chapter, you should be able to:

1. Discuss legal and ethical requirements regarding the use, dispensation, and administration of medications.

2. Explain how the need for drug control evolved.

3. Discuss the poisoning disaster that led to legislation requiring testing for the purity, strength, effectiveness, safety, and packaging quality of drugs.

4. Explain the major points of the thalidomide disaster of 1962.

5. List the provisions of the Controlled Substances Act.

6. Differentiate between each of the five schedules for controlled substances.

7. Define *orphan drug* and then list some examples.

8. Discuss the federal regulatory agencies that deal with food, drugs, and disease control.

9. Explain which level of government primarily controls pharmacy licensure.

10. Define *ethics* as it relates to pharmacology.

Key Terms

abuse potential (p. 54)
anabolic steroids (p. 56)
controlled substances (p. 52)
designer drugs (p. 54)

ethics (p. 61)
interstate commerce (p. 52)
legend drugs (p. 53)
nuclear pharmacy (p. 57)

orphan drugs (p. 56)
reimportation (p. 56)

Introduction

All health care workers who deal with dispensing, preparing, and administering medications must be familiar with the legal and ethical requirements that relate to these procedures. In the United States, the early 1900s marked the beginnings of drug legislation. Today, federal regulations are in place to help protect consumers from the harmful effects of improper use of drugs; however, drug-related adverse effects still occur even with "approved" over-the-counter (OTC) and prescription drugs. The use of dangerous or illicit drugs is prohibited by state and federal governments. The sale and distribution of drugs in the United States is controlled primarily by two major legislative acts: the federal Food, Drug, and Cosmetic Act (FDCA) and the federal Controlled Substances Act (CSA). These acts give the Food and Drug Administration (FDA) and other federal and state agencies the power to enforce legislative decisions. The FDCA is predominantly concerned with fixing the rules and regulations by which drugs are imported, manufactured, distributed, and sold in the United States. The CSA is part of the Comprehensive Drug Abuse Prevention and Control Act of 1970, which, as the title suggests, is concerned with the prevention and control of the abuse of certain drugs called **controlled substances**—or drugs whose possession and use are controlled by the act.

The CSA is administered and enforced by the Department of Justice under the attorney general and is a unit of the Federal Bureau of Investigation (FBI) known as the Drug Enforcement Administration (DEA). Although the two agencies have separate missions, they do cooperate in the administration of the federal drug abuse treatment program. The DEA is required to obtain the expert scientific advice of the FDA when seeking to add a substance to the list of controlled substances.

These two acts are supplemented on the federal level by a series of legislative acts designed to address specific problems, including the Poison Prevention Packaging Act of 1970 and the federal Hazardous Substances Act.

The Need for Drug Control

During the nineteenth century, there was virtually no regulation of the sale of drugs in the United States. Opium was readily and legally available over the counter in pharmacies, in grocery and general stores, and from mail-order houses. The medications containing opium were advertised extensively in newspapers. Labels often did not reveal the contents. No law required that the contents of a drug be stated.

Case after case of addiction to opiates and fatal delay in seeking medical treatment—caused by reliance on the claims of charlatans or drug-clouded perceptions—occurred (Figure 5-1 ■). To combat this

Figure 5-1 ■ During the nineteenth century in the United States, over-the-counter opium could be purchased at pharmacies and grocery stores. As a result, addiction became a problem, leading to programs such as the one advertised in this poster. However, in 1906, the Pure Food and Drug Act put an end to the sale of unsafe and untested drugs, such as opium.

situation, Congress passed the first Pure Food and Drug Act in 1906.

Federal Law

Congress found the authority to pass drug legislation within its constitutional right to control **interstate commerce**—that is, the commerce, traffic, transportation, and exchange between states of the United States. The purpose of the FDCA of 1938 was the same then as it still is today: to limit interstate commerce of drugs to those that are safe and effective.

Whereas the act (which is described more completely later in this chapter) requires that drugs comply with the standards of safety and efficacy, the earlier Pure Food and Drug Act of 1906 focused on standards of strength and purity as well as proper labeling that indicated the kind and amount of ingredients present. In 1912, Congress passed the Sherley Amendment, prohibiting the use of fraudulent therapeutic claims.

To fulfill the obligation undertaken in 1912, Congress adopted the Federal Narcotic Drug Act in 1914. This law became popularly known as the Harrison Narcotic Act.

SULFANILAMIDE DISASTER OF 1937

A manufacturer decided to market the antimicrobial sulfanilamide in a liquid form for sore throats and mixed the sulfanilamide with diethylene glycol, which is the same ingredient used today as antifreeze in car radiators. Because sulfanilamide was poorly soluble in known solvents, drug marketers rushed to be the first to find a suitable solvent and develop a liquid version of the drug, particularly for use in young children. Diethylene glycol was chosen because of its pleasant color and taste.

However, it was a deadly poison, and because no clinical safety or efficacy studies were required before marketing, this fact went overlooked until patients started dying. There were 107 reported deaths from this product. The 1938 FDCA, which followed this disaster, prevented the marketing of new drugs before they had been properly tested for purity, strength, effectiveness, safety, and packaging quality. This act gave the FDA the authority to approve or deny new drug applications. As a result of this law and further legislation, the FDA now approves the investigational use of drugs on humans and ensures that all approved drugs are safe and effective.

The Durham-Humphrey Amendment of 1951

The Durham-Humphrey Amendment of 1951 exempted certain drugs from the requirement that their labeling must contain adequate directions for use. These drugs, which could be taken safely only under medical supervision, were exempted provided they were sold pursuant to the order of a licensed physician or administered under a prescriber's supervision. The Durham-Humphrey Amendment of 1951 prohibits the dispensing of legend drugs without a prescription. Federal law requires **legend drugs** (prescription drugs) to bear the following statement: "Caution: Federal law prohibits dispensing without prescription." Nonlegend, or OTC, drugs were not restricted for sale and use under a physician's supervision. They were deemed safe for the public for self-limited use in minor conditions. Their sale is not restricted, and their use is thought, in most cases, to require neither prescription nor medical supervision.

THALIDOMIDE DISASTER OF 1962

In 1962, thalidomide, used as a sleeping pill and antinausea agent during pregnancy, was being used widely abroad. Before it could be approved for use in the United States, its adverse effects on developing fetuses were discovered. Meanwhile, women in other countries who took thalidomide during their first trimester of pregnancy delivered babies with severe deformities, including malformed or missing limbs.

These events led to the passage of the Kefauver-Harris Amendment in 1962. Currently, thalidomide has limited availability in the United States for the treatment of leprosy, bone marrow transplantation, acquired immunodeficiency syndrome (AIDS), and several other conditions.

Focus on Pediatrics

Drugs and Birth Defects

Thalidomide is not the only drug known to cause birth defects if taken by pregnant women. Studies have proven that drinking alcohol while pregnant can cause fetal alcohol syndrome, characterized by abnormalities of the face and head, growth disturbances, and mental deficiency. Smoking during pregnancy has been linked to smaller birth-weight babies and to abnormal infant reflexes.

* Apply Your Knowledge 5.1

The following questions focus on what you have just learned about drug control, federal law, and early legislation that related to drug control.

CRITICAL THINKING

1. What law was passed in Congress to combat the lack of drug regulation in the United States?
2. Which law gave the FDA the authority to approve or deny new drug applications and what happened that caused Congress to pass this law?
3. What was the thalidomide disaster of 1962?
4. Describe legend and nonlegend drugs.
5. Define the DEA and then describe its requirements.

DRUG ABUSE CONTROL AMENDMENT OF 1965

This amendment, the effective precursor of the Drug Abuse Control Act, permitted only certain authorized registrants to manufacture stimulant drugs. This drug abuse control legislation provided the first guidelines for determining the classifications of drugs subject to abuse. By and large, they were incorporated into the 1970 act, which follows.

COMPREHENSIVE DRUG ABUSE PREVENTION AND CONTROL ACT OF 1970

One of the primary functions of this act was to encompass all federal laws dealing with narcotic drugs, stimulants, depressants, and abused **designer drugs** that did not fit the historical classifications. (Designer drugs are defined as drugs produced by a minor modification in the chemical structure of an existing drug, resulting in a new substance with similar pharmacologic effects. Scientists also call these drugs *analogues*.) This act also served to consolidate the government's enforcement activities that had previously been handled by various competing agencies. For example, the Bureau of Narcotics and the Bureau of Drug Abuse Control became the Bureau of Narcotics and Dangerous Drugs (BNDD). Finally, in 1973, all agencies involved in drug abuse control and the enforcement of drug abuse laws were combined into one agency: the DEA. The DEA, housed within the Department of Justice, became the nation's sole legal drug enforcement agency.

The Comprehensive Drug Abuse Prevention and Control Act of 1970, also called the CSA, became effective on May 1, 1971. This law was designed to:

✳ Provide increased research into and prevention of drug abuse and drug dependence.

✳ Provide for the treatment and rehabilitation of drug abusers and drug-dependent persons.

✳ Improve the administration and regulation of the manufacture, distribution, and dispensing of controlled substances by legitimate handlers of these drugs to help reduce their widespread dispersion into illicit markets.

Drugs covered by this act have a potential for causing drug dependence, abuse, or both and are classified according to their use and **abuse potential** (possibility of causing abuse or dependence in a user).

Drugs with the potential for abuse are classified into five schedules: I, II, III, IV, and V. Drugs in Schedule I have the highest potential for abuse and addiction, and those in Schedule V have the least potential.

Schedule I: These drugs have a high potential for abuse, and they are not accepted for medical use in the United States. Properly registered individuals

Figure 5-2 ■ Amphetamines, Schedule II drugs, have a high abuse potential and are sold illegally under many street names.

may use Schedule I substances for research, analysis, or instruction purposes.

Schedule II: These drugs also have a high potential for abuse, but they are currently accepted for medical use in the United States. The abuse of these drugs may result in severe psychological or physical dependence. The quantity of the substance in a drug product often determines the schedule that will control it. For example, amphetamines (Figure 5-2 ■) and codeine are usually classified in Schedule II; however, specific products containing smaller quantities of Schedule II substances, most often manufactured in combination with a noncontrolled substance, are controlled by Schedules III and IV. An example is Tylenol mixed with codeine, which is considered a Schedule III drug.

Schedule III: These drugs have less abuse potential than those in Schedules I and II and cause only low to moderate physical dependence if abused. They have accepted medical uses in the United States. Schedule III drugs contain limited quantities of certain narcotic and nonnarcotic agents.

Schedule IV: These drugs have only slight abuse potential and accepted medical uses in the United States. They are still more potent than Schedule V drugs and require a prescription.

Schedule V: These drugs have the lowest abuse potential of all the controlled substances and consist of preparations containing limited quantities of certain narcotic drugs that are generally used for antitussive and antidiarrheal purposes. Schedule V drugs are OTC preparations that may be sold without a prescription to individuals 18 years or older. Diphenoxylate with atropine (Lomotil), which is listed as a Schedule V drug, is an exception; it requires a prescription. The generic-only drug paregoric (a drug that causes emesis, or vomiting) is now restricted to prescription sales only and is included in Schedule III (Table 5-1 ■).

Focus Point

Keeping Medications Safe in the Hospital

In the hospital, all restricted substances must be stored in locked storage facilities to prevent access by unauthorized persons. The nurse in charge of the shift or the pharmacy technician working directly under the supervision of the in-charge pharmacist carries the keys to the locked storage. Likewise, restricted substances kept in other medical settings, such as physicians' offices, must be kept in locked storage facilities.

Table 5-1 ■ Drug Schedules

SCHEDULE	ABUSE POTENTIAL	PRESCRIPTION REQUIREMENTS	EXAMPLES
I	High abuse potential; no accepted medical use	No prescription permitted	Heroin, lysergic acid (LSD), marijuana, mescaline, and peyote
II	High abuse potential; accepted medical use	Prescription required; no refills permitted without a new written prescription	Cocaine, codeine, methamphetamine (Desoxyn), methadone (Methadose), morphine (Astramorph), opium (deodorized), methylphenidate (Ritalin), and secobarbital (Seconal)
III	Low to moderate abuse potential; accepted medical use	Prescription required; five refills permitted in 6 months	Certain drugs compounded with small quantities of narcotics; also other drugs with high potential for abuse (Tylenol with codeine tablets) and certain barbiturates
IV	Low abuse potential; accepted medical use	Prescription required; five refills permitted in 6 months	Barbital, chloral hydrate (Somnote), diazepam (Valium), chlordiazepoxide (Librium), and pentazocine (Talwin)
V	Low abuse potential; accepted medical use	No prescription required for patients 18 years or older	Cough syrups with codeine, diphenoxylate with atropine (Lomotil)*

*This Schedule V drug *does* require a prescription.

Focus Point

Ensuring Specificity of Orders

An order or prescription must clearly state the specific circumstances and conditions under which the drug may be given. Health care providers must not accept conditions that are nonspecific (e.g., "if needed," "if indicated," or "as warranted").

ORPHAN DRUG ACT OF 1983

Substantial evidence of both safety and effectiveness is required before a new drug can be marketed in the United States; this requirement causes the drug development process to be extremely expensive, lengthy, and difficult. Therefore, because drug companies are businesses trying to make money, they are more likely to invest the millions of dollars and years of research necessary to secure approval for drugs that would be used to treat millions of people with common diseases and disorders. This means that effective new drugs for rare diseases would likely go undeveloped. Recognizing this as a problem in drug research and development, the government passed the Orphan Drug Act of 1983, which offers federal financial incentives to nonprofit and commercial organizations to develop and market drugs to treat rare diseases that affect fewer than 200,000 people in the United States—that is, **orphan drugs**.

This act offers a 7-year patent exclusivity on drug sales and tax breaks to induce drug companies to undertake development and manufacturing of such drugs. Since going into effect, more than 100 orphan drugs have been approved, including those used to treat AIDS, cystic fibrosis, blepharospasm (uncontrolled, rapid blinking), and snake bites.

PRESCRIPTION DRUG MARKETING ACT OF 1987

This act prohibits the **reimportation** (importation of a drug into the United States that was originally manufactured here) of a drug by anyone but the manufacturer. It also deals with safety and competition issues raised by secondary drug markets and prohibits the trading or sale of drug samples, the distribution of samples except by mail or common carrier, and the distribution of samples to persons other than those licensed to prescribe them.

SAFE MEDICAL DEVICES ACT OF 1990

This act requires that medical device users report to manufacturers and the FDA occurrences in which a

medical device has contributed to or caused the death or illness of or serious injury to a patient. The illness or injury must be life-threatening or result in permanent impairment of body function or permanent damage to body structures. Medical devices may include dialyzers, electronic equipment, implants, monitors, restraints, syringes, catheters, in vitro diagnostic test kits and reagents, disposables, components, parts, accessories, related software, thermometers, ventilators, and other types of devices.

ANABOLIC STEROIDS CONTROL ACT OF 1990

Anabolic steroids are hormonal substances related to estrogen, progestins, testosterone, and corticosteroids, which promote muscle growth. Athletes sometimes use these agents to increase their physical performance. This act, which became effective in February 1991, placed anabolic steroids under the CSA's regulatory provisions. It is important because it reflects an essential change of direction for drug abuse control. Anabolic steroids may lead to cardiovascular problems, including heart attack or endocarditis, as well as liver cancer, depression, suicidal thoughts, and a higher risk of viral or bacterial infections. This act was amended in 2004 to modify the definition of the term *anabolic steroids* to include additional related chemicals. Frequently, abusers take both oral and injectable anabolic steroids in doses that are up to 100 times higher than those used for medical conditions.

Focus Point

Ensuring Clarity of Orders

Health care providers must ensure that orders and prescriptions clearly include in writing the drug's name, dosage, route, and frequency of administration. The order must be signed with clear notation of the prescribing physician's name.

OMNIBUS BUDGET RECONCILIATION ACT (OBRA) OF 1990

This act requires that pharmacists offer to counsel Medicaid and Medicare patients about drug information and potential adverse effects for all new and refilled prescriptions. OBRA '90 reduced state entitlements to reimbursement from the federal government and requires states that seek such reimbursement to adopt programs directly affecting the pharmacy profession. Only costs for drugs approved as "safe and

effective" are reimbursed—with just a few exceptions. States must require pharmacists who provide services under this program to give consulting services. These pharmacists may discuss with their patients dosage form, dosage, route of administration, duration of drug therapy, name and description of medication, interactions with other drugs or food, therapeutic contraindications, common adverse effects, proper storage, self-monitoring of medication therapy, special directions for and precautions to be taken, and action in the event of a missed dose.

Focus on Geriatrics

Checklists for Elderly Patient Care

The OBRA was implemented by many nursing home–care facilities to establish a checklist for patients, including:

- Yearly re-evaluation of health; memory; hobbies; habits; and the ability to walk, talk, comprehend, communicate, dress, and bathe

- Assistance in finding a doctor, if needed, plus the right to be informed about treatment programs, which can be refused if desired

✳ Apply Your Knowledge 5.2

The following questions focus on what you have just learned about orphan drugs and recent drug legislation.

CRITICAL THINKING

1. Describe orphan drugs and then give two examples.

2. What was the purpose of the Controlled Substances Act?

3. Describe the classifications of scheduled drugs and determine which class has a high potential for abuse but is currently accepted for medical use in the United States.

4. Why is the abuse of anabolic steroids dangerous?

5. What law mandates that pharmacists offer to counsel Medicaid and Medicare patients about drug information and potential adverse effects for all prescriptions?

Focus Point

Maintaining Reasonable Standards of Care

The law requires all health care professionals to maintain reasonable standards regarding medication management duties—always mindful of the patient's care.

OCCUPATIONAL SAFETY AND HEALTH ACT OF 1970 (REVISED IN 1992)

This act, originally signed in 1970 by President Richard M. Nixon, is administered by the Occupational Safety and Health Administration (OSHA), which is part of the Department of Labor. In the late 1980s, the medical industry became involved with OSHA-related publicity surrounding the threat of human immunodeficiency virus (HIV) infection as it extended to health care workers. OSHA's mission is to ensure workplace safety and a healthy workplace environment. The HIV/AIDS crisis provoked improvements in protection of health care workers who cared for patients with the disease. Before HIV/AIDS, OSHA had focused more directly on viral hepatitis and other pathogens as they affected medical staff members. In July 1992, OSHA's Final Ruling on Bloodborne Pathogens became fully effective. Medical facilities must now comply with the Bloodborne Pathogens Standard and be able to prove their compliance to OSHA inspectors (Figure 5-3 ■). Common OSHA violations include missing or improper labeling of hazardous chemicals, lack of eyewash facilities, inadequate documentation of annual and initial employee training, lack of proof of destruction of hazardous waste, deficient records of the required Written Exposure Control Plan and Emergency Action Plan, missing records of hepatitis B vaccinations on declaration forms, inadequate annual hazard assessment, and neglected posting of OSHA Form 300A during the required time period.

The first specialty area in the pharmacy profession, for which a special regulation at the state level has been established, is the area of **nuclear pharmacy** (a specialty area of pharmacy dealing with radioactive materials for nuclear studies). In nuclear medicine, exposure to

Figure 5-3 ■ In 1992, the Occupational Safety and Health Administration's Final Ruling on Bloodborne Pathogens became law. Safety measures, such as sharps containers for the disposal of needles and syringes, were implemented to stem the spread of HIV/AIDS and other bloodborne diseases.

Michal Heron/Pearson Education/PH College

chemotherapy requires safety procedures and special precautions. Most regulations make it unlawful for any persons to provide nuclear pharmaceutical services unless they are under a qualified nuclear pharmacist's supervision.

HEALTH INSURANCE PORTABILITY AND ACCOUNTABILITY ACT (HIPAA) OF 1996

This act, known as HIPAA, was signed into law in August 1996 by President Bill Clinton, amending the Internal Revenue Service Code of 1986 (also known as the Kassebaum-Kennedy Act). Each of its four administrative simplification parts has generated various standards and rules, with different compliance deadlines from 2000 to 2005. The four parts are:

1. **Electronic health transaction standards**—Standard code sets must be adopted by health organizations and used in all health transactions. All parties to any transaction must use and accept the same coding systems, which describe diseases, injuries, and other health problems (as well as their symptoms, causes, and actions taken). The goal is to reduce mistakes, duplication, and costs.

2. **Unique identifiers**—HIPAA aims to reduce multiple identification numbers when organizations deal with each other to reduce confusion, errors, and costs.

3. **Security and electronic signature standards**—Physical storage and maintenance, transmission, and individual health information access standards were improved by this section, governing all individual health information that is maintained or transmitted (Figure 5-4 ■). The loophole is that this

Figure 5-4 ■ The electronic transmission and storage of medical records is protected by the Health Insurance Portability and Accountability Act.

Mike Gallitelli/Pearson Education/PH College

section applies only to transactions adopted under HIPAA.

4. **Privacy and confidentiality standards**—This section limits nonconsensual use and release of private health information (now called *protected health information*). It gives patients new rights to access their medical records and to be informed of others who have accessed them. It also restricts most disclosure of health information to the minimum required for the intended purpose. This section also developed new civil and criminal sanctions for the improper use or disclosure of health information and new requirements for access to records by researchers and others.

FDA MODERNIZATION ACT OF 1997

The FDA Modernization Act of 1997 reformed the regulation of cosmetics, food, and medical products by focusing mostly on safe pharmacy compounding, user fees, food safety, and medical devices. Under this act, patients now have increased access to experimental drugs and devices. It also gave manufacturers 6-month extensions on new pediatric drugs, with drug trial test data on file, and mandated risk assessment reviews of any foods or drugs containing mercury. This act, also known as the FDAMA, changed the promotion of off-label drugs and required legend drugs to be packaged with the "Rx" symbol included. This act was intended to speed up the drug approval process and address changing technologies and drug marketing.

MEDICARE PRESCRIPTION DRUG, IMPROVEMENT, AND MODERNIZATION ACT OF 2003

The Medicare Prescription Drug, Improvement, and Modernization Act of 2003 is also known as the Medicare Modernization Act (MMA), and it overhauled Medicare more than any other act. It introduced subsidies for prescription drugs as well as tax breaks. It presented new Medicare "Advantage" plans that offered patients better choices about care, providers, coverage, and federal reimbursements. It also established a partially privatized Medicare system, offered pretax medical savings accounts, and raised certain fees for older adults whose net worth is over a certain amount. Overall, this act was designed to help senior citizens by reducing drug costs and to help employers offer drug benefits to their employers.

This act established Medicare Part D, which may be obtained either by joining a prescription drug plan (PDP) or a Medicare Advantage (MA) plan. This is a voluntary program that operates on an annual renewal basis, with varied plans and co-payment amounts. Part D only covers drugs that are approved by the FDA and does not cover people who already have Medicare Part A or B coverage.

COMBAT METHAMPHETAMINE EPIDEMIC ACT OF 2005

The Combat Methamphetamine Epidemic Act of 2005 is focused on the provisions of the Patriot Act extension that dealt with methamphetamine provisions. It was designed to stop illegal use of methamphetamine and regulated trafficking of this drug (and certain others, such as crack cocaine) when these activities are used to finance terrorism. The government can now confiscate the personal property of anyone involved in such activities. Drugs that fall under this act's jurisdiction must be kept behind a counter or in a locked case. It also limits sales of ingredients used to manufacture methamphetamine (ephedrine or pseudoephedrine) to only 9 grams per month per person. To buy these drugs, a customer must provide identification and sign a sales log. Sellers of these drugs must be registered with the U.S. Attorney General's office and receive specialized training.

CHILDREN'S HEALTH INSURANCE PROGRAM REAUTHORIZATION ACT OF 2009

The Children's Health Insurance Program Reauthorization Act expanded the State Children's Health Insurance (SCHIP) program to include approximately 4 million more children, including coverage of illegal immigrants, with no waiting period for the first time ever in history. This expansion was funded by increased taxes on cigarettes, chewing tobacco, and other tobacco products. The SCHIP program has now been simplified to be called the Children's Health Insurance Program (CHIP). It is administered by the Department of Health and Human Services and provides matching funds to states for health insurance to families with children. It was designed to cover uninsured children in families with incomes that were considered "modest," but still too high to qualify for Medicaid.

FAMILY SMOKING PREVENTION AND TOBACCO CONTROL ACT OF 2009

The Family Smoking Prevention and Tobacco Control Act gave the FDA the power to regulate the tobacco industry. It imposed new warnings and labels on tobacco packaging and advertisements to discourage minors and young adults from smoking. It also banned flavored cigarettes, placed limits on advertising of tobacco products to minors, and required tobacco companies to seek FDA approval for new tobacco products.

PATIENT PROTECTION AND AFFORDABLE CARE ACT OF 2010

The Patient Protection and Affordable Care Act (PPACA) is commonly known as the Affordable Care Act (ACA), as well as "ObamaCare." Along with the Health Care and Education Reconciliation Act amendment, it represented the most significant regulatory overhaul of the United States health care system since the passage of Medicare and Medicaid. It was enacted to increase quality and affordability of health insurance, lower the uninsured rate by expanding public and private insurance coverage, and reduce costs of health care for individuals and the government. The act also introduced mandates, subsidies, and insurance exchanges, and required insurance companies to cover all applicants within new minimum standards, offering the same rates regardless of preexisting conditions or gender. This act lost popularity since it resulted in much higher rates for many people. Some states experienced rate increases that were as low as 25% and as high as 116%. Several large insurance companies announced that they would stop selling insurance through the exchanges created by the act. President Trump promised to repeal this act and replace it with something much more affordable and effective.

HEALTH CARE AND EDUCATION RECONCILIATION ACT OF 2010

The Health Care and Education Reconciliation Act was designed to amend the Patient Protection and Affordable Care Act. It includes the Student Aid and Fiscal Responsibility Act, which was attached as a rider. This act was signed into law only 7 days after the Affordable Care Act. It increased tax credits to buy insurance, eliminated kickbacks, lowered the penalty for not buying insurance, closed Medicare Part D loopholes while giving seniors a rebate, required doctors treating Medicare patients to be reimbursed at the full rate, set up a Medicare tax on unearned incomes of families earning more than $250,000 per year, offered more generous subsidies to lower-income people, and made many other changes. Its Student Aid and Fiscal Responsibility Act ended government subsidies to private banks giving out federally insured loans, increased Pell Grant scholarships, initiated loan caps, loosened loan forgiveness rules, simplified federal student loans obtained by parents, and helped fund poor and minority schools while increasing community college funding.

HEALTHY, HUNGER-FREE KIDS ACT OF 2010

The Healthy, Hunger-Free Kids Act helped reauthorize funding for child nutrition and free lunch programs in school. It set new nutrition standards for schools and allocated billions of dollars for their implementation. Since its enactment, millions of American children have received free or reduced-price lunches at school. Across the country, the school lunch program varies by state.

Federal Regulatory Agencies

The three most important federal regulatory agencies concerning pharmacology include the Food and Drug Administration (FDA), Drug Enforcement Administration (DEA), and Centers for Disease Control and Prevention (CDC).

FOOD AND DRUG ADMINISTRATION

The FDA, a branch of the U.S. Department of Health and Human Services, is responsible for cosmetics, medicines, medical devices, radiation-emitting products, food and drugs used for farm animals, domestic and imported food, bottled water, and wine beverages that contain less than 7% alcohol. All drug administration laws are initiated, implemented, and enforced by the FDA.

DRUG ENFORCEMENT ADMINISTRATION

The DEA enforces controlled substance laws and regulations and investigates and prosecutes individuals (and organizations) who grow, manufacture, or distribute illegal substances. It also targets people who use violence in the coercion of others to help them in their illegal activities and distributes information about illegal substances to educate the public. The DEA also works with other governments to assist global drug trafficking enforcement.

CENTERS FOR DISEASE CONTROL AND PREVENTION

The CDC provides statistics and information to health professionals about the treatment of common and rare diseases worldwide. Its services include investigating, identifying, preventing, and controlling disease. The CDC's primary function is to issue infection control regulations. Established in 1946 as the Communicable Disease Center, the CDC changed its name to the Centers for Disease Control in 1970, with the words "and Prevention" added in 1992. However, Congress requested that the initials "CDC" remain the same. This agency has been actively involved in the war against AIDS and HIV.

✺ Apply Your Knowledge 5.3

The following questions focus on what you have just learned about OSHA, HIPAA, and federal regulatory agencies.

CRITICAL THINKING

1. Why must all health professionals obey OSHA guidelines?
2. Describe HIPAA and its four parts.
3. Compare the functions of the FDA, DEA, and CDC.
4. Explain the four parts of Medicare.
5. Describe the Combat Methamphetamine Epidemic Act.

State Law

State governments, not the federal government, are the main regulators of laws that regulate pharmacy practice. Each state is concerned with protecting the health, safety, and welfare of its citizens. Pharmacy laws, although differing from state to state, are based on the same goals, objectives, and principles of pharmaceutical practice.

State law requires minimal qualifications for individuals involved with pharmacy practice—no one may practice pharmacy without a license except those exempted by the state legislation that creates the licensing requirement. Licensed individuals must successfully complete state board of pharmacy requirements. These boards are part of the licensing division of state health departments.

Pharmacy licensure is difficult to gain and not easily revoked. After due process and for just cause as set out in the appropriate legislation, the state can suspend, revoke, or terminate a pharmacist's license. The practice of licensed pharmacists is safeguarded by federal and state constitutions as a property right. Certificates of registration are granted for 1 or 2 years in most states.

Health care providers must use prescription pads only for writing prescriptions for medications. Prescription pads must be secured at all times. Some states allow medication administration by allied health professionals; other states do not. Therefore, health care workers must know the laws of the state in which they work. It is also important to understand the rulings that apply to phoning in prescriptions to pharmacists.

Certificates of registration, or pharmacy licenses, can be cancelled or revoked only under special circumstances. Depending on the type of state law violation, a pharmacist's license may be suspended or revoked permanently. An example is the dispensing of a scheduled drug without a prescription or proper documentation. The National Association of Boards of Pharmacy (NABP) developed a Model State Pharmacy Practice Act (MSPPA), which offers flexibility to the states that adopt it but provides a greater degree of uniformity between states.

Ethics in Clinical and Pharmacy Practice

Ethics are standards of behavior and include concepts of right and wrong beyond what legal considerations are in any given situation. Health care professionals are expected to act in ways that reflect society's ideas of right and wrong even if such behavior is not enforced by law. Allied health professionals must use confidentiality in all areas concerning medications and their administration.

Although drug companies, by law, may provide free supplies of medications to physicians for promoting sales (Figure 5-5 ■), these samples may not be sold. A sample drug is marked "sample," bears a federal legend (℞), and requires a prescription. Some manufacturers may also provide drug coupons that discount the price of a specific prescribed drug, but these coupons cannot be sold or traded. Samples should be stored immediately where they are not accessible to patients and organized by indication and expiration date. Health care professionals may not legally supply medicine samples to family, friends, or themselves. Other ethical considerations cover pharmacists' or other health care providers' professional relationships with their patients and dispensing of medications that may be against their personal beliefs.

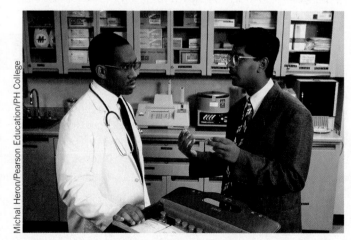

Michal Heron/Pearson Education/PH College

Figure 5-5 ■ Pharmaceutical company representatives provide drug samples to physician offices. These samples may not be sold.

PRACTICAL SCENARIO 1

Anabolic steroids are very popular among today's athletes who want to gain a competitive edge over others by building muscle. The evening news often contains stories of professional athletes testing positive for anabolic steroids. One such 20-year-old male athlete illegally obtained anabolic steroids from another athlete at his school and began injecting them regularly to improve his performance in college football. During the season, he collapsed on the field and later died.

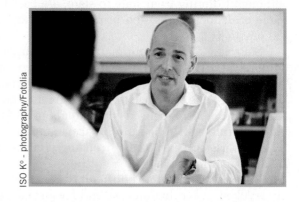

Laima Druskis/Pearson Education/PH College

Critical Thinking Questions

1. What are the most important side effects of using anabolic steroids?
2. What types of heart conditions are linked to the use of anabolic steroids?

PRACTICAL SCENARIO 2

Paula, a medical assistant, has worked for a family practitioner for 7 years. In the past, she has been allowed to contact the pharmacy for prescription refills for patients. Her boyfriend has been experiencing back pain after a disc herniation. Paula, wanting to help, writes several prescriptions over a 6-month period for a scheduled drug to relieve his pain. The pharmacist notices the frequency of these prescriptions and calls the family practitioner to ask if he is aware of this patient. The family practitioner says he is not. He confronts Paula, who admits the patient is her boyfriend and that she has been writing the prescriptions herself and stamping them with the family practitioner's signature.

ISO K° - photography/Fotolia

Critical Thinking Questions

1. What are the likely consequences of Paula's actions?
2. What organization or agency oversees scheduled drugs?

Chapter Capsule

This section repeats the objectives from the beginning of the chapter and then provides a summary of the most important concepts for that objective. Use this section as a quick review and to check your knowledge.

Objective 1: Discuss legal and ethical requirements regarding the use, dispensation, and administration of medications.

- Federal regulations protect consumers from potential for harm from both legal and illicit drugs
- The FDA controls all drug administration laws

Objective 2: Explain how the need for drug control evolved.

■ Absence of laws requiring drug testing or drug labeling in the early nineteenth century

■ The Pure Food and Drug Act of 1906 was developed to require safety and efficacy of drugs

Objective 3: Discuss the poisoning disaster that led to legislation requiring testing for the purity, strength, effectiveness, safety, and packaging quality of drugs.

■ Sulfanilamide mixed with diethylene glycol, sold to the public in liquid form for upper respiratory infections, resulted in 107 reported deaths

■ The Food, Drug, and Cosmetic Act, created in 1938, gave the FDA authority to approve or deny new drug applications

■ The FDA approves investigational use of drugs on humans and ensures safety and efficacy of all approved drugs

Objective 4: Explain the major points of the thalidomide disaster of 1962.

■ Thalidomide (used in other countries) was tested for marketing in the United States as a sleeping pill or antinausea medication for pregnant women

■ Discovery of birth defects (severe deformities) in the children of many women of other countries who took thalidomide during their first trimester of pregnancy

■ Kefauver-Harris Amendment, passed in 1962, limited thalidomide use to treatment of leprosy, bone marrow transplantation, AIDS, and some other conditions

Objective 5: List the provisions of the Controlled Substances Act.

■ Provides increased research into and prevention of drug abuse and drug dependence

■ Provides treatment and rehabilitation of drug abusers and drug-dependent persons

■ Regulates the manufacture, distribution, and dispensing of controlled substances

■ Applies schedules to drugs with potential for causing drug dependence, abuse, or both

Objective 6: Differentiate between each of the five schedules for controlled substances.

■ Schedule I—High abuse potential; not accepted for medical use in the United States

■ Schedule II—High abuse potential; accepted for medical use in the United States

■ Schedule III—Low to moderate abuse potential; accepted for medical use in the United States

■ Schedule IV—Slight abuse potential; accepted for medical use in the United States

■ Schedule V—Lowest abuse potential of all; includes OTC preparations

Objective 7: Define *orphan drug* and then list some examples.

■ Used to treat diseases that affect fewer than 200,000 people in the United States

■ Provides a 7-year monopoly on the sale and breaks on taxes given to manufacturers

■ 100 orphan drugs approved, including those used to treat AIDS, cystic fibrosis, uncontrolled rapid blinking, and snake bites

Objective 8: Discuss the federal regulatory agencies that deal with food, drugs, and disease control.

■ The Food and Drug Administration controls drugs for legal use

■ The Drug Enforcement Administration enforces controlled substance laws, regulations, and more

■ Centers for Disease Control and Prevention:

❑ Provides statistics and information about the treatment of common and rare diseases worldwide

❑ Provides facilities and services for investigating, identifying, preventing, and controlling disease

❑ Issues infection control regulations

Objective 9: Explain which level of government primarily controls pharmacy licensure.

■ States are the main regulators of laws governing pharmacy practice

■ Licensing required of practicing pharmacies except if exempted by state legislation that creates licensing requirements

Objective 10: Define *ethics* as it relates to pharmacology.

■ Expectation of health care professionals to act in ways that reflect society's ideas of right and wrong even if such behavior is not enforced by law

■ Guarantee of confidentiality in all areas that concern medications and their administration

■ Security and proper use of prescription pads

 Internet Sites of Interest

■ The National Institutes of Health (NIH) website provides information on ethical considerations in research studies. Search for "ethics." **www.nlm.nih.gov**

■ The abuse of pain medications has led some health care providers to limit the appropriate use of pain medications in patients who need them. For a discussion among government agents about this issue: **www.usdoj.gov/dea/pubs/press-rel/pr102301.html**

■ Read about laws enforced by the FDA: **www.fda.gov/RegulatoryInformation/Legislation/default.htm**

■ Find information about the Orphan Drug Act: **http://www.fda.gov/ForIndustry/DevelopingProductsforRareDiseasesConditions/HowtoapplyforOrphanProduct Designation/ucm364750.htm**

■ Access an overview of the FDA: **www.emedicinehealth.com/script/main/art.asp?articlekey=8468**

Chapter 6

Terminology, Abbreviations, Drug Forms, and Dispensing Prescriptions

Chapter Objectives

After completing this chapter, you should be able to:

1. Define the suffixes *-ism*, *-itis*, *-pathy*, and *-tomy*.
2. Explain abbreviations used in pharmacology.
3. Define *chemical, generic*, and *trade names* of drugs.
4. Describe five sources of drug derivation.
5. Explain black box warnings.
6. List various solid drug forms.
7. Describe topical drugs.
8. Explain gaseous drugs.
9. List seven component parts of a prescription.
10. Define *standing orders*.

Key Terms

alkaloids (p. 68)

chemical name (p. 68)

generic name (p. 68)

glycoside (p. 68)

parenteral (p. 71)

sustained-release (SR) (p. 71)

trade name (p. 68)

Introduction

Learning the language of medicine is essential for all fields of the health care industry. Medical terminology originated primarily from Greek and Latin prefixes, roots, and suffixes, which are known as *word parts*. There are also new terms that are derived from the universal language of English. A majority of terms related to surgery and diagnosis have Greek origins, and most anatomic terms come from Latin origins. To learn medical terminology, it is very helpful to memorize word parts and rules for creating words. By understanding how word parts are combined, it is possible to determine the meanings of medical words.

Health care professionals who are involved with pharmacology must be familiar with word building, common medical terms, and abbreviations. They must understand general pharmacology terms and concepts. Drug names include complex chemical names, simpler generic names, and trade names provided by drug manufacturers. There may be multiple trade name versions of the same generic drug.

In this chapter, terminology and abbreviations, sources of drugs, drug forms, and drug dispensing are reviewed in detail. Further information is provided about how a drug may be removed from the market and the use of black box warnings, which are the most serious types of drug information issued by the Food and Drug Administration.

Pharmaceutical Terminology

Allied health care professionals who must deal with pharmaceutical agents need to be familiar with medical and pharmaceutical terminology. They must understand roots, prefixes, suffixes, and combining vowels.

A *root* is the main part of a word that gives the word its central meaning. It is the basic foundation of a word that can be made more complex through the addition of other word parts. A *prefix* is a structure at the beginning of a word that modifies the meaning of the root; Table 6-1 ■ shows some common general prefixes. A *suffix* is a word ending that modifies the meaning of the root; Table 6-2 ■ gives some common general suffixes.

Medical terms are formed from many different word parts. These parts are often joined by vowels known as *combining vowels*. The most common combining vowel is the letter *o* and, occasionally, the letter *i*. For example, *o* serves as a combining vowel in the term *hyperlipoproteinemia* (hyper / lip / o / protein / emia).

Abbreviations Used in Pharmacology

Abbreviations are shortened forms of words representing commonly used medical terms. Many such abbreviations are used in all areas of health care practice. It is essential for health care professionals to be familiar with the most common abbreviations used for writing prescriptions (Table 6-3 ■), the abbreviations associated with various measurements (Table 6-4 ■), and general medical abbreviations (Table 6-5 ■).

Table 6-1 ■ Some Common General Prefixes

PREFIX	MEANING	EXAMPLE
alb-	white	albinism
ante-	before	antepartum
anti-	against	antibiotic
bi-	two, both	bilateral
bio-	life	biology
ecto-	outside	ectopic
endo-	into, within	endoscopic
epi-	upon, above	epidermic
multi-	many	multinuclear
myo-	muscle	myocarditis
poly-	many	polyarthritis
semi-	half	semiconscious
ultra-	beyond, excessive	ultrasound

Table 6-2 ■ Some Common General Suffixes

SUFFIX	MEANING	EXAMPLE
-ectomy	excision, removal	hysterectomy
-emesis	vomit	hyperemesis
-gram	record	electrocardiogram
-ism	condition	cryptorchidism
-itis	inflammation	appendicitis
-logy	study of	microbiology
-oma	tumor	carcinoma
-pathy	disease	hemopathy
-phobia	abnormal fear	photophobia
-stomy	surgical creation of a new opening	colostomy
-tomy	incision, cutting	phlebotomy

✳ Apply Your Knowledge 6.1

The following questions focus on what you have just learned about pharmaceutical terminology.

CRITICAL THINKING

1. List the most common combining vowels.
2. Define the terms *prefix*, *root*, and *suffix*.
3. Identify the meanings of the terms *cryptorchidism*, *hemopathy*, *photophobia*, and *colostomy*.
4. Describe the meanings of the prefixes *ante-*, *alb-*, *semi-*, *epi-*, and *ecto-*.

Table 6-3 ■ Abbreviations Commonly Used in Prescriptions

ABBREVIATION	MEANING	ABBREVIATION	MEANING
āā, aa	of each	per	through or by
Ac	before meals	p.m., PM	afternoon
Ad	to, up to	po, PO	by mouth
ad lib	as desired	PR	through the rectum
a.m., AM	morning	prn, PRN	as needed
amt	amount	PULV	powder
aq	water	q	every
bid, BID	twice a day	q2h	every 2 hours
bin	twice a night	qh	every hour
c̄	with	qid, QID	four times a day
cap, caps	capsule	QN	every night
comp	compound	qs, qv	as much as you wish (sufficient quantity)
d	day	s̄	without (sine)
dil	dilute	Sig	write on label
disp	dispense	sol	solution
elix	elixir	sos	if necessary
hr	hour	sp	spirits
IM	intramuscular	stat	immediately
inj, INJ	inject	supp	suppository
IV	intravenous	syr	syrup
liq	liquid	tab	tablet
mixt	mixture	tid	three times a day
noct	at night	top	topically
non rep	do not repeat, no refills	tr., tinct	tincture
NPO	nothing by mouth (*nulla per os*)	vo	verbal order
oint	ointment	x	multiplied by
pc	after meals		

Note: See the "Internet Sites of Interest" section at the end of this chapter for the Institute for Safe Medical Practices (ISMP) website, which provides a list of medical abbreviations that are frequently misinterpreted and involved in harmful errors and thus should not be used.

Table 6-4 ■ Abbreviations Commonly Used for Measurements

ABBREVIATION	MEANING	ABBREVIATION	MEANING
°C	degrees Celsius	mEq	milliequivalent
cm	centimeter (2.5 cm = 1 in.)	mg	milligram
°F	degrees Fahrenheit	mL	milliliter
fl	fluid	No. or \#	number
g, gm	gram	oz	ounce
gtt	drop or drops	T	temperature
kg	kilogram (1 kg = 2.2 lb)	Tbs, Tbsp	tablespoon
L	liter	tsp	teaspoon
lb	pound	w/v	weight in volume
mcg	microgram		

Drug Names

Each drug may have three different types of names: the **chemical name** (describing the chemical makeup of a drug), the **generic name** (also called *approved name*, *official name*, or *nonproprietary name*), and the **trade name** (also called the *brand name* or *proprietary name*). For example, hydroxybenzyl penicillin is the chemical name of the generic drug called amoxicillin. This drug is a commonly prescribed antibiotic. All drugs have a generic name, which is not protected by trademark. Amoxicillin is marketed under dozens of proprietary names, including Alphamox and Amoxil. Proprietary names are assigned by various manufacturers and are protected by trademark. Because there is only one generic name per drug, the use of a drug's generic name is encouraged over trade names to avoid confusion. Drugs are also classified by their therapeutic use. For example, Tylenol is the brand name of the generic drug acetaminophen, which is classified as an analgesic and an antipyretic agent.

Sources of Drug Derivation

There are basically five sources of drugs: (1) plants, (2) animals (including humans), (3) minerals or mineral products, (4) synthetics (chemical substances), and (5) engineered (investigational) sources. Today, chemicals and even human tissues, such as those used in stem-cell therapy, can be manipulated to create new drug sources.

PLANTS

Plant sources are grouped by their physical and chemical properties. **Alkaloids** are organic nitrogen-containing compounds that are alkaline and usually bitter tasting. They are combined with acids to make a salt. Atropine, nicotine, and morphine are examples of these chemical compounds. An important cardiac **glycoside** (an organic compound that yields sugar and nonsugar substances when hydrolyzed) is digoxin. Digoxin is made from digitalis, a derivative of the foxglove plant.

�֎ Apply Your Knowledge 6.2

The following questions focus on what you have just learned about abbreviations used in pharmacology.

CRITICAL THINKING

1. Identify what each of the following abbreviations represent: Ad, aq, liq, per, QN, supp, and x.
2. Identify the terms that correspond to these abbreviations: gtt, fl, mcg, kg, Bx, CVA, Dx, and HBV.
3. Find the abbreviations for the terms *potassium*, *nitrogen*, *sodium*, *iodine*, and *iron*.
4. Find the abbreviations for the terms *catheter*, *electrocardiogram*, *genitourinary*, and *hemoglobin*.
5. Find the abbreviations for the terms *intrauterine device*, *weight*, *chest x-ray*, and *microgram*.

Table 6-5 ■ General Medical Abbreviations

ABBREVIATION	MEANING	ABBREVIATION	MEANING
AP	anterior–posterior	Hg	mercury
BE	barium enema	Hgb	hemoglobin
BP	blood pressure	Hib	*Haemophilus influenzae* type B
Bx	biopsy	Hx, hx	history
C	carbon	I	iodine
C&S	culture & sensitivity	IM	intramuscular
c/o	complains of	IUD	intrauterine device
Ca	calcium, cancer, or carcinoma	IV	intravenous
CAD	coronary artery disease	K	potassium
cath.	catheter	LMP	last menstrual period
CBC	complete blood count	MI	myocardial infarction
CHF	congestive heart failure	MMR	measles–mumps–rubella
CO	carbon monoxide	N	nitrogen
COPD	chronic obstructive pulmonary disease	Na	sodium
CVA	cerebrovascular accident	OB	obstetrics
CXR	chest x-ray	P	pulse
D&C	dilatation & curettage	PERRLA	pupils equal, round, reactive to light and accommodation
DOB	date of birth	PO	orally
DPT	diphtheria–pertussis–tetanus	Pt	patient
Dx	diagnosis	R	respirations, right
ECG	electrocardiogram	R/O	rule out
EEG	electroencephalogram	RBC	red blood cell
EENT	eyes, ears, nose, throat	ROM	range of motion
FBS	fasting blood sugar	SOB	shortness of breath
Fe	iron	T	temperature
FUO	fever of unknown origin	TIA	transient ischemic attack
GI	gastrointestinal	Tx	treatment
GU	genitourinary	UA	urinalysis
Gyn	gynecology	UTI	urinary tract infection
H	hydrogen	VS, vs	vital signs
H&P	history and physical	WBC	white blood cell
HBV	hepatitis B virus	WNL	within normal limits
HCT	hematocrit	wt	weight

HUMANS AND OTHER ANIMALS

Animal sources, such as the body fluids and glands of animals, can act as drugs. The drugs obtained from animal sources include such hormones as adrenaline, insulin, and thyroid. Enzymes such as pancreatin and pepsin are also from animal sources.

MINERALS

Minerals from the earth and soil are used to provide inorganic materials unavailable from plants and animals. They are used as they occur in nature. Examples include sodium, iodine, potassium, iron, and gold, which are used to prepare medications. Sodium chloride (table salt) is one of the best-known examples in this group. Gold is prescribed to prevent severe rheumatoid arthritis, and coal tar is used to treat seborrheic dermatitis and psoriasis.

SYNTHETIC SOURCES

Certain drugs may come from living organisms (organic substances) or nonliving materials (inorganic substances). These drugs are known as synthetic or manufactured drugs. They have evolved from the application of chemistry, biology, and computer technology. Because they do not exist in nature, these medications come from artificial substances. Examples of synthetic drugs include oral contraceptives, meperidine (Demerol), and sulfonamides. Certain organic drugs, such as penicillin, are semisynthetic and are made by altering their natural compounds or elements. Some drugs are both organic and inorganic, such as propylthiouracil, which is an antithyroid hormone.

ENGINEERED SOURCES

The newest area of drug origin is gene splicing, or *genetic engineering*. The newer forms of insulin for use in humans have been produced by this technique. A tissue plasminogen activator for heart attack victims is also being developed via this method. Growth hormones (bovine or porcine somatotropin) are being produced from bacteria that have received the appropriate gene (human, cow, or pig). Another new and experimental treatment is gene therapy, which involves replacing a gene that is missing or not functioning correctly with the correct gene. The first successful gene therapy was used in 1990 to treat an immune system defect in children. Genetically engineered products, featuring modified DNA, are being produced to treat malignant brain tumors, cystic fibrosis, and HIV. The public seems to be greatly interested in this new way of developing a wide range of new drugs.

Removal of a Drug from the Market

In certain situations, the FDA may require that a drug be removed from the market and its use be discontinued. This may be because of a variety of reasons, including improper manufacturing, harmful ingredients, the development of adverse effects not seen in the drug development process, or lack of effectiveness. A drug may be recalled at any time after it has been approved. On an annual basis, the FDA holds public meetings to address comments from health professionals and patients concerning the safety and effectiveness of drugs.

Black Box Warnings

A *black box warning* is the most severe warning from the FDA about a drug. It appears on the prescription label to alert all health care providers and patients about potentially harmful adverse effects of the drug. The FDA requires a black box warning for each of the following situations:

✱ The medication may cause serious undesirable effects (such as a fatal, life-threatening, or permanently disabling adverse reaction) compared with the potential benefit from the drug.

✱ A serious adverse reaction can be prevented, reduced in frequency, or reduced in severity by proper use of the drug. For example, a medication may be safe for adults but not for children.

Drug Forms

Pharmaceutics is the science of formulating drugs into such different types of preparations as tablets, ointments, injectable solutions, or eye drops. It also includes studying the ways in which various drug forms influence pharmacokinetic and pharmacodynamic activities of the active drug.

Many drugs are available in different formulations. This variety assists the prescriber in choosing a formulation that is best suited for the individual patient and route of administration. Formulations, such as oral pills and tablets, injectable medications, or rectally or vaginally administered drugs, also determine whether a drug acts locally or is absorbed into the systemic circulation. Failure to administer the drug in the correct form results in a medication error. Using an incorrect form can also cause damage to body cells. Therefore, allied health care professionals need to learn about the various drug preparations and their uses. Drug dosage forms are classified according to their physical state (e.g., liquid or solid) and chemical composition. Various forms of drug preparations allow for oral, topical, mucous membrane, or **parenteral** use (introduction of a drug outside of the gastrointestinal [GI] tract; generally in injectable form) and for miscellaneous drug delivery systems.

Some substances can undergo a change of state or phase—from solid to liquid (melting) or from liquid to gas (vaporization). Certain drugs are soluble in water, some are soluble in alcohol, and others are soluble in a mixture of liquids.

PREPARATIONS FOR ORAL USE

An oral drug may appear in solid form (e.g., tablets, capsules, or powders) or liquid form (solutions, elixirs, or suspensions). Disintegration of the solid dose form must occur before *dissolution*, a process by which a drug goes into solution and becomes available for absorption. The form of drug dose is important because the more rapid the rate of dissolution, the more readily the compound crosses the cell membrane and is absorbed into the systemic circulation to be circulated to the site where it acts. Oral drugs in liquid form are therefore more rapidly available for GI absorption than those in solid form.

SOLID DRUGS

The route for administering a medication depends on its form, its properties, and the effect desired. Solid forms of drugs are widely used in drug treatment. The solid forms are also a convenient way to take unpleasant-tasting or irritating drugs. Solid drugs include pills, tablets, capsules, **sustained-release (SR)** tablets and capsules (that are specially coated so they dissolve at specific times), enteric-coated tablets and capsules, caplets, gelcaps, powders, granules, and troches or lozenges (Figure 6-1 ■). Some plasters are also considered to be solid drugs, although they are generally semisolids.

Pills

A single-dose unit of medicine made by mixing the powdered drug with a liquid, such as syrup, and rolling it into a round or oval shape is called a *pill*.

Tablets

A *tablet* is a pharmaceutical preparation made by compressing the powdered form of a drug and bulk-filling material under high pressure (Figure 6-2 ■). Tablets may appear as simple white disks or may be multilayered or coated with a film to mask an unpleasant taste. Special forms of tablets include sublingual tablets and enteric-coated tablets. Most tablets are intended to be swallowed whole for dissolution and absorption in the GI tract. Some are intended to be dissolved in the mouth, dissolved in water, or inserted as suppositories. Many times, tablets are mistakenly called pills. Tablets come in various sizes, shapes, colors, and compositions. The various forms of tablets include chewable, sublingual, buccal, enteric-coated, and buffered tablets. Chewable tablets contain a flavored or sugar base and must be chewed. They are commonly used for antacids and antiflatulents and for children who cannot swallow medication. Sublingual tablets must be dissolved under the tongue for rapid absorption; an example is nitroglycerin for angina pectoris. Buccal tablets are placed between the cheek and the gum until they are dissolved and absorbed.

Capsules

A *capsule* is a medication dosage form in which the drug is contained in an external shell (Figure 6-3 ■).

Figure 6-1 ■ Solid drug forms.

Figure 6-2 ■ Examples of tablets.

Sommai/Fotolia

Figure 6-3 ■ Examples of capsules.

Capsule shells are usually made of a hard cylindrical gelatin and enclose or encapsulate powder, granules, liquids, or some combinations of these. Liquids may be placed in soft gelatin capsules; examples are vitamin E capsules and cod liver oil capsules. They are used when medications have an unpleasant odor or taste. Capsules can be pulled apart, and the entire contents can be added as powder to food for individuals who have difficulty swallowing. Some forms of capsules come with a controlled-release dosage and are used over a defined period of time (sustained-release or timed-release capsules). These drugs should *never* be crushed or dissolved because this would negate their timed-release action.

Focus on Geriatrics

Coated Aspirin Tablets

Some patients, particularly older adults who have stomach ulcers, cannot take certain medications, such as aspirin. Therefore, these patients should be given enteric-coated aspirin tablets.

Sustained-Release Tablets and Capsules

Sustained-release drug forms contain several doses of a drug. The doses have special coatings that dissolve at different rates; therefore, the drug is released into the digestive system gradually. Sustained-release drugs are referred to as *delayed release* and *timed release*. An example is diltiazem (Cardizem SR), a calcium channel blocker used in the treatment of angina pectoris and hypertension.

Enteric-Coated Tablets and Capsules

Some tablets and capsules are covered by a special coating that keeps them from dissolving in the stomach, which contains hydrochloric acid. These drugs do not dissolve until they reach the intestine. Therefore, the strength of these drugs remains undiluted as they pass through the stomach, providing a delayed action that is desirable. An example is Ecotrin, a nonnarcotic analgesic used for pain, an antipyretic used for fever, and a nonsteroidal anti-inflammatory used in the treatment of arthritis. Also important is the fact that enteric coatings may prevent nausea and vomiting that some drugs can induce from dissolving in the stomach. Furthermore, enteric coatings prevent decomposition of chemically sensitive drugs (e.g., penicillin G and erythromycin) by gastric secretions. These two drugs are examples of substances that are unstable in the acid pH of the stomach.

Focus Point

Administering Enteric-Coated Tablets

Do not crush or mix enteric-coated tablets or capsules into liquids or foods because it will destroy the enteric coating. This would result in the drug's being released into the stomach instead of the small intestine.

Caplets

A *caplet* is shaped like a capsule but has the form of a tablet. The shape and film-coated covering make swallowing easier.

Gelcaps

A *gelcap* is an oil-based medication that is enclosed in a soft gelatin capsule (Figure 6-4 ■).

Figure 6-4 ■ Examples of gelcaps.

Powders

A drug that is dried and ground into fine particles is called a *powder*. An example is potassium chloride powder (Gen-K or Klor-con).

Granules

A small pill, usually accompanied by many others encased within a gelatin capsule, is called a *granule*. In most cases, granules within capsules are specially coated to gradually release medication over an extended period.

Troches or Lozenges

A hard or semisolid dosage form containing a medication intended for local application in the mouth or throat is called a *troche* or *lozenge*. These are flattened disks. Typically, a troche is placed on the tongue or between the cheek and gum and left in place until it dissolves. The medications most commonly administered by means of troches include cough suppressants and treatments for sore throat.

LIQUID DRUGS

Liquid preparations include drugs that have been dissolved or suspended. Examples of liquid drugs are syrups and linctuses, solutions, emulsions, spirits or essences, liniments, gels or jellies, lotions, most aerosols, and magmas.

Focus on Pediatrics

Liquid Drugs

Infants and young children are not able to take solid drug forms, such as tablets or capsules. Therefore, they should be given liquid drugs.

Syrups and Linctuses

Aqueous solutions containing a high concentration of sugars, syrups, and linctuses may or may not have medical substances added (e.g., simple syrup and ipecac syrup).

Solutions

A *solution* is a drug or drugs dissolved in an appropriate solvent. Examples of solutions include elixirs, fluidextracts, mixtures and suspensions, and tinctures, which are highly concentrated forms of drugs.

ELIXIRS

A drug vehicle that consists of water, alcohol, and sugar is known as an *elixir*. It may or may not be aromatic and may or may not have active medical properties. Their alcohol content makes elixirs convenient liquid dosage forms for many drugs that are only slightly soluble in water. In these cases, the drug is first dissolved in alcohol, and the other elixir components are added. All elixirs contain alcohol (e.g., terpin hydrate elixir and phenobarbital elixir). Elixirs differ from tinctures in that they are sweetened. They should be used with caution in patients with diabetes or a history of alcohol abuse. Some pediatric medications retain the name of elixirs, although they no longer contain alcohol.

FLUIDEXTRACTS

A concentrated solution of a drug removed from a plant source by mixing ground parts of the plant with a suitable solvent, usually alcohol, and then separating the plant residue from the solvent is called a *fluidextract*. Typically, 1 mL contains 1 g of the drug. Fluidextracts are not intended to be administered directly to a patient. Instead, they are prescribed to provide a source of drug in the manufacture of final dosage forms. Only vegetable drugs are used (e.g., glycyrrhiza fluidextract).

MIXTURES AND SUSPENSIONS

In a *mixture* or a *suspension*, an agent is mixed with a liquid but not dissolved. These preparations must be shaken before being taken by or administered to the patient. Examples include chlorpheniramine/pseudoephedrine (mixture) and betamethasone (suspension).

Focus Point

Storing Drugs That Contain Alcohol

Elixirs, spirits, tinctures, and fluidextracts contain alcohol. They must be kept tightly sealed so the alcohol cannot evaporate. They should be stored in a dark place, as specified on the labels.

TINCTURES

A *tincture* is an alcoholic preparation of a soluble drug, usually from a plant source. In some cases, the solution may also contain water (e.g., digitalis tincture and iodine tincture).

Emulsions

A pharmaceutical preparation in which two agents that cannot ordinarily be combined or mixed is called an *emulsion*. In the typical emulsion, oil is dispersed inside water. Most creams and lotions are emulsions (e.g., Kondremul Plain).

Spirits or Essences

An alcohol-containing liquid that may be used pharmaceutically as a solvent is called a *spirit* or *essence* (e.g., essence of peppermint and camphor spirit).

Liniments

Liniments are liquid suspensions for external application to the skin to relieve pain and swelling. One example is Watkins Liniment Pain Relief Spray.

Gels or Jellies

A *gel* is a jellylike, semisolid substance in a nonfatty base that may be used for topical application and contains fine particles. Examples include Dermarest psoriasis medicated treatment gel and Mentholatum Acnes medicated sealing jell acne treatment jelly.

Lotions

Lotions are suspensions of drugs in a water base for external use. They are patted onto the skin rather than rubbed in. Lotions tend to settle in their containers and thus must be shaken before use. An example is calamine lotion, an antipruritic (anti-itch medication) used to treat exposure to poison ivy.

Aerosols

Aerosol medications are frequently delivered by oral inhalers or nebulizers that allow for rapid absorption into the blood circulation. An example is albuterol (Proventil), a bronchodilator used in asthma. Aerosols are generally classified as liquid drugs because they often contain a mist. Those that contain dry powders are considered to be semisolid drugs.

Magmas

Magmas contain particles suspended in a liquid and exhibit a more pasty quality in their consistency than other suspensions. The most popular example of a magma is probably Phillips Milk of Magnesia.

INJECTABLE DRUGS

When a rapid response time to medication is desired or if the patient is not able to take the medication orally, parenteral forms of medication can be selected. Injectable drug forms may be available as powders or solutions. A powder consists of dry particles of medications. Because the powder itself cannot be injected, it must be reconstituted to a liquid for injection. A diluent, such as sterile water, is added to the powder and then mixed well. A solution, as previously explained, is a mixture of one or more substances that are dissolved in another substance. Most solutions are fluids that form a homogeneous mixture. There are a variety of administration routes for parenteral medications, including intra-articular, epidural (into the subarachnoid space), intradermal, subcutaneous, IM, and IV.

OTHER FORMS OF MEDICATIONS

There are also other forms of drugs, including topical; semisolid; transdermal patches; gaseous (inhalation); ophthalmic, otic, and nasal; vaginal; and rectal.

Topical Drugs

Drugs that are applied to the skin are known as *topical* drugs. They usually provide a local effect. Topical medications include transdermal patches, lotions, ointments, and liniments. Some topical drugs are used to deaden nerves, control itching, or relieve pain and congestion in muscles and joints.

Semisolid Drugs

Semisolid drugs are often used for topical application. These drugs are soft and pliable. Semisolid drugs include creams, ointments, most plasters, and dry-powder aerosols.

CREAMS

A *cream* is a semisolid preparation that is usually white and contains a drug incorporated into both an aqueous base and an oily base. Creams may be applied externally or intravaginally. Examples include benzoyl peroxide (Clearasil, to treat acne topically) and terconazole (Terazol, to treat vulvovaginal candidiasis).

OINTMENTS

An *ointment* is a semisolid preparation in an aqueous or oily base for local protective, soothing, astringent, or transdermal application for systemic effects. Ointments can also be used as anti-inflammatory drugs, topical anesthetics, and antibiotics. Examples are zinc oxide ointment and Bengay ointment.

PLASTERS

A *plaster* is a composition of liquid and powder that hardens when dry. Plasters may be solid but are generally semisolid drugs (e.g., salicylic acid plaster used to remove corns).

Transdermal Patches

For a constant, time-released systemic effect, some medications can be absorbed slowly through the skin. Transdermal patches release a very small amount of a drug at a consistent rate, which is absorbed into the skin and then carried off by the capillary blood supply. Examples of drugs used transdermally include nicotine, estrogen, and nitroglycerin.

Gaseous Drugs (Inhalation Drugs)

Pharmaceutical gases include such anesthetic agents as nitrous oxide and halothane. Compressed gases comprise oxygen or carbon dioxide. Most of the oxygen administered in hospitals for therapy is provided from a central source, where it is stored as a gas or liquid oxygen. Inhalation medications, such as bronchodilators, can be administered through metered-dose inhalers (MDIs) or handheld nebulizers (HHNs). Inhalation medications are discussed in Chapter 35.

Ophthalmic, Otic, and Nasal Drugs

Ophthalmic drugs include drops and ointments that are instilled in the eye for a local effect. They must be sterile and isotonic so they do not cause infections or burning. Ophthalmic medications may be antibiotics, anesthetics, antiviral agents, decongestants, or formulations that provide artificial tears. For the ears, otic medications can control localized infections or inflammation and require very low dosages to be effective. Nasal solutions can treat minor congestion or infection and act locally. They may be in the form of drops or sprays (Figure 6-5A–C ■).

Vaginal Drugs

Vaginal drugs come in a variety of forms, including solutions, creams, tablets, and suppositories. Commonly used vaginal drugs include anti-infectives and contraceptives.

Rectal Drugs

Rectal medications are used for patients with nausea, vomiting, or constipation or for those who may be unconscious and therefore unable to take drugs by mouth. Rectal medications are usually available as cocoa butter or gelatin-based suppositories or as enemas. Most rectal drugs offer systemic effects.

Figure 6-5 ■ Examples of (**A**) otic, (**B**) ophthalmic, and (**C**) nasal drops.

Focus Point

Safe Storage of Drugs

In general, medicines should not be exposed to sunlight, bright light, moisture, or extremes in temperature. Insulin and vaccine preparations should be stored in a refrigerator according to the manufacturer's directions.

✳ Apply Your **Knowledge** 6.3

The following questions focus on what you have just learned about sources of drug derivation and drug forms.

CRITICAL THINKING

1. List at least 10 examples of solid drugs.
2. Compare caplets, gelcaps, and capsules.
3. Differentiate between syrups and linctuses.
4. Compare emulsions with liniments.
5. Differentiate between creams and lotions.
6. Identify the meaning of *sustained-release*.
7. Explain the differences between tablets and pills.
8. Identify the meaning of *enteric-coated tablets* and *capsules*.
9. Give another name for troches, and identify an example.
10. Explain fluidextracts, tinctures, and magmas.
11. Discuss the difference between emulsions and lotions.
12. Give three examples of transdermal patches.

Dispensing Drugs

There are two methods of dispensing drugs: (1) over the counter (OTC) and (2) by prescription. OTC drugs are available to the public for self-medication without a prescription.

An allied health care professional who is directly involved in patient care should have an understanding of some basic facts regarding OTC drugs. Today, patients are better informed about their personal health care and want to be active participants in health care decisions. They need facts to make informed choices when using OTC preparations. Most OTC preparations are safe if used as directed on their packages.

Prescription drugs are issued by a licensed prescriber (medical practitioner, dentist, or veterinary surgeon). In some states, nurse practitioners and even pharmacists can write prescriptions with certain restrictions. According to legal terminology, prescription drugs are those that federal law lists as dangerous, powerful, or habit forming and illegal to use except

under a prescriber's order. A *prescription* is an order written by an authorized health care professional for the compounding or dispensing and administration of drugs to a particular patient. A prescription must be signed by a physician or the order cannot be carried out. These drugs have the legend "Caution: Federal law prohibits dispensing without a prescription" printed on the label. Sometimes, a prescription can be sent by a fax machine, electronically from a physician's computer, or by telephone to a pharmacist. Controlled substances and Schedule I–V drugs are discussed in Chapter 5.

COMPONENTS OF PRESCRIPTIONS

A prescription must be clear, concise, and correct. It has elements that can be correlated with five of the seven nursing rights of medication administration (see Chapter 7 for all seven rights): the patient's name and address (right patient); date written; generic or proprietary drug name (right drug); drug strength and dosage (right dose); route of administration (right route); dosage instruction or frequency of administration (right time); and signature, name, and address of the prescriber (Figure 6-6 ■). Therefore, the component parts of a prescription include:

✳ Name and address of the patient

✳ Address of the prescriber's office

✳ Date

✳ Names and quantities of the prescribed medication (*inscription*)

✳ Rx symbol (*superscription*) (℞)

✳ Dispensing directions to pharmacist (*subscription*)

✳ Directions for the patient (*signa*)

✳ Refill and special labeling

✳ The prescriber's signature and license or Drug Enforcement Administration (DEA) number

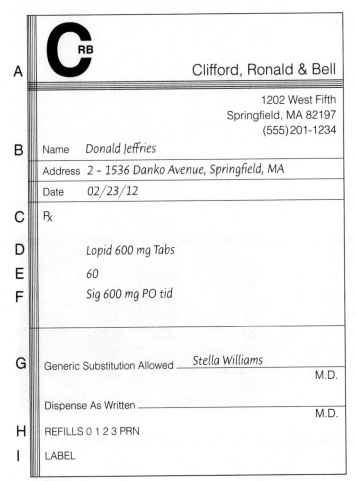

Figure 6-6 ■ Example of a physician's prescription. (**A**) The prescriber's office name, address, and phone number. (**B**) The patient's name, address, and date of prescription. (**C**) The superscription (℞). (**D**) The inscription (names and quantities of ingredients). (**E**) The subscription (tells the pharmacist how many units of medication are needed). (**F**) The signa (Sig), which tells the patient how to take the medication. (**G**) Signature blank(s), where the prescriber signs. (**H**) The repetatur (which tells how many refills are allowed). (**I**) A sample prescription.

TELEPHONE ORDERS AND STANDING ORDERS

Medications are also sometimes prescribed by physicians who are not present or will not be present when the medication is administered. For example, a physician may telephone a drug prescription (called *telephone orders*) to a pharmacist, who is legally entitled to dispense the prescription, or to a nurse, who is entitled to administer it on oral instructions. In some states, medical assistants are also allowed to do this. The physician must then, as soon as is practicable, write the drug order on a prescription pad, sign it, and post or deliver it to the pharmacy or use the hospital drug chart (see the next section). A faxed prescription copy can confirm an oral order but is not legally acceptable because the signature has to be original (i.e., in the physician's handwriting); the pharmacist must see the original prescription before releasing the drug to the patient. *Standing orders* are written orders sometimes left by physicians as ongoing prescriptions in a hospital, nursing home, or residential-care setting. These orders have no legal validity unless they are properly written, dated, and signed—just as is true for any normal prescription.

HOSPITAL DRUG CHARTS

Prescriptions in hospitals are usually written on a drug chart or physician order sheet and transcribed onto a medication administration record (MAR; Figure 6-7 ■). These can become quite complicated and may run to many pages

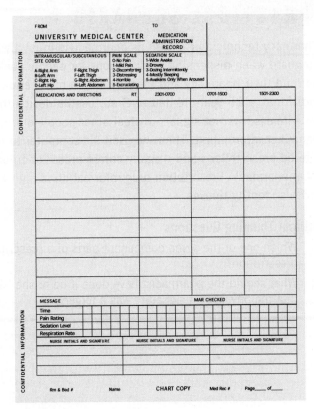

Figure 6-7 ■ Medical administration record as used in many hospitals.

in a patient's medical record because patients in hospitals are frequently prescribed 10–15 drugs during one stay. In the sample chart, note that the users are instructed:

✳ To use approved names for drugs

✳ Not to alter existing orders

✳ To record all instances when drugs are administered or when drugs were not administered, giving reasons

✳ To record IV fluid orders on a separate IV orders chart

✳ To have nurse-initiated therapy (e.g., mild analgesics, laxatives, antacids) countersigned by a physician

Today, the majority of hospitals in the United States (and those in some other countries) use computer charting.

✳ Apply Your **Knowledge 6.4**

The following questions focus on what you have just learned about dispensing drugs.

CRITICAL THINKING

1. What are the components of prescriptions?

2. Define the terms *inscription*, *superscription*, and *subscription*.

3. What are standing orders?

4. What are the meanings of the Rx symbol (Rx) and the term *signa*?

5. What does the abbreviation MAR stand for, and how is this type of paperwork used?

PRACTICAL SCENARIO 1

Pharmacy technicians as well as pharmacists must always be on guard when dispensing prescriptions for people seeking to defraud their pharmacy and illegally obtain medications. One such individual, a 25-year-old named Brad, used a device that scanned for wireless Internet signals to steal other people's prescription painkiller information. Then, he used his computer to print out altered prescriptions and illegally obtain prescription drugs at his local pharmacy. Prescription drug information is highly prized by today's identity thieves.

Darryl Bush/Pearson Education/PH College

Critical Thinking Questions

1. Which one of the seven component parts of a prescription could Brad not provide in his computer-generated prescription?

2. What should the pharmacist have done if he or she had any suspicions about the prescription itself or suspected that the physician's signature was a forgery?

PRACTICAL SCENARIO 2

A medical assistant gives some samples of a medication in capsule form to the mother of a 5-year-old patient. Originally, the physician had ordered the powdered form of this medication, which could be dissolved in water or juice. Because the powdered form is unavailable, the medical assistant gives the capsules to the mother and instructs her to simply open and empty them into water or juice for her child.

SergiyN/Fotolia

Critical Thinking Questions

1. Do you think that capsules can be opened so their contents can be used in this manner?

2. What was wrong with this medical assistant's actions?

Chapter Capsule

This section repeats the objectives from the beginning of the chapter and then provides a summary of the most important concepts for that objective. Use this section as a quick review and to check your knowledge.

Objective 1: Define the suffixes *-ism*, *-itis*, *-pathy*, and *-tomy*.

- ■ -ism = condition
- ■ -itis = inflammation
- ■ -pathy = disease
- ■ -tomy = incision, cutting

Objective 2: Explain abbreviations used in pharmacology.

- ■ Abbreviations are shortened forms of words representing commonly used medical terms; terms used for writing prescriptions; and terms associated with various measurements

Objective 3: Define *chemical*, *generic*, and *trade names* of drugs.

- ■ Each drug may have three different types of names:
  - ❑ The *chemical name* (describing the chemical makeup of a drug); this is the most complex type of name
  - ❑ The *generic name* (also called *approved name*, *official name*, or *nonproprietary name*); this is much simpler than the chemical name
  - ❑ The *trade name* (also called the *brand name* or *proprietary name*); this is issued by the drug's manufacturer and is trademarked

Objective 4: Describe five sources of drug derivation.

- ■ Plants
- ■ Animals (including humans)
- ■ Minerals or mineral products

- Synthetics
- Engineered (investigational) sources

Objective 5: Explain black box warnings.

- A *black box warning* is the most severe warning from the FDA about a drug. It appears on the prescription label to alert all health care providers and patients about potentially harmful adverse effects of the drug. The FDA requires a black box warning for medications that may cause serious undesirable effects compared with potential benefits, and when a serious adverse reaction can be prevented, reduced in frequency, or reduced in severity by proper use of the drug.

Objective 6: List various solid drug forms.

- Pills are powdered drugs mixed with liquids and rolled into a round or oval shape
- Tablets are powdered drugs compressed with bulk-filling materials under high pressure
- Capsules are drugs contained in an external shell
- Sustained-release tablets and capsules contain several doses of a drug with special coatings that dissolve at different rates, thereby releasing the drug gradually
- Enteric-coated tablets and capsules are covered by a special coating that keeps the drugs from dissolving in the stomach; these drugs do not dissolve until they reach the intestines
- Caplets are drugs shaped like capsules but in the form of tablets, with film coatings
- Gelcaps are oil-based medications enclosed in soft gelatin capsules
- Powders are drugs that are dried and ground into fine particles
- Granules are small pills accompanied by many others, encased within gelatin capsules
- Troches or lozenges are flattened disks placed on the tongue or between the cheek and gum and left in place until they dissolve

Objective 7: Describe topical drugs.

- Semisolid are soft and pliable and often used for topical applications
- Creams are semisolid preparations that are usually white and contain a drug incorporated into both an aqueous base and an oily base
- Ointments are semisolid preparations in an aqueous base or an oily base for local protective, soothing, astringent, or transdermal application for systemic effects
- Plasters are compositions of liquid and powder that harden when dry; may be solid or semisolid
- Transdermal patches are used for a constant, time-released systemic effect, as their medications are absorbed slowly through the skin

Objective 8: Explain gaseous drugs.

- Pharmaceutical gases include such anesthetic gases as nitrous oxide and halothane
- Compressed gases include therapeutic oxygen or carbon dioxide
- Inhalation medications, such as bronchodilators, can be administered through metered-dose inhalers (MDIs) or handheld nebulizers (HHNs)

Objective 9: List seven component parts of a prescription.

- The component parts of a prescription may include the following:
    - ❑ Name and address of the patient
    - ❑ Address of the prescriber's office
    - ❑ Date written
    - ❑ Names and quantities of the prescribed medication (*inscription*)
    - ❑ Rx symbol (superscription) (℞)
    - ❑ Dispensing directions to pharmacist (subscription)
    - ❑ Directions for the patient (signa)
    - ❑ Refill and special labeling
    - ❑ The prescriber's signature and license or Drug Enforcement Administration (DEA) number

Objective 10: Define *standing orders*.

- Orders given by physicians who may not be present at a later time when the medication is needed or ongoing prescriptions for patients in a hospital, nursing home, or residential-care setting; valid only when written, signed, and dated by the physician or other health care provider with prescribing authority

Internet Sites of Interest

- Information on the parts of a prescription: **www.mapharm.com/prescr_parts.htm**
- A list of medical abbreviations, symbols, and dosage designations that are frequently misinterpreted and involved in harmful errors, along with their approved substitutions: **www.ismp.org/Tools/errorproneabbreviations.pdf**
- Search for any medical abbreviation or term: **www.medilexicon.com**
- A list of drugs from "A" to "Z": **www.rxlist.com/drugs/alpha_a.htm**
- Information about black box warnings: **www.drugwatch.com/2012/01/18/ fda-black-box-warnings/**

Chapter 7

Administration of Medications

Chapter Objectives

After completing this chapter, you should be able to:

1. Summarize patient assessment factors that have an impact on medication administration.
2. Identify the seven rights of drug administration.
3. Define *percutaneous administration*.
4. Describe when a nasogastric tube should be used.
5. Explain the reasons why sublingual or buccal administration may be chosen for certain medications.
6. List and describe the various routes of medication administration.
7. Identify equipment and supplies required for parenteral administration of medications.
8. Define terms related to needles used in the parenteral administration of medications.
9. Identify sites used for intradermal, subcutaneous, and intramuscular injections.
10. Explain how to administer an intradermal, subcutaneous, and intramuscular injection.

Key Terms

aseptic (p. 86)
bevel (p. 87)
cannula (p. 87)
gastrostomy tube (p. 85)

gauge (p. 87)
hub (p. 87)
hypodermic (p. 87)
invasive (p. 86)

nasogastric (NG) tube (p. 85)
stat (p. 84)
wheal (p. 88)

Introduction

It is important to remember that medications have the potential to cause serious harm to a patient. Therefore, the process of dispensing and administering medication orders must always be treated with great care. When you are involved in medication administration, you must be constantly vigilant to prevent errors and deliver quality patient care.

No matter what types of medications are to be administered, the order must come from the physician. If a physician delegates drug administration to a medical assistant, it must be allowable under state laws. Every state has a *medical practice act* that defines whether a medical assistant or other caregiver (besides a nurse) can administer drugs under the supervision of a physician. Some states permit medical assistants to administer only certain types of medications; some prohibit medical assistants from giving injections. To ensure patient safety in drug administration, health care professionals must perform certain procedures every time a medication is ordered. These procedures are discussed in this chapter.

Principles of Drug Administration

The health care professionals who may be administering medications should always assess a patient's health status and obtain a medication history before giving any medication. The extent of the assessment depends on the patient's illness or current condition, the intended drug, and the route of administration. For example, if a patient has dyspnea, the nurse or medical assistant must assess respirations carefully before administering any medication that might affect breathing. It is important to determine whether the route of administration is suitable. For example, a patient who is nauseated may not be able to tolerate a drug taken orally. In general, the health care professional assesses the patient before administering any medication to obtain baseline data for evaluating the effectiveness of the medication.

The medication history includes information about the drugs the patient is taking currently or has taken recently. This includes prescription drugs; such over-the-counter (OTC) drugs as antacids, alcohol, and tobacco; and illegal drugs, such as marijuana. Sometimes, an incompatibility with one or more of these drugs affects the choice of a new medication.

Many patients, especially older adults, often take vitamins, herbs, and food supplements or use folk remedies that they do not list in their medication history. Because many of these have unknown or unpredictable actions and side effects, the health care professional should always ask about their use and note it in the patient history, with close attention paid to possible incompatibilities with other prescribed medications.

Any problems the patient may have in self-administering a medication must also be identified. For example, a patient with poor eyesight may require special labels for the medication container; elderly patients with unsteady hands may not be able to hold syringes or inject themselves or another person. Obtaining information about how and where the patient stores medications is also important. If the patient has difficulty opening certain containers, he or she may change containers but leave the old labels on, which increases the risk of medication errors.

Socioeconomic factors need to be considered for all patients but especially for older adults. Two common problems are lack of transportation to obtain medications and inadequate finances to purchase medications. If the health care professional is aware of these problems, proper resources can be obtained for the patient.

THE SEVEN RIGHTS OF DRUG ADMINISTRATION

Safeguarding the patient during drug administration involves using the seven rights of proper drug administration. (The first five rights were introduced in Chapter 6.) Two more have been added since the original five were created:

1. **The *right* patient.** The easiest way to make sure the drug is being given to the right patient is to ask the patient his or her name or call the patient by name before administering the medication. You cannot assume that the person to whom you are administering a medication is the correct person without verifying his or her name in this manner. Patients can be confused or anxious and may not hear what you say. Therefore, check the patient's chart.

   Always check for allergies before administering medications. Ask the patient directly because recent allergic reactions might not be listed in the record. You should explain the medication's name, dosage, desired action, potential effects, and any precautions that need to be taken.

2. **The *right* drug.** Determining the right drug begins with clarifying the physician's order if needed. Each time a drug is dispensed, the medication label must be checked three times during its preparation to confirm the right drug, right dose, and right strength. Compare the physician's written order with the label. The first check is done when the medication is taken from the storage area. The second is performed just before removing the medication from its container. The third check is performed when the medication is returned to the storage area or just before administration.

   Also check the expiration date to ensure that the medication is still effective. If it has expired, dispose of it appropriately. It is appropriate to flush certain outdated medication into the sewer line.

For controlled substances, you must ask someone to witness and document the disposal, referred to as "wasting the medication."

3. **The *right* dose.** If the dose ordered does not match the dose available, perform appropriate dosage calculations to determine the accurate dose (see Chapter 8). Remember to have a colleague check your calculations if you doubt the dose accuracy. Many facilities require health care workers who set up insulin or heparin doses to check them with a coworker. After you have calculated the amount to be administered, measure it out carefully. Medication errors are significantly reduced by using unit-dose systems because the medications are already in the correct dose.

4. **The *right* route.** Check the physician's order to clarify the route of administration for the medication—whether it is oral, topical, or parenteral. Many drugs can be given by a variety of routes. Because the route of administration can affect the medication's absorption, it is important that the drug is given by the correct route. If you are not sure what route is intended, confirm it with the physician.

5. **The *right* time.** In the ambulatory care setting, most medications are ordered **stat** (see Chapter 6). However, it is important to check the physician's order to clarify the appropriate time for medications to be administered. Some medications must be taken on an empty stomach (30 minutes before or 2 hours after a meal), but others should be taken with food.

6. **The *right* technique.** A health care professional must be familiar with the proper techniques for all routes of administration. If there are any doubts about the ability to administer a particular drug, always ask for help.

7. **The *right* documentation.** Immediately after giving the drug to the patient, document the date and time of administration; the drug's name, strength, dose, and route of administration; any patient reactions to the medication; and details of patient education regarding the drug. If the patient requests a prescription refill, document all pertinent information on the patient chart. The medical record is the legal document recording the order for the medication and its administration. If the medication ordered was not given or the patient refused it, the reason must be included in the record. If the patient refuses to take medication you have prepared, do not return it to its original container. Dispose of it and notify the physician.

SAFETY IN DRUG ADMINISTRATION

Every time a medication is ordered, certain procedures must be performed to ensure patient safety. The physician's order must be completely understood and clearly read; any questions about the medication and its dose,

Focus Point

Administering Medications

Nurses or medical assistants must be extremely knowledgeable when administering medications in the physician's office. Follow all physician orders exactly as written. If you are unsure about an order, ask for clarification before proceeding. Administer a medication only after the order is written in the patient's chart. This helps eliminate errors and possible omissions in medication therapy. Always implement the seven rights and perform three drug order and label checks when dispensing and administering medications.

✳ Apply Your Knowledge 7.1

The following questions focus on what you have just learned about the seven rights of drug administration.

CRITICAL THINKING

1. Describe the principles of drug administration.

2. Identify the seven rights of drug administration.

3. Discuss the problems commonly seen in elderly patients when self-administering a medication.

4. Explain why medication history is important.

5. Identify the most important factors to keep in mind concerning drug administration.

route of administration, and strength must be answered by the physician. When questions arise, the drug should be looked up in a pharmacology reference book (such as a drug handbook) to review its possible side effects, precautions, purpose, and recommended dose. Only after all these steps are taken should the drug be dispensed and administered.

Routes of Drug Administration

Medications may be delivered to the body by different methods. The method of administration depends on the purpose of the medication. Medication may be administered in a variety of ways, but some must be given in specific and limited ways to be effective. Each route has its advantages and disadvantages. Drugs are administered either *enterally* (for absorption through the gastrointestinal [GI] tract) or *parenterally* (by injection) to produce systemic effects. If medications are placed in direct contact with the skin or mucous membranes to be absorbed for a local effect, this is called *percutaneous administration*. When choosing the route and technique of medication administration, the most reliable method of delivery ensures expected results.

ENTERAL ROUTES

The enteral route is the route of drug administration through the GI tract. This method of administration of drugs is safe and convenient for most patients and is relatively economical. Administration of medication through the GI tract may be by the oral, nasogastric or gastrostomy tube, sublingual, or buccal routes.

Oral Route

The oral route is the most common route. It is the easiest and most economical way for a patient to take medication. As long as a patient can swallow and retain the drug in the stomach, this is the route of choice. Medications given by the oral route are absorbed from the stomach and small intestine, traveling first to the liver, where they may be metabolized before they ever reach their target tissues or organs. This process, called first-pass metabolism, is discussed in Chapter 3.

Oral medications are contraindicated when a patient is vomiting, has gastric or intestinal suction, or is unconscious and unable to swallow. Generally, oral medications should be taken with enough water to ensure the drug reaches the stomach. Liquid medications are ideal for children. Solid drugs should not be given to children until they are old enough to safely swallow them without the danger of aspiration.

Nasogastric and Gastrostomy Routes

For patients who cannot take anything by mouth and have a nasogastric or gastrostomy tube in place, an alternative route for administering medications is through the tube. A **nasogastric (NG) tube** is inserted by way of the nasopharynx (the part of the pharynx that lies above the soft palate and opens into the nasal cavity) and is placed into the patient's stomach for the purpose of feeding the patient or removing gastric secretions. A **gastrostomy tube** is surgically placed directly into the patient's stomach and provides another route for administering medications and nutrition.

Sublingual Route

Medications given via the sublingual route are held under the tongue until completely dissolved (Figure 7-1 ■). This method is used when rapid action is desired because the mucosa of the oral cavity contains a very rich blood supply, offering fast absorption of certain drugs. Absorption via this route bypasses the GI tract, and the medication goes directly from the oral mucosa to the systemic circulation. Medications administered via the sublingual route are not destroyed by digestive enzymes, and they do not undergo first-pass metabolism in the liver. Examples of medications that can be administered by the sublingual route include nitroglycerin (Nitrostat) for angina pectoris and ergotamine tartrate (Ergomar) for migraines.

Tablet

Figure 7-1 ■ Medication given via the sublingual route.

Focus on Geriatrics

Medications May Stain Teeth and Dentures

Advise elderly patients who have dentures to remove them before taking certain medications. Some oral liquid drugs, such as liquid iron or iodides, may stain the teeth.

Buccal Route

For the administration of drugs via the buccal route (a type of percutaneous route), the medication is placed between the gum and cheek and left there until it dissolves (Figure 7-2 ■). Buccal medications are available in the form of tablets, capsules, lozenges, and troches. These medications should not be swallowed. They are absorbed more slowly from the buccal mucosa than the sublingual area. The buccal route is preferred over the sublingual route for sustained-release delivery because of its greater mucosal surface area.

Tablet

Figure 7-2 ■ Administration of drugs via the buccal route.

Focus Point

Buccal and Sublingual Medications

Patients should not drink or eat anything when buccal or sublingual medications are administered until the medication has dissolved completely.

✴ Apply Your Knowledge 7.2

The following questions focus on what you have just learned about enteral routes of drug administration.

CRITICAL THINKING

1. Explain the safest method of medication administration.
2. Compare the nasogastric and gastrostomy routes.
3. What is the buccal route and when should it be used?
4. Name three drugs administered via the sublingual route.
5. What is the enteral route?

PARENTERAL ROUTES

Parenteral administration, as noted in Chapter 6, refers to the injection of a drug into the body with a needle and syringe. Parenteral administration of medications is a common procedure in medical offices, hospitals, ambulatory centers, home-care centers, and other facilities by certain medical workers. Parenteral medications may be given via intradermal (ID), subcutaneous (SC), intramuscular (IM), or intravenous (IV) routes. The IV route may be more dangerous than the others because of the possibility of injecting a drug incorrectly into a vein, which may cause serious harm or even death. Because these medications are absorbed more quickly than oral medications and are irretrievable after being injected, the allied health worker must prepare and administer them carefully and accurately. The parenteral route is especially used in emergencies when a drug effect is needed immediately. Administering parenteral drugs requires

an **invasive** procedure (one that requires insertion of an instrument or device through the skin or a body orifice), and an **aseptic** technique must be used (handwashing and other techniques to minimize the risk of infection).

Equipment

Syringes, needles, ampules, and vials are used to administer parenteral medications. Ampules and vials contain medications; syringes and needles are used to withdraw the medication and then administer it to the patients.

SYRINGES

Three parts make up a standard syringe: the barrel (the outside part), which has printed scales used to measure medication amounts; the plunger, which fits inside the barrel; and the tip, which connects with the needle (Figure 7-3 ■). The outside of the barrel and the handle of the plunger may be touched, but no unsterile object

Figure 7-3 ■ The plunger and barrel of a standard syringe, attached to a needle, with its shaft portion identified.

should ever come into contact with the tip or the inside of the barrel, the plunger's shaft, or the needle's shaft or tip. Syringes are available in many sizes, and are calibrated according to how they will be used. For example, the common 3-mL syringe is divided into tenths of a milliliter. It is used to measure most drugs.

Insulin syringes are commonly calibrated in 50- or 100-unit sizes. Unlike other syringes, insulin syringes have permanently attached needles and no *dead space* (fluid that remains in the needle or syringe after the plunger is depressed fully). These differences help the patient self-administer the correct amount of insulin.

Tuberculin syringes hold 1-mL, and are calibrated in hundredths of milliliters. Figure 7-4 ■ shows examples of tuberculin, insulin, and 3-mL **hypodermic** syringes.

Figure 7-4 ■ Examples of tuberculin, insulin, and 3-mL hypodermic syringes.

Hypodermic syringes are available in 2-, 2.5-, 3-, and 5-mL sizes. They are commonly used to administer IM injections.

Injectable medications are often available in disposable prefilled unit-dose systems:

✳ Prefilled syringes, ready to use

✳ Prefilled sterile cartridges and needles that must be attached to a reusable holder (injection system) before use

Examples of prefilled unit-dose systems are shown in Figure 7-5 ■.

NEEDLES

Most needles are disposable and are made of stainless steel. Special-procedure needles may be reusable and need to be repeatedly sharpened because their points can become dull with use. Dull or damaged needles should never be used.

There are three parts that make up a needle:

✳ **Bevel**—the slanted part at the needle's tip

✳ **Cannula** or shaft—the actual metal length that makes up the majority of the needle; it is attached to the hub

✳ **Hub**—the part of the needle that fits onto the syringe

There are three variable characteristics in needles used for injections:

✳ **Gauge** (or diameter of the shaft)—the gauge varies from #18 to #28. The larger the gauge, the smaller the shaft's diameter. Larger gauges are required for thicker medications, such as penicillin.

✳ Length of the shaft—common lengths range from 1/2 to 2 inches. The correct shaft length is determined by the type of injection, the patient's weight, and the patient's muscle development.

✳ Slant or length of the bevel—longer bevels cause less discomfort and provide the sharpest needles (these are commonly used for IM and SC injections). Short bevels are used for IV or ID injections.

Figure 7-5 ■ Prefilled unit-dose systems.

AMPULES AND VIALS

Sterile parenteral medications are often packaged in either ampules or vials. An ampule is made of clear glass and usually contains a single dose of a drug. It ranges in size from 1 mL to 10 mL or larger. Ampules have a distinctive neck that is tight or constricted; most ampule necks are prescored to be easily opened and are marked with a colored ink at the point at which they are to be opened.

Ampules are broken open at the constricted neck by using a plastic cap over the top of the ampule (to prevent injury from broken glass) and a cutter within the cap that further scores the neck of the ampule when it is rotated. After being broken open, the medication is aspirated into a syringe by using a filter needle, which prevents aspiration of any glass particles. Figure 7-6 ▪ shows an example of drawing medication from a vial.

Figure 7-6 ▪ Drawing medication from a vial with a syringe.

A *vial* consists of a small glass bottle that is sealed with a rubber cap and may range from single to multi-dose sizes. Vials must be pierced with a needle to access the medication. Air is injected into the vial before the medication can be withdrawn from it. The air prevents a vacuum from building up within the vial, allowing easier withdrawal of medication.

Drugs that are dispensed as powders in vials (for reconstitution with solvents, such as sterile water or sterile normal saline, or diluents) include penicillin.

Intradermal Injection

ID injections are usually given just below the epidermis into the dermis in the inner forearm or upper back—areas that have little hair growth (Figure 7-7A ▪). The ID route is commonly used for tuberculin or allergy skin tests or for the administration of local anesthetics. One method of tuberculin screening is the tine test, which is administered with individually packaged disposable sterile stamps with four prongs on the end that have been treated with tuberculin solution. However, the tine test is not as accurate as the Mantoux (purified protein derivative [PPD]) ID screening test. Absorption via this route is slow. A 15-degree angle is used when the needle is inserted between the skin's upper layers (Figure 7-8A ▪), and the injection of a substance should produce a small **wheal** (a slightly reddened, raised lesion) on the skin's outer surface. With the Mantoux test, a 0.1-mL solution of PPD is injected using a needle gauge of #26 to #27.

Figure 7-7 ▪ **(A)** Intradermal injection. **(B)** Subcutaneous injection. **(C)** Intramuscular injection.

Figure 7-8 ■ Angles and depths of injection for intradermal (**A**), subcutaneous (**B**), and intramuscular (**C**) injections.

Subcutaneous Injection

Subcutaneous injections are usually given into subcutaneous tissue below the dermis in the upper arms, upper back, or upper abdomen (Figure 7-7B ■). The subcutaneous route is commonly used for heparin and insulin injections. Absorption via this route is slower than via IM injections. A 45-degree angle is usually used, although this depends on the patient's body weight, which also influences the length of needle used (Figure 7-8B ■). Small volumes of medication (between 0.5 and 1 mL) are given subcutaneously.

Intramuscular Injection

IM injections are usually given into the deltoid (upper arm), vastus lateralis (thigh), and ventrogluteal or

Focus Point

Heparin Injections

For subcutaneous heparin injections, make sure that 0.1 to 0.2 mL of air is in the syringe to prevent heparin leakage into tissue, thus avoiding localized hemorrhaging.

dorsogluteal (hip) muscles (Figure 7-7C ■). The IM route is commonly used for drugs that are irritating to subcutaneous tissue. Absorption via this route is more rapid than other methods because of the rich blood supply found in the muscles. A 90-degree angle is used most commonly (Figure 7-8C ■), although the *Z-track method of IM injection* is also used. To avoid irritation to the skin and subcutaneous tissues, the Z-track injection method prevents any leakage back from the deep muscle into the upper subcutaneous layers by displacing the upper tissue laterally before the needle is inserted. Larger volumes of medication (1–3 mL) can be given at one site using IM injections.

Intravenous Injection

Intravenous injections are given directly into the veins—most commonly those of the arms. The IV route is used for many varieties of drugs and fluids, and distribution via this route is almost immediate. Drugs given via the IV route may be administered slowly, rapidly (IV push); by piggyback infusions (drugs are mixed with compatible fluids and administered over 30–90 minutes); into an existing IV line (the IV port); into an intermittent venous access device, such as a heparin lock; or by adding them to an IV solution. IV needles are inserted into veins at short angles (of about 25 degrees) to the skin.

Focus Point

Self-Administration of Insulin

Teach diabetic patients who must self-administer insulin at home to rotate insulin administration sites.

Focus on Pediatrics

Injections in Infants and Young Children

Infants and young children usually require smaller, shorter needles (#22 to #25 gauge, 5/8- to 1-inch long) for IM injection. The gluteal muscles are developed by walking. Therefore, do not use the dorsogluteal site in children younger than 3 years unless the child has been walking for at least 1 year. The vastus lateralis site is recommended as the site of choice for IM injections for infants 7 months or younger.

Focus on Geriatrics

Injections in Older Patients

Older patients may have decreased muscle mass, or muscle atrophy. A shorter needle may be needed. Assessment of appropriate injection site is critical. Absorption of medication may occur more quickly than expected.

Focus Point

Z-Track Technique of Injection Used for Certain Medications

Some specific medications, such as iron, are irritating or may stain the skin. Therefore, use the Z-track technique of injection for these medications.

✳ Apply Your Knowledge 7.3

The following questions focus on what you have just learned about parenteral routes of drug administration.

CRITICAL THINKING

1. Describe a Z-track injection.
2. Why is the vastus lateralis muscle the preferred injection site for infants?
3. Describe a cartridge syringe and its advantages.
4. Explain a tine test and the abbreviation *PPD*.
5. Compare ampules with vials.
6. Describe the parts of a needle.
7. Define the term *hypodermic*.
8. Describe the three parts of a syringe.

OTHER ROUTES OF DRUG ADMINISTRATION

Drugs may be applied to skin and mucous membranes either topically (on the skin's outer layers) or via the eyes (using instillations or irrigations), the ears (using drops of medicated solution), the nose (using drops and sprays), inhalation (drawing breath, vapor, or gas into the lungs), the vagina (using instillations), and the rectum (using suppositories).

Transdermal Applications

Topical skin preparations include creams, ointments, pastes, lotions, powders, sprays, and patches. Transdermal patches allow drugs to be absorbed slowly through the skin to create a constant, time-released systemic effect (Figure 7-9 ■). For example, the nitroglycerin patch is particularly useful for patients with frequent attacks of angina. Other drugs administered via transdermal patches include nicotine (to assist in smoking cessation) and estrogen. The rate of delivery of the drug is controlled and varies with each product (12 hours to 1 week).

Figure 7-9 ■ Examples of transdermal patches.

Focus Point

Use of Transdermal Patches

Instruct patients to shower with the transdermal patch in place. If the patch is to remain on for 24 hours, a new patch should be applied every day at the same time. Advise patients to rotate sites to prevent skin irritation and to avoid placing the patch on scars and areas with a large amount of body hair.

Ophthalmic Route

Medications are administered to the eye by using instillations or irrigations in the form of liquids or ointments. Eye drops and ointments are used to administer medication by sterile technique. For example, prescribed liquids are usually diluted to less than 1% strength. An eye irrigation is administered to wash out the conjunctival sac to remove secretions or foreign bodies or to remove chemicals that may injure the eye. Figures 7-10 ■ and 7-11 ■ show the instillation of eye ointments and eye drops into the lower conjunctival sac.

Figure 7-10 ■ Instillation of eye ointment.

Figure 7-11 ■ Instillation of eye drops.

Otic Route

Localized infection or inflammation of the ear or ears is treated by dropping a small amount of a sterile medicated solution into them. In children younger than 3 years of age, gently pull the earlobe down and back; in adults, gently pull the earlobe up and out (Figure 7-12 ■). The patient must remain lying on his or her opposite side for 5 minutes to allow the medication to run into and coat the surface of the inner ear canal.

Figure 7-12 ■ Instillation of ear medication.

Nasal Route

Nose drops and sprays are generally used to shrink swollen mucous membranes or to loosen secretions and facilitate drainage. Sometimes, nasal medications are prescribed to treat infections of the nasal cavity or sinuses. Nasal decongestants are the most common nasal instillations. Many of these medications are OTC drugs. The medication should be drawn up into a dropper and held over one nostril at a time. Then, the required number of nose drops are administered. Nasal drops are usually used with the patient in the supine position—with the head tilted back (Figure 7-13 ■).

Figure 7-13 ■ Administration of nasal medications.

Inhalation Route

Inhalation is the act of drawing breath, vapor, or gas into the lungs. Inhalation therapy may involve the administration of medicines; water vapor; and such gases as oxygen, carbon dioxide, and helium. The medication must be inhaled to achieve local effects within the respiratory tract through aerosols (Figure 7-14A–C ■), nebulizers, Spinhalers, or *metered-dose inhalers* (MDIs). Some inhaled medications are intended to alter the condition of

Focus Point

Otic and Ophthalmic Drops

Otic and ophthalmic drops can be easily confused. Emphasize to patients that otic medications cannot be put in the eyes because they can cause pain and irritation.

Focus Point

Self-Administration of Medication by Patients

Correct administration of medications by patients at home requires patient education by the health care professional. Make sure the patient understands the purpose of the drug; the time, frequency, and amount of the dose; any special storage requirements; and the typical side effects that may occur. Emphasize to the patient the possible serious adverse effects of the medication. Advise the patient to quickly report adverse effects to the physician.

A

B

C

Figure 7-14 ■ **(A)** A girl breathes mist through a nebulizer, with a bite piece in her mouth. **(B)** A breath-actuated inhaler. **(C)** An inhaler with a face mask.

of inhaled oxygen causes alveolar collapse, intra-alveolar hemorrhage, hyaline membrane formation, disturbance of the central nervous system, and retrolental fibroplasias in newborns.

By far, the predominant use of inhaled medications is for the treatment of asthma or other pulmonary disorders. In treating patients with asthma, a common method of administering medications is by nebulizer (see Figure 7-14A). A nebulizer is used to deliver a fine spray (fog or mist) of medication or moisture to a client. There are two kinds of nebulization: *atomization* and *aerosolization*. In atomization, a device called an *atomizer* produces rather large droplets for inhalation. In aerosolization, the droplets are suspended in a gas, such as oxygen. The smaller the droplets, the farther they can be inhaled into the respiratory tract.

The MDI is a handheld nebulizer (Figure 7-15 ■), which is a pressurized container of medication that the patient can use to release the medication through a nosepiece or mouthpiece.

the mucous membranes (albuterol and anti-inflammatory medications), to alter the character of the secretions in the respiratory system (acetylcysteine), or to treat infections of the respiratory tract (antibiotics such as tobramycin).

Oxygen is another medication that is administered by the inhalation route. Because oxygen is a drug, it needs to be prescribed according to the flow rate, concentration, method of delivery, and length of time for administration. Oxygen is prescribed as liters per minute (LPM) and as percentage of oxygen concentration (%). Oxygen toxicity may develop when 100% oxygen is breathed for a prolonged period. A high concentration

Figure 7-15 ■ Metered-dose inhaler.

Focus Point

Oxygen Precautions

Delivery of oxygen requires specific precautions. Be alert to the flammability of oxygen and make sure no open flames (including lighters, matches, or candles) are being used in the area near the oxygen.

Vaginal Route

Vaginal medications, or instillations, are inserted as creams, jellies, foams, or suppositories to treat infections or to relieve vaginal discomfort, such as pain or itching. Vaginal creams, jellies, and foams are applied by using a tubular applicator with a plunger. Suppositories are designed to melt at body temperature, so they are usually kept in a refrigerator (Figure 7-16A ■). Vaginal suppositories are gelatin or cocoa butter based and are instilled by using an applicator (Figure 7-16B ■).

Rectal Route

Rectal medications are commonly given in suppository form. The rectal route is useful if the patient is nauseated, vomiting, or unconscious. Manufacturers supply rectal medications in the form of gelatin- or cocoa butter–based suppositories, which melt in the warmth of the rectum and release the medication, or in the form of enemas as a solution. The rectal route of administration is shown in Figure 7-17 ■.

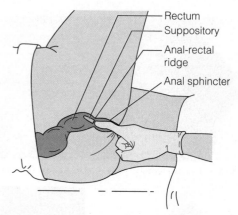

Figure 7-17 ■ Inserting a rectal suppository into the anus.

Figure 7-16 ■
(**A**) Instilling vaginal suppositories.
(**B**) Instilling vaginal cream by using an applicator.

✳ Apply Your Knowledge 7.4

The following questions focus on what you have just learned about other routes of drug administration.

CRITICAL THINKING

1. When may oxygen toxicity occur in patients because of the inhalation route?
2. Compare how the otic route of drug administration is used for infants and adults.
3. Compare the terms *transdermal* and *topical*.
4. What position is the best for administering drugs via the nasal route?
5. What are the most common nasal instillations?
6. What are the indications of the rectal route?

PRACTICAL SCENARIO 1

A 72-year-old woman had a vaginal infection. Her physician prescribed vaginal suppositories for the condition. His medical assistant was busy and did not completely explain how the patient should administer the medication, assuming that she knew. The patient purchased the prescription and administered the suppositories for the 10-day period. After 3 weeks, she returned to her physician and complained that the condition was the same with no relief. Her physician asked her exactly how she was using the suppositories. The patient replied that she had been inserting the suppositories rectally every 12 hours.

Kenneth Sponsler/Shutterstock

Critical Thinking Questions

1. What mistake did this patient make in administering the suppositories?
2. What should the medical assistant have made sure the patient knew about the proper administration of these suppositories?

PRACTICAL SCENARIO 2

A medical assistant was instructed to give an iron supplement via injection to a pregnant woman who had severe iron-deficiency anemia. She injected the medication subcutaneously. After 3 days, the patient returned with discoloration at the site of injection and complained to the physician.

Blaj Gabriel/Shutterstock

Critical Thinking Questions

1. For injectable iron supplementation, what injection technique must be used?
2. What is the result of subcutaneous injection of this medication?

Chapter Capsule

This section repeats the objectives from the beginning of the chapter and then provides a summary of the most important concepts for that objective. Use this section as a quick review and to check your knowledge.

Objective 1: Summarize patient assessment factors that have an impact on medication administration.

- Depends on patient's illness or current condition, intended drug, and route of administration
- Includes other factors, such as breathing problems, nausea, history of or current medication use, and vitamins or food and herbal supplements being taken

Objective 2: Identify the seven rights of drug administration.

- The *right* patient
- The *right* drug
- The *right* dose
- The *right* route
- The *right* time
- The *right* technique
- The *right* documentation

Objective 3: Define *percutaneous administration*.

- Percutaneous administration involves medications being placed in direct contact with the skin or mucous membranes to be absorbed for a local effect.

Objective 4: Describe when a nasogastric tube should be used.

- A nasogastric tube should be used to administer medications for patients who cannot take anything by mouth. The tube is inserted by way of the nasopharynx (the part of the pharynx that lies above the soft palate and opens into the nasal cavity) and is placed into the patient's stomach for the purpose of feeding the patient or removing gastric secretions.

Objective 5: Explain the reasons why sublingual or buccal administration may be chosen for certain medications.

- The sublingual route is used when rapid action is desired because the mucosa of the oral cavity contains a very rich blood supply, offering fast absorption of certain drugs. Absorption via this route bypasses the GI tract, and the medication goes directly from the oral mucosa to the systemic circulation.

- The buccal route is a type of percutaneous route, in which a medication is placed between the gum and cheek and left there until it dissolves. It is used for medications that should not be swallowed. They are absorbed more slowly from the buccal mucosa than the sublingual area. The buccal route is preferred over the sublingual route for sustained-release delivery because of its greater mucosal surface area.

Objective 6: List and describe the various routes of medication administration.

- Enteral—through the GI tract
  - ❏ Oral—via the mouth
  - ❏ Nasogastric or gastrostomy tube—through the nasopharynx or stomach
  - ❏ Sublingual (percutaneous)—under the tongue
  - ❏ Buccal (percutaneous)—between the gum and cheek

- Parenteral—injected
- Topical (percutaneous)—through the skin
- Skin application
- Ophthalmic route—eye
- Otic route—ear
- Nasal route—nose
- Inhalation—through the airways
- Vaginal—vagina
- Rectal—rectum

Objective 7: Identify equipment and supplies required for parenteral administration of medications.

- Syringes, needles, ampules, and vials

Objective 8: Define terms related to needles used in the parenteral administration of medications.

- Bevel—the slanted part at the needle's tip
- Cannula—the metal needle shaft
- Gauge—the needle shaft's diameter
- Hub—the part of the needle that fits onto the syringe

Objective 9: Identify sites used for intradermal, subcutaneous, and intramuscular injections.

- Intradermal—given within the skin layers of the inner forearm or upper back
- Subcutaneous—given into the upper arms, upper back, or upper abdomen
- Intramuscular—given into the upper arm or the thigh or hip

Objective 10: Explain how to administer an intradermal, subcutaneous, or intramuscular injection.

- Intradermal—a 15-degree angle is used; volumes less than 0.1 mL
- Subcutaneous—a 45-degree angle is used; only small volumes of medication
- Intramuscular—a 90-degree angle, or the Z-track method, is used; larger volumes of medication

Internet Sites of Interest

- The Institute for Safe Medication Practices provides a list of look-alike or sound-alike drugs that are commonly confused: **www.ismp.org/Tools/confuseddrugnames.pdf**
- Article about strategies to reduce medication errors offered by the U.S. Food and Drug Administration: **www.fda.gov/forconsumers/consumerupdates/default.htm**. Search for "medical errors."
- About Senior Health offers much health and medical information for older adults: **http://seniorhealth.about.com**. Search for "taking medications."

- Good teaching information provided for parents of pediatric patients: **www.fda
  .gov/forconsumers/consumerupdates/default.htm**. Search "how to give medicine
  to children."

- The Joint Commission provides an index of articles, such as *Using Medication
  Reconciliation to Prevent Errors, Medication Errors Related to Potentially
  Dangerous Abbreviations, Infusion Pumps: Preventing Future Adverse Events*,
  and others: **www.jointcommission.org/sentinel_event.aspx**

Checkpoint Review 1

Select the best answer for the following questions.

1. The half-life is the major determinant of which of the following?

   a. The adverse effects of a drug after a single dose

   b. The interaction with another single dose

   c. The duration of elimination of a drug after administration of multiple doses

   d. The duration of action of a drug after a single dose

2. *Hypersensitivity* is often used synonymously with which of the following terms?

   a. Immunogen

   b. Allergy

   c. Antigen

   d. Allergen

3. Which of the following agencies oversees controlled substances and prosecutes individuals who illegally distribute them?

   a. HIPAA

   b. FDA

   c. DEA

   d. CDC

4. Which of the following federal laws offers a 7-year monopoly on drug sales and tax breaks to induce drug companies to undertake development and manufacturing of drugs used for rare diseases that affect small numbers of people in the United States?

   a. Orphan Drug Act of 1983

   b. Prescription Drug Marketing Act of 1987

   c. Durham–Humphrey Amendment of 1951

   d. Comprehensive Drug Abuse Prevention and Control Act of 1970

5. Which of the following phases of drug approval evaluates toxicology data?

   a. Phase I

   b. Phase II

   c. Phase III

   d. Phase IV

6. The angle of insertion for intradermal injections is which of the following degrees?

   a. 30

   b. 90

   c. 15

   d. 45

7. Which of the following is the route of administration of a drug that is placed between the gums and the cheek?

   a. Buccal

   b. Topical

   c. Sublingual

   d. Transdermal

8. Which of the following is a drug that was withdrawn after postmarketing surveillance?

   a. Penbutolol

   b. Atenolol

   c. Furosemide

   d. Celecoxib

9. The proprietary drug name is also called the:

   a. Chemical name

   b. Generic name

   c. Trade name

   d. None of the above

10. The study of drugs derived from herbal and other natural sources is called:

    a. Pharmacodynamics

    b. Pharmacotherapy

    c. Pharmacognosy

    d. Pharmacology

11. Which of the following drugs carries a black box warning?

    a. Rifampin

    b. Rofecoxib

    c. Valdecoxib

    d. Celecoxib

12. Herbal products and dietary supplements are controlled by the

    a. Center for Disease Control and Prevention

    b. Center for Biologics Evaluation and Research

    c. Center for Food Safety and Applied Nutrition

    d. Center for Drug Evaluation and Research

13. Which of the following can determine the dose-effect relationship?

    a. Pharmacodynamics

    b. Pharmacokinetics

    c. Both A and B

    d. Pharmacology

14. Which of the following represents the number of patients that respond to the actions of a drug?

    a. Frequency distribution curve
    b. Median effective dose
    c. Median lethal dose
    d. Dose-effective relationship

15. Bioavailability of a drug means:

    a. The determination of whether two or more drug products release their contents in equal amounts over the same absorption
    b. The degree to which a drug releases itself from its dosage form to become accessible for its intended effect
    c. The process of drug movement into the systemic circulation
    d. The study of the chemical reactions that occur within a living organism

16. The abbreviation *qid*, as used in prescriptions, means:

    a. Every hour
    b. Every 4 hours
    c. Every other day
    d. Four times a day

17. The therapeutic index of a drug is used to predict whether a certain

    a. Drug has any side effects
    b. Dosage is toxic for pregnant women
    c. Dosage is safe for a specific patient
    d. Dosage is lethal for a specific patient

18. Which of the following schedule of drugs has the lowest abuse potential of all the controlled substances?

    a. Schedule IV
    b. Schedule III
    c. Schedule V
    d. Schedule II

19. Orphan drugs are used to treat which of the following diseases or conditions?

    a. Shark bite
    b. AIDS
    c. Asthma
    d. Cancer

20. Coal tar is used to treat which of the following disorders?

    a. Rheumatoid arthritis
    b. Scarlet fever
    c. Psoriasis
    d. AIDS

21. The affinity for a target receptor is its

    a. Transcription factor
    b. Enzyme activation
    c. Target molecule
    d. Attractive force

22. Which of the following is an enzyme embedded in cell membranes?

    a. Serotonin
    b. Gamma-aminobutyric acid
    c. Insulin
    d. Acetylcholine

23. How long does preclinical investigation usually take?

    a. Between one and six months
    b. Between three and nine months
    c. Between one and three years
    d. Between three and nine years

24. Competitive antagonists are also referred to as

    a. Partial agonists
    b. Agonist-antagonists
    c. Surmountable antagonists
    d. Insurmountable antagonists

25. Which of the following parts of a prescription is also known as the subscription?

    a. Medication prescribed
    b. Dispensing directions to the pharmacist
    c. Directions for patient
    d. Refill and special labeling

26. Which of the following carries blood directly to the liver?

    a. A biochemical pathway
    b. Renal portal circulation
    c. Hepatic portal circulation
    d. Lymphatic portal circulation

27. Short needles are used for which of the following routes of drug injections?

    a. Intravenous or intradermal
    b. Intramuscular and subcutaneous
    c. Intradermal and subcutaneous
    d. Intravenous and intramuscular

28. Faster drug excretion via the kidneys occurs by converting

    a. Lipid-soluble drugs into more water-soluble forms
    b. Water-soluble drugs into more lipid-soluble forms
    c. The color of urine
    d. Urea to amino acids

29. Total clearance of a drug is directly affected by the

    a. Dosage of the drug
    b. Drug plasma concentration
    c. Amount of blood flow to the organs of elimination
    d. Age, sex, and race of the patient

30. All drug administration laws are initiated, implemented, and enforced by which of the following laws?

    a. MSPPA
    b. OSHA
    c. FDA
    d. HIPAA

31. All the following are examples of the transdermal patch except:

    a. Estrogen
    b. Testosterone
    c. Nicotine
    d. Nitroglycerin

32. A comparatively large dose given at the beginning of treatment to quickly obtain therapeutic effects is called a

    a. Loading dose
    b. Maintenance dose
    c. Plateau
    d. Half-life

33. Programmed cell death that allows cells to self-destruct is called

    a. Necrosis
    b. Ascites
    c. Toxicosis
    d. Apoptosis

34. Which of the following medications may stain and irritate the skin and for which you should use the "Z-track technique" of injection?

    a. Penicillin
    b. Protein plasma
    c. Iodine
    d. Iron

35. Which of the following is an abbreviation meaning "immediately"?

    a. Sig
    b. SOS
    c. Syr
    d. Stat

36. Any components inside the body to which drugs bind are called

    a. Drug targets
    b. Pathogens
    c. Genomes
    d. Autosomes

37. The DEA is a branch of which department that became the nation's sole legal drug enforcement agency?

    a. U.S. Department of Health
    b. U.S. Department of Labor
    c. U.S. Department of Health and Human Services
    d. U.S. Department of Justice

38. The interferon lambda-3 enzyme is encoded by the IFNL3 gene, which is linked to which of the following infections?

    a. Pancreatitis
    b. Meningitis
    c. Hepatitis E
    d. Hepatitis C

39. Which of the following abbreviations means "by mouth"?

    a. pc
    b. po
    c. prn
    d. pm

40. Which of the following laws was passed to prevent the marketing of new drugs before they had been properly tested for purity, strength, effectiveness, safety, and packaging quality?

    a. Durham-Humphrey Amendment
    b. Food, Drug, and Cosmetic Act
    c. Safe Medical Devices Act
    d. Controlled Substances Act

41. The generic name of "Lipitor" is

    a. Valproic acid
    b. Atorvastatin
    c. Pravastatin
    d. Rifampin

42. Which of the following types of allergic drug reactions causes anaphylaxis?

    a. I
    b. II
    c. III
    d. IV

43. A list of officially recognized drug names is known as the:

    a. U.S. Drug Code
    b. National Formulary
    c. National pharmacopeia
    d. International pharmacopeia

44. Stevens-Johnson syndrome may cause severe damage to which organ?

    a. Liver
    b. Pancreas
    c. Brain
    d. Heart

45. A drug's adverse effects are based on its

    a. Margin of safety
    b. Manufacturing process
    c. Date of expiration
    d. Frequency of use

46. Which of the following drugs has been associated with Reye's syndrome in children?

    a. Ibuprofen
    b. Naproxen
    c. Aspirin
    d. Phenobarbital

47. The dose that produces a given toxicity in 50% of patient is known as the

    a. Dose effect
    b. Median lethal dose
    c. Median toxicity dose
    d. Median effective dose

48. If a drug has a half-life of one day, in how many days would plateau be reached?

    a. Two days
    b. Three days
    c. Four days
    d. Seven days

49. Most drugs bind to which of the following plasma proteins?

    a. Globulin
    b. Gamma globulin
    c. Insulin
    d. Albumin

50. In which of the following organs does biotransformation mostly occur?

    a. Kidneys
    b. Stomach
    c. Mouth
    d. Liver

For questions 51–55, match the lettered drug schedule to the numbered drug.

DRUG

51. _____ Diphenoxylate hydrochloride with atropine sulfate (Lomotil)

52. _____ Certain drugs compounded with small quantities of narcotics

53. _____ Marijuana

54. _____ Diazepam (Valium)

55. _____ Morphine

DRUG SCHEDULE

    a. Schedule I
    b. Schedule II
    c. Schedule III
    d. Schedule IV
    e. Schedule V

For questions 56–60, match the lettered abbreviation to the numbered meaning.

MEANING

56. _____ As directed

57. _____ As needed

58. _____ Four times a day

59. _____ After meals

60. _____ Three times a day

ABBREVIATION

    a. tid
    b. qid
    c. pc
    d. prn
    e. ud

For questions 61–62, please answer in sentences.

CASE STUDIES

61. A 13-year-old girl is picked up at the medical office by her father. Her parents are divorced, and her mother has legal custody. Her father would like to see the girl's medical records. Can he see the medical records by law? Explain.

_____

_____

_____

_____

_____

62. A physician prescribed marijuana for a 35-year-old man who has advanced AIDS. Before the pharmacy technician dispenses the prescription, a health care professional wants to know in which schedule of drugs the marijuana is. On the Internet, the technician should search under which federal law?

UNIT 2

Mathematics and Dosage Calculations

It is the health care professional's responsibility to ensure the patient receives the proper dose of medication and to educate the patient about the proper measurement of doses.

Chapter 8

Principles of Math in Medicine

Chapter Objectives

After completing this chapter, you should be able to:

1. Describe the difference between Arabic numbers and Roman numerals.
2. Convert an improper fraction to a mixed fraction.
3. Add fractions that have the same denominator.
4. Subtract fractions that have the same denominator.
5. Multiply fractions and mixed fractions.
6. Divide fractions and mixed fractions.
7. Add, subtract, multiply, and divide decimals.
8. Define *ratios*, *proportions*, and *percents*.

Key Terms

Arabic number (p. 107)
common fraction (p. 109)
decimals (p. 111)
denominator (p. 108)
extremes (p. 114)
fraction (p. 108)

improper fraction (p. 109)
means (p. 114)
minuend (p. 112)
mixed fraction (p. 109)
multiplicand (p. 112)
multiplier (p. 112)

numerator (p. 108)
percent (p. 113)
ratio (p. 113)
Roman numeral (p. 107)
subtrahend (p. 112)

Introduction

The ability to make accurate dosage calculations requires allied health professionals to have skills in adding, subtracting, multiplying, and dividing whole numbers. It is essential that you have a knowledge of basic mathematics—such as Arabic numbers, Roman numerals, fractions, decimals, percents, and ratios—to be able to calculate dosages accurately and quickly.

Arabic System and Roman Numeral System

The **Arabic number** system is commonly used in expressing quantity and value, such as 0, 1, 2, 3, 4, 5, 6, 7, 8, and 9. Any number may be represented by combining these numbers. Arabic numbers can be written as whole numbers, decimals (e.g., 0.6), and fractions (e.g., 3/4). The **Roman numeral** system consists of letters that represent number values—most commonly of numbers between 1 and 100. When working with numbers that range from 1 to 30, only three Roman numerals—I (1), V (5), and X (10)—are required and are used in various combinations.

Example

$$IV = 4$$
$$XXI = 21$$

Roman numerals are commonly used to express units of the apothecary system of weights and measures in writing prescriptions. The most common Roman numerals and their values are shown in Table 8-1 ■.

READING ROMAN NUMERALS

Roman numerals are read by adding or subtracting the value of the letters. When a letter appears twice in a row, the value of the letter is counted twice, and so on (Example 1). If a lower-valued letter follows a larger-valued letter, the letters should be added. The letter representing the largest possible number should be used to represent a value. If a lower-valued letter is placed before a higher-valued letter, the lower letter is subtracted from the higher letter (Example 2).

Example 1

$$VII = 5 + 1 + 1 = 7$$
$$III = 1 + 1 + 1 = 3$$
$$XIV = 10 + 4 = 14$$
$$XXI = 10 + 10 + 1 = 21$$
$$XXXIV = 10 + 10 + 10 + 4 = 34$$

Example 2

$$IV = 5 - 1 = 4$$
$$IX = 10 - 1 = 9$$
$$XL = 50 - 10 = 40$$

Table 8-1 ■ The Most Common Roman Numerals and Their Arabic Values

ROMAN NUMERAL	ARABIC VALUE
I	1
II	2
III	3
IV	4
V	5
VI	6
VII	7
VIII	8
IX	9
X	10
XV	15
XX	20
XXV	25
XXX	30
XL	40
L	50
LX	60
LXX	70
LXXV	75
LXXX	80
XC	90
C	100
D	500
M	1,000

Using Numbers for Calculations

In pharmacology, various types of numbers are used to perform calculations. Basically, fractions are expressed as a certain number being part of a total number of parts, and with the numbers in the fraction divided by a *fraction bar*. Decimals are used to express fractions within the metric system, and they are based on the number 10 or multiples of 10. Percentages symbolize parts per hundred, and they may also be expressed as fractions or decimals, and even ratios. Ratios compare two numbers

❋ Apply Your **Knowledge 8.1**

The following questions focus on what you have just learned about Arabic numbers and Roman numerals.

DO THE MATH
Convert these Roman numerals to Arabic numbers.

1. VIII = _8_
2. XXV = _25_
3. XV = _15_
4. VI = _6_
5. XXI = _21_

Add or subtract the Roman numerals.

6. VI + VIII = _XIV_
7. XI + IV = _XV_
8. VII + IX = _XVI_
9. XXI + VI = _XXVII_
10. XIX − XII = _XVII_
11. XVII − VI = _XI_
12. XVIII − XII = _VI_
13. XXIV − XIV = _X_

MATCHING
Match the lettered term to the numbered description. Lettered terms may be used more than once.

DESCRIPTION	TERM
1. ____ Commonly used to express units of the apothecary system of weights and measures in prescriptions	a. Arabic numbers
2. _b_ Read by adding or subtracting the value of letters	b. Roman numerals
3. _A_ Commonly used in expressing quantity and value	
4. _A_ Can be written as whole numbers, decimals, and fractions	
5. _b_ Only three of these are needed to express numbers from 1 to 30	

or a part of a whole number, and they are written using a colon to separate the numbers. A proportion shows the relationship between two ratios, utilizing either a double colon or an equal sign between the two ratios.

FRACTIONS

Health care workers who deal with administering medications and dispensing drugs need to understand fractions to interpret and act on practitioners' orders, read prescriptions, and understand patients' records. Fractions are used in apothecary and household measures for dosage calculations. A **fraction** is one or more equal parts of a unit. It is written as a divided number, with one portion considered to be a part of the whole amount,

such as 1/2 or 3/4 (one part out of a total of two parts or three parts out of a total of four).

The two parts of a fraction are called the *numerator* and the *denominator*. The **numerator** is the top number of the fraction. The **denominator** is the bottom number and indicates how many equal parts the whole has been divided into. In 3/4, the number 3 is the numerator and the number 4 is the denominator. The numerator shows how many of the parts are used. For example, the fraction 3/4 is read as "three-fourths" and indicates three parts out of the four parts that make up the whole. The fraction bar that separates the numerator and the denominator also means "divided by." Thus, 3/4 can be read as "three divided by four" or "3 ÷ 4." This definition is important when one changes fractions to decimals.

Classification of Fractions

Fractions are generally classified into two groups: common fractions and decimal fractions. A **common fraction** represents equal parts of a whole. A decimal fraction is commonly referred to simply as a *decimal*. Common fractions are subclassified as proper, improper, mixed, and complex.

PROPER FRACTIONS

A proper fraction has a numerator that is smaller than the denominator and designates less than one whole unit. For example, $3/4 < 1$.

IMPROPER FRACTIONS

An **improper fraction** has a numerator that is greater than or the same as the denominator. The number 5/3 is an improper fraction because the numerator 5 is greater than the denominator 3.

Example

$$\frac{5}{3} > 1 \quad \text{or} \quad \frac{5}{5} = 1$$

MIXED FRACTIONS

A **mixed fraction** is a whole number and a proper fraction combined. The value of the mixed fraction is always greater than 1.

Example

$$5\frac{2}{3} = 5 + \frac{2}{3} > 1$$

A mixed fraction can be converted to an improper fraction by converting the whole number to a fraction and adding (see the section "Adding and Subtracting Fractions with Dissimilar Denominators").

COMPLEX FRACTIONS

A complex fraction has the numerator or the denominator or both as a whole number, proper fraction, or mixed fraction. The value may be less than, greater than, or equal to 1.

Example

$$\frac{\frac{3}{5}}{\frac{1}{2}}, \frac{\frac{1}{3}}{50}, \text{ and } \frac{25}{\frac{1}{8}}$$

Adding Fractions

If fractions have the same denominator, simply add the numerators and keep the value of the common denominator the same. Then, reduce the numbers to the lowest terms by dividing the numerator and denominator by the same common divisor (in this case, 2). Remember, by dividing both by 2, you are essentially dividing by 1 because

$$\frac{2}{2} = 1$$

Example 1

$$\frac{1}{10} + \frac{3}{10} = \frac{4}{10} = \frac{2}{5}$$

Example 2

$$\frac{4}{18} + \frac{3}{18} + \frac{6}{18} = \frac{13}{18}$$

Subtracting Fractions

If fractions have the same denominator, subtract the smaller numerator from the larger numerator. Keep the denominator the same and then reduce to the lowest terms to obtain the final answer.

Example

$$\frac{6}{8} - \frac{2}{8} = \frac{4}{8} = \frac{1}{2}$$

Adding and Subtracting Fractions with Dissimilar Denominators

If fractions do not have the same denominator, change the fractions so they have the smallest common denominator, subtract (or add) the numerators, and leave the denominator the same.

Example

$$\frac{10}{24} - \frac{4}{12} = ?$$

Because 12 is a multiple of 24 ($24 \div 2 = 12$), divide 24 by 2 to reach the smallest common denominator of 12:

$$\frac{10}{24} \div \frac{2}{2} = \frac{5}{12}$$

Then, complete the subtraction:

$$\frac{5}{12} - \frac{4}{12} = \frac{1}{12}$$

Sometimes, however, the common denominator is not the smallest number even though both could be divided by 2. In the next example, the numerator 13 cannot be evenly divided by 2. Therefore, multiply the smaller denominator (12) by 2 to get a common denominator of 24. You will also need to multiply the numerator by 2. Remember, by multiplying the numerator and the denominator by 2, you are essentially multiplying by 1.

Example

$$\frac{13}{24} - \frac{2}{12} = ?$$

$$\frac{2}{12} \times \frac{2}{2} = \frac{4}{24}$$

$$\frac{13}{24} - \frac{4}{24} = \frac{9}{24} = \frac{3}{8}$$

As noted in the section on mixed fractions, you can convert a mixed fraction to an improper fraction by using the following steps:

Example

$$5\frac{2}{3}$$

First, convert the whole number to a fraction:

$$5 = \frac{5}{1}$$

Then, find a common denominator:

$$\frac{5}{1} + \frac{2}{3} = \frac{15}{3} + \frac{2}{3}$$

Finally, add the fractions:

$$\frac{15}{3} + \frac{2}{3} = \frac{17}{3}$$

Multiplying Fractions

To multiply fractions, first multiply the numerators; second, multiply the denominators; then, place the product of the numerators over the product of the denominators; and finally, reduce to lowest terms.

Example

$$\frac{3}{5} \times \frac{2}{4} = \frac{6}{20} = \frac{3}{10}$$

Dividing Fractions

To divide fractions, first invert (or turn upside down) the divisor, reduce to lowest terms, and then multiply the numerators and divisors.

Example

$$\frac{4}{8} \div \frac{2}{8} = ?$$

Invert the divisor:

$$\frac{4}{8} \times \frac{8}{2} = ?$$

Reduce to lowest terms and then multiply the numerators and then the denominators:

$$\frac{1}{2} \times \frac{4}{1} = \frac{4}{2} = \frac{2}{1} = 2$$

✳ Apply Your Knowledge 8.2

The following questions focus on what you have just learned about fractions.

FILL IN THE BLANK

Select terms from your reading to fill in the blanks.

1. A proper fraction has a numerator that is __<__ than the denominator.

2. The numerator is the of the _____ fraction.

3. A mixed fraction is a whole number and a proper fraction that are _____.

4. If fractions have the same denominator, subtract the _____ numerator from the _____ numerator.

5. To divide fractions, first _____ the divisor and then _____.

6. The numerator in 35/10 is _____.

7. The denominator in 42/100 is _____.

8. The numerator in 88/99 is _____.

9. The denominator in 14/60 is _____.

10. Twelve is the _____ in 12/5.

MULTIPLE CHOICE

Select the correct answer from choices a–d.

1. Determine the proper fraction from the following examples:

   a. 11/11 = 1

   b. 32/68 =

   c. 90/72 =

   d. 48/38 =

2. Determine the improper fraction from the following examples:

   a. 14/6

   b. 3/9

   c. 27/45

   d. 17/35

3. Determine the mixed fraction from the following examples:

   a. 2/6

   b. 101/16

   c. 11.238

   d. $6\dfrac{2}{4}$

DECIMALS

Decimal fractions, or **decimals**, are used with the metric system. Each decimal fraction has a denominator of 10 or a multiple of 10. Instead of writing the denominator, a decimal point is added to the numerator.

Example

$$\frac{3}{4} = \frac{75}{100} = 0.75$$

In writing a decimal fraction, always place a zero to the left of the decimal point so the decimal point can be readily seen.

Example

Fraction	Decimal Fraction
$\dfrac{2}{10}$	0.2
$\dfrac{19}{100}$	0.19
$\dfrac{256}{1,000}$	0.256

Decimals increase in value from right to left (Figure 8-1 ■); they decrease in value from left to right. Decimals increase in value in multiples of 10. Each column in a decimal has its own value—it depends on where it is situated in relation to the decimal point.

Figure 8-1 ■ Decimal values as they relate to the location of the decimal point.

Focus Point

Zeros in Decimals

When writing decimals, *eliminate* unnecessary zeros ("trailing" zeros) at the end of a decimal figure (e.g., write 2.0 as 2) to avoid confusion. For example, if a 1-mg dose of a medication is written as "1.0 mg," the decimal point may not be seen, resulting in a 10-mg dose being administered. This is 10 times the desired dose and may result in a dangerous overdose. However, you should *always* insert a 0 before the decimal point of numbers less than 0 (e.g., 0.25 instead of .25). For example, if a 0.5-mg dose of a medication is written as ".5 mg," the decimal point may not be seen, resulting in a 5-mg dose being administered. Again, this is 10 times the desired dose—with the potential to result in a dangerous overdose.

Adding and Subtracting Decimal Fractions

To add decimals, write the decimals in a column, placing the decimal points directly under each other. Then, add as in the addition of whole numbers and place the decimal point in the sum directly under the decimal points in the addends.

Example

$$0.2 + 0.5 + 0.7 = 1.4$$

Align the figures as follows:

$$
\begin{array}{r}
0.2 \\
0.5 \\
+0.7 \\
\hline
1.4
\end{array}
$$

To subtract decimals, write the decimals in columns, keeping the decimal points under each other. Then, subtract as whole numbers (zeros may be added after the decimal without changing the value) and place the decimal point in the remainder—directly under the decimal point in the **subtrahend** (the number that is deducted) and **minuend** (the number from which another number is deducted).

Example

$$0.525 - 0.30 = 0.225$$

Align the figures as follows:

$$
\begin{array}{rl}
0.525 & \text{(minuend)} \\
-0.30 & \text{(subtrahend)} \\
\hline
0.225 & \text{(difference)}
\end{array}
$$

Multiplying and Dividing Decimal Fractions

To multiply decimal fractions, multiply the two numbers and count off from right to left as many decimal places in the product (answer) as there were in the **multiplier** (the number that multiplies another number) and **multiplicand** (the number that is multiplied by another number).

Example

$$
\begin{array}{rl}
33.86 & \text{(multiplicand)} \\
\times 5.4 & \text{(multiplier)} \\
\hline
182.844 & \text{(product)}
\end{array}
$$

Because the multiplicand has two decimal places and the multiplier has one decimal place, you must count off three places from right to left and then insert the decimal point at this spot in the answer.

To divide decimal fractions, first move the decimal point in the divisor (the number that divides another number) enough places to the right to make it a whole number. Then, move the decimal point in the dividend (the number that is being divided) as many places as it was moved in the divisor. Place the decimal point in the answer directly above the one in the dividend.

Example

$$4.75 \div 0.5 = ?$$

$$\frac{4.75}{0.5} = \frac{\text{dividend}}{\text{divisor}}$$

In this example, 4.75 becomes 475 (the decimal point is moved two places). Therefore, 0.5 becomes 50 (the decimal point is moved two places). Now the problem may be divided as follows:

$$475 \div 50 = 9.5$$

✳ Apply Your Knowledge 8.3

The following questions focus on what you just learned about decimals.

DO THE MATH

Calculate these problems.

1. $0.12 + 5.77 + 9.06 + 18 =$ _____
2. $9.75 + 4.6 + 0.21 + 43.4 =$ _____
3. $14.006 - 0.5 =$ _____
4. $7.192 + 0.077 =$ _____
5. $28.4 - 0.188 =$ _____
6. $\$8.12 - \$0.97 =$ _____
7. $\$17.52 - \$1.93 =$ _____
8. $6 + 2.93 + 0.63 + 0.009 =$ _____
9. $5 + 7.2 + 0.07 + 9.33 =$ _____
10. $600 - 275.97 =$ _____
11. $3.002 \times 0.05 =$ _____
12. $16.1 \times 25.04 =$ _____
13. $75.1 \times 1000.01 =$ _____
14. $23.2 \times 15.025 =$ _____
15. $1.14 \times 0.014 =$ _____
16. $45 \div 0.15 =$ _____
17. $73 \div 13.40 =$ _____
18. $25.3 \div 6.76 =$ _____
19. $515 \div 0.125 =$ _____
20. $16 \div 0.04 =$ _____

PERCENTAGES

The term **percent**, or the symbol %, means "hundredths." Thus, a percentage may also be expressed as a fraction, as a decimal fraction, or as a ratio.

Example

40% means *40 parts per hundred* or $\dfrac{40}{100}$

75% means *75 parts per hundred* or $\dfrac{75}{100}$

Example

Percent		Fraction		Decimal		Ratio
60%	=	$\dfrac{60}{100}$	=	0.60	=	60:100

Note: To change a percent to a decimal, move the decimal point two places to the left. In the example, the decimal point comes before the whole number 60. To change a fraction to a percent, divide the numerator by the denominator and then multiply the results by 100. Then, add a percent symbol (%).

Example 1

To convert $\dfrac{6}{10}$ to a percent:

$$6 \div 10 = 0.6$$
$$0.6 \times 100 = 60\%$$

Example 2

To convert $\dfrac{1}{5}$ to a percent:

$$1 \div 5 = 0.2$$
$$0.2 \times 100 = 20\%$$

✳ Apply Your Knowledge 8.4

The following questions focus on what you have just learned about percentages.

FILL IN THE BLANK

Select terms from your readings to fill in the blanks.

1. To convert a percent to a decimal, the decimal point comes before the _____.
2. The symbol % for *percent* means *hundredths*
3. The *fraction* 25/100 is equivalent to 25%.
4. To change a fraction to a percent, divide the numerator by the *denominator* and multiply by 100.
5. To change a _____ to a decimal, move the _____ point two places to the left.

DO THE MATH

Convert these percentages to decimals. Convert these decimals to percentages.

1. 2% = *.02*
2. 18% = *.18*
3. 40% = *.4*
4. 106% = *1.06*
5. 0.8% = _____
6. $24\frac{1}{2}\%$ = _____
7. 150.75% = _____
8. 4.5% = _____
9. 0.08 = _____
10. 32 = _____
11. 0.44 = _____
12. 0.5 = _____
13. 0.019 = _____
14. 5.7 = _____
15. 13 = *13.00%*
16. 0.99 = *99%*

RATIOS

A **ratio** is a mathematical expression that compares the relationship of one number with another number or expresses a part of a whole number. When written, the two quantities are separated by a colon (:). The colon means "division." The expression 3:4 means there are *three parts to four parts*. Ratios are frequently used to show concentrations of a medication in a solution. They are also used to express measurement equivalents and dosages of medications per unit (such as tablet or capsule). For example, 1 grain is equal to 15 g, which in a ratio would be expressed as 1 grain:15 g. One tablet containing 500 mg of a medication can be expressed as 1 tablet:500 mg. When measuring insulin, 100 units are contained in 1 mL, which can be written as 100 units:1 mL.

Example

$\frac{2}{5}$ may be expressed as a ratio: 2:5.

✳ Apply Your **Knowledge** 8.5

The following questions focus on what you have just learned about ratios.

FILL IN THE BLANK
Select terms from your reading to fill in the blanks.

1. In a ratio, the two quantities are separated by a ___colon___ or ___:___ (symbol).
2. Ratios are frequently used to show concentrations of medication in a _____.
3. A 100-unit insulin syringe contains 100 units in 1 mL, which can be written as a ratio of _____.
4. In administering medications, you can use ratios to express measurement equivalents and dosages of drug per _____.

DO THE MATH
Change the ratios to fractions and then reduce to lowest terms.

1. 0.05:0.15 = _____
2. 6:8 = ___6/8 = 3/4___
3. 3:150 = _____
4. 6:10 = ___6/10 = 3/5___
5. 4:7 = ___4/7___
6. 9:18 = ___9/18 = 1/2___

Proportions

A *proportion* is a way of expressing a relationship of equality between two ratios. A proportion may be expressed as:

$$1:4 \;\; :: \;\; 3:12$$

or

$$1:4 = 3:12$$

or

$$\frac{1}{4} = \frac{3}{12}$$

In the examples above, the relationship of 1 to 4 is the same as the relationship of 3 to 12. In a proportion, these terms have names. The **means** are the two inside terms, and the **extremes** are the two outside terms. This relationship is shown in Figure 8-2 ■.

In a proportion, the product of the means is equal to the product of the extremes, which in turn equals 1. To prove this, convert the proportion into fractions and then cross-multiply the numerators and denominators.

Figure 8-2 ■ The means and extremes of a proportion.

Example

$$1:5 \;\; :: \;\; 2:10$$

Convert to fractions.

$$\frac{1}{5} = \frac{2}{10}$$

Cross-multiply the numerators and the denominators of the fraction.

$$\frac{1}{5} \times \frac{2}{10} = \frac{10}{10} = 1$$

✱ Apply Your Knowledge 8.6

The following questions focus on what you have just learned about means and extremes.

DO THE MATH
Determine the missing means or extremes values.

1. 10:X :: 5:8 = __16__
2. 3:12 :: X:36 = __9__ $\frac{3}{12} \times \frac{9}{36}$
3. 33:39 :: 55:X = _____
4. 10:4 :: 20:X = __8__ $\frac{10}{4} \times \frac{20}{8} = \frac{180}{180}$
5. 100:X :: 50:2 = __4__
6. 21:27 :: X:45 = __35__
7. X:15 :: 100:75 = __20__ $\frac{20}{15} \times \frac{100}{75}$
8. 4:25 :: 16:X = __100__

$\frac{4}{25} \times \frac{16}{100}$

PRACTICAL SCENARIO 1

Pharmacy technicians must always be careful when using mathematical equations for compounding. Phil, a pharmacy technician who only recently began working in a pharmacy, is asked by the pharmacist to mix a powdered drug with a solution so the amount of drug is 3%. Phil converts 3% to a decimal (0.03) so he can more easily mix the proper amount. He then mixes 0.03 g of the powdered drug into 100 mL of solution. When the pharmacist checks Phil's calculations, she finds that the mixture is much too weak.

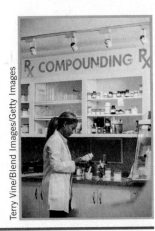

Terry Vine/Blend Images/Getty Images

Critical Thinking Questions

1. What miscalculation did Phil make when mixing the solution?
2. What is a good preventative measure when performing calculations for compounding?

PRACTICAL SCENARIO 2

A respiratory care technician was attempting to calculate a 60% solution as a decimal. He calculates this as a 0.06 solution.

Phase4Photography/Fotolia

Critical Thinking Questions

1. What decimal would have been correct to represent a 60% solution?
2. What would be the ratio of 60% of medication to the solution containing it?

Chapter Capsule

The section repeats the objectives from the beginning of the chapter and then provides a summary of the most important concepts for that objective. Use this section as a quick review and to check your knowledge.

Objective 1: Describe the difference between Arabic numbers and Roman numerals.

- Arabic uses numbers, decimals, and fractions to express values
- Roman uses letters that represent number values

Objective 2: Convert an improper fraction to a mixed fraction.

- 5/3—5 is the numerator and 3 is the denominator
- To convert it to a mixed fraction, divide the numerator by the denominator
- Answers: 1 and 2/3

Objective 3: Add fractions that have the same denominator.

- $\dfrac{1}{4} + \dfrac{2}{4} = \dfrac{3}{4}$

- $\dfrac{2}{5} + \dfrac{2}{5} = \dfrac{4}{5}$

- $\dfrac{3}{10} + \dfrac{6}{10} = \dfrac{9}{10}$

Objective 4: Subtract fractions that have the same denominator.

- $\dfrac{8}{12} - \dfrac{7}{12} = \dfrac{1}{12}$

- $\dfrac{9}{20} - \dfrac{6}{20} = \dfrac{3}{20}$

- $\dfrac{27}{45} - \dfrac{19}{45} = \dfrac{8}{45}$

Objective 5: Multiply fractions and mixed fractions.

- $\dfrac{1}{4} \times 1\dfrac{3}{4} = \dfrac{1}{4} \times \dfrac{7}{4} = \dfrac{7}{16}$

- $\dfrac{3}{10} \times 2\dfrac{7}{10} = \dfrac{3}{10} \times \dfrac{27}{10} = \dfrac{81}{100}$

- $\dfrac{3}{7} \times 1\dfrac{2}{7} = \dfrac{3}{7} \times \dfrac{9}{7} = \dfrac{27}{49}$

Objective 6: Divide fractions and mixed fractions.

- $1\dfrac{1}{12} \div \dfrac{9}{12} = \dfrac{13}{12} \times \dfrac{12}{9} = \dfrac{156}{108} = 1\dfrac{48}{108} = 1\dfrac{4}{9}$

- $2\dfrac{1}{3} \div \dfrac{2}{3} = \dfrac{7}{3} \times \dfrac{3}{2} = \dfrac{21}{6} = \dfrac{7}{2} = 3\dfrac{1}{2}$

- $5\dfrac{1}{2} \div \dfrac{1}{2} = \dfrac{11}{2} \times \dfrac{2}{1} = \dfrac{22}{2} = 11$

Objective 7: Add, subtract, multiply, and divide decimals.

- $0.2 + 7.13 + 3.067 = 10.397$
- $9.77 - 2.9 - 1.38 = 5.49$
- $1.6 \times 0.77 \times 7.1 = 8.7472$
- $12.33 \div 3.6 \div 1.5 = 2.283333 =$ (rounds to 2.283)

Objective 8: Define *ratios*, *proportions*, and *percents*.

- Ratios—compare one number with another or express a part of a whole number (e.g., 3:4 means "three parts to four parts")
- Proportions—express a relationship of equality between two ratios (e.g., 1:4 :: 3:12 means the relationship of 1 to 4 is the same as the relationship of 3 to 12)
- Percents—mean "hundredths"; may also be expressed as a fraction, a decimal, or a ratio (e.g., 40% means "40 parts per hundred," or 40/100)

 ## Internet Sites of Interest

- Get online help with math calculations at S.O.S. Math: **www.sosmath.com**
- On The Math Page, you can click on a chapter in an online textbook to find instructions and plenty of examples for the arithmetic or algebra problem that is confounding you: **www.themathpage.com**
- Fractions, decimals, and percents are covered by clicking on each topic: **www.math.com**
- Medical mathematics tutorial: **http://becps.net**
- Drug calculations quiz page: **www.testandcalc.com/quiz/index.asp**
- Dosage calculations tutorial: **www.dosagehelp.com**

Chapter 9

Measurement Systems and Their Equivalents

Chapter Objectives

After completing this chapter, you should be able to:

1. Name the basic units of the metric system for weight, volume, and length.

2. Understand metric abbreviations used in pharmacy and clinical settings.

3. Identify major apothecary system units.

4. Identify major household system units.

5. Convert units of measure to equivalent units of measure within the same system of measurement.

6. Recognize the difference between the Celsius and Fahrenheit temperature scales.

7. Explain the difference between the 12-hour and 24-hour clocks.

8. Discuss milliequivalents and International Units.

9. Determine the equivalents in the apothecary and household systems for the following amounts: 1 mL, 1 mg, 1 g, and 1 kg.

10. Determine the equivalents in the metric system for the following amounts: 1 dr, 1 cup, 1 qt, and 1 lb.

Key Terms

apothecary system (p. 121)
drams (p. 121)
grain (p. 121)
gram (p. 119)
household system (p. 121)

International Units (p. 125)
liter (p. 119)
meter (p. 119)
metric system (p. 119)
milliequivalents (p. 125)

minims (p. 121)
ounces (p. 119)
unit (p. 119)

Introduction

Health care professionals who deal with the administration of medications prescribed for patients must ensure the accuracy and correctness of drug dosages. They must have a complete knowledge of the weights and measures used in drug administration for prescribed amounts.

Units of Measure

Three systems of measurement are used in pharmacology and the calculation of drug dosages: (1) metric, (2) apothecary, and (3) household. Today, however, household and apothecary measures, such as teaspoons and **ounces** (equivalent to 437.5 grains or 28.35 g), are used less commonly. The most common, most accurate, and safest system of measurement in all countries is the **metric system**—a system based on the decimal system. Medications are administered with three parameters in mind: (1) weight, (2) volume, and (3) length. Weight is the most used parameter and is essential as a dosage **unit** (a unit is defined as a standard of measure, weight, or any other similar quality). Measurement of volume is the next most important parameter and is used for liquids. Length is the least used parameter for dosage calculations.

METRIC SYSTEM

The basic units of weight and volume in the metric system are based on units of "10," as in the decimal system. The metric system uses the basic units of **gram** (g) as the unit of weight (equivalent to 15.432358 grains), **liter** (L) as the unit of volume (equivalent to 1.056688 quarts), and **meter** (m) as the unit of length (equivalent to 39.37007874 inches). In medicine, it is common to use weight for determining medication doses based in kilograms and volume to express liquid amounts. Parts of these basic units are named by adding prefixes that describe multiples or fractions of the standard measures for weight, volume, and length based on units of 10. The prefixes usually relate to Latin and Greek measures. Table 9-1 ■ shows Latin prefixes. Table 9-2 ■ shows Greek prefixes.

Table 9-1 ■ Latin Prefixes

PREFIX*	VALUE	EQUIVALENTS
micro- (mc):	1/1,000,000	= 0.000001
milli- (m):	1/1,000	= 0.001
centi- (c):	1/100	= 0.01
deci- (d):	1/10	= 0.1

*Remember: Latin prefixes denote fractions.

Table 9-2 ■ Greek Prefixes

PREFIX*	VALUE
deca- (da):	10
hecto- (h):	100
kilo- (k):	1,000
mega- (M):	1,000,000

*Remember: Greek prefixes denote multiples.

A system for international standardization of metric units was established throughout the world in 1960 with the introduction of the International System, or SI (from the French *Système International*). Table 9-3 ■ shows SI standardized abbreviations.

Table 9-3 ■ SI Standardized Abbreviations (Metric System)

PARAMETER	UNIT	ABBREVIATION	EQUIVALENTS
Weight	gram (basic unit)	g	1 g = 1,000 mg
	milligram	mg	1 mg = 1,000 mcg = 0.001 g
	microgram	mcg	1 mcg = 0.001 mg = 0.000001 g
	kilogram	kg	1 kg = 1,000 g
Volume	liter (basic unit)	L	1 L = 1,000 mL
	milliliter	mL	1 mL = 1 cc* = 0.001 L
Length	meter (basic unit)	m	1 m = 100 cm = 1,000 mm
	centimeter	cm	1 cm = 0.01 m = 10 mm
	millimeter	mm	1 mm = 0.001 m = 0.1 cm

*This abbreviation should not be used in clinical practice to avoid medication errors.

Focus Point

Use of the Metric System

The United States does not use the metric system as its standard method for measurement, unlike the rest of the world. The opposition to the metric system began in the 1870s because manufacturers did not want to spend large amounts of money to replace their machinery, which was calibrated in inches. However, all fields of science including medicine use the metric system, and metric unit dosing is much more precise than household measurements.

✱ Apply Your Knowledge 9.1

The following questions focus on what you have just learned about the metric system.

FILL IN THE BLANK
Rewrite the following metric numbers by using numerals and abbreviations.

1. Twenty-five grams _25,000 mg /25g_
2. Eight milliliters _8mL_
3. Fifty-five hundredths of a milligram _____
4. One hundred micrograms _____
5. Seven and two-tenths micrograms _____
6. Sixteen liters _16 L_
7. Two thousand milliliters _2000 mL_
8. Four meters _4m_
9. Nineteen millimeters _19mm_
10. Three and one-half centimeters _3 1/2 cm_

MULTIPLE CHOICE
Select the correct answer from choices a–d.

1. The metric system is based on which of the following?
   a. Units
   b. Fractions
   c. Decimals ⓒ
   d. Proportions

2. Which of the following is the least used parameter for dosage calculations?
   a. Volume
   ⓑ Length
   c. Unit
   d. Weight

3. In medicine, it is common to use weight for determining medication doses in which of the following increments?
   a. Ounces
   ⓑ Kilograms
   c. Pounds
   d. International Units

4. The abbreviation for the International System is:
   a. INS
   b. IS
   ⓒ SI
   d. SIN

5. The value of the prefix *hecto-* is:
   a. 10
   ⓑ 100
   c. 1,000
   d. 1,000,000

APOTHECARY SYSTEM

The **apothecary system** is a very old English system that has slowly been replaced by the metric system. The apothecary system uses **minims** (the basic unit of volume), **drams** (fluidrams—equivalent to 1/8 ounce), ounces (fluid ounces), pints, quarts, and gallons to measure volume. It measures weight by grains, drams, ounces, and pounds. The apothecary system also uses Roman numerals to indicate the amount of drug. The basic unit of weight is the **grain**. Today, the apothecary system is used for only a few drugs, such as acetaminophen, aspirin, and phenobarbital. Table 9-4 ■ shows common apothecary equivalents.

Table 9-4 ■ **Apothecary System**

PARAMETER	UNIT	ABBREVIATION	EQUIVALENTS
Weight	grain (basic unit)	gr	
	dram	dr or ʒ*	
	ounce	oz or ʒ*	1 oz = 16 dr = 437.5 gr
	pound	lb	1 lb = 16 oz = 7000 (gr)
Volume	minim (basic unit)	M or m*	
	fluidram	fl dr	
	fluid ounce	ʒ*	pt i = ʒ* 16
	pint	pt	qt i = ʒ* 32
	quart	qt	qt i = pt ii
	gallon	gal	

*These abbreviations should not be used in clinical practice to avoid medication errors.

Note: There are no essential equivalents of weight or length to learn for this system.

✳ Apply Your **Knowledge** 9.2

The following questions focus on what you have just learned about the apothecary system of measurements.

FILL IN THE BLANK
Select abbreviations or symbols for the apothecary system to fill in the blanks.

1. fluid ounce _____
2. grain _____
3. dram _____
4. quart _____
5. pint _____
6. minim _____

HOUSEHOLD SYSTEM

The **household system** is used in most American homes. This system of measurement is important for a patient at home who has no knowledge of the metric or apothecary systems. However, household measurements, consisting of teaspoons and tablespoons, are not precisely accurate, so they should never be used in the medical setting. The only household units of measurement used to measure drugs are units of volume. These include the drop, teaspoon, tablespoon, ounce (fluid), cup, pint, quart, and gallon. Table 9-5 ■ shows common household units, abbreviations, and equivalents.

Table 9-5 ■ Household Measurements

UNIT	ABBREVIATION	EQUIVALENTS
drop	gtt	15 gtt = 1 mL
teaspoon	t (tsp)	1 tsp = 5 mL
tablespoon	T (tbsp)	1 T = 3t
ounce (fluid)	oz	2 T = 1 oz
cup	cup	1 cup = 8 oz
pint	pt	1 pt = 2 cups
quart	qt	1 qt = 4 cups = 2 pt
gallon	gal	1 gal = 4 qt

Note: Cups, quarts, and gallons are commonly used to measure medications.

✳ Apply Your Knowledge 9.3

The following exercises focus on what you have just learned about conversions among measurement systems.

FILL IN THE BLANK
Select terms from your reading to fill in the blanks.

1. How many cups equal 2 pints? __4__
2. Forty-five teaspoons are equivalent to how many tablespoons? __15__
3. How many cups are equivalent to 8 ounces? __1__
4. How many teaspoons are equivalent to 1 ounce? __6__
5. How many drops are equivalent to 2 tablespoons? _____
6. How many tablespoons are equivalent to 1 ounce? _____
7. How many pints are equivalent to 8 cups? _____
8. How many ounces are equivalent to 4 tablespoons? _____
9. A meter is a metric unit that measures _____.
10. A liter is a metric unit that measures _____.
11. A gram is a metric unit that measures _____.
12. 3 cups = __24__ oz
13. 220 drops = _____ tsp

Temperature Conversions

Two scales of temperature are used throughout the world: the Celsius (Centigrade) and Fahrenheit scales. The Fahrenheit scale is still used in the United States; the Celsius scale is used in most other parts of the world. The abbreviation used in the Fahrenheit scale is an *F*, and in the Celsius scale, it is a *C*.

Water freezes at 32°F and at 0°C. This difference of 32 degrees is used in converting temperature from one scale to the other. It can also be determined that water boils at 212°F and at 100°C.

There is a 180-degree difference between the freezing and boiling points on the Fahrenheit scale and a 100-degree difference between these two points on the Celsius scale. The difference between the boiling point and the freezing point on the Fahrenheit scale and the Celsius scale can be set as a ratio of each Celsius degree being 9/5 times greater than each Fahrenheit degree, as seen in the following formula:

$$180:100 = \frac{180}{100} = \frac{9}{5}$$

If the fraction 9/5 is expressed as a decimal, it can be stated that each Celsius degree is 1.8 times greater than each Fahrenheit degree. To convert a given temperature from one scale to the other, you may use one of the following formulas:

$$°F = 18°C + 32$$
$$°F = 9/5°C + 32$$

Example 1
Convert 100°C to Fahrenheit.

$$°F = 1.8 \times 100°C + 32 \qquad °F = 9/5 \times 100°C + 32$$
$$°F = 180 + 32 \qquad\qquad °F = 180 + 32$$
$$°F = 212 \qquad\qquad\quad °F = 212$$

Example 2
Convert 212°F to Celsius. (*Note:* Subtract 32 from both sides of the equation.)

$$212°F = 1.8°C + 32$$
$$212°F - 32 = 1.8°C + 32 - 32$$
$$180°F = 1.8°C$$
$$°C = 100$$

or

$$212°F = 9/5°C + 32$$
$$212°F - 32 = 9/5°C + 32 - 32$$
$$180°F = 1.8°C$$
$$°C = 180°F ÷ 9/5$$
$$°C = 180°F \times 5/9$$
$$°C = 100°F$$

Figure 9-1 ■ indicates that water freezes at 32°F and at 0°C.

Figure 9-1 ■ Thermometer showing the temperatures at which water freezes (0°C and 32°F) and boils (100°C and 212°F).

✱ Apply Your **Knowledge 9.4**

The following questions focus on what you have just learned about temperature conversions.

FILL IN THE BLANK
Convert these to the Celsius or Fahrenheit scale.

1. 13°C _____
2. 21°C _____
3. 34°C _____
4. 45°C _____
5. 67°C _____
6. 97°C _____
7. 99.9°C _____

8. 106°C _____
9. 38°F _____
10. 52°F _____
11. 76°F _____
12. 98°F _____
13. 104°F _____
14. −16°F _____

Time Conversions

The majority of countries, but not the United States in general, recognize the *International Standard ISO 8601* in regard to calculating the time of day. This universal standard is used in the United States military, by scientific organizations, in hospitals, and in the computer industry. Under this standard, the hours, minutes, and seconds of the current time are expressed as *hhmmss*, meaning that two digits are used to express the day, the hour, and the seconds. The *hh* means the total and complete hours passed since midnight. For example, the time of 11:38 A.M. and 42 seconds would be written as *113842*. The time of 11:38 P.M. and 42 seconds, however, would be written as *233842*, since the hour of 11 P.M. is expressed as the 23rd hour of the day.

It is important to understand that actual *seconds* are usually not documented in most cases. Therefore, for the same times described above, 11:38 A.M. would be expressed as *1138*, whereas 11:38 P.M. would be expressed as *2338*. You can see that in most countries there is no need to use "A.M." or "P.M." because the 24-hour clock format clearly expresses which hour of the day is being referenced. The hours occurring between midnight and noon range from 0 to 11, whereas the hours occurring between noon and midnight range from 12 to 23. The only time an hour of "24" would be used would be to signify midnight itself, as *2400 hours.*

The 12-hour clock has been used since the dark ages, during which time Roman numerals were used, and there was no symbol signifying "zero." Since the 12-hour clock has only the numbers 1 through 12, this means that "A.M." and "P.M." must be used to signify the actual time of day. To convert time, you must first understand that beginning at 12:00 midnight (A.M.), the corresponding figure on the 24-hour clock is either *0000* or *2400*, depending on what you are expressing. If the time you need to express is 12:00 noon (P.M.) or after, you convert to the 24-hour format by increasing one digit past 12 for every hour. You can see that this would mean that 1:00 P.M. on the 12-hour clock equals *1300* on the 24-hour clock, and 2:00 P.M. on the 12-hour clock equals *1400* on the 24-hour clock, and so on. Table 9-6 ■ lists the equivalent numbers for every hour of the day on both clocks.

With minutes being written following each hour, it is easy to see that 3:45 A.M. would be written as 0345 and that 3:45 P.M. would be written as 1545. The advantages of using the 24-hour clock include less chance for human error when documenting important times that events occurred in medicine or in writing instructions for medication dosages during a given day. There is another way to remember how to convert a specific time from the 12-hour clock to the 24-hour clock. This involves drawing a circle within a circle, symbolizing a clock face, replacing the standard numbers that appear on the 12-hour clock. Instead of the numbers 12, 1, 2, 3, etc. that normally appear, these should be replaced with 1200, 0100, 0200, 0300, etc. Then it is easy to visualize that with each increasing position on the clock face, you consider that (after noon) you are simply adding one more digit to the hour, beginning with 1200 (signifying noon). Therefore, 1200 plus one, signifying 1:00 P.M., becomes 1300; 1200 plus two, signifying 2:00 P.M., becomes 1400; and 1200 plus three, signifying 3:00 P.M., becomes 1500.

Table 9-6 ■ Time Conversions

12-HOUR CLOCK TIME	24-HOUR CLOCK TIME
12:00 midnight (A.M.)	0000 (2400)
1:00 A.M.	0100
2:00 A.M.	0200
3:00 A.M.	0300
4:00 A.M.	0400
5:00 A.M.	0500
6:00 A.M.	0600
7:00 A.M.	0700
8:00 A.M.	0800
9:00 A.M.	0900
10:00 A.M.	1000
11:00 A.M.	1100
12:00 noon (P.M.)	1200
1:00 P.M.	1300
2:00 P.M.	1400
3:00 P.M.	1500
4:00 P.M.	1600
5:00 P.M.	1700
6:00 P.M.	1800
7:00 P.M.	1900
8:00 P.M.	2000
9:00 P.M.	2100
10:00 P.M.	2200
11:00 P.M.	2300

✳ Apply Your Knowledge 9.5

The following questions focus on what you have just learned about time conversions.

FILL IN THE BLANK

Convert the given time into either international standard time or 12-hour (English) time, as required).

1. 5:50 A.M. = _0550_
2. 8:18 A.M. = _0818_
3. 7:36 P.M. = ~~0736~~ _1936_
4. 4:44 P.M. = _1644_
5. 10:03 A.M. = _1003_
6. 1:33 P.M. = _1333_

7. 2020 = _820 pm_
8. 1246 = _1246 pm_
9. 1514 = _314 pm_
10. 1706 = _506 pm_
11. 0209 = _209 am_
12. 0034 = _1234 am_

Milliequivalents and Units

Milliequivalents and units are measurements used to indicate the strength of certain drugs. Pharmacists and chemists define *milliequivalent* measures as an expression of the number of grams of equivalent weight of a drug contained in 1 mL of a normal solution. Electrolytes, such as sodium and potassium, are usually measured in milliequivalents (mEq). Examples of drugs that are prescribed in milliequivalents include potassium chloride, sodium bicarbonate, and sodium chloride. Because the dosage is individualized, no calculations are involved.

Units mainly measure the potency of heparin, insulin, penicillin, and some vitamins. A unit is the amount of a medication required to produce a specific effect. The size of a unit varies for each drug. Vitamins are measured in standardized units called **International Units**, which show the amount of drug required to produce a certain effect, but they are standardized by international agreement. The International Unit does not measure a medication in terms of its physical weight or volume. Units and milliequivalents cannot be directly converted into the metric, apothecary, or household systems.

Conversion Within and Between Systems

Drug doses are usually ordered in metric system amounts, such as grams, milligrams, liters, and milliliters. Sometimes, you need to convert drug dosages between the metric, apothecary, and household systems of measurement. First, you must know how the measure of a quantity in one system compares with its measure in another system. For example, you learned the relationships between gram and kilogram, milliliter and liter, and teaspoon and tablespoon. To convert between systems, you may also need to know the relationship between milliliter and teaspoon. For example, 1 tsp = 5 mL or 1 kg = 1,000 g. Most prescriptions and medication orders are written in the metric system. Medications are usually ordered in a unit of weight measurement, such as grams or grains. You must be able to convert between units of measurement within the same system or convert units of measurement from one system to another. Table 9-7 ■ summarizes equivalent measures for volume in three different systems.

Table 9-7 ■ Approximate Equivalents for Volume and Weight

	METRIC	APOTHECARY	HOUSEHOLD
Volume	5 mL	1 dr	1 tsp
	15 mL	4 dr	1 T
	30 mL	1 fl oz	2 T
	240 mL	8 fl oz	1 cup
	480 mL	16 fl oz	1 pt
	960 mL	32 fl oz	1 qt

(continued)

Table 9-7 ■ **Approximate Equivalents for Volume and Weight** (*continued*)

	METRIC	APOTHECARY	HOUSEHOLD
Weight	1.3 mg	gr 1/50 (1/50 grain)	3/100,000 oz
	16.2 mg	gr 1/4 (1/4 grain)	5/10,000 oz
	32.4 mg	gr ss 1/2 grain)	1/1,000 oz
	64.8 mg	gr i (1 grain)	1/500 oz
	0.518 g	gr viii (8 grains)	2/100 oz
	972 mg	gr xv (15 grains)	2/1,000 lb
	1 kg	15,432 grains	2.2 lbs

✳ Apply Your Knowledge 9.6

The following questions focus on what you have just learned about conversion between different systems for volume and weight.

FILL IN THE BLANK
Convert the following amounts.

1. 5 L = _____ oz
2. 0.25 L = _____ oz
3. 20 oz = _____ L
4. 12 oz = _____ L
5. 4 oz = _____ mL
6. 8-1/2 oz = _____ mL
7. 1/2 oz = _____ mL
8. 60 mL = _____ oz
9. 150 mL = _____ oz
10. 15 mL = _____ oz
11. 5 g = _____ gr

12. 0.5 g = _____ gr
13. 0.1 g = _____ gr
14. 3 gr = _____ g
15. 1-1/2 gr = _____ g
16. 4 gr = _____ mg
17. 1-1/2 gr = _____ mg
18. 7-1/2 gr = _____ mg
19. 150 mg = _____ gr
20. 30 mg = _____ gr
21. 15 mg = _____ gr

PRACTICAL SCENARIO 1

Tara is a 7-month-old girl who is brought to her doctor's office by her mother. Her body temperature is 103.4°F. Her pediatrician orders acetaminophen 7 mL every 4 hours while her fever is above 101°F. You, the medical assistant, advise Tara's mother about carefully following the physician's order. Tara's mother, who grew up in England and only recently relocated to the United States, asks if you can convert the temperature of 101°F into Celsius degrees, and you agree to do this.

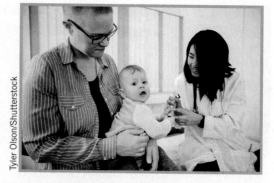

Tyler Olson/Shutterstock

Critical Thinking Questions

1. Which formula should you use to convert 101°F into Celsius degrees?
2. What is the answer that you give to Tara's mother?
3. What type of measuring instrument should you instruct Tara's mother to use?

PRACTICAL SCENARIO 2

A physician instructs a mother to give her child 10 milliliters of a medication every 6 hours. The mother of the child asks the nurse if she can use a teaspoon to administer the ordered dose.

Photographee.eu/Shutterstock

Critical Thinking Questions

1. How many teaspoons constitute 10 milliliters?
2. How many drops are equal to 10 milliliters?

Chapter Capsule

This section repeats the objectives from the beginning of the chapter and then provides a summary of the most important concepts for that objective. Use this section as a quick review and to check your knowledge.

Objective 1: Name the basic units of the metric system for weight, volume, and length.

- Weight—gram (g)
- Volume—liter (L)
- Length—meter (m)

Objective 2: Understand metric abbreviations used in pharmacy and clinical settings.

- Grams (g)
- Milligrams (mg)
- Micrograms (mcg)
- Kilograms (kg)
- Liters (L)
- Milliliters (mL)

Objective 3: Identify major apothecary system units.

- Major apothecary system units include minims, drams (fluidrams), ounces (fluid ounces), pints, quarts, gallons, grains, drams, pounds

Objective 4: Identify major household system units.

- Major household system units include drops, teaspoons, tablespoons, ounces (fluid), cups, pints, quarts, gallons

Objective 5: Convert units of measure to equivalent units of measure within the same system of measurement.

- For example: 1 kg = 1,000 g; 1 g = 1,000 mg; 1 mg = 1,000 mcg
- 1 L = 1,000 mL
- 1 m = 1,000 mm; 1 cm = 10 mm
- 1 lb = 16 oz = 7,000 gr
- 1 pt = 16 fluid ounces

- 2 pt = 1 qt
- 1 T = 3 tsp
- 2 T = 1 oz
- 1 cup = 8 oz

Objective 6: Recognize the difference between the Celsius and Fahrenheit temperature scales.

- Celsius—used in most parts of the world besides the United States; abbreviation for Celsius is C; water freezes at 0°C; water boils at 100°C
- Fahrenheit—used in the United States; abbreviation for Fahrenheit is F; water freezes at 32°F; water boils at 212°F; °F = 1.8°C + 32 or °F = 9/5°C + 32

Objective 7: Explain the difference between the 12-hour and 24-hour clocks.

- In the 12-hour clock, the times of day are expressed as either between midnight and noon (as A.M.), or between noon and midnight (as P.M.). For example, 3:33 A.M. occurs after midnight but before noon, whereas 3:33 P.M. occurs after noon but before midnight. In this clock system, the each numbered hour occurs twice per day. This clock is primarily used by the public in the United States.
- In the 24-hour clock, the times of day are expressed uniquely, with hours and minutes being written as follows: 3:33 A.M. is expressed as 0333; 3:33 P.M. is expressed as 1533. Therefore, a unique number (01 through 24) is used to express the 24 hours of the day. Note that when midnight falls, the minutes during the 12:00 A.M. hour are actually expressed as "00", not "24." Therefore, 12:33 A.M. would be written as "0033," not "2433." This clock is used in nearly every country throughout the world, and in the United States by scientists, the military, and other professionals.

Objective 8: Discuss milliequivalents and International Units.

- Milliequivalents and units are measurements used to indicate the strength of certain drugs.
- Milliequivalent measures are defined as expressions of the number of grams of equivalent weight of a drug contained in 1 mL of a normal solution.
- Electrolytes, such as sodium and potassium, are usually measured in milliequivalents.
- Other drugs ordered in milliequivalents include potassium chloride, sodium bicarbonate, and sodium chloride.
- Units mainly measure the potency of heparin, insulin, penicillin, and some vitamins.
- A unit is the amount of a medication required to produce a specific effect, and the size of a unit varies for each drug.
- Vitamins are measured in standardized units (per international agreement) called International Units.
- International Units do not measure a medication in terms of its physical weight or volume.

Objective 9: Determine the equivalents in the apothecary and household systems for the following amounts: 1 mL, 1 mg, 1 g, and 1 kg.

- 1 mL = 16.23 minims, 0.27 fluidrams, 0.2 teaspoons, 15.42 drops, 0.03 fluid ounces
- 1 mg = 0.02 grains, 0.00003 ounces
- 1 g = 15.43 grains, 0.04 ounces
- 1 kg = 15,432.36 grains, 35.27 ounces, 2.2 pounds

Objective 10: Determine the equivalents in the metric system for the following amounts: 1 dr, 1 cup, 1 qt, and 1 lb.

- 1 dr = 3.7 milliliters, 3.7 cubic centimeters
- 1 cup = 236.59 milliliters, 23.66 centiliters, 0.24 liters
- 1 qt = 946.35 milliliters, 94.64 centiliters, 0.95 liters
- 1 lb = 453.59 grams, 0.45 kilograms

Internet Sites of Interest

- Quick check of common weights and measures used by pharmacy technicians and other medical professionals: **www.rxtrek.net/weights.htm**

- Click on the appropriate calculator at **www.sciencelab.com/data/conversion.shtml** and then convert between different units of measure for weight and mass, metric weight, temperature, length, distance, volume, speed, pressure, area, force, energy, frequency, power, torque, and astronomical units.

- Online 12- to 24-hour converter: **www.onlineconversion.com/date_12-24_hour.htm**

- Milliequivalent calculations and conversions: **www.wellness.com/reference/ health-and-wellness/milliequivalent-and-millimole-calculations-and-conversions**

Adult and Pediatric Dosage Calculations

Chapter Objectives

After completing this chapter, you should be able to:

1. Discuss the differences between dosage ordered, desired dose, and dose on hand.

2. Explain how to use the formula $D/H \times Q = X$ to calculate drug doses.

3. Explain the fraction proportion method and the formula used in this method.

4. Discuss how to calculate parenteral medications and the formula used.

5. Calculate intramuscular doses.

6. Name the most common types of insulin used in the United States.

7. Explain the steps required for the proper injection of insulin.

8. Convert physician orders of heparin to the volume of solution that contains the amount of heparin ordered.

9. Calculate whether the amount of a prescribed pediatric dosage is the safe or appropriate amount for a particular patient.

10. Define the most accurate method of calculating a child's dose and perform correct calculations by using this method.

Key Terms

calibrated (p. 131)
capsules (p. 133)
conversion (p. 131)
desired dose (p. 131)
dilutions (p. 132)
dose (p. 131)
elixirs (p. 134)

heparin (p. 132)
injectable (p. 137)
insulin (p. 138)
loading dose (p. 131)
maintenance doses (p. 131)
nomogram (p. 143)

prophylactic dose (p. 131)
scored (p. 133)
spirits (p. 134)
suspensions (p. 134)
syrups (p. 134)
tablet (p. 133)

Introduction

The ability to accurately calculate drug dosages is an essential skill in health care. Serious harm to patients may result from a mathematical error during a calculation and the subsequent administration of a drug dosage. It is the responsibility of those administering drugs to carry out medical orders precisely and efficiently.

General Dosage Calculations

The **dose** of a drug is the amount a patient takes for the intended therapeutic effect, and the *dosage regimen* is the schedule of dosing for a drug. Many factors contribute to determining the dose and dosage regimen, including the potency of the drug and route of administration as well as such patient factors as weight, disease state, and tolerance. A **loading dose** may be required for some drugs to produce an adequate blood level that yields the desired therapeutic effect; this dose would then be followed by smaller **maintenance doses** to maintain an adequate blood level. A **prophylactic dose** of a drug may be given to prevent a disease, but a *therapeutic dose*, which is usually higher than the prophylactic dose, is given to treat an ongoing disease. The dose for most drugs is given in units of weight (e.g., 500 mg), but the dose for some drugs, such as biologics, is given based on activity.

The doses for many drugs, such as antihypertensives, are general and usually not patient-specific. However, the doses for some drugs require patient data, such as body surface area (BSA), clinical laboratory values, or pharmacokinetic parameters.

It is the health care professional's responsibility to ensure that the patient receives the proper dose of medication and to educate the patient about the proper measurement of doses. For solid-dosage forms, the correct dose is easily administered in premeasured tablets or capsules. However, if the drug is a liquid, the dose is usually a volume that must be accurately measured by using a standardized 5-mL teaspoon, **calibrated** dropper (a dropper that is marked with graduated measurements), or syringe. If the pharmacist compounds a specific product for a patient, it is also his or her responsibility to ensure that the correct amount of drug is delivered in each dose.

As a health care professional, you must also be familiar with the following terms to understand dosage calculations:

✳ Amount to administer—The volume of a medication that contains the desired dose; the number of tablets (or milliliters of a solution) administered once to provide the desired amount of a drug.

✳ **Desired dose**—The amount to be administered at one time. It must be in the same unit of measurement as the dosage unit.

✳ Dosage ordered—The total amount of ordered drug, along with the frequency it is to be administered. Its measurement units may not be the same as the dosage unit.

✳ Dosage strength—The dose on hand per the dosage unit. If the dose on hand is 100 mg per capsule and the dosage unit is one capsule, the dosage strength is 100 mg/capsule.

✳ Dosage unit—The volume of medication that contains a quantity of drug as listed on the drug label. If a drug contains 50 mg of drug per capsule, the dosage unit is one capsule.

✳ Dose on hand—The amount of drug in a dosage unit. If a drug has 150 mg of drug per capsule, the dose on hand is 150 mg.

CALCULATING DOSAGES

The first step in computing medication dosage, regardless of the method used, is to make certain the strength of the drug ordered and the strength of the drug available are in the same unit of measure. If necessary, **conversion** (changing) to a single unit must be carried out. After this is done, the problem can be set up by using this formula:

$$\frac{D}{H} \times Q = X$$

The answer is most commonly signified by the letter X. In this formula, D represents the desired dosage of the drug to be administered. H represents the dosage of the drug available. D and H must always be in the same unit of measure. Q represents the number of tablets, capsules, milliliters, minims, and so forth, that contains the available dosage. X represents the number of tablets, capsules, milliliters, minims, and so on, of the desired dose (the amount to be administered). Q and X must always be in the same unit of measure. Make certain that all the terms in the formula are labeled with the correct units of measure.

Several formulas can be used to calculate drug dosages. One formula uses ratios:

$$\frac{\text{Dose on hand } (H)}{\text{Quantity on hand } (Q)} = \frac{\text{Desired dose } (D)}{\text{Quantity desired } (X)}$$

Example 1
Amoxil 500 mg is ordered. It is supplied in a liquid form containing 250 mg in 5 mL. To calculate the dosage, use this formula:

$$\frac{250 \text{ mg } (H)}{5 \text{ mL } (Q)} = \frac{500 \text{ mg } (D)}{X}$$

Then, cross-multiply:

$$250 \, X = 5 \text{ mL} \times 500 \text{ mg}$$

$$X = \frac{5 \times 500}{250}$$

Therefore, the dose ordered is 10 mL.

You can also use the formula above to calculate dosages:

$$\text{Amount to administer } (X) = \frac{\text{Desired dose } (D)}{\text{Dose on hand } (H)} \times \text{Quantity on hand } (Q)$$

Example 2

Heparin, an anticoagulant, is often distributed in vials in prepared **dilutions** (less concentrated mixtures) of 10,000 units/mL. If the order calls for 2,500 units, you can use the previous formula to calculate:

$$X = \frac{2,5000 \text{ units}}{10,000 \text{ units/mL}} \times 1$$

$$X = 0.25 \text{ or } 1/4 \text{ mL}$$

Focus Point

Double-Checking Calculations

Any health care professional who is unsure about a dosage calculation should have another health care professional double-check the calculation before the administration of medication.

✱ Apply Your Knowledge 10.1

The following questions focus on what you have just learned about general dosage calculations.

MATCHING

Match the lettered terms to the numbered descriptions. The lettered terms may be used more than once.

DESCRIPTION

1. ____ The amount to be administered at one time
2. ____ The amount of drug in a dosage unit
3. ____ The volume of medication that contains a quantity of drug
4. ____ The volume of medication that contains the desired dose
5. ____ The total amount of ordered drug, along with the frequency it is to be administered
6. ____ The dose on hand per the dosage unit

TERM

a. Dosage unit
b. Dosage strength
c. Dosage ordered
d. Desired dose
e. Dose on hand
f. Amount to administer

DRUG DOSAGE CALCULATIONS

Calculate the drug dosages.

1. Ordered: cimetidine (Tagamet) 0.2 g PO qid

   On hand: Tagamet 400 mg is available

   How many tablet(s) would you administer per dose? _____

2. Ordered: methyldopa (Aldomet) 150 mg PO tid

   On hand: Aldomet 250 mg/5 mL is available

   How many milliliters would you administer per dose? _____

3. Ordered: lorazepam (Ativan) 1 mg PO tid

   On hand: Ativan 0.5 mg is available

   How many tablet(s) would you administer? _____

4. Ordered: clarithromycin (Biaxin) 100 mg PO qid

   On hand: Biaxin 125 mg/5 mL is available

   How many milliliters (mL) should the patient receive per dose? _____

CALCULATING ORAL DOSAGES

Oral medications are divided into solid types (such as tablets and capsules) and liquids. The **tablet** is the most common form of solid oral medication. Certain tablets are specially designed to be administered sublingually (under the tongue) or buccally (between the cheek and gum). Some tablets are chewable; others dissolve in water to make a liquid that the patient can drink. Always check the drug label to find out how a tablet is meant to be administered. **Capsules** are usually oval-shaped gelatin shells that contain medication in powder or granule form. Some tablets and capsules are available in sustained-release form. This allows increased duration of drug action and therefore the patient does not have to take as many doses of the drug.

Solid Doses

Tablets may be broken into parts only if they are **scored** (notched), and they must be broken only along the line of the scoring. Unscored tablets must *not* be broken into parts.

Before administering medication to a patient, you need to determine how many tablets or capsules will deliver the *desired dose*. If necessary, convert the *dosage ordered* to the *desired dose* by using the same unit of measurement as the dose on hand. Then, you can calculate the *amount to administer* by using the fraction proportion method.

$$\frac{\text{Dose on hand } (H)}{\text{Dosage unit } (Q)} = \frac{\text{Desired dose } (D)}{\text{Amount to administer}}$$

or

$$\text{Desired dose } (D) \times \frac{\text{Dosage unit } (Q)}{\text{Dose on hand } (H)}$$
$$= \text{Amount to administer}$$

Example 1

Ordered: Zocor 40-mg bid
On hand: Zocor 20-mg tablets
The dosage ordered is 40 mg, the dose on hand is 20 mg, and the dosage unit is 1 tablet. The units of the dosage ordered and the dose on hand are the same, so no conversion is needed. The desired dose is 40 mg.
Use the formula:

$$D \times \frac{Q}{H} = X$$

$$40 \text{ mg} \times \frac{1 \text{ tablet}}{20 \text{ mg}} = X$$

$$X = 2 \text{ tablets}$$

Example 2

Ordered: doxazosin mesylate 4 mg PO daily
The label is shown in Figure 10-1 ■. How many tablets will you administer to the patient?

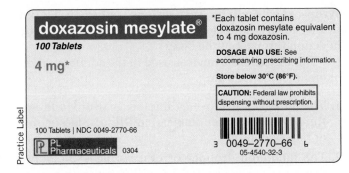

Figure 10-1 ■ Drug label for doxazosin mesylate.

Use this formula:

$$D \times \frac{Q}{H} = X$$

$$4 \text{ mg} \times \frac{1 \text{ tablet}}{4 \text{ mg}} = 1 \text{ tablet}$$

Example 3

Ordered: amlodipine besylate 5 mg PO daily
The label is shown in Figure 10-2 ■. How many tablets will you administer to the patient?
Use the formula:

$$D \times \frac{Q}{H} = X$$

$$5 \text{ mg} \times \frac{1}{2.5 \text{ mg}} = X$$

$$\frac{5}{2.5} = 2 \text{ tablets}$$

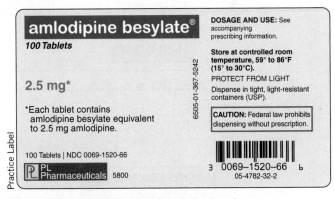

Figure 10-2 ■ Drug label for amlodipine besylate.

Liquid Doses

Liquid medications can be measured in small units of volume. Therefore, a greater range of doses can be ordered and administered. They are commonly used for children and elderly patients. Liquid medications can also be given via feeding tubes. Many medications are given as liquids, which are supplied initially as powders. Liquid preparations are drugs that have been dissolved or suspended. Examples of liquid drugs are

syrups, **spirits**, **elixirs**, **suspensions**, and so on. Liquid drugs can be administered systemically by mouth or by injection throughout the body.

Three measuring devices used in the administration of oral medications are:

1. The measuring cup—calibrated in fluid ounces, fluidrams, cubic centimeters, milliliters, teaspoons, or tablespoons

2. The medicine dropper or oral syringe—medicine droppers are calibrated in milliliters, minims, or drops, whereas oral syringes are usually calibrated in cubic centimeters

3. The calibrated spoon—usually calibrated in teaspoons and cubic centimeters

To calculate oral liquid doses, this formula can be used:

$$D \times \frac{H}{Q} = X$$

Example 1

The physician orders 400 mg of the antibiotic cefdinir (Omnicef). Figure 10-3 ■ shows the availability of the drug. Calculate how many milliliters you will administer. The label on the bottle indicates that 5 mL contains 125 mg of cefdinir. Therefore,

$$\frac{5 \text{ mL}}{125 \text{ mg}}$$

$$400 \times \frac{5}{125} = \frac{2,000}{125} = 16 \text{ mL}$$

Example 2

The pediatrician orders erythromycin 375 mg. Figure 10-4 ■ shows the availability of this drug. Calculate how many milliliters you will administer:

$$375 \times \frac{5 \text{ mL}}{200} = \frac{1,875}{200} = 9.375 \text{ mL} = 9.4 \text{ mL}$$

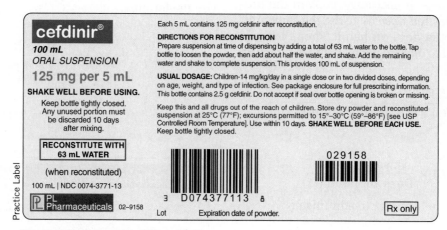

Figure 10-3 ■ Drug label for cefdinir.

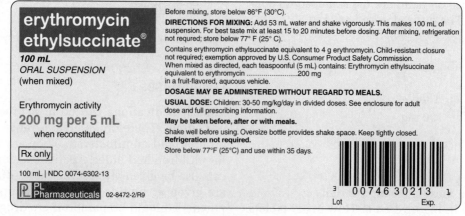

Figure 10-4 ■ Drug label for erythromycin ethylsuccinate.

Focus on Pediatrics

Administering Medicine to Young Children

Dosage cups are convenient for children who know how to drink from a cup without spilling, but for children who cannot drink from a cup, the following options are available:

- *Syringes* are convenient for infants who cannot drink from a cup. A parent can squirt the medicine into the back of the child's mouth, where it is less likely to spill out, or can measure out a dosage for a babysitter to use with the child later.

- *Droppers* are safe and easy to use with pediatric patients but must be measured at eye level and administered quickly to avoid losing any of the medication.

- *Cylindrical dosing spoons* have long handles that can be held easily by small children, with small cups that fit easily into their mouths.

Focus on Geriatrics

New Medication-Dispensing Systems Help Elderly Patients

Advances in communication and artificial intelligence are examples of the ways that medication-dispensing systems are improving care for elderly patients. Some systems help to manage home administration of complex, multiple-drug regimens by offering "smart" bottles arranged on a tray that alert the patient when it is time to take a medication. The bottles release the correct amount of medication doses and offer a self-locking feature to prevent accidental overdose. When supplies get low, the system alerts the pharmacist or caregiver. A complete record of all medications dispensed is retained by the system for future reference.

✳ Apply Your Knowledge 10.2

The following questions assess your knowledge about calculating oral drug doses.

LABELING

Calculate the drug dosages by using the labels shown.

1. Erythromycin (EryPed)
   245 mg = _____ mL

(continued)

Apply Your Knowledge 10.2 (continued)

2. Amlodipine (Norvasc)

   2.5 mg = _____ tab

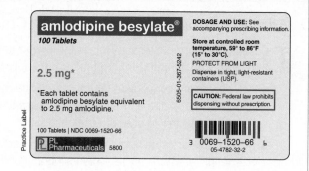

3. Simvastatin (Zocor)

   80 mg = _____ tab

4. Glipizide (Glucotrol XL)

   0.01 g = _____ tab

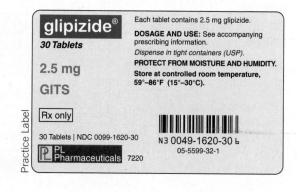

DRUG DOSAGE CALCULATIONS

Calculate the solid or liquid doses to be administered.

1. Ordered: nifedipine (Procardia) 20 mg PO tid

   On hand: Procardia 10 mg is available

   How many capsule(s) would you administer? _____

2. Ordered: levothyroxine (Synthroid) 0.3 mg PO daily

   On hand: Synthroid 0.15 mg is available

   How many tablet(s) would you administer? _____

3. Ordered: Keflex 500 mg PO bid

   On hand: Keflex 250 mg/5 mL

   How many milliliters would you administer per dose? _____

4. Ordered: Augmentin 1 g PO bid

   On hand: Augmentin 400 mg/5 mL is available

   How many milliliters would you administer per dose? _____

5. Ordered: Singulair 5 mg PO daily

   On hand: Singulair 5 mg is available

   How many tablet(s) would you administer per dose? _____

CALCULATING PARENTERAL MEDICATIONS

Injections are mixtures that contain the drug dissolved in an appropriate liquid. Medication can be administered by injection intradermally (within the skin), subcutaneously (into fatty tissue under the skin), intramuscularly (IM; into the muscle), and intravenously (IV; into the vein). Such **injectable** medications are prescribed in grams, milligrams, micrograms, grains, or units. The injectable drugs can be prepared in packages as solvents (diluents or solutions) or in powdered form. Drug solutions for injection are commercially premixed and stored in vials and ampules for immediate use.

Intradermal Injection

An intradermal injection is usually used for skin testing to diagnose the cause of an allergy or to determine the presence of a microorganism. The common syringe that is used for intradermal testing is the tuberculin syringe with a 25-gauge needle.

The inner portion of the forearm is usually used for diagnostic testing because there is less hair in that area and the test results are more visible. The upper back may also be used as a testing site. Test results are read 48–72 hours after the intradermal injection. A reddened or raised area is a positive reaction.

Subcutaneous Injection

Drugs injected into the subcutaneous tissue are absorbed slowly because there are fewer blood vessels in fatty tissue. The amount of drug solution administered subcutaneously is generally 0.5–1 mL at a 45-degree angle.

The two types of syringes used for subcutaneous injections are the tuberculin syringe (1 mL), calibrated in 0.1-mL and 0.01-mL increments, and the 3-mL syringe, calibrated in 0.1-mL increments. To calculate dosages for subcutaneous or IM injections, use the basic formula of $D/H \times V$, or the ratio and proportion method. Heparin is a drug commonly administered subcutaneously.

Medications given by IM injection are absorbed more rapidly than those given by subcutaneous injection. The volume of solution for IM injections is 0.5–3.0 mL. For calculating IM doses, the following examples can be used:

Example 1

Ordered: gentamicin 60 mg IM

On hand: gentamicin is available 80 mg/2 mL in a vial

To calculate, use this formula:

$$\frac{D}{H} \times V = \frac{60}{80} \times 2 = \frac{120}{80} = 1.5 \text{ mL}$$

or

$$H:V :: D:V$$

$$80 \text{ mg}:2 \text{ mL} :: 60 \text{ mg}:X \text{ mL}$$

$$80X = 120$$

$$X = \frac{120}{80} = 1.5 \text{ mL}$$

Example 2

Ordered: atropine 0.2 mg subcutaneously stat

On hand: atropine 400 mcg/mL (0.4 mg/mL)

By using the same formula, you can calculate the amount of atropine to be given.

$$\frac{D}{H} \times V = \frac{0.2 \text{ mg}}{0.4 \text{ g}} \times 1 \text{ mL} = \frac{0.2}{0.4} \times 1 = 0.5 \text{ mL}$$

Insulin Injection

Insulin is a pancreatic hormone that stimulates glucose metabolism. Patients who have insulin-dependent diabetes often need regular injections of insulin to keep their blood glucose from rising to levels that could be life-threatening. These regular injections must be rotated to various sites of the body to prevent scarring of the tissue at a single injection site. Different forms of insulin are available, and insulin may be administered several ways depending on the form. These ways include subcutaneous injections, IV administration, and continuous administration through an insulin pump.

There are four types of insulin: (1) rapid-acting, (2) short-acting, (3) intermediate-acting, and (4) long-acting types. (See Chapter 32 for complete information on insulins.) Insulin is packaged in two ways: (1) vials containing 10 mL of solution with 100 units of insulin per milliliter and (2) prepackaged syringes that contain smaller amounts of insulin. In the United States, insulin is usually standardized to 100 units/mL. Insulin vials can combine NPH (neutral protamine Hagedorn; Humulin N) and regular insulin (Humulin R, Novolin R) in one solution. The most common is 70/30, but 50/50 is also available (Figure 10-5 ■). It is important to always use *insulin syringes* to administer insulin and no other types of syringes.

The three types of insulin syringes are: (1) 100-unit syringes, (2) 50-unit syringes, and (3) 30-unit syringes (Figure 10-6 ■)

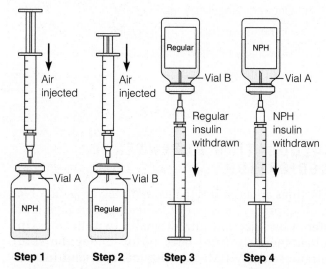

Figure 10-5 ■ Mixing regular and NPH (neutral protamine Hagedorn) insulins in one syringe.

Figure 10-6 ■ Insulin syringes: 100 unit **(A)**, 50 unit **(B)**, and 30 unit **(C)**.

Focus Point

Preparing Insulin Injections

For more accurate measurements, use a 30-unit insulin syringe for insulin doses less than 30 units and a 50-unit insulin syringe for insulin doses less than 50 units if a standard 100-unit syringe is not available. To successfully remove insulin from a vial for injection, first draw up the same quantity of air as the ordered insulin volume before withdrawing the appropriate insulin quantity. If the physician orders two types of insulin to be administered, they may be combined in one syringe to allow for one injection. Draw up the shorter-acting insulin first.

The size of the syringe depends on the size of the dose to be administered. For example, if you needed to give 18 units of regular insulin and 11 units of NPH insulin, you would select a 30-unit syringe. Similarly, if you needed 35 units of regular and 40 units of NPH, you would select a 100-unit syringe to administer these larger unit sizes. The smallest-size syringe that will contain the number of units required is best because it is easier to see the unit markings on the syringe.

Figure 10-7 ■ Tuberculin syringe.

Example 2

Figure 10-8 ■ shows a 100-unit insulin syringe. In this type of syringe, 100 units is equivalent to 1 mL. Each measurement line on the syringe measures 2 units, or 0.02 mL.

Figure 10-8 ■ 100-unit insulin syringe.

Example 3

Figure 10-9 ■ shows a 50-unit insulin syringe. In this type of syringe, each measurement line only measures 1 unit, or 0.01 mL.

Figure 10-9 ■ 50-unit insulin syringe.

Example 4

Figure 10-10 ■ shows a 30-unit insulin syringe, also known as a "Lo-Dose syringe." In this type of syringe, the measurement lines are the same as in the 50-unit insulin syringe, measuring just 1 unit, or 0.01 mL.

Example 1

Find how much liquid is in the tuberculin syringe in Figure 10-7 ■.

You can see that the top ring of the plunger is even with one line above 0.60 mL. Each marking line represents 0.01 mL, so the amount of liquid in this syringe is 0.61 mL.

Figure 10-10 ■ 30-unit insulin syringe.

Example 5

Figure 10-11 ■ shows a partially filled 50-unit insulin syringe. You can see that the top ring of the plunger is even with three lines above the number 25. Because each line represents 1 unit, this syringe contains 28 units of liquid.

Figure 10-11 ■ A partially filled 50-unit insulin syringe.

Example 6

Figure 10-12 ■ shows a partially filled 100-unit insulin syringe. You can see that the top ring of the plunger is even with one line above 70. Because each line represents 2 units, this syringe contains 72 units of liquid.

Figure 10-12 ■ A partially filled 100-unit insulin syringe.

Focus Point

Safe Insulin Practices

Avoid keeping insulin on top of medication carts or counters or under pharmacy compounding hoods because it could be confused with heparin (which is also measured in units). Immediately return insulin to the proper storage area after use. If insulin concentration is not 100 units/mL, apply *bold warning labels* to alert the user about the concentration. Always use single standard concentration for all adult IV insulin infusions. Prescribers should order insulin cartridges for outpatients to help ensure correct dispensing.

Heparin Calculation

The anticoagulant heparin is measured in USP (United States Pharmacopoeia) units. It is given to patients to reduce or prevent the blood from clotting. Heparin can be administered to a patient by subcutaneous injection or IV injection.

The abbreviation *U* should be avoided in practice to prevent medication errors. Vials of heparin are prepared by the manufacturer in a variety of strengths. The vials come in 1,000-unit, 5,000-unit, 20,000-unit, and 40,000-unit sizes. Ampules are supplied in 1,000-unit, 5,000-unit, and 10,000-unit sizes.

Heparin is also available in premixed IV solutions—for example, 12,500 units in 250 mL of 5% dextrose in water (D_5W); or 25,000 units in 500 mL of 0.45% saline solution. With a premixed parenteral solution, you have to convert the physician's order to the volume of solution that contains the amount of heparin ordered.

Example 1

Ordered: heparin 5,000 units subcutaneously q8h
On hand: heparin is available as 10,000 units/mL
You need to convert units to milliliters.

$$10,000 \text{ units} = 1 \text{ mL} = 5,000 \text{ units}:X \text{ mL}$$

$$10,000 \, X = 5,000$$

$$X = \frac{5,000}{10,000} = \frac{1}{2} = 0.5 \text{ mL}$$

Example 2

Ordered: 1,000 mL of D_5W containing 20,000 units of heparin, which is to be infused at 30 mL/h
How much heparin should be given to the patient per hour?

$$20,000 \text{ units}:1,000 \text{ mL} = X \text{ units}:30 \text{ mL}$$

$$1,000 \, X = 20,000 \times 30$$

$$\frac{1,000 \, X}{1,000} = \frac{600,000}{1,000}$$

$$X = 600 \text{ units/h}$$

Intravenous Calculation

IV fluid therapy is used to administer fluids that contain water, dextrose, vitamins, electrolytes, and drugs. Medications for IV administration are usually available in small-volume vials that are mixed in a large-volume solution by the pharmacist before administration to the patient. The drug added to a parenteral solution is often available in a solution. Therefore, the additive amount is calculated in terms of volume—usually in milliliters.

The amount of drug in a parenteral solution is clearly stated on the label, but the pharmacist must be careful to notice whether the amount is given in terms of concentration (e.g., 5 mg/mL) or amount of drug in the vial (e.g., 80 mg in a 2-mL vial). The concentration is used to calculate the correct volume to be mixed with a parenteral diluent to produce the prescribed dose.

IV fluids and drugs may be administered by intermittent or continuous IV infusion. Intermittent IV infusion, such as IV piggyback and IV push infusions, are used for IV administration of drugs and supplement fluids. Continuous IV infusions are used to replace fluid or to help maintain fluid levels and electrolyte balance and to serve as vehicles for drug administration. Detailed discussions of IV solutions, equipment, and calculations are not suitable for this pharmacology book. Therefore, for more information, it is advisable to refer to a pharmaceutical calculations textbook.

✱ Apply Your **Knowledge** 10.3

The following questions assess your knowledge of calculating doses of parenteral medications.

LABELING

Answer the drug labeling questions by using the labels depicted below.

1. What is the usual daily adult dose of hydroxyzine pamoate? _____

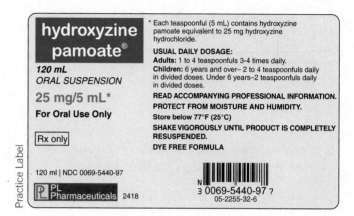

2. How many milligrams of ritonavir are contained in this package? _____

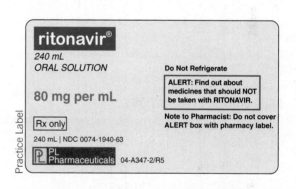

3. How many milligrams of indomethacin are there in 2.5 mL of solution? _____

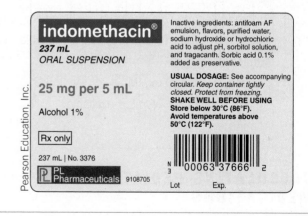

(continued)

Apply Your Knowledge 10.3 (*continued*)

4. How many milliliters of zidovudine are needed for a 150-mg dose? _____

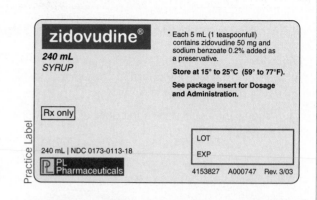

5. If only half the indomethacin suspension was used, how many milliliters would be left? _____

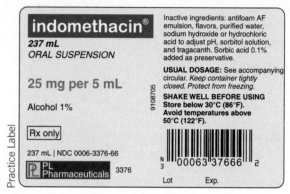

DRUG DOSAGE CALCULATIONS

Calculate the amount of medications you should administer.

1. Ordered: Humulin R U-500 insulin in 80 units

   Administer: _____

2. Ordered: 150 units Humulin R, IV stat

   Administer: _____

3. Ordered: Heparin 5,000 units subcutaneously q8h

   On hand: Heparin 10,000 units/mL is available

   Administer: _____

4. Ordered: Valium 10 mg IM

   On hand: Valium 5 mg/mL is available

   Administer: _____

5. Ordered: Lidocaine 25 mg subcutaneously

   On hand: Lidocaine 5% solution

   Administer: _____

6. Ordered: Lanoxin 300 mcg IM stat

   On hand: Lanoxin (digoxin) 500 mcg in 2 mL

   Administer: _____

7. Ordered: Zantac 50 mg IM qid

   On hand: Zantac 25 mg/mL

   Administer: _____

CALCULATING PEDIATRIC MEDICATIONS

The pediatrician must determine the proper kind and amount of medication for a child. Dosages for infants and children are usually less than the adult dosages for the same medication. The body mass in children is smaller, and their metabolism is different from that of adults. Therefore, dosage calculations for pediatric patients (infants or children) must be precise.

For many years, pediatric dosage calculations used such pediatric formulas as Clark's rule, Young's rule, or Fried's rule (see page 144). These formulas are based on the weight of the child in pounds or on the age of the child in months, and they aid in determining how much medication should be prescribed for a particular child.

Today, the most accurate methods of determining an appropriate pediatric dose are by weight and body area. You must know whether the amount of a prescribed pediatric dosage is the safe or appropriate amount for a particular patient. If this information is not on the drug label, it can be found on the package insert, in the *Physician's Desk Reference* (*PDR*), on a hospital formulary, in the *United States Pharmacopoeia*, or in pharmacology texts.

Focus Point

Questions to Ask When a Child Is Prescribed Medication

Encourage parents or caregivers of children to ask their physician the following questions:

- What is the drug, and what is it used for?
- Will it cause a problem with other drugs my child is taking?
- How often and for how many days or weeks should I give my child this medicine?
- What if I miss giving my child a dose?
- How soon will the drug start working?
- What side effects does it have, and what should I do if my child has any of these side effects?
- Should I stop giving the medicine when my child gets better?
- Is there a less expensive generic version I can use?

Drug Dosage Calculation by Body Surface Area

BSA is determined by using a **nomogram** (a numerical relationship chart) and the child's height and weight. This is considered to be the most accurate method of calculating a child's dose. Standard nomograms give a child's BSA according to weight and height (Figure 10-13 ■).

The calculation formula is the ratio of the child's BSA to the surface area of an average adult (1.7 square meters, or 1.7 m²) multiplied by the normal adult dose of the drug:

Example 1

$$\text{Child's dose} = \frac{\text{Surface area of child (m}^2)}{1.7 \text{ m}^2} \times \text{Normal adult dose}$$

A child who weighs 12 kg and is 60 cm tall has a BSA of 0.4 m². Therefore, a child's dose of ampicillin that corresponds to an adult dose of 250 mg would be:

$$\text{Child's dose} = \frac{0.4 \text{ m}^2}{1.7 \text{ m}^2} \times 250 \text{ mg} = 0.23 \times 250$$
$$= 58.32 \text{ mg}$$

Example 2

The pediatrician ordered: digoxin 0.64 mg/m² PO daily The child's BSA is 0.9 m². How many milligrams would you administer to this child as a loading dose?

First, you need to convert BSA to dose in milligrams:

$$0.9 \text{ m}^2 = X \text{ mg}$$

$$0.9 \text{ m}^2 \times \frac{? \text{ mg}}{? \text{ m}^2} = X \text{ mg}$$

Figure 10-13 ■ Pediatric nomogram used for determining body surface area.

Because 0.64 mg = 1 m², the equivalent fraction is:

$$\frac{0.64 \text{ mg}}{1 \text{ m}^2}$$

You then cancel the square meters and obtain the dose in milligrams.

$$0.9 \text{ m}^2 \times \frac{0.64 \text{ mg}}{1 \text{ m}^2} = 0.576 \text{ mg or } 0.58 \text{ mg}$$

Therefore, the child should receive 0.58 mg of digoxin.

Drug Dosage Calculation by Body Weight

Drug manufacturers sometimes recommend a dosage based on the weight of the child. This method uses a specific number of milligrams, micrograms, or units for each kilogram of body weight (mg/kg, mcg/kg, and units/kg, respectively). Usually, drug data for pediatric dosage (mg/kg) is supplied by manufacturers in a drug information insert.

Example
Ordered: amoxicillin 60 mg PO tid
On hand: 125 mg/5 mL
Child's weight: 12-1/2 lb
   To calculate, first change pounds to kilograms.

$$\frac{12.5 \text{ lb}}{2.2 \text{ kg}} = 5.7 \text{ kg}$$

The pediatric dosage for a child who weighs 20 kg is 20–40 mg/kg/day in three equal doses.

$$20 \text{ mg/kg/day} \times 5.7 \text{ kg} = 114 \text{ mg/day}$$

$$40 \text{ mg/kg/day} \times 5.7 \text{ kg} = 228 \text{ mg/day}$$

$$60 \text{ mg} \times 3 = 180 \text{ mg}$$

Because 180 mg falls within the recommended daily dose range for amoxicillin, it is considered a safe dose.

CLARK'S RULE
Clark's rule is based on the weight of the child, which is much more accurate than Young's or Fried's rules.

Clark's rule uses average adult weight (usually considered to be 150 lb or 70 kg) and assumes that the child's dose is proportionately less. To calculate pediatric dose by Clark's rule, use the following formula.

Example
Calculate the dose of cortisone for a 42-lb child (adult dose = 100 mg).

$$\text{Pediatric dose} = \frac{\text{Child's weight in lb}}{150 \text{ lb}} \times \text{Adult dose}$$

$$\frac{42 \text{ lb}}{150 \text{ lb}} \times 100 \text{ mg} = 28 \text{ mg}$$

YOUNG'S RULE
Young's rule is used for children older than 1 year of age.

Example

$$\text{Pediatric dose} = \frac{\text{Child's age in years}}{\text{Child's age in years} + 12} \times \text{Adult dose}$$

Calculate the dose of Tylenol for a 5-year-old child (adult dose + 1,000 mg):

$$\frac{5 \text{ years}}{5 \text{ years} + 12} \times 1,000 \text{ mg} = 294 \text{ mg}$$

FRIED'S RULE
Fried's rule is a method of estimating the dose of medication for infants younger than 1 year of age.

$$\frac{\text{Child's age in months}}{150 \text{ lb}} \times \text{Average adult dose}$$

Example
Calculate the dose of phenobarbital for an 8-month-old infant (adult dose = 400 mg).

$$\frac{8 \text{ mo}}{150 \text{ lb}} \times 400 \text{ mg} = 21 \text{ mg}$$

✷ Apply Your Knowledge 10.4

The following questions focus on what you have just learned about dosage calculations for pediatric patients.

MULTIPLE CHOICE

Choose the correct answer from choices a–d.

1. The most accurate methods of determining an appropriate pediatric dose are:

   a. Clark's rule and Young's rule

   b. Young's rule and Fried's rule

   c. By weight and body area

   d. By weight and Clark's rule

2. Which of the following methods of pediatric dosage calculations is used for children older than 1 year of age?

   a. Clark's rule

   b. Fried's rule

   c. Freud's rule

   d. Young's rule

3. Body surface area is determined by using the child's height and weight and a:

   a. Nomogram

   b. Sonogram

   c. Child's dose of a similar medication

   d. Loading dose

4. Drug manufacturers sometimes recommend doses based on the:

   a. Height of the child

   b. Weight of the child's parents

   c. Usual daily dosage

   d. Weight of the child

5. Which of the following dosage calculation methods is the most accurate?

   a. Clark's rule

   b. Young's rule

   c. Fried's rule

   d. The child's height

DO THE MATH

Convert these weights (in pounds) to kilograms.

1. 55 lb = _____

2. 11 lb = _____

3. 157 lb = _____

4. 18 lb = _____

5. 209 lb = _____

6. 27 lb = _____

7. 93 lb = _____

8. 135 lb = _____

PRACTICAL SCENARIO 1

A physician orders a medication in the amount of 250 mg per 5 mL for a patient's upper respiratory tract infection. Before dispensing the medication, the medical assistant calculated the amount of medication required as 125 mg/mL. This would have meant the patient might have received 625 mg/5 mL instead of what the physician ordered. A second person in the medical office checked the calculation and found the error before administration. Therefore, it is essential for allied health care professionals to accurately calculate dose calculations and always consult another coworker or physician to verify accuracy.

Keith Brofsky/Photodisc/Getty Images

Critical Thinking Questions

1. What is the formula the medical assistant should have used to calculate the proper dose?
2. Besides checking that the dose calculation was right, what other "rights" does the assistant need to check?

PRACTICAL SCENARIO 2

A physician ordered Keflex 500 mg PO bid. A pharmacy technician has Keflex 250 mg per mL.

Robert Kneschke/Shutterstock

Critical Thinking Questions

1. If the pharmacy technician wants to dispense this medication, how many milliliters will be needed to contain each required dose?
2. How many milliliters should the patient receive per day?

Chapter Capsule

This section repeats the objectives from the beginning of the chapter and then provides a summary of the most important concepts for that objective. Use this section as a quick review and to check your knowledge.

Objective 1: Discuss the differences between dosage ordered, desired dose, and dose on hand.

- Dosage ordered: total amount ordered and its frequency of administration
- Desired dose: amount to be administered at one time
- Dose on hand: amount of drug in a dosage unit

Objective 2: Explain how to use the formula $D/H \times Q = X$ to calculate drug doses.

- D = desired dose
- H = dose available
- D and H: must always be in the same unit of measure

- ■ Q = number of tablets, milliliters, or other units that contain H
- ■ X = number of capsules, minims, or other units that D will be contained in (also known as the "amount to be administered")

Objective 3: Explain the fraction proportion method and the formula used in this method.

- ■ The fraction proportion method uses the dose on hand (H), dosage unit (Q), desired dose (D), and amount to administer to calculate doses. The formula that is used in this method is:

$$\frac{\text{Dose on hand } (H)}{\text{Dosage unit } (Q)} = \frac{\text{Desired dose } (D)}{\text{Amount to administer}}$$

This can also be expressed in this formula:

$$\text{Desired dose } (D) \times \frac{\text{Dosage unit } (Q)}{\text{Dose on hand } (H)} = \text{Amount to administer}$$

Objective 4: Discuss how to calculate parenteral medications and the formula used.

- ■ For parenteral medications, a drug is dissolved in an appropriate liquid. These medications are commonly prescribed in grams, milligrams, micrograms, grains, or units. To calculate parenteral medications, use this formula:

$$\frac{\text{Desired dose } (D)}{\text{Dose on hand } (H)} \times \text{Volume of parenteral solution } (V)$$

Objective 5: Calculate intramuscular doses.

- ■ $D/H \times V = X$
- ■ Or: $H{:}V :: D{:}X$

Objective 6: Name the most common types of insulin used in the United States.

- ■ Rapid-acting insulin
- ■ Short-acting insulin
- ■ Intermediate-acting insulin
- ■ Long-acting insulin

Objective 7: Explain the steps required for the proper injection of insulin.

- ■ Step 1: Inject the same quantity of air as the ordered insulin volume into the vial.
- ■ Step 2: Withdraw the appropriate quantity of insulin.
- ■ Step 3: Draw up the shorter-acting insulin first if using two types of insulin.
- ■ Step 4: Inject the insulin per the physician's instructions.

Objective 8: Convert physician orders of heparin to the volume of solution that contains the amount of heparin ordered.

- ■ If required, convert units to milliliters: 10,000 units = 1 mL
- ■ Then, use this formula: X mL = ordered units/available units
- ■ Or: 10,000 units:1 mL :: ordered units: X mL

Objective 9: Calculate whether the amount of a prescribed pediatric dosage is the safe or appropriate amount for a particular patient.

- For the calculation, use either the child's weight or body area
- To find safe pediatric dosages, check drug labels, package inserts, the *PDR*, hospital formularies, the *USP*, or pharmacology texts

Objective 10: Define the most accurate method of calculating a child's dose and perform correct calculations by using this method.

- Most accurate method is the body surface area (BSA) method
  - To find the child's body surface area, use a nomogram, which compares the child's weight and height
- Use this formula:
  - Child's dose = m^2 (child's BSA) ÷ $1.7\ m^2$ × normal adult dose

Internet Sites of Interest

- *Diabetes Health* magazine presents an article at **www.diabeteshealth.com** that discusses errors in calculation of insulin dosage by adolescents and the impact of using an insulin dosage calculator (IDC). Search "insulin dosage calculator adolescents."
- Calculators for math, including equations and formulas: **www.rncalc.com**
- Targeted to medical assistants' needs, the Medical Office Pharmacology Review for Medical Assistant Students and Professionals website at **www.mapharm.com/dosage_calc.htm** provides an overview of dosage calculations.
- A discussion about the need to correctly split pills in order for safe dosing: **www.webmd.com/a-to-z-guides/features/pill-splitting-when-is-it-safe-when-is-it-unsafe**
- Prescription Drug Info offers dosages for regular insulin: **www.medschat.com/drugs/regular-insulin**
- Safe pediatric dosage and examples: **www.drugguide.com/ddo/ub/view/Davis-Drug-Guide/109514/0/Pediatric_Dosage_Calculations**

Chapter 11

Medication Errors and Prevention

Chapter Objectives

After completing this chapter, you should be able to:

1. Explain why errors can occur in three stages in the medication process.
2. Describe factors that cause medication errors.
3. Explain general recommendations to reduce medication errors.
4. Describe the legal and ethical responsibility of health care professionals to report all medication errors.
5. Explain the role of the Food and Drug Administration in medication errors.
6. Describe the role of The Joint Commission in preventing medication errors.
7. Explain the steps that may be taken to avoid medication errors and ensure safe administration of medication.
8. Define *polypharmacy*.
9. Describe why medication reconciliation is important.
10. Explain the importance of patient education concerning medications.

Key Terms

medication error (p. 150)

medication reconciliation (p. 155)

polypharmacy (p. 154)

risk management departments (p. 154)

root cause analysis (RCA) (p. 152)

sentinel events (p. 153)

Introduction

Medication errors occur in small and large communities across the United States. Tens of thousands of Americans die each year from various medical errors while they are receiving care. Errors in quality of care by physicians, nurses, pharmacists, and other allied health professionals routinely harm patients, causing disability, permanent damage, and even death. A system of true quality would greatly help to prevent these occurrences. The current system does not make the best use of its resources. On a daily basis, medical errors, medication errors, lack of access to clinical information, duplication of services, delays, and overuse of medications and natural supplements all combine to increase the risks of patient harm. All health care professionals must take their responsibilities seriously in order to help prevent medical and medication errors. Also, patients and their families must be educated about potential errors that can happen at home and take steps to reduce or prevent these errors.

Medication Errors

A **medication error** is the inappropriate or incorrect administration of a drug that should be preventable through effective system controls involving physicians, pharmacists, nurses, risk management personnel, legal counsel, administrators, and patients. Medication errors can occur because of manufacturing mistakes. Thousands of medication errors occur each year in hospitals throughout the United States. These errors often result in pain, injury, and even death. According to the Institute of Medicine (IOM), medical errors have caused up to 98,000 deaths annually in the United States. The IOM suggests that this should be considered a national epidemic. Another study conducted by HealthGrades has shown as many as 195,000 deaths per year in American hospitals because of preventable medical errors.[1]

Medication errors usually occur more frequently than they are reported and are the result of either human error or a flawed system within a health care facility. Errors can occur in three stages within the medication process:

1. *The first stage involves prescribing or ordering medication.* During this stage, physicians or other persons prescribing the medication may be distracted or interrupted and as a result provide incomplete orders—greatly increasing the risk of errors. Medication errors are most prevalent when choosing a medication, its dosage, and the schedule.

2. *The second stage is when the medication is dispensed to patients or consumers.* Dispensing errors can occur as a result of insufficient or inexperienced staffing and a lack of adequate time for patient counseling and can lead to confusion about how to take the medication or how to assist the patient in taking it. It is an extremely important and effective practice for all health-care professionals to double-check medications against the medication administration record (MAR). This practice helps those who are dispensing the medication to catch errors before medications are dispensed.

3. *The third stage is when the medication is administered and monitored for side effects.* At this stage, medication administration errors are most commonly attributed to nurses or others who are legally allowed to handle administration. Those who administer medications may be accountable for medication errors that can be attributed to poor communication or misread prescriptions, orders, or drug labels. Other factors that contribute to errors include similar labeling and packaging of products and medications with similar names (see Appendix C for a list of medications with similar-sounding names). After administering medication, health care professionals must also ensure that the patient does not have a reaction to the medication.

The most common error is dosage; errors also often involve antibiotics and analgesics. For example, a community pharmacist misreads a handwritten prescription for 10 mg of Metadate ER and instead dispenses 10 mg of methadone for a 7-year-old boy. Fortunately, the boy's mother reads the information that accompanies the prescription and realizes the error.

A medication error may occur when dealing with outpatients because of the increasing number of prescriptions in the United States and because pharmacists do not adequately counsel patients. In addition, there is a shortage of pharmacists and pharmacy technicians, which contributes to medication errors. Increased usage of over-the-counter (OTC) drugs and herbals and the availability of drugs through the Internet also cause medication errors.

A medication error must be reported as soon as it is noticed, and the patient must be monitored to see if

Focus Point

Medication Errors

Factors that may result in medication errors include handwriting misinterpretation, verbal or phone order misunderstandings, inaccurate administrations, and miscalculations.

any undesirable effect or injury from the medication develops. Medication errors must be documented in the medical record with the signature of the individual who made the error. If allied health professionals who are involved with prescribing, dispensing, or administering medication follow the seven rights of medication administration (see Chapter 7) and adhere to dispensing guidelines, medication errors should not occur.

Causes of Medication Errors

A number of factors cause medication errors, including:

* Use of incorrect abbreviations: Many abbreviations may be mistaken for different units and different dosages

* Miscommunication: Poor handwriting, similar drug names, dosing unit confusion

* Missing information: Lack of patient information, such as allergies, diseases, drug history, laboratory information, and drug information or warnings

* Lack of appropriate labeling: By the manufacturer or the pharmacist

* Environmental factors: Noise, lighting, stress, and fatigue affecting health care providers

* Poor management: Unhealthy health care facility culture

Medication errors may occur in such inpatient settings as hospitals and nursing homes or in such outpatient settings as physicians' offices or clinics. They can also happen during the manufacturing process and include errors in formulation, packaging, labeling, and distribution. They may be the result of undiscovered toxicity. Medication errors are preventable and are the single largest source of all medical errors.

Medication errors may occur as a result of the following:

* Wrong patient
* Incorrect route
* Incorrect drug
* Incorrect dose
* Incorrect time
* Incorrect technique
* Incorrect information on the patient chart

Focus Point

Medical Errors During the Prescribing Process

The three most common forms of prescribing errors include dosing errors, prescribing medications to which the patient has had an allergic response, and errors involving the prescribing of inappropriate dosage forms.

Focus Point

Administering Medications

Nurses and medical assistants must be extremely knowledgeable when administering medications in the physician's office. Follow all physician orders exactly as written. If unsure about an order, ask for clarification before proceeding. Administer a medication only after the order is written in the patient's chart. This helps eliminate errors and possible omissions in medication therapy. Always implement the seven rights and perform three drug order and label checks when dispensing and administering medications.

Results of Medication Errors

Medication errors may occur anywhere, at any time. In hospitals, medication errors are the most common causes of morbidity and preventable death. Medication errors affect not only patients but also their families and responsible health care professionals. Medication errors may result in extended stays in the hospital, higher costs, and increased separation from family and normal activities. Each health care professional involved in medication errors may experience serious emotional trauma because of his or her responsibility for the patient's welfare. High error rates can seriously harm the representations of health care staff members and entire facilities. Financial penalties may be assessed, and legal cases may result.

The goal of every health care facility should be to reduce medication errors to the lowest number possible.

✳ Apply Your **Knowledge 11.1**

The following questions focus on what you have just learned about medication errors.

CRITICAL THINKING

1. Define the term *medication errors*.
2. Describe what most medication errors involve.
3. Identify how the Internet may cause medication errors.
4. Explain the risk factors for medication errors.
5. Describe when medication errors can occur.

Each error should be thoroughly investigated and documented. This can help greatly in the prevention of future errors. Investigations should be conducted so they encourage the correct reporting of what occurred and not under threat of penalties. After error patterns have been identified, steps can be taken to eradicate activities that lead to the error occurring.

Documentation of Medication Errors

Documentation of medication errors should be clear and factual, following the facility's policies and procedures guidelines. Blame and judgment should be put aside with the goal being to determine the causes of the error so they can be eradicated in the future. Documentation of medication errors must include the interventions that were undertaken to counteract the error. The patient's medical record should be updated with complete information about the error. If the patient is hospitalized, the MAR should also be fully updated.

After updating the specific records about a medication error, the person who made the error or the person who observed its occurrence should complete a separate written report (often called an "incident report" or "occurrence report"). A factual, objective recording of the specific details of the error should be assembled. These reports are used by risk management personnel for quality improvement and assurance.

For legal reasons, accurate documentation in a medical record and in an error report is required. These documents help to improve medication administration processes and verify that patient safety was protected. If there is any attempt to delay corrective action or to hide a mistake, the legal ramifications may be much more severe. This is also true if interventions are not documented in the patient's chart.

Quality and improvement programs are used by hospitals and other health care facilities to monitor medication errors. These may alert practitioners about trends in medication errors and help to create specific solutions. Many facilities use **root cause analysis (RCA)** to prevent future mistakes, asking exactly what happened, why it happened, and what can be done to prevent its recurrence. RCA may also be used to determine whether risk of recurrence has actually been reduced.

Reporting Medication Errors

It is the legal and ethical responsibility of staff members to report all occurrences of medication errors. Patients who were harmed seriously enough may have had to undergo lifesaving interventions and may need follow-up supervision and treatments. At the federal level, the Food and Drug Administration (FDA) coordinates the reporting of medication errors by using its MedWatch program. Also known as the FDA Safety Information and Adverse Event Reporting Program, MedWatch provides timely information that is clinically important regarding medical products. This includes information about safety issues for prescription drugs, OTC drugs, biologics, medical devices, radiation-emitting devices, and special nutritional products. Health care professionals are encouraged to use the MedWatch database to report medication errors and situations that may lead to errors. This reporting may be done anonymously, directly to the FDA, either by the Internet or telephone. MedWatch may be contacted at www.fda.gov/Safety/MedWatch/default.htm or by calling (800) 332-1088.

The National Coordinating Council for Medication Error Reporting and Prevention (NCC MERP) provides assistance with medication errors. This organization has helped to standardize the medication error reporting system. The NCC MERP coordinates medication error information and provides preventive education. They may be contacted at www.nccmerp.org/home or (800) 233-7767.

The Institute for Safe Medication Practices (ISMP) publishes *Safe Medicine*, a consumer newsletter about medication errors. The ISMP accepts consumer and health care professional reports that relate to medication safety. The ISMP may be contacted at www .ismp.org/newsletters/consumer/default.aspx. The U.S. Pharmacopeia's MEDMARX medication error reporting program is used by hospitals. Contact www .medmarx.com.

The Joint Commission (TJC) has established patient safety standards that address many significant patient safety issues. These include patient safety programs; management practices that focus on safety; and regular analysis of the ordering, preparation, and dispensing of medications. The Joint Commission requires that hospitals inform patients when they have been harmed because of hospital errors. Continually attempting to standardize practices in hospitals nationwide, The Joint Commission has established National Patient Safety Goals (NPSGs). Because of their efforts, the use of bar coding for medication administration is now standard in all hospitals. The Joint Commission's website is www .jointcommission.org.

Sentinel Events

Sentinel events are unexpected occurrences involving death or serious physical or psychological injury or risk thereof. They are recognized by The Joint Commission and are always investigated so interventions may be used to ensure zero recurrence. RCA is used to identify causes and the needed type of intervention.

Focus Point

Over-the-Counter Drugs

Patient use of OTC drugs and herbal substances may cause adverse reactions and medication errors.

✳ Apply Your Knowledge 11.2

The following questions focus on what you have just learned about reporting and documenting medication errors.

CRITICAL THINKING

1. Explain why each medication error must be thoroughly investigated and documented.
2. Identify the federal agency that coordinates the reporting of medication errors.
3. Briefly explain the MedWatch program.
4. Explain which organization assists in standardizing the medication error reporting system.
5. Identify the advantages of documenting medication errors.

Reducing and Preventing Medication Errors

Medication errors may relate to professional practice, health care products, procedures, and systems. The following statements are guidelines for communication, education, and policy to assist in decreasing the rate of medication errors. To reduce medication errors, general recommendations include:

✳ Using an adequate number of allied health staff (nurses, medical assistants, and pharmacy technicians) who are trained to prepare, dispense, and administer medications to patients

✳ Using standardized measurement systems for both inpatients and outpatients

✳ Using prospective error-tracking systems that are run on a consistent basis to target and monitor common patient errors

✳ Clearly defining a system for drug administration, ordering, and dispensing that includes reviews of original drug orders

✳ Compiling medication profiles for inpatients, outpatients, and ambulatory patients with updated allergy histories after each encounter

✳ Providing suitable work environments for safe, effective drug preparation

✳ Electronic medical records and e-prescribing offer automatic surveillance measures that seek out potential medication errors, especially when information is lacking or conflicting with other information.

REDUCING ERRORS IN HEALTH CARE FACILITIES

In many health care facilities, medications are stored in locked, automated, and computerized cabinets. Each nurse is given a specific code for accessing these cabinets. Automation allows the cabinets to maintain an accurate inventory of medication supplies. In larger facilities, **risk management departments** are used to minimize medication errors and examine risks that may cause them. Risk management specialists track data, investigate incidents, identify problems, and provide recommendations to help improve the accuracy of patient care. Collaboration between nurses and risk management specialists helps to modify the facility's policies and procedures. Errors can be reduced by a variety of methods, including correct storage of medications, avoiding use of expired medications, avoiding transfer of medications between containers, avoiding overstocking, avoiding dangerous abbreviations, and keeping reference materials up to date.

Strategies for Handling Medication Errors

Many medication errors are related to certain populations such as children or older adults and types of health care facilities. Administering the wrong dosage or an incorrect drug and using the wrong route of administration are all common examples of medication errors. Since children receive dosages that are based on weight, they are more likely to experience medication errors than adults due to miscalculations. Also, older adults are at increased risk because **polypharmacy**, age-related physiological changes, and more than one physician are common factors. The following steps can help in avoiding medication errors and promoting safe administration of medications:

1. *Assessment:* asking patients about allergies, health condition, use of medications and herbal supplements in correct doses and routes—taken at the right times; educating the patient about all medications he or she needs; and assessing body system functions to determine if pharmacotherapy impairments exist.
2. *Planning:* avoiding abbreviations that can be misunderstood, questioning orders that are unclear, refusing verbal orders, and following all policies and procedures exactly. Patients should restate dosing directions, including dosage amounts, routes, and times. The patient should be asked to explain the goals of the medication therapy.
3. *Implementation:* eliminating distractions during medication administration (including noise, talking, and other events); ensuring that the right patient, time, frequency, dose, route, and drug are all exact; and identification verification, correct procedures and techniques, exact dose calculations, correct and timely opening of medications, correct documentation of procedures, confirmation (if an oral medication) that the patient has completely swallowed the dose, and double-checking for long-acting oral dosage forms.
4. *Evaluation:* assessing the patient for correct outcomes and determining any adverse effects.

There are nine various categories of medication errors, and health care professionals should be familiar with all of them. These categories are:

✳ Category A: circumstances or events that have the capacity to cause errors
✳ Category B: errors that occurred but did not reach the patient
✳ Category C: errors that reached the patient but did not cause any harm
✳ Category D: errors that occurred, reached the patient, and required monitoring to ensure no patient harm or that required intervention to prevent patient harm
✳ Category E: errors that occurred and may have contributed to or resulted in temporary harm to the patient (and required intervention)
✳ Category F: errors that occurred that might have contributed to or resulted in temporary harm to the patient (and required initial or prolonged hospitalization)
✳ Category G: errors that occurred that might have contributed to or resulted in permanent patient harm
✳ Category H: errors that occurred that required intervention necessary to sustain life
✳ Category I: errors that occurred that might have contributed to or resulted in the patient's death

Most types of medication errors involve administration of an improper dose (41%). Nearly half of fatal medication errors occur in patients older than 60 years of age (Figure 11-1 ■). As previously mentioned, this is likely because older adults often need many different medications, have multiple health care providers, or experience age-related physiologic changes. Children are also more likely to experience medication errors because doses are based on body weight, which increases the likelihood of calculation errors. Up-to-date drug information must be available so health care practitioners can verify correct data on the medications they are administering.

Focus on Geriatrics

Physiologic Changes Impact Medication Effects

The physiologic changes associated with aging include altered memory, poorer vision, decreased renal function, less complete and slower absorption from the gastrointestinal tract, and decreased liver function. These changes can increase the possibility of cumulative and possibly toxic effects of medications.

Figure 11-1 ■ Nearly half of fatal medication errors occur in patients older than 60 years of age.

Reconciling Medications

In older adults, multiple medications may be taken concurrently. *Polypharmacy* is defined as "receiving multiple medications, sometimes for the same condition, that have conflicting pharmacologic actions." Polypharmacy is most prevalent in the older age groups but may occur in all ages. It is hard to keep track of multiple medications and health care providers, but this is made even more difficult by poor medication information, documentation, and reporting.

Keeping track of a patient's medications as they change health care providers is called **medication reconciliation**. This involves accurately listing all medications a patient takes in order to reduce duplications, dosing errors, omissions, and drug interactions. When a patient is hospitalized, nurses document all medications previously being taken at home, including the dose, frequency, and route. This list is maintained and used whenever the patient is admitted to other facilities or transferred to different hospital units and is checked during the hospital discharge procedure. Many potential medication errors have been caught during medication reconciliation procedures. Medications being taken by a patient should be considered to include prescription medications, OTC medications, herbal supplements, and even vitamins.

The Joint Commission has identified many serious medication errors related to medication reconciliation and has developed recommendations for their prevention. The Joint Commission encourages hospitals to completely document all medications used by each patient during the admission process. Prescription medications, OTC medications, vitamins, and herbal supplements must all be documented. These patient medication lists must be communicated to all providers of service, both inside and outside the hospital. After a patient is discharged, he or she should receive a complete list of medications to be taken as well as instructions on the use of any newly prescribed medications.

Patient Education About Medications

The importance of educating patients about their medications cannot be overstated. They must have at least a basic understanding about medication risks and benefits and how to administer medications safely and appropriately. Patients should receive counseling to ensure that they fully understand the information concerning this subject. Studies have shown that most patients prefer to receive this information from their physicians. When patients do not receive appropriate, direct education, they often resort to relying on printed information included on drug labels or package inserts, which they may not fully comprehend.

It is best to provide thorough spoken instruction to each patient, which can then be followed up by providing complete written information. Poor health literacy is a barrier to adequate patient care. A common example of a lack of understanding occurs in elderly patients, who may not know exactly why it is important to take certain medications at specific times of the day. When the physician communicates this information directly to them, or to their caregivers, the reasons behind specific dosing times are better understood, resulting in higher percentages of dosing regimen compliance.

Regarding their medications, patients should be provided with age-appropriate written information, audiovisual teaching aids when available, and contact information of the professionals to be notified in the case of an adverse reaction. Patients should know the names of all medications they are taking as well as the uses of these medications and dosages and when and how they should be taken. They should understand potential adverse effects that need to be reported immediately. Patients should always use specified medication devices to administer their medications and not household utensils, such as spoons, which may be inaccurate. They should be instructed to carry a list of all their prescription and OTC medications (as well as vitamins and herbal supplements) with them at all times and to use one pharmacy for all their prescriptions. They should be encouraged to ask questions so they can partner in maintaining safe medication principles.

✳ Apply Your Knowledge 11.3

The following questions focus on what you have just learned about strategies for handling and reconciling medications.

CRITICAL THINKING

1. Identify the steps that may help in avoiding medication errors.
2. Discuss the age group of individuals that makes up nearly half of those who experience fatal medication errors.
3. Explain the meaning of *polypharmacy*.
4. Define *medication reconciliation*.
5. Explain why older adults often need many different medications.

PRACTICAL SCENARIO 1

A physician wrote a prescription for ".5 mg IM morphine for postoperative pain" for a 9-month-old infant. The unit secretary recorded the order in the MAR as "5 mg." An inexperienced nurse followed the directions on the MAR without question and gave the baby 5 mg of IM morphine initially and another 5-mg dose 4 hours later. About 2 hours after the second dose, the baby stopped breathing and experienced respiratory arrest. If the physician had written "0.5 mg," the unit secretary would probably not have had any misunderstanding of the intended amount and the nurse would have administered the correct dose.

Marlon Lopez MMG1 Design/Shutterstock

Critical Thinking Questions

1. Although the initial error was not the nurse's, what steps should he or she have taken to avoid this medication error?
2. What measures could the facility implement to curtail future medication errors?
3. Explain how using a standardized written measurement system would have prevented this adverse drug event.

PRACTICAL SCENARIO 2

A 75-year-old man was taking several different medications for hypertension, hyperplasia of the prostate, and rheumatoid arthritis. Four of his medications were to be taken before bed, and three were to be taken in the morning. One night, he recalled that he had forgotten to take one of his medications. He got out of bed, went into his kitchen, and avoided turning on the light so as not to disturb his son-in-law, who was sleeping in the adjacent family room. In the darkness, he inadvertently took one of the medications he had already taken earlier. After 2 hours, he woke up to go to the bathroom and felt chest pain and dizziness, which caused him to collapse, awakening his wife.

Monkey Business Images/Shutterstock

Critical Thinking Questions

1. Which of his medications would cause lower blood pressure, chest pain, and dizziness?
2. What are the disadvantages of taking several drugs at the same time?

Chapter Capsule

This section repeats the objectives from the beginning of the chapter and then provides a summary of the most important concepts for that objective. Use this section as a quick review and to check your knowledge.

Objective 1: Explain why errors can occur in three stages in the medication process.

- ■ First-stage errors can occur during prescribing or ordering if practitioners are distracted or interrupted.

- ■ Second-stage errors can occur during dispensing because of inexperience, insufficient staff, lack of time for patient counseling, and not double-checking medications against a MAR or other paperwork.

- ■ Third-stage errors can occur during administration and monitoring because of poor communication, misread paperwork, similar labeling and packaging of products, medications with similar names, and not monitoring patients for reactions to medications.

Objective 2: Describe factors that cause medication errors.

- ■ Factors that cause medication errors include use of incorrect abbreviations, miscommunication, missing information, lack of appropriate labeling, environmental factors, and poor management.

Objective 3: Explain general recommendations to reduce medication errors.

- ■ In general, to reduce medication errors, there should be an adequate amount of staff members; standardized measurement systems in place; consistently used error-tracking systems; a clearly defined system for drug administration, ordering, and dispensing with a review of the original drug orders; compilation of medication profiles; and a suitable work environment.

Objective 4: Describe the legal and ethical responsibility of health care professionals to report all medication errors.

- The legal and ethical reporting of medication errors by all health care professionals is of utmost importance in protecting patients. The FDA and other organizations offer systems for reporting medication errors. Health care professionals are encouraged to use these systems to report medication errors and situations that may lead to errors.

Objective 5: Explain the role of the Food and Drug Administration in medication errors.

- On a federal level, the FDA coordinates the reporting of medication errors via its MedWatch program. This program provides timely information that is clinically important regarding medical products. Reporting to the FDA may be done anonymously, directly to the FDA, either via the Internet or telephone.

Objective 6: Describe the role of The Joint Commission in preventing medication errors.

- The Joint Commission has established patient safety standards that address many significant patient safety issues. They require that hospitals inform patients when they have been harmed because of hospital errors. Continually attempting to standardize practices in hospitals nationwide, The Joint Commission has established National Patient Safety Goals (NSPGs). The use of bar coding for medication administration is now standard in all hospitals.

Objective 7: Explain the steps that may be taken to avoid medication errors and ensure safe administration of medication.

- *Assessment:* asking patients about allergies, health condition, use of medications and herbal supplements in correct doses and routes—taken at the right times; educating the patient about all medications needed; and assessing body system functions to determine if pharmacotherapy impairments exist.
- *Planning:* avoiding abbreviations that can be misunderstood, questioning orders that are unclear, refusing verbal orders, and following all policies and procedures exactly.
- *Implementation:* eliminating distractions during medication administration, ensuring the seven rights, identification verification, correct procedures and techniques, exact dose calculations, correct and timely opening of medications, correct documentation of procedures, confirmation that the patient has completely swallowed an oral dose of medication, and double-checking for long-acting oral dosage forms.

Objective 8: Define *polypharmacy*.

- Polypharmacy is defined as receiving multiple medications—sometimes for the same condition—that have conflicting pharmacologic actions.

Objective 9: Describe why medication reconciliation is important.

- Keeping track of a patient's medications as they change health-care providers is called medication reconciliation. It involves accurately listing all medications a patient takes in order to reduce duplications, dosing errors, omissions, and drug interactions. It is important because many potential medication errors have been caught during medication reconciliation procedures.

Objective 10: **Explain the importance of patient education concerning medications.**

■ Patients must understand medication risks and benefits and how to administer medications safely and appropriately. They should receive counseling to ensure that they fully understand the information concerning this subject. Most patients prefer to receive this information from their physicians. Without appropriate, direct education, patients often resort to relying on printed information included on drug labels or package inserts, which they may not fully comprehend. Thorough spoken instruction should be provided to each patient, which can then be followed up by written information. Poor health literacy is a barrier to adequate patient care. When a physician communicates directly with patients or their caregivers, dosing instructions are better understood, resulting in better compliance.

 Internet Sites of Interest

■ The most common medication errors: **www.medicinenet.com/script/main/art .asp?articlekey=55234**

■ Medication errors: **www.fda.gov/Drugs/DrugSafety/MedicationErrors/default.htm**

■ Polypharmacy: **www.rightdiagnosis.com/medical/polypharmacy.htm**

■ Reducing medication errors: **www.fda.gov/Drugs/ResourcesForYou/Consumers/ ucm143553.htm**

■ Reporting medication errors: **https://www.ismp.org/errorreporting/reporterrortoISMP .aspx**

Checkpoint Review 2

IDENTIFYING FRACTIONS

1. Circle the *improper* fraction(s).

$$\frac{3}{4} \quad 2\text{-}\frac{5}{8} \quad \frac{4}{4} \quad \frac{9}{7} \quad \frac{18}{19} \quad \frac{\frac{1}{5}}{\frac{2}{3}}$$

2. Circle the *complex* fraction(s).

$$\frac{3}{5} \quad 1\text{-}\frac{3}{4} \quad \frac{6}{6} \quad \frac{7}{6} \quad \frac{8}{9} \quad \frac{\frac{1}{100}}{\frac{1}{160}}$$

3. Circle the *proper* fraction(s).

$$\frac{1}{3} \quad \frac{1}{12} \quad \frac{12}{1} \quad \frac{16}{16} \quad \frac{132}{12}$$

4. Circle the *mixed* number(s) *reduced to lowest terms.*

$$\frac{2}{5} \quad 1\text{-}\frac{1}{6} \quad \frac{5}{7} \quad 1\text{-}\frac{2}{9} \quad \frac{2}{3} \quad 7\text{-}\frac{7}{9}$$

Change the following proper or improper fractions to fractions, whole numbers, or mixed numbers and reduce to lowest terms.

5. $\frac{12}{16} = $ _____

6. $\frac{4}{4} = $ _____

7. $\frac{30}{9} = $ _____

8. $\frac{44}{16} = $ _____

9. $\frac{100}{75} = $ _____

Change the following mixed numbers to improper fractions.

10. $6\text{-}\frac{1}{2} = $ _____

11. $7\text{-}\frac{5}{6} = $ _____

12. $1\text{-}\frac{1}{5} = $ _____

13. $10\text{-}\frac{2}{3} = $ _____

14. $102\text{-}\frac{3}{4} = $ _____

Circle the correct answer.

15. Which is smaller? $\frac{1}{100}$ or $\frac{1}{1,000}$

16. Which is larger? $\frac{1}{15}$ or $\frac{1}{10}$

17. Which is smaller? $\frac{3}{10}$ or $\frac{5}{10}$

18. Which is larger? $\frac{2}{9}$ or $\frac{5}{9}$

Add and then reduce your answers to lowest terms.

19. $\frac{3}{4} + \frac{2}{3} = $ _____

20. $\frac{3}{4} + \frac{1}{8} + \frac{1}{6} = $ _____

21. $\frac{1}{7} + \frac{2}{3} + \frac{11}{21} = $ _____

22. $\frac{1}{4} + \frac{5}{33} = $ _____

23. $\frac{12}{17} + 5 - \frac{2}{7} = $ _____

24. $7\text{-}\frac{4}{5} + \frac{2}{3} = $ _____

Multiply and then reduce your answers to lowest terms.

25. $\frac{30}{10} \times \frac{1}{12} = $ _____

26. $\frac{1}{100} \times 3 = $ _____

27. $\frac{3}{4} \times \frac{2}{3} = $ _____

28. $\frac{5}{8} \times 1\text{-}\frac{1}{6} = $ _____

29. $\frac{3}{4} \times \frac{1}{8} = $ _____

30. $12\text{-}\frac{1}{2} \times 20\text{-}\frac{1}{2} = $ _____

Divide and then reduce your answers to lowest terms.

31. $\frac{1}{60} \div \frac{1}{2} = $ _____

32. $\frac{1}{8} \div \frac{7}{12} = $ _____

33. $2\text{-}\frac{1}{2} \div \frac{3}{4} = $ _____

34. $\frac{1}{150} \div \frac{1}{50} = $ _____

FILL IN THE BLANK

Select terms from your reading to fill in the blanks.

35. Liters and milliliters are metric units that measure _____.

36. 1 mg is _____ of a gram.

37. 1 liter = _____ mL.

38. 1,000 mcg = _____ mg.

39. There are _____ mL in a liter.

40. Which is smallest: a kilogram, gram, or milligram? _____

41. Which is largest: a kilogram, gram, or milligram? _____

42. Milligrams are metric units that measure _____.

METRIC NOTATION

Circle the correct metric notation.

43. 4 kg   4.0 kg   kg 04   4 kG   4 KG

44. .6 g   0.6 Gm   0.6 g   .6 Gm   0.60 g

45. 2.5 mm   2-1/2 mm   2.5 Mm   2.50 MM   2-1/2 MM

46. mg 20   20 mG   20.0 mg   20 mg   20 MG

FILL IN THE BLANK

Write the term for these abbreviations.

47. g _____

48. mm _____

49. cm _____

50. kg _____

51. mcg _____

52. mL _____

Write the terms for these abbreviations and symbols.

53. qt _____

54. gr _____

55. ℥ _____

56. ʒ _____

Write the terms for these equivalencies.

57. 16 oz = pt _____

58. qt i = oz _____

Write the following apothecary quantities using abbreviations and proper notation.

59. ten grains _____

60. two pints _____

61. one-half ounce _____

62. sixteen pints _____

63. four ounces _____

64. three grains _____

Write these measurements using abbreviations.

65. 3 tablespoons _____

66. 10 teaspoons _____

67. 6 drops _____

68. 25 milliequivalents _____

Convert these measurements to the units shown.

69. 1 oz = _____ T

70. 16 oz = _____ lb

71. 4 T = _____ oz

72. 24 oz = _____ cups

Write the terms for these abbreviations.

73. 20 mEq _____

74. 15 lb _____

75. 50 gtt _____

76. 8 T _____

CALCULATIONS

Calculate the amounts to administer and then write them in the blank spaces.

77. Ordered: Lanoxin 0.125 mg PO daily

    On hand: Lanoxin 0.25 mg tablets

    Administer: _____ tablet(s)

78. Ordered: Duricef 1 g PO bid

    On hand: Duricef 500 mg capsules

    Administer: _____ capsule(s)

79. Ordered: Synthroid 0.1 mg PO daily

    On hand: Synthroid 50 mcg tablets

    Administer: _____ tablet(s)

80. Ordered: Diabinese 0.1 g PO daily

    On hand: Diabinese 100 mg tablets

    Administer: _____ tablet(s)

81. Ordered: amoxicillin 100 mg PO qid

    On hand: 80 mL bottle of Amoxil (amoxicillin) Oral pediatric suspension 125 mg for 5 mL

    Administer: _____ mL

82. Ordered: Septra-DS suspension 200 mg PO bid

    On hand: Septra-DS suspension 400 mg for 5 mL

    Administer: _____ mL

83. Ordered: Esidrix solution 100 mg PO bid

    On hand: Esidrix solution 50 mg for 5 mL

    Administer: _____ t

84. Ordered: digoxin elixir 0.25 mg PO daily

    On hand: digoxin elixir 50 mcg/mL

    Administer: _____ mL

85. Ordered: Tylenol 0.5 g PO q4h PRN pain

    On hand: Tylenol 500 mg for 5 mL

    Administer: _____ t

86. Ordered: Pathocil 125 mg PO q6h

    On hand: Pathocil suspension 62.5 mg for 5 mL

    Administer: _____ t

87. Ordered: erythromycin 1.2 g PO q8h

    On hand: erythromycin 400 mg per 5 mL

    Administer: _____ mL

88. Ordered: cephalexin 375 mg PO tid

    On hand: cephalexin 250 mg per 5 mL

    Administer: _____ t

89. Ordered: Demerol syrup 75 mg PO q4h PRN pain

    On hand: Demerol syrup 50 mg for 5 mL

    Administer: _____ mL

90. Ordered: Coumadin 7.5 mg PO daily

    On hand: Coumadin 2.5 mg tablets

    Administer: _____ tablet(s)

91. Ordered: Urecholine 50 mg PO tid

    On hand: Urecholine 25 mg tablets

    Administer: _____ tablet(s)

92. Ordered: V-Cillin K 300,000 units PO qid

    On hand: V-Cillin K 200,000 units for 5 mL

    Administer: _____ mL

93. Ordered: codeine gr 1/4 PO daily

    On hand: codeine 30 mg tablets

    Administer: _____ tablet(s)

94. Ordered: Orinase 250 mg PO bid

    On hand: Orinase 0.5 g tablets

    Administer: _____ tablet(s)

95. Ordered: Ceclor suspension 225 mg PO bid

    On hand: Ceclor suspension 375 mg for 5 mL

    Administer: _____ mL

96. Ordered: Aspirin gr v PO daily

    On hand: Aspirin 325 mg tablets

    Administer: _____ tablet(s)

97. Ordered: Levaquin 0.5 g PO daily

    On hand: Levaquin 500 mg tablets

    Administer: _____ tablet(s)

98. Ordered: atropine gr 1/100 IM on call to OR

    On hand: atropine 0.4 mg/mL

    Administer: _____ mL

99. Ordered: lidocaine 50 mg IV stat

    On hand: lidocaine 2%

    Administer: _____ mL

100. Ordered: heparin 3,500 units subcutaneous q12h

    On hand: heparin 5,000 units/mL

    Administer: _____ mL

101. Ordered: Lasix 60 mg IV stat

    On hand: Lasix 20 mg for 2 mL ampule

    Administer: _____ mL

FORMULAS

Using the formula $D \times Q/H = X$, answer the following:

102. (*D*) represents _____.

103. (*Q*) represents _____.

104. (*H*) represents _____.

105. (*X*) represents _____.

FILL IN THE BLANK

Select terms from your reading to fill in the blanks.

106. The common syringe that is used for intradermal testing is the _____.

107. The volume of solution for IM injection is 0.5 to _____ mL.

108. The most common insulin combining NPH and regular insulin is _____, but 50/50 insulin is also available.

109. The anticoagulant heparin is measured in _____ units.

110. Intravenous fluids and drugs may be administered by intermittent or _____ IV infusion.

111. Body surface area is determined by using a _____ and the child's height and weight.

112. Dosage calculations use such pediatric formulas as Clark's rule, _____ rule, and _____ rule.

113. Clark's rule is based on the _____ of the child.

114. _____ rule is used for children older than 1 year of age.

115. _____ rule is a method of estimating the dose of medication for infants younger than 1 year of age.

116. The most common medication errors occur because of _____ _____.

117. In the hospital, _____ _____ are the most common cause of morbidity and preventable death.

118. Health care professionals may report medication errors to the _____.

119. _____ and improvement programs are used by hospitals and other health care facilities to monitor medication errors.

120. Strategies for handling medication errors involve four steps: assessment, planning, implementation, and _____.

121. According to the _____ _____ _____, medical errors have caused up to 98,000 deaths annually in the U.S.

122. The most common error is _____; errors often involve antibiotics and analgesics.

123. Medication errors may occur _____ and at any time.

124. Many facilities use root cause analysis to prevent future _____, asking what happened and why it happened.

125. Sentinel events are _____ occurrences involving death or serious physical or psychological injury, or risk thereof.

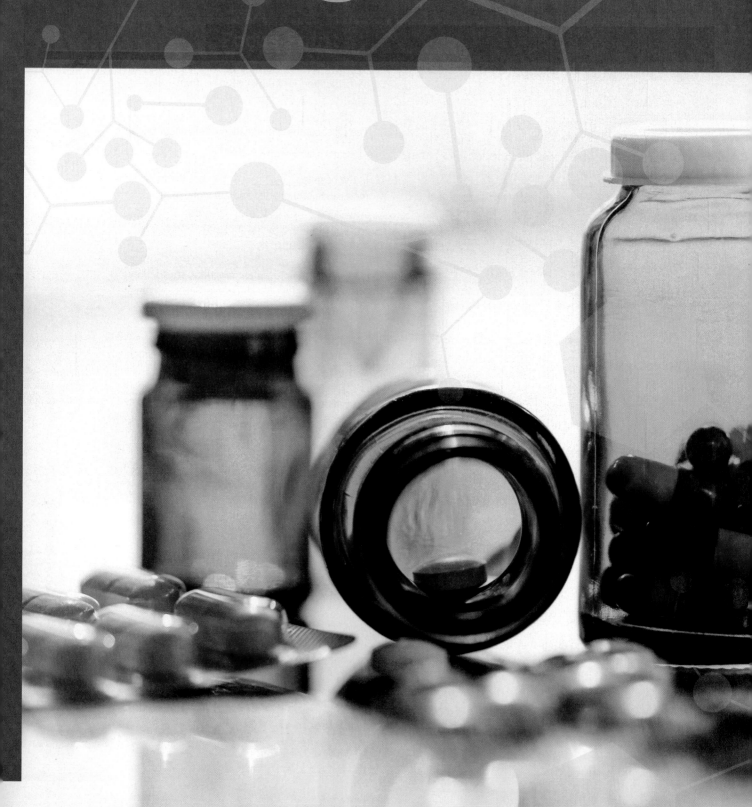

UNIT 3

Drug Effects on Multiple Systems

" Antibiotic use has had a tremendous impact on the way microorganisms respond to various agents. Subtherapeutic doses or overuse can affect microorganism resistance. "

Chapter 12

Nutritional Aspects of Pharmacology

Chapter Objectives

After completing this chapter, you should be able to:

1. Identify the seven basic food components and explain their major functions.
2. Differentiate the classifications of nutrients.
3. Explain the role of calories in the diet.
4. Define the role of essential fatty acids in optimal health.
5. List the water-soluble vitamins.
6. Discuss the toxicity of vitamin A.
7. Indicate the significance of vitamin E deficiency in infants.
8. List the five essential trace minerals and the symptoms of their toxicity.
9. Explain general indications for total parenteral nutrition.
10. Describe the benefits of food additives.

Key Terms

additives (p. 181)
alpha tocopherol (p. 173)
anemia (p. 172)
antioxidant (p. 174)
ascorbic acid (p. 169)
beriberi (p. 174)
calciferol (p. 174)
calcitonin (p. 174)
calcitriol (p. 174)
carbohydrates (p. 168)
carotene (p. 173)

cholecalciferol (p. 173)
cholesterol (p. 168)
cobalamin (p. 172)
congenital hypothyroidism (p. 177)
essential amino acids (p. 167)
fatty acids (p. 167)
fiber (p. 168)
goiter (p. 177)
hypervitaminosis (p. 174)
macrominerals (p. 167)
major minerals (p. 176)

microminerals (p. 177)
nutrition (p. 167)
pellagra (p. 171)
phylloquinone (p. 173)
recommended dietary allowances (RDAs) (p. 179)
rickets (p. 174)
spina bifida (p. 172)
total parenteral nutrition (TPN) (p. 178)

Introduction

Nutrition is the process of how the body takes in and uses food and other sources of nutrients for growth and repair of tissues. This process has five parts: intake, digestion, absorption, metabolism, and elimination. This chapter gives you an understanding of how a well-planned diet can lead to optimal health and well-being for your patients, and it provides important information about food and drug interactions.

Nutrients

The human body needs a variety of nutrients for energy, growth, repair, and basic processes. Seven basic food components provide these nutrients and work together to help keep the body healthy:

1. Proteins
2. Fatty acids (also called *lipids* or *fats*)
3. Carbohydrates
4. Fiber
5. Vitamins
6. Minerals
7. Water

Only proteins, fats, and carbohydrates contain calories and provide the body with energy. The remaining four food components perform a variety of other essential functions. The nutritional sciences study the nature and distribution of nutrients in food, their metabolic effects, and the consequences of inadequate food intake.

A *nutrient* is any element or compound from the diet that supports normal metabolism, growth, reproduction, or other normal body functioning. Some nutrients are called *essential* because they are needed by the body for normal functioning. Essential nutrients cannot be synthesized by the body and thus must be derived from the diet. Essential nutrients include vitamins, minerals, amino acids, fatty acids, and some carbohydrates. On the other hand, *nonessential* nutrients are those the body can synthesize from other compounds, although they may also be derived from the diet. Another way that nutrients are subdivided is into *macronutrients* and *micronutrients*.

Focus Point

Malnourishment

Nutritional deficiencies are very common, especially among elderly and hospitalized patients. In a 30-month study conducted in two U.S. hospitals, blood tests found that 55% of patients were malnourished. Another study of elderly patients showed that 100% had low folic acid levels, 87% had low zinc levels, 83% had deficient vitamin B_6 levels, and 62% had low vitamin D levels.

Macronutrients

Macronutrients are needed by the body in relatively large amounts and constitute the bulk of the diet. They supply energy as well as essential nutrients needed for growth, maintenance, and activity. Carbohydrates, fats (including essential fatty acids), proteins, **macrominerals** (dietary minerals needed by the human body in high quantities), and water are macronutrients. Carbohydrates are converted to glucose (a simple sugar) and other monosaccharides (carbohydrates that cannot form any simple sugar), fats are converted to fatty acids and glycerol, and proteins are converted to peptides and amino acids. These macronutrients are interchangeable as sources of energy; fats yield 9 kilocalories of energy per 1 g consumed (9 kcal/g); proteins and carbohydrates yield 4 kcal/g.

The macrominerals—such as sodium, chloride, potassium, calcium, phosphorus, and magnesium—are required by humans in relatively large quantities (i.e., grams) per day. Water is also considered a macronutrient because it is required in the amount of 1 mL/kcal of energy expended, or about 2,500 mL/day.

ESSENTIAL AMINO ACIDS

Essential amino acids are those components of proteins that cannot be synthesized by the body and must be provided by the diet. Of the 20 amino acids in proteins, nine are essential. The requirement for dietary protein correlates with the growth rate, which varies at different times in the life cycle. The amino acid composition of proteins varies widely.

ESSENTIAL FATTY ACIDS

Essential **fatty acids** (such as linoleic acid and linolenic acid) are required in amounts equaling 6–10% of fat intake (5–10 g/day). These fatty acids must be provided by the diet; for example, vegetable oils provide linoleic acid and linolenic acid. Essential fatty acids are required for the formation of prostaglandins (hormone-like substances) and thromboxanes (biochemically related to the prostaglandins). Fatty acids, particularly omega-3 fatty acids, appear to play a role in decreasing the risk of coronary artery disease. Research has shown that consumption of omega-3 fatty acids decreases triglyceride levels and the growth rate of atherosclerotic plaque, slightly lowers blood pressure, and decreases the risk of arrhythmias.

Fatty acids can be either saturated or unsaturated. The chemical structure of a *saturated* fatty acid contains all the hydrogen possible and therefore is dense, heavy, and solid at room temperature. Examples of saturated fats are the fats found in dairy products and meats.

Unsaturated fatty acids can take on more hydrogen and are less heavy and less dense. Unsaturated fats are usually liquid at room temperature. If fatty acids have one unfilled hydrogen bond, the fat is called *monounsaturated*. Olives, olive oil, and peanut oil contain monounsaturated fats. *Polyunsaturated* fats, such as corn, safflower, and soy oils, have two or more unfilled hydrogen bonds. All essential fatty acids are polyunsaturated fatty acids, but not all polyunsaturated fatty acids are essential fatty acids.

Cholesterol, a natural lipid found in cell membranes, is found in highest concentrations in animal muscles and organ cells. Cholesterol does not exist in plants. It is essential for certain cell structures; however, excess cholesterol can deposit in blood vessels, form atherosclerotic plaque, and lead to cardiovascular disease.

CARBOHYDRATES

Carbohydrates in food provide about two-thirds of an individual's fuel for daily energy needs. They aid in fat metabolism and help reserve protein for uses other than supplying energy, such as repairing and building our bodies. The daily requirement for carbohydrates is 50–60% of total caloric intake. Carbohydrate deficiency leads to weight loss, protein loss, and fatigue.

There are two basic types of carbohydrates: *simple sugars*, which are found in fruits, some vegetables, milk, and table sugar, and *complex carbohydrates*, which are found in such grain foods as pastas, breads, and rice and such fruits and vegetables as potatoes, broccoli, corn, apples, and pears. The two types of carbohydrates have a function in health and consist of many variations. With the exception of fibers, carbohydrates are easily digested and absorbed into the body. Simple sugars are quickly absorbed, but complex carbohydrates must be processed before they can be absorbed in the intestinal tract. A small amount of glucose is stored in the liver and muscles as glycogen (starch). This stored glucose is available to supplement dietary supplies of carbohydrates. Excess amounts of carbohydrates are stored in the body as fat or *adipose* tissue. Carbohydrates are also needed to regulate protein and fat metabolism.

Focus Point

Blood Glucose Levels

The central nervous system (CNS) requires a constant minute-to-minute supply of glucose to function properly. Sustained low blood glucose levels, which can be caused by an excessively low intake of carbohydrates, can result in brain damage and death.

Focus on Pediatrics

Lactose Sensitivity

Lactose is the sugar contained in human and animal milk. It must be broken down in the body by the enzyme lactase to enable the body to digest dairy products. Many infants and children have trouble digesting foods that contain lactose and must eliminate those foods from their diets. Children who are especially sensitive to dietary lactose are often referred to as being *lactose-intolerant*. Generally, removing milk products from the diet is recommended for lactose-intolerant children. Lactose-free milk can be substituted, as can sources of calcium, such as yogurt, buttermilk, and cheese, which contain less lactose than milk.

FIBER

Fiber is a type of complex carbohydrate that does not supply energy or heat to the body. Fiber is the tough, stringy part of vegetables and grains. It can be classified as soluble or insoluble. *Soluble fiber*, found in foods such as oats, dry beans, barley, and some fruits and vegetables, tends to absorb fluid and swell when eaten. Water-soluble fiber helps to lower blood cholesterol levels. It also may stabilize blood sugar levels in the body by slowing the absorption of carbohydrates into the blood. *Insoluble fiber*, which is found in the bran of whole wheat and brown rice, primarily promotes regular bowel movements by contributing to stool bulk, which stimulates peristalsis. It also helps to prevent colon cancer (the stool bulk scours the intestines of waste matter as it passes through) and seems to reduce the risk of heart attack. Although insoluble fiber is not absorbed by the body, it serves to increase and soften the bulk of the stool, promoting normal defecation. Therapeutically, insoluble fiber can help treat and prevent constipation, diverticular disease, and irritable bowel syndrome. It is linked to reduction in gallstone formation and risks of certain types of cancer, especially colon cancer, and other diseases.

The recommended amount of daily dietary fiber intake for adults is 25–40 g/1,000 kcal. Because fiber works with other substances and nutrients, it is advisable to get dietary fiber from a variety of food sources. Adequate water intake is especially important for fiber to work properly. Without adequate water intake, constipation and bloating may occur. Water also stimulates peristalsis in the intestine.

✳ Apply Your Knowledge 12.1

The following questions focus on what you have just learned about macronutrients and their role in health.

CRITICAL THINKING

1. Describe essential nutrients.
2. Name two essential fatty acids and describe the indications of omega-3 fatty acids.
3. Describe cholesterol.
4. Explain the indication of water-soluble fiber.
5. Classify carbohydrates and name an example for each.
6. Discuss macronutrients.
7. Identify six macrominerals.
8. Describe the effect of insoluble fiber in the human body.

Micronutrients

Vitamins and essential trace minerals comprise *micronutrients*—a group of nutrients that are required in very small amounts by the human body for normal functioning. Foods contain small amounts of these micronutrients. However, if any of these micronutrients is lacking in the diet, biochemical alterations—such as changes in the structure and function of tissues and organs—result and possibly cause deficiency or disease.

VITAMINS

Vitamins are organic (carbon-containing) compounds required for normal human growth, development, and maintenance of normal body function; however, the amount needed by the body is very small. The total volume of vitamins that a healthy individual normally requires per day would barely fill a teaspoon! Thus, vitamin requirements are measured in milligrams or micrograms—exceedingly small and difficult units to visualize. Deficiencies of vitamins occur when a special condition or disorder creates an increased need in a particular person at a particular time.

Vitamins are classified by their solubility; they are soluble in either water or fat. This difference has importance in bodily storage of vitamins and in vitamin deficiency or toxicity.

Water-Soluble Vitamins (B and C Vitamins)

Water-soluble vitamins include eight members of the vitamin B group (Table 12-1 ■) and vitamin C (**ascorbic acid**). All members of the B-vitamin group act as *coenzymes* (organic chemicals that must combine with an enzyme in order for the enzyme to function)—usually after being processed. The coenzymes are frequently grouped together because many are found in similar foodstuffs.

THIAMINE (VITAMIN B_1)

Also called *vitamin B_1*, thiamine is converted into a pyrophosphate, which functions as a coenzyme in some important carbohydrate metabolic processes. For example, the metabolism of alcohol depends on thiamine pyrophosphate. People with alcoholism frequently experience thiamine deficiency because heavy consumption of alcohol interferes with the body's ability to absorb the vitamin from food.

The main natural dietary sources of thiamine are whole grains (especially wheat germ), lean meats, fish, soybeans, and other beans. Processed foods are often fortified with thiamine.

Deficiency of thiamine leads to the disease **beriberi**, which is characterized by edema, cardiovascular abnormalities, and neurologic symptoms.

Table 12-1 ■ Water-Soluble Vitamins

GENERIC NAME	TRADE NAME	FUNCTIONS	HYPOVITAMINOSIS (*DEFICIENT INTAKE*)	HYPERVITAMINOSIS (*EXCESSIVE INTAKE*)
B_1 (thiamine)	Betalins, Bewon, Biamine	Metabolic reactions coenzyme	Anorexia, depression, dyspnea, loss of muscle strength, loss of memory, and peripheral neuritis	Very little toxicity; in extreme overdosage, symptoms include hypotension, neuromuscular or ganglionic blockage, and respiratory depression
B_2 (riboflavin)	Riboflavin, B_2-400	Metabolic reactions coenzyme	Anemia, dermatitis of the face, sore throat and mouth, and swollen tongue	Low toxicity levels, but in extreme overdosage, symptoms include dark urine, nausea, and vomiting
B_3 (nicotinamide, niacin, or nicotinic acid)	Niac, Nicobid	Metabolic reactions coenzyme	Dementia, diarrhea, dizziness, headache, impaired memory, insomnia, skin eruptions, and sore mouth	Diarrhea, dizziness, dry skin, dysrhythmias, flushing, muscle pain, nausea, pruritus, and vomiting
B_5 (pantothenic acid)	(Generic only)	Metabolic reactions coenzyme	Induced in humans via a metabolic antagonist; symptoms include cardiac instability, depression, frequent infections, and neurologic disorders	None (except in unusually high doses, diarrhea)
B_6 (pyridoxine)	Pyri-500, Rodex, Vitabee-6	Amino acid metabolic coenzyme	Peripheral neuritis, seborrheic-like skin lesions, seizures, and sore mouth	Low toxicity (except in chronic overuse, then neurotoxicity, including clumsiness, lack of muscle coordination, and numbness)
B_7 (biotin)	(Generic only)	Metabolic reactions coenzyme	Anorexia, depression, dry skin, fine and brittle hair, fungal infections, hair loss, muscle pain, nausea and vomiting, rashes, and seborrheic dermatitis	No documented cases of overdosage
B_9 (folate, folic acid, or pteroylglutamic acid)	Folacin-800, Folvite, FA-8	Amino acid and nucleic acid metabolic coenzyme	Megaloblastic anemia	Allergic reactions, fever, pruritus, rashes, and redness of skin

GENERIC NAME	TRADE NAME	FUNCTIONS	HYPOVITAMINOSIS (*DEFICIENT INTAKE*)	HYPERVITAMINOSIS (*EXCESSIVE INTAKE*)
B_{12} (cobalamin, cyanocobalamin, or hydroxocobalamin)	LA-12, B12, Cobal, Vitabee 12	Nucleic acid metabolic coenzyme	Abnormal blood cell production, confusion, dementia, memory loss, and nervous system damage	No toxic effects; overdosage is extremely rare but may cause a deficiency of the other B vitamins
Choline	(Generic only)	Metabolic reactions coenzyme	Liver damage in adults, alterations in memory, and increased fetal brain cell death	None listed for choline alone, but when used in combination preparations, symptoms of overdosage include confusion, diarrhea, dizziness, drowsiness, headache, hearing impairment, respiratory changes, sweating, and vomiting
C (ascorbic acid)	Acerola, Cecon, Ascot	Coenzyme and antioxidant	Anemia, gingivitis, and scurvy	Dizziness, kidney stones; in high doses, diarrhea, nausea and vomiting, and redness of skin

Note: For any trade name versions of vitamins that use only the same exact name as the vitamin in a capitalized trade name, no "registering" of the name is possible.

RIBOFLAVIN (VITAMIN B_2)

Riboflavin—also called *vitamin B_2*—is important in the metabolism of fats, carbohydrates, and proteins. The main dietary sources of riboflavin are dairy products, yeast products, and liver. Almonds are also a good source, and many other plant products contain reasonable amounts.

A deficiency of riboflavin causes cheilosis (fissures on the lips) and stomatitis (cracks in the angles of the mouth). Glossitis (inflammation of the tongue) and seborrheic dermatitis—mainly of the face and scrotum—can occur, as can a decreased resistance to infections. There is no known danger of excessive consumption of riboflavin. However, patients using riboflavin supplements should be warned that their urine may be bright yellow.

Riboflavin is sensitive to light and other foods; therefore, vitamin supplements containing riboflavin should be kept out of direct sunlight.

NICOTINAMIDE (VITAMIN B_3)

Nicotinamide is also known as *niacin*. Humans can actually make some of this vitamin from the amino acid tryptophan. The main food sources of nicotinamide are liver, yeast products, peanuts, whole-grain cereals, and fish (tuna is exceptionally high in this vitamin). Deficiency of nicotinamide causes **pellagra**—a condition marked by "the four Ds": dementia, dermatitis, diarrhea, and death.

Nicotinamide is therefore used chiefly in the treatment of patients with pellagra. It has also been found to be useful with thiamine and riboflavin in the treatment of those with nutritional deficiency in chronic alcoholism because these patients also have deficiencies of thiamine and riboflavin. Large doses lower cholesterol, triglycerides, and free fatty acids. Therefore, nicotinamide is used in the treatment of patients with hypercholesterolemia (high blood cholesterol level)—mostly in combination with the cholesterol-lowering drugs cholestyramine, colestipol, or clofibrate (see Chapter 29). Toxicity associated with high doses of niacin includes hepatic impairment, severe hypotension, and various skin conditions.

PANTOTHENIC ACID (VITAMIN B_5)

The term *pantothenic* derives from the Greek, meaning "all over the place." This vitamin is needed for the formation of the important coenzyme A, which is required for numerous biochemical processes. A deficiency syndrome has been experimentally induced in human

Focus Point

Pharmacologic Doses of Niacin

At high doses, niacin decreases blood levels of low-density lipoprotein cholesterol (the bad cholesterol) and triglyceride levels—both of which are linked with cardiovascular disease. In addition, pharmacologic doses of niacin improve high-density lipoprotein cholesterol (the good cholesterol) levels. When niacin is used in this sense, it functions more as a drug than a vitamin and should be used only under medical supervision.

volunteers and results in vomiting, cramps, abdominal pains, and personality changes. Pantothenic acid is readily available in many plant and animal sources. It is very difficult for individuals to have a deficiency of this vitamin.

PYRIDOXINE (VITAMIN B₆)

Vitamin B₆ does not denote a single substance but rather is a collective term for a group of naturally occurring pyridines that are metabolically and functionally interrelated: pyridoxine, pyridoxal, and pyridoxamine. The various forms of pyridoxine are widely distributed in animal and plant products, making deficiency rare.

Vitamin B₆ reputedly has several therapeutic uses. It is used routinely in patients on isoniazid therapy to prevent neuritis. Pyridoxine is also prescribed to treat women with hyperemesis gravidarum (nausea during pregnancy), particularly when given parenterally, and to suppress lactation when given orally.

BIOTIN (VITAMIN B₇)

Biotin is widely available in the foods we eat, and deficiency is almost unknown. It is also made by the natural flora of the intestine. Biotin does not seem to produce any toxicity if taken in excess, and abuse of this vitamin does not seem to be common.

FOLATE (VITAMIN B₉)

The name *folate* comes from the Latin word *falium*, meaning "leaf." The name was given to this vitamin because a major source is from dark green leafy vegetables. *Folate* is now used as the common, generic name for this vitamin that exists in many chemical forms. The most stable form of folate is folic acid, which is rarely found in food but is the form usually used in vitamin supplements and fortified food products. In its basic coenzyme role, folate is essential to the formation of all body cells because it takes part in the creation of DNA, the important cell nucleus material that transmits genetic characteristics. Folate is also essential to the formation of hemoglobin and synthesis of amino acids.

A direct deficiency of folate causes a special type of **anemia** (a deficiency of hemoglobin, red blood cell number, or red blood cell volume) called *megaloblastic anemia*, which is a particular risk during pregnancy

because of increased fetal growth demands for folate. Rapidly growing adolescents—especially those following fad diets—and those who smoke develop low levels of folate in the blood, risking anemia.

The role of adequate folate in reducing the serious public health problem of neural defects during pregnancy has received increasing study and public awareness in recent years. Neural tube defects, such as **spina bifida** (a condition wherein the spinal column is imperfectly closed, resulting in protrusion of the meninges or spinal cord) and *anencephaly* (the congenital absence of most of the brain and spinal cord), are the most common birth defects involving the brain and spinal cord. Therefore, increased folic acid intake is recommended for all women who are capable of becoming pregnant. Adverse effects of excess consumption of folate from foods have not been observed.

COBALAMIN (VITAMIN B₁₂)

Vitamin B₁₂ is also known as **cobalamin**, which promotes normal function of all cells, especially normal blood formation. It is also necessary for proper nervous system function.

Although it is essential, the amount of dietary vitamin B₁₂ needed for normal human metabolism is very small. Vitamin B₁₂ deficiency is responsible for pernicious anemia. A component of the digestive gastric secretions called *intrinsic factor* is necessary for absorption of vitamin B₁₂ into the bloodstream. Gastrointestinal (GI) disorders that destroy the cell lining can disrupt the secretion of intrinsic factor and thus inhibit vitamin B₁₂ absorption. If the vitamin cannot be absorbed to make hemoglobin, pernicious anemia occurs. In such cases, vitamin B₁₂ must be given by injection to bypass the absorption defect. Deficiency is much more common in older adults because of a lack of either intrinsic factor or hydrochloric acid in the stomach, not because of insufficient dietary intake.

Although small amounts of vitamin B₁₂ are stored in the liver, excess intake of vitamin B₁₂ does not produce adverse effects in healthy individuals; therefore, no toxicity has been established. This vitamin is naturally found only in animal products (it is originally made by bacteria in the intestine of herbivores), such as fish, meat, poultry, eggs, milk, and milk products; breakfast cereals are often fortified with vitamin B₁₂.

VITAMIN B FACTORS (CHOLINE)

Choline is a water-soluble nutrient associated with the B-complex vitamins. Although it is synthesized in the human body, choline plays an important role as a structural component of cell membranes. Choline is an essential component in the production of acetylcholine, which is a neurotransmitter involved in memory storage, muscle control, and many other functions. A deficiency of choline from food sources appears to be associated with liver damage. This occurs because very-low-density lipoproteins cannot be synthesized, causing fat to accumulate in the liver and resulting in liver damage. Choline deficiency can affect healthy nerve function and may play a role in the development of Huntington's chorea, Parkinson's disease, and Alzheimer's disease.

Choline is found naturally in a wide variety of foods, especially milk, eggs, liver, and peanuts.

Excess choline rarely causes toxicity. Adverse effects have only been observed in cases in which choline intake was several times greater than normal intake from food. Very high doses of choline have been associated with lowered blood pressure, fishy body odor, sweating, excessive salivation, and reduced growth rate.

ASCORBIC ACID (VITAMIN C)

Vitamin C (ascorbic acid) is required for building and maintaining strong tissues for wound healing, resistance to infection, and enhanced iron absorption. Vitamin C has several critical functions in the body. It acts as a protective agent (antioxidant) and plays a role in many metabolic and immunologic activities—perhaps as a preventative agent in many cancers and cardiovascular disease. Ascorbic acid is thought to lower the incidence of atherosclerosis by aiding the conversion of cholesterol to bile acids. It enhances iron bioavailability, promotes calcium absorption, and aids in wound healing and tissue repair. Ascorbic acid is also essential for the body's constant production of collagen in connective tissue as part of normal tissue turnover.

A deficiency of ascorbic acid can result in scurvy—a serious and severe disease caused by the degeneration of connective tissue. Scurvy is marked by anemia, edema of the gums, and bleeding into the skin and mucous membranes.

The two best sources of vitamin C are capsicums and guavas—not citrus fruits, as is commonly believed. Kiwi fruit is also very high in ascorbic acid. If large doses of ascorbic acid are used, plenty of water should be taken at the same time to avoid the formation of kidney stones. Diarrhea and gastritis can occur with large doses.

Focus on Geriatrics

Vitamin C and Cataracts

Vitamin C may be protective against the development of cataracts. The body concentrates vitamin C in the lenses of the eyes in higher levels than what is present in the blood plasma. The use of vitamin C supplements for 10 or more years is associated with a 77–83% lower prevalence of early to moderate lens opacities (cataracts).

Fat-Soluble Vitamins

Fat-soluble vitamins include retinol (vitamin A), **cholecalciferol** (vitamin D_3), ergocalciferol (vitamin D_3), **alpha tocopherol** (vitamin E), and **phylloquinone** (vitamin K_1) and menaquinone (vitamin K_1). Unlike water-soluble vitamins, fat-soluble vitamins are stored in the body. This storage can create an excess of these vitamins and may lead to toxicities. Excess amounts of vitamin A, in particular, can cause toxicity.

RETINOL (VITAMIN A)

The major function of vitamin A, or retinol, is in the retina of the eye. Retinol is an essential part of rhodopsin, which is a pigment in the eye commonly known as visual purple. A mild deficiency of vitamin A may cause night blindness, slow adaptation to darkness, or glare blindness. Adequate intake of retinol prevents two eye conditions: *xerophthalmia* (blindness) and *xerosis* (burning and itching).

Retinol also maintains healthy *epithelial tissue* (the vital outside layer of protective cells covering open surfaces of the body), such as skin and the inner mucous membranes in the nose, throat, eyes, GI tract, and genitourinary tract. These tissues provide our primary barrier to infection. Retinol is essential to the growth of skeletal and soft tissues and influences the stability of cell membranes and protein synthesis. Vitamin A is also important in the production of immune cells responsible for fighting bacterial, parasitic, and viral attacks.

Fish liver oils, butter, egg yolk, liver, and cream are sources of natural vitamin A. Although vitamin A only occurs naturally in the fat part of milk, the FDA requires that all milk—including nonfat milk—be fortified with vitamin A. **Carotene** is found in dark green and yellow vegetables and fruits. Beta-carotene (one of three carotenes: alpha, beta, and gamma) is important to human nutrition because the body can convert it to vitamin A, thus making it a primary source of the vitamin. Some good sources of beta-carotene are turnip greens, spinach, carrots, sweet potatoes, mangos, pumpkins, and apricots.

The liver can store large amounts of retinol. In healthy individuals, the storage efficiency in the liver of ingested retinol is more than 50%, and the liver contains about 90% of the body's total store. Thus, large amounts of supplemental retinol added to normal dietary sources can cause toxicity. Excess vitamin A intake is called **hypervitaminosis** A. Symptoms of this toxicity include loss of hair, jaundice, joint pain, and thickening of the long bones. Liver injury and *ascites* (fluid accumulation in the abdominal cavity) may occur.

Focus on Pediatrics

Vitamin A Deficiency

Dietary vitamin A deficiency is the number one cause of blindness in children worldwide.

Focus Point

Overconsumption of a Vitamin or Mineral

Nutrition experts suggest that individuals who suspect they have been taking too much of a vitamin (or mineral) should not stop taking it completely but rather should cut back to about half the current dosage. This is because the body has adjusted itself to the overly large dose, and stopping it altogether could trigger a deficiency. Individuals should consult their doctors or a registered dietician in these cases, especially if they have diabetes or high blood pressure.

CHOLECALCIFEROL (VITAMIN D₃)

Vitamin D is not actually a true vitamin because it is made in our own bodies with the help of the sun's ultraviolet rays. Today, we know that the compound made in our skin by sunlight is actually a *prohormone* (an intraglandular chemical substance that can be processed to become a hormone). This compound, when distributed in the skin, has been given the name *cholecalciferol* (vitamin D_3)—often shortened to **calciferol**, which controls calcium metabolism in bone building. The initial compound produced in the skin by sunlight is a cholesterol base. Calciferol is activated by cholesterol in the liver and then in the kidney, becoming the active vitamin D hormone called **calcitriol**. There are actually five forms of vitamin D, but cholecalciferol is the form that is most clinically significant.

Calcitriol acts physiologically with two other hormones: the parathyroid hormone (PTH), which is critical to calcium and phosphorus balance, and **calcitonin**, a thyroid hormone that lowers blood levels of calcium and phosphate and promotes bone formation. In balance with these two hormones, vitamin D stimulates absorption of calcium and phosphorus in the small intestine. A deficiency of calcitriol causes **rickets**, a condition characterized by malformation of skeletal tissue in growing children. Children with rickets have soft long bones that bend under their own weight.

Only yeast and fish liver oils are natural sources of vitamin D. Therefore, the only regular food sources of vitamin D are those that have been fortified with the vitamin.

Excess intake of vitamin D, especially in infants, can be toxic. Symptoms of toxicity, or hypervitaminosis D, include calcification of soft tissue, such as in the kidneys, lungs, and fragile bones. A deficiency of vitamin D leads to rickets, osteomalacia, and osteoporosis. Hypoparathyroidism may also occur because calcium cannot be absorbed for use by the body without vitamin D. (For a discussion of osteoporosis, see Chapter 36; for hypoparathyroidism, see Chapter 32.)

TOCOPHEROL (VITAMIN E)

Early vitamin studies identified a substance necessary for animal reproduction that was chemically an alcohol. This substance was named *tocopherol*. The most vital function of tocopherol is its action as an antioxidant. An **antioxidant** is an agent that prevents cellular structure from being broken down by oxygen. Vitamin E can protect fragile red blood cell walls (mainly in premature infants) from breaking down—a condition that is termed *hemolytic anemia*.

A deficiency of vitamin E in young infants, especially premature infants who miss the final 1–2 months of gestation when tocopherol stores are normally built up, are particularly vulnerable to hemolytic anemia. In older children and adults, a deficiency of tocopherol disrupts the normal synthesis of *myelin* (the protective fat covering of nerve cells that helps them pass messages along specific tissue, such as spinal cord fibers) and affects physical activity, such as walking and vision.

The richest sources of tocopherol are vegetable oils (wheat germ, soybean, and safflower oil), nuts, fortified cereals, and avocado.

Tocopherol from food sources has no known toxic effect in humans. Supplemental intake of tocopherol that exceeds the normal dose may interfere with vitamin K activity and blood clotting.

VITAMIN K

Vitamin K is composed of a group of substances with similar biologic activity in blood clotting. The major form found in plants and initially isolated from alfalfa is phylloquinone, or vitamin K_1, because of its chemical structure. Whereas phylloquinone is our dietary form of vitamin K, menaquinone, or vitamin K_2, is synthesized by intestinal bacteria.

Vitamin K is known to have two metabolic functions in the body: blood clotting and bone development.

Vitamin K is essential for maintaining normal levels of some blood-clotting factors, particularly the factor prothrombin. Phylloquinone can serve as an antidote for the excess effects of anticoagulant drugs, such as warfarin (Coumadin). Phylloquinone is often used in the control and prevention of certain types of hemorrhages.

Because intestinal bacteria synthesize menaquinone, a constant supply is normally available to back up dietary sources. Therefore, deficiency of vitamin K is not usually found in humans. Only some clinical conditions related to blood clotting, malabsorption, or lack of intestinal bacteria to synthesize the vitamin lead to deficiency. Green leafy vegetables are clearly the best dietary sources of vitamin K. Small amounts of phylloquinone are found in milk and dairy products, meats, fortified cereals, fruits, and vegetables.

Toxicity from vitamin K—even when large amounts are taken over extended periods—has not been observed.

Focus on Pediatrics

Vitamin K

Because the intestinal tract of a newborn is sterile, phylloquinone is routinely given to prevent hemorrhage when the umbilical cord is cut. The "vitamin K shot" given at birth has the trade names of Aqua-Mephyton and Vitamin K.

Focus on Natural Products

Mineral and Vitamin Interactions

Caution patients to adhere to the following guidelines when taking vitamin and mineral supplements:

- Insufficient vitamin D intake hinders the uptake of calcium.
- High amounts of supplemental vitamin C reduce copper levels in the body.
- Vitamin C can increase iron absorption as much as 30%.
- Excessive amounts of vitamin E interfere with iron absorption.
- Vitamin B_6 is required to metabolize magnesium and zinc.

✸ Apply Your **Knowledge 12.2**

The following questions focus on what you have just learned about vitamins and their role in health.

CRITICAL THINKING

1. Describe the fat-soluble vitamins, and list their various actions.
2. Describe how scurvy occurs.
3. Discuss the result of thiamine deficiency.
4. Name the generic forms of vitamins B_1, B_3, B_5, B_6, and B_{12}. Explain the functions of each.

(*continued*)

Apply Your Knowledge 12.2 (continued)

5. Describe pellagra, spina bifida, and pernicious anemia as well as their causes.

6. Explain rickets, and list its signs and symptoms.

7. Discuss antioxidants, and give two examples.

Focus Point

Proper Dosage of Vitamins

Anurse or medical assistant should advise patients about vitamins to prevent deficiency or toxicity. Patients should be told that vitamins are non-caloric essential nutrients found in a wide variety of foods that are needed in very small amounts for specific metabolic control and disease prevention. They should be warned that certain health problems are related to inadequate or excessive vitamin intake.

MINERALS

The body requires stores of minerals in varying amounts. For example, the body stores relatively large quantities of calcium, mostly in bone tissues. Adults who weigh 150 pounds have about 3 pounds of calcium in their bodies. On the other hand, about 3 g of iron is stored in adults of similar weight. In both cases, the amount of each mineral is essential for its specific task. Minerals are inorganic and do not contain carbon.

Major Minerals

Elements called **major minerals**, such as calcium, occur in large amounts in the body. The daily requirements of the major minerals—including calcium, phosphorus, sodium, potassium, magnesium, and chlorine—are more than 100 mg/day.

CALCIUM

Calcium and phosphorus deficiencies are usually caused by metabolic rather than nutritional deficits. Calcium acts in bone formation, impulse conduction, myocardial and skeletal muscle contractions, and blood clotting. The major sources of calcium are milk, cheese, salmon, green leafy vegetables, and whole grains.

Calcium absorption is dependent on vitamin D, the amount of phosphorus in the blood, and PTH. Such bone deformities as rickets, osteomalacia, and osteoporosis occur with calcium deficiency. Excess amounts of calcium in the blood, or hypercalcemia, may cause constipation, hypotension, nausea and vomiting, kidney stones, and cardiac arrhythmias.

PHOSPHORUS

Phosphorus is also needed for bone formation as well as tooth formation and energy. Fat storage and metabolism of other nutrients depend on this mineral. The best sources of phosphorus are milk, cheese, legumes, beef, fish, and pork.

Phosphorus supplements may cause electrolyte imbalances, GI upsets, and bone or joint pain. Phosphorus deficiency can cause anemia, bone brittleness, confusion, and weakness. The toxic effects of excessive phosphorus may cause hypocalcemia and kidney stones.

SODIUM

Sodium is the major electrolyte in the extracellular fluid (ECF). It helps body fluid balance and acid–base balance. Sodium also regulates nerve transmission and cell membrane irritability. The primary source of sodium is table salt. Other sources include meat, milk, celery, and carrots.

Deficiency of sodium may cause headache, confusion, nausea, weakness, anxiety, muscle spasms, and hypotension. Sodium toxicity produces hypertension and edema.

POTASSIUM

Potassium is a major electrolyte of intracellular fluid. It is found in blood, nerve tissue, and muscle fibers. Potassium is necessary for normal cardiac and muscle function. The best sources for potassium are oranges, bananas, red meats, vegetables, yams, milk products, and coffee.

Potassium deficiency can cause loss of muscle tone, weakness, paralysis, cardiac arrhythmias, and digitalis toxicity. Excessive potassium may produce muscle weakness, diarrhea, severe dehydration, abdominal pain, hypotension, and cardiac arrest.

MAGNESIUM

Magnesium is required to form proteins. It stimulates muscle contraction and nerve transmission, activates enzymes, and aids in bone formation. Good sources of magnesium include green leafy vegetables, whole grains, and legumes.

An excess or deficit in magnesium may cause tetany, convulsions, or muscle spasms.

CHLORINE

Chlorine is a major electrolyte, along with sodium, in the ECF. It is a component of gastric hydrochloric acid. Its sources include table salt, meat, milk, and processed foods. A deficiency in chlorine is rare, and toxic levels do not occur.

Essential Trace Minerals

Essential trace minerals, also called **microminerals**, are defined as those having a required intake of less than 100 mg/day. They are not less important than major minerals; rather, they are needed in smaller amounts. These minerals include iron, iodine, fluoride, zinc, chromium, selenium, manganese, molybdenum, and copper. Fluoride forms a compound with calcium (CaF_2) that stabilizes the binding substances in bones and teeth and prevents tooth decay. Except for deficiencies of iron and zinc, other deficiencies of microminerals are uncommon in clinical practice in industrialized countries. Therefore, in the following section, only iron, zinc, fluoride, and copper are discussed.

IRON

Although essential for life, iron is toxic in excess. Thus, the body has developed systems for balancing iron intake and excretion and for efficiently transporting iron into and out of cells to maintain health. Iron functions in the synthesis of hemoglobin and in the body's general metabolism. The human body contains about 45 mg of iron per kilogram of body weight.

Iron is widely distributed in the U.S. food supply, mainly in meat, eggs, vegetables, and cereals. The body absorbs iron more readily when it is ingested with vitamin C.

The major condition caused by iron deficiency is anemia. Iron-deficiency anemia is the most prevalent nutritional problem in the world today. Women and children are affected more than others. Iron deficiency may result from several causes, including:

✳ Inadequate supply of dietary iron

✳ Excessive blood loss

✳ Inability to form hemoglobin because of the absence of other necessary factors such as vitamin B_{12} (e.g., pernicious anemia)

✳ Lack of gastric hydrochloric acid necessary to help liberate iron for absorption

On the other hand, iron toxicity can occur from a single large dose (20–60 mg/kg) and can be fatal.

Focus on Pediatrics

Iron Toxicity

In the United States, iron overdose from supplements is the leading cause of poisoning among young children. Symptoms include nausea, vomiting, and diarrhea. If not treated immediately, several organ systems may be adversely affected, such as the brain, kidneys, liver, and heart.

IODINE

In humans, the basic function of iodine is to participate in the thyroid gland's synthesis of the hormone thyroxine, which in turn controls the body's basal metabolic rate. After thyroxine is used to stimulate metabolic processes in cells, it is broken down in the liver, and the iodine portion is excreted in bile as inorganic iodine. The average adult body contains only 20–50 mg of iodine. Seafood provides a good amount of iodine, although the major reliable source is iodized table salt.

A lack of iodine in the diet contributes to several deficiency diseases, such as **goiter** (a swelling of the thyroid gland), **congenital hypothyroidism** (a condition of extreme hypothyroidism characterized by physical deformity, dwarfism, and mental retardation), and *myxedema* (a life-threatening complication of hypothyroidism, marked by coma, hypothermia, and respiratory depression). Goiter is a classic condition that often occurs in areas where the water and soil contain little iodine.

Intake of iodine through supplementation may result in toxicity for some individuals. Excess iodine may result in acne-like skin lesions or may worsen the preexisting acne of adolescents or young adults.

Focus on Pediatrics

Congenital Hypothyroidism

Congenital hypothyroidism is a serious condition that occurs in children born to mothers who had limited iodine intake during adolescence and pregnancy. During pregnancy, the mother's iodine need takes precedence over that of the developing child. Thus, the fetus experiences iodine deficiency and continues to do so after birth. These children are retarded in their physical and mental development.

ZINC

Zinc is an essential trace element with wide clinical significance. It is especially important during growth periods, such as pregnancy, lactation, infancy, childhood, and adolescence. Zinc is more abundant in the adult body than any of the other microminerals—about 1.5 g in women and 2.5 g in men. Zinc is present in minute quantities in all body organs, tissues, fluids, and secretions.

Zinc is very important during periods of rapid tissue growth, such as childhood and adolescence. Retarded physical growth (such as dwarfism) and retarded sexual maturation (especially in men) have been observed in some populations in whom dietary intake of zinc is low. Zinc deficiency commonly causes poor wound healing, hair loss, diarrhea, and skin irritation. Impaired taste and smell are improved with increased zinc intake if previous dietary intake has been inadequate.

The greatest source of dietary zinc in the United States is meat, which supplies about 70% of the zinc consumed. Seafood, particularly oysters, is another excellent source of zinc.

Zinc toxicity from food sources is uncommon. However, prolonged supplementation in excess of recommendations can cause such adverse effects as nausea and vomiting and decreased immune function. Excess zinc inhibits the absorption of copper, resulting in copper deficiency.

FLUORIDE

Fluoride forms a strong bond with calcium, which means that fluoride accumulates in calcified body tissues, such as bones and teeth. Fluoride's main function in human nutrition is to prevent dental caries. Fluoride strengthens the ability of the tooth structure to withstand the erosive effect of bacterial acids. The continuous intake of fluoride throughout life maximizes the protective effect of fluoride on teeth and maintains an adequate level of fluoride in tooth enamel. Fish products and tea contain the highest concentration of fluoride in foods.

Because fluoride stimulates new bone formation, it has become an experimental drug in the treatment of patients with osteoporosis. Presently, no evidence supports fluoride's ability to prevent osteoporosis. There is also no recommendation to increase fluoride intake during pregnancy and lactation.

Focus on Pediatrics

Fluoride

Fluoridated toothpaste and other tooth products containing fluoride should not be swallowed; therefore, children younger than 6 years of age should not use these products because they are unable to avoid swallowing them.

COPPER

This trace element has frequently been called the "iron twin" because the two are metabolized in much the same way and share functions as components of cell enzymes. Both are also related to energy production and hemoglobin synthesis. Severe copper deficiency is rare. However, copper depletion that causes low blood levels has been observed during **total parenteral nutrition (TPN)** and in cases of anemia. An increase in copper intake is recommended for pregnant or lactating women to meet their increased needs.

The richest food sources of copper are organ meats, especially liver, followed by seafood, nuts, seeds, legumes, and grains.

Wilson's disease is a genetic disorder causing excess storage of copper in the body. Without treatment, Wilson's disease can result in liver and nerve damage.

✳ Apply Your Knowledge 12.3

The following questions focus on what you have just learned about essential trace minerals and their role in health.

CRITICAL THINKING

1. Identify the outcomes of iodine deficiency, and explain the disorders it may cause.

2. Explain essential trace elements.

3. Discuss which major minerals exist in the highest quantities in the human body, and describe their major functions.

4. Compare the function of zinc with that of fluoride in the human body.

5. Identify the causes of iron deficiency.

6. Differentiate between sodium and potassium.

7. Explain the cause of Wilson's disease, and identify the organs of the body that this disease usually damages.

Nutritional Requirements

The objective of a proper diet is to achieve and maintain a desirable body composition and a high potential for physical and mental work. The daily dietary requirements for essential nutrients, including energy sources, depend on age, sex, height, weight, and metabolic and physical activity. The Food and Nutrition Board of the National Academy of Sciences/National Research Council and the U.S. Department of Agriculture periodically review the scientific literature on human requirements for the 45 essential nutrients. Every 5 years, the Food and Nutrition Board issues **recommended dietary allowances (RDAs)**, which are computed to meet the needs of all healthy individuals. For vitamins and minerals, about which less is known, safe and adequate daily dietary intakes have been estimated.

For good health, body composition must be kept within reasonable limits. This requires balancing energy intake with energy expenditure. If energy intake exceeds expenditure or expenditure decreases, body weight increases, resulting in obesity. Conversely, if energy intake is less than expenditure, body weight decreases.

Female patients need to know about the importance of nutrition during pregnancy. Pregnant women should be advised to gain about 25–35 pounds during pregnancy. The rate of weight gain should be 2–5 pounds per week in the first trimester and about 1 pound per week thereafter. Gaining too little weight contributes to the risk of having a small baby; gaining too much weight may cause an early delivery or a very large baby as well as health issues for the woman, such as gestational diabetes, high blood pressure, and varicose veins.

Focus on Pediatrics

Nutritional Requirements

During the first year of life, an infant grows and develops more rapidly than at any other time during the lifespan. Breast milk and commercially prepared formula contain the balance of nutrients that infants' bodies need during that period. Cow's milk does not meet these standards.

Nutritional Support

Oral supplementation with energy- and protein-rich foods is indicated for patients on modified consistency diets that require continued diet therapy, those with chronic disease and anorexia, and those with chronic inflammatory disease or terminal malignancy. *Modified consistency diets* are those that provide foods in a physically altered form (such as chopped, ground, or pureed). Some conditions that warrant the use of modified consistency diets include tooth problems and gum conditions. Other indications result from head or neck injuries or surgeries.

ENTERAL NUTRITION

Enteral tube nutrition may be used in patients with a functioning GI tract to supplement or completely replace oral feeding. Complete replacement of oral feeding is indicated for patients who require intensive protein and

caloric support and who are unable or unwilling to take oral supplementation. Enteral nutrition is safer and less expensive than TPN and is the preferred route when the integrity of the GI tract is preserved. General indications include severe protein-energy malnutrition, trauma to the head and neck or neurologic disorders preventing satisfactory oral feeding, coma or depressed mental state, hepatic failure, and serious illness (such as burns), in which metabolic requirements are high. Specific indications may include preparation of the bowel for surgery in seriously ill or malnourished patients.

PARENTERAL NUTRITION

Parenteral nutrition is administered intravenously and can be partial or total. Partial parenteral nutrition supplies only part of the patient's daily nutritional requirements to supplement oral intake. Many hospitalized patients receive dextrose or amino acid solutions by this method as part of their routine care.

Total parenteral nutrition supplies all the patient's daily nutritional requirements. A peripheral vein may be used for short periods, but when concentrated solutions are used for prolonged periods, thrombosis can occur.

Therefore, central venous access is usually required. TPN is used not only in the hospital for long-term administration but also at home, enabling many persons who have lost small intestine function to lead useful lives.

Focus Point

Cachexia

Cachexia is a specific profound syndrome caused by malnutrition and a disturbance in glucose and fat metabolism. It is usually seen in patients with terminal cancer or AIDS and in patients who are in generally poor health. It is indicated by an emaciated appearance.

✳ Apply Your Knowledge 12.4

The following questions focus on what you have just learned about nutrition.

CRITICAL THINKING

1. Explain cachexia.
2. Compare cow's milk with breast milk.
3. Describe total parenteral nutrition.
4. Explain how total parenteral nutrition is administered.
5. Explain the normal range of weight gain during pregnancy, as well as the risk of too little weight gain in this period.

Nutrient–Drug Interactions

The concept of drug interaction is often extended to include situations in which food or certain dietary items influence the activity of a drug. For example, drug interactions with foods, herbs, or other natural substances may alter the activity of a drug.

Foods can influence the absorption of a number of drugs. In some situations, absorption may be delayed but not reduced. In other circumstances, the total amount of drug absorption may be the result of slowed gastric emptying. However, food may also affect absorption by binding with a drug, decreasing the access of drugs to sites of absorption, altering the dissolution rate of drugs, or altering the pH of GI contents.

The presence of food in the GI tract reduces the absorption of many anti-infective agents. However, there are some exceptions, such as penicillin V (Beepen-VK), amoxicillin (Amoxil), doxycycline (Doryx, Vibramycin), and minocycline (Dynacin, Minocin). With these drugs, it is generally recommended that they be given at least 1 hour before or 2 hours after meals to achieve optimum absorption.

There have been reports of serious reactions (hypertensive crises) occurring in people being treated with monoamine oxidase inhibitors (MAOIs), such as phenelzine (Nardil) and isocarboxazid (Marplan), after ingesting certain foods containing a high amount of tyramine.

Tyramine is metabolized by MAOIs; normally, enzymes in the intestinal wall and liver protect against the pressor actions of amines in foods. However, when these enzymes are inhibited, large quantities of unmetabolized tyramine can accumulate and act to release norepinephrine from adrenergic neurons. Among the foods having the highest tyramine content are aged cheeses (such as cheddar; in contrast, cottage and cream cheeses contain little or no tyramine and need not be restricted). Other foods with very high amounts of tyramine include certain alcoholic beverages (such as Chianti wine), pickled fish (such as herring), concentrated yeast extracts, and broad bean pods.

The consumption of grapefruit juice has been reported to increase the serum concentration and activity of a number of medications, such as certain calcium channel blockers (such as amlodipine [Norvasc], nisoldipine [Sular], and cyclosporine [Neoral]). The bioavailability of most of these agents is generally low, primarily as a result of extensive first-pass metabolism. It has been suggested that components of grapefruit juice reduce the activity of the cytochrome P450 enzymes (a group of enzymes involved in the metabolism of many drugs).

Certain drugs, such as laxatives, colchicine, cholestyramine (Questran), and colestipol (Colestid), have been reported to cause malabsorption problems that result in decreased absorption of vitamins and nutrients

Table 12-2 ■ Drugs That Affect Appetite, Absorption, and Tissue Metabolism

DRUGS OR DRUG CLASSIFICATIONS	DRUG EFFECTS
Alcohol, antihistamines, insulin, some psychoactive drugs, steroids, sulfonylureas, thyroid hormone	Increased appetite
Bulk agents (guar gum, methylcellulose), cyclophosphamide, digitalis, glucagon, indomethacin, morphine	Decreased appetite
Chlortetracycline, indomethacin, kanamycin, methotrexate, neomycin, para-aminosalicylic acid, phenindione	Malabsorption
Warfarin, narcotic analgesics, phenothiazines, phenytoin, probenecid, thiazide diuretics	Hyperglycemia
Aspirin, barbiturates, beta-blockers, monoamine oxidase inhibitors, phenacetin, phenylbutazone, sulfonamides	Hypoglycemia
Aspirin and p-aminosalicylic acid, chlortetracycline, colchicine, dextrans, fenfluramine, glucagon, L-asparaginase, phenindione, sulfinpyrazone, trifluperidol	Reduced plasma lipids
Adrenal corticosteroids, chlorpromazine, ethanol, growth hormone, oral contraceptives (estrogen–progesterone type), thiouracil, vitamin D	Increased plasma lipids
Chloramphenicol, tetracycline	Decreased protein metabolism

from the GI tract. It should be recognized that these agents can also alter the absorption of other drugs that are administered simultaneously.

Many drugs affect appetite, which in turn can lead to deficiencies of certain nutrients. Drugs may also affect absorption and tissue metabolism (Table 12-2 ■).

Certain drugs affect mineral metabolism. Diuretics, especially thiazide diuretics, and corticosteroids, such as prednisone, hydrocortisone, methylprednisolone, and others, can cause potassium depletion, which increases the risk of digitalis-induced cardiac arrhythmias. Potassium depletion may also result from the regular use of *purgatives* (agents that promote bowel movements). Corticosteroids and aldosterone cause marked sodium and water retention, which also occur with estrogen–progestin oral contraceptives (Ortho-Novum, Norinyl). Sulfonylureas (used to treat type 2 diabetes) and lithium (Eskalith) can impair the uptake or release of iodine by the thyroid gland; oral contraceptives can lower plasma zinc levels and elevate copper levels. Prolonged use of corticosteroids, which reduces the work of the construction cells in the bones, causing bone loss, can lead to osteoporosis (see Chapters 36 and 38 for more information about osteoporosis).

Vitamin metabolism is also affected by some drugs. Ethanol alcohol impairs thiamine absorption, and isoniazid is a pyridoxine (vitamin B_6) antagonist. Ethanol and oral contraceptives inhibit folic acid absorption. Anticonvulsant-induced vitamin D deficiency is well recognized. Vitamin B_6 malabsorption has been reported with salicylic acid, potassium iodide (Pima, ThyroShield), colchicine, ethanol, and oral contraceptive use.

Food Additives and Contaminants

The addition of chemicals to foods to facilitate their processing and preservation, to enhance their restorative or stimulating properties, and to control natural contaminants is stringently regulated. Only food **additives** that have passed exacting laboratory testing are permitted to be used at specific levels.

Reported health problems suspected to be caused by some food additives have been trivial and largely anecdotal. Adverse health effects of approved additives and contaminants in the long term have not been established.

The benefits of additives, including reducing waste and providing the public with a greater variety of attractive foods than would otherwise be possible, must be weighed against known risks. The issues involved are frequently complex. The use of nitrite in cured meats is an example. Nitrite inhibits the growth of *Clostridium botulinum* and imparts a desired flavor. However, evidence indicates that nitrite is converted in the body to nitrosamines, which are known carcinogens in animals. On the other hand, the amount of nitrite added to cured meat is small compared with the amount that may be ingested from naturally occurring good nitrates that are converted to nitrite by the salivary glands. In addition, dietary vitamin C can reduce nitrite formation in the GI tract.

Patients need to know about the role of nutrition in helping to prevent specific medical conditions. Health care professionals should emphasize to patients that careful reading of food packaging is a good habit and that nutrient–drug interactions can create adverse effects. Therefore, patients should always tell their health care providers what nutrient supplements they are taking on a regular basis and ask about nutrient–drug interactions when prescribed a new medication.

 Apply Your Knowledge 12.5

The following questions focus on what you have just learned about nutrient–drug interactions.

CRITICAL THINKING

1. Identify the benefits of additives in food.
2. Name two drugs that affect mineral metabolism and can cause potassium depletion.
3. Name five foods that contain the highest amounts of tyramine.
4. Explain the concept of drug interaction.
5. Discuss the adverse health effects of approved food additives in the long term.

PRACTICAL SCENARIO 1

Kate, an abnormally thin 15-year-old girl, is taken to the emergency room by her mother, who reports that the girl is dizzy and shaky, complaining of a pounding heartbeat, and has been having crying spells for the past 2 weeks. Medical records indicate that Kate was diagnosed at age 12 years with bulimia nervosa, an eating disorder associated with emotional distress that is characterized by frequent episodes of *binge eating* (eating an amount of food within 1 hour that is significantly larger than normal for most people) and *purging* (self-induced vomiting and abuse of diuretics or laxatives). For the past 6 months, Kate has been eating small quantities of only a few foods and exercising excessively because she believes she is still too fat. Her
mother fears that Kate's illness has evolved into anorexia nervosa, a common progression. The medical examination finds that Kate has lost 30% of her body weight in 1 year, her electrolytes are seriously imbalanced, and she is hypoglycemic and has protein-energy malnutrition. She is admitted to the hospital for immediate treatment.

Critical Thinking Questions

1. Assuming Kate's gastrointestinal tract is functional, what would be the most efficient method of reversing her physiologic and nutritional starvation?
2. Which of Kate's nutritional deficits is the probable cause of her cardiac arrhythmia?

PRACTICAL SCENARIO 2

A 3-year-old child was brought to his pediatrician's office. While the medical assistant was taking the history of the patient from his mother, she noticed that the child's legs appeared to be "bowing." His mother asked the medical assistant about the cause of this condition in her child.

Critical Thinking Questions

1. What is the most common cause of deformity of the leg bones in children?
2. What is the most appropriate treatment for a patient with this condition?

Chapter Capsule

This section repeats the objectives from the beginning of the chapter and then provides a summary of the most important concepts for that objective. Use this section as a quick review and to check your knowledge.

Objective 1: Identify the seven basic food components and explain their major functions.

■ Proteins, lipids (fats), carbohydrates, fiber, vitamins, minerals, and water

■ Provide energy, promote growth and repair of the body, and ensure the basic processes for life by keeping the body healthy

Objective 2: Differentiate the classifications of nutrients.

■ Generally classified as macronutrients and micronutrients

■ Macronutrients (needed by the body in relatively large amounts): carbohydrates, fats, proteins, macrominerals, and water

■ Micronutrients (required by the body in small amounts): vitamins and essential trace minerals

Objective 3: Explain the role of calories in the diet.

■ Supply the body with energy

■ About two-thirds of total calories come from carbohydrates

Objective 4: Define the role of essential fatty acids in optimal health.

■ Linoleic and linolenic acid (provided by vegetable oils): required for the formation of prostaglandins (hormone-like substances) and thromboxanes (biochemically related to the prostaglandins)

Objective 5: List the water-soluble vitamins.

■ The B and C vitamins are water soluble, whereas the rest are fat soluble.

Objective 6: Discuss the toxicity of vitamin A.

■ Called *hypervitaminosis A*

■ Marked by loss of hair, jaundice, joint pain, and thickening of the long bones

■ May also cause liver injury and fluid accumulation in the abdominal cavity (ascites)

Objective 7: Indicate the significance of vitamin E deficiency in infants.

■ Causes infants to be particularly vulnerable to hemolytic anemia

Objective 8: List the five essential trace minerals and the symptoms of their toxicity.

■ Iron: nausea and vomiting, diarrhea

■ Iodine: acne-like skin lesions, worsening of preexisting acne

■ Zinc: nausea and vomiting, decreased immune function

■ Fluoride: discolored teeth, brittle tooth enamel and bones, brain damage, heartburn, and pain in the extremities

■ Copper: liver and nerve damage

Objective 9: Explain general indications for total parenteral nutrition.

- Inability to use the oral route
- Coma or depressed mental state
- Severe burns or serious illness, with high metabolic requirements
- Severe protein-energy malnutrition

Objective 10: Describe the benefits of food additives.

- Reduce waste.
- Provide greater variety of attractive foods.
- Inhibit bacterial growth.
- Impart desired flavor.
- Enhance restorative or stimulating properties.
- Control natural contaminants.

 Internet Sites of Interest

- Medline Plus, a service of the U.S. National Library of Medicine and the National Institutes of Health (NIH), provides information about the latest vitamin- and mineral-related studies: **www.nlm.nih.gov/medlineplus/vitamins.html**
- The American Dietetic Association provides a wealth of nutrition fact sheets: **www.eatright.org**
- Nutritional tips for pregnant women are available at the website of the Weight-Control Information Network, a service of the National Institute of Diabetes and Digestive and Kidney Diseases: **www.niddk.nih.gov/health-information/health-topics/weight-control/tips-for-two-pregnancy/Pages/fit-for-two.aspx**
- The American Heart Association provides tips for reading food labels at **www.heart.org**. Search for "reading food nutrition labels."
- Guidelines for good nutrition for older adults available at the website of the National Institute on Aging: **www.nia.nih.gov/health/publication/healthy-eating-after-50**

Chapter 13

Dietary Supplements and Alternative Therapies

Chapter Objectives

After completing this chapter, you should be able to:

1. Describe the use of herbal supplements.
2. Explain why the Dietary Supplement Health and Education Act was established.
3. Discuss the lack of controls in the dietary supplement industry.
4. Identify herbal supplements that must be avoided during pregnancy.
5. Differentiate between herbal and nonherbal supplements.
6. List over-the-counter supplements and how they may interact with prescription medications.
7. Define various alternative therapies.
8. Explain how certain cultures have differing views on the use of supplements and alternative therapies.
9. Identify "home remedies" used for alternative therapies.
10. Identify supplements known to have antitumor or cancer-fighting properties.

Key Terms

complementary and alternative medicine (CAM) (p. 186)

dietary supplements (p. 187)
herbal supplements (p. 186)

nonherbal supplements (p. 191)
phytomedicine (p. 186)

Introduction

Herbal and nonherbal supplements are used regularly by more than 158 million Americans, and are easily purchased over-the-counter (OTC) without any prescription being required. This is an important consideration in pharmacology because many of these supplements can interact with a variety of other commonly used substances. There may be potentially dangerous interactions between many supplements and prescription medications, as well as with OTC medications, foods, and even other supplements. Consumers who use these supplements often state that they believe they contain more concentrated healing agents than are found in synthetically created medications. Another factor in their popularity is overall lower cost.

Phytomedicine is the use of plants or plant parts for therapeutic treatments. Approximately 80% of the population of the world uses herbal remedies as their primary form of health care. The use of herbal substances is often aimed at restoring normal balance to the body. They usually offer lower cost, easy availability, and additional advantages such as being able to be used without a prescription. However, problems include the use of herbs that originate from foreign countries, which may not have adequate safety controls in place to ensure that they will be effective, yet harmless. It is vital that every patient using herbal supplements, nonherbal supplements, or alternative therapies discuss these with a physician in order to avoid interactions with prescribed and OTC medications, as well as potential adverse effects.

Herbal Supplements

An **herbal supplement** may be defined as any mixture of ingredients based on plant sources that is designed for the improvement of health or treatment of certain conditions. However, herbal supplements are not considered by the FDA to be drugs but, rather, food products. They are often used by individuals to supplement traditional medical therapies. This practice has led to undesired medical outcomes, interactions with drugs, and toxicity. Patients must understand that the taking of herbal supplements should not occur without consulting their physician. There should be an open dialogue about which supplements are being taken, and in what quantities, especially when prescription drugs are also being used. Because the FDA does not regulate these supplements, there is no independent verification of their quality and effectiveness or the quantity of ingredients they contain. For example, some herbs contain substances that are toxic to all body systems or, most often, the liver. Others have known carcinogenic, mutagenic, or teratogenic properties.

Herbal supplements are available in many different forms, including capsules, liquids, and powders. Many people believe that herbal supplements, because they are "natural," contain stronger healing properties than "synthetic" drugs. The lack of real testing of these supplements means that proof of actual effectiveness is not well documented. The term *herb* is defined as a *botanical* product without stems or bark. Botanicals have been used for thousands of years to treat many different conditions. Their popularity has continually increased and decreased over time. **Complementary and alternative medicine (CAM)** involves different healing systems and therapies, including herbal therapies, nutritional supplements, and special diets.

There are many differences between herbal supplements and prescription or OTC drugs. Perhaps most important is that most modern drugs contain only one active ingredient that is standardized and measured with accuracy. However, many herbal supplements contain a variety of active ingredients, in widely varying quantities and strengths. It is quite possible that they contain large amounts of active chemicals that may not work well together for a controlled effect. There have been recent attempts to standardize certain herbal extracts, including ginkgo biloba and ginseng root. Figure 13-1 ■ shows two ginkgo biloba labels and Figure 13-2 ■ shows various ginkgo biloba formulations.

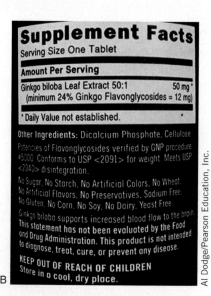

Figure 13-1 ■ Two ginkgo biloba labels: note the lack of standardization in (**A**) 60 mg of extract, 24% ginkgo flavone glycosides and 6% terpenes; and (**B**) 50:1 ginkgo leaf extract, 24% ginkgo flavone glycosides.

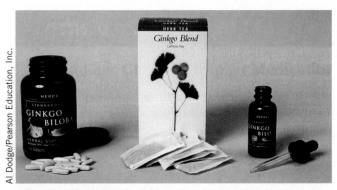

Figure 13-2 ■ Three different ginkgo formulations: tablets, tea bags, and liquid extract.

History of Supplements

The terms *herb* and *botanical* have been used throughout history to refer to plant products that may contain healing properties, flavor-enhancing properties, or food enhancement properties. Herbs have been used for thousands of years, with one of the first recorded uses occurring in 3000 B.C., when garlic was prescribed to treat a medical condition. Thousands of herbs, alone or in various combinations, have been used in both Western and Eastern medicine.

The use of herbs began to decline in the late 1800s, as the pharmaceutical industry experienced widespread development. It soon became easier for manufacturers to formulate, standardize, and distribute their products in comparison to natural herbal products. With increased regulation, many herbal products were removed from the market. Health care became more focused on treating diseases instead of promoting wellness in an attempt to prevent the eventual development of disease.

However, in the 1970s, there was a resurgence of interest in herbal products and alternative therapies. Today, most Americans take these types of products regularly, or state that they have taken them previously. With the gradual aging of the population, and the fact that people are simply living longer, many older Americans have looked for additional treatments that were possibly less expensive yet more effective than standard prescription medications.

Legislation Concerning Supplements

The Dietary Supplement Health and Education Act (DSHEA) of 1994 attempted to regulate herbal supplements as part of its overall description of **dietary supplements**. These supplements are defined as products that are intended to enhance or supplement the diet. They include botanicals, vitamins, minerals, and other extracts or metabolites not already approved as drugs by the FDA. As a result of this act, the FDA can now remove any supplement that it determines poses a significant or unreasonable risk to the public. Manufacturers of these products must label them clearly as "dietary supplements." However, the act is lacking in its regulatory capacity.

The DSHEA also established the Office of Dietary Supplements (ODS), a part of the National Institutes of Health (NIH). The ODS coordinates research on dietary supplements and publishes information about legal and regulatory issues. The National Center for Complementary and Alternative Medicine (NCCAM) is a newer part of the NIH. It coordinates research and training in research methods that concern CAM. It also publishes information about CAM to health care providers and consumers.

There is still no real standardization in the dietary supplement industry. Manufacturers do not have to demonstrate the effectiveness of these products before they can be sold. They also do not have to prove the safety of these supplements. The labeling of these products is required to state that the product is not intended to diagnose, treat, cure, or prevent any disease, but the labels can still make other claims. For example, it is legal for manufacturers to state that their supplements promote healthy immune systems, reduce anxiety and stress, help maintain cardiovascular function, and reduce pain and inflammation. The labels may say that the product contains certain substances, but this claim may or may not be correct, and the included amounts of ingredients may or may not be factual. It is important to remember that just because a supplement is described as "natural," this is no guarantee of its safety.

The Dietary Supplement and Nonprescription Drug Consumer Protection Act took effect in 2007. It required that manufacturers must include contact information on product labels for consumers so that they can report adverse effects of the products. If a manufacturing company is alerted to such an event, it must inform the FDA of the occurrence within 15 days after receiving a consumer complaint. Manufacturers must keep records of these events for at least 6 years, subject to FDA inspection. The FDA now also requires manufacturers to evaluate the identity, potency, purity, and composition of their products, with labels accurately reflecting this information.

Patient medical histories should always include complete listings of herbal supplements so that their effects and/or interactions can be tracked over time. Also, these products have a potential for causing allergic reactions because of ingredients that may be either not listed on the labels or not noticed by the consumer. Patients taking medications such as insulin, warfarin, or digoxin should be educated about never taking supplements without first discussing them with their physicians because these drugs have great potential for interactions.

The American Herbal Products Association (AHPA; http://ahpa.org) assigns safety ratings to all herbal products in four categories, as follows:

❋ Class 1—Those that may be safely consumed if used appropriately

❋ Class 2—Those that carry usage restrictions, unless otherwise directed by a qualified expert:
  • 2a—for external use only
  • 2b—not to be used during pregnancy
  • 2c—not to be used during lactation and nursing
  • 2d—other specific use restrictions, as noted

❋ Class 3—Those that have significant data resulting in the label, "To be used only under the supervision of an expert qualified in the appropriate use of this substance." The label of a Class 3 herbal product must include:
  • Dosage
  • Contraindications
  • Potential adverse effects
  • Potential drug interactions
  • Any other relevant information related to safe use

❋ Class 4—Those that have insufficient data available for classification

Table 13-1 ■ lists the most commonly used herbal supplements and their uses and potential interactions.

Figure 13-3 ■ shows two labels of black cohosh, which is primarily used for menstrual and menopausal symptoms, as well as for headaches.

Table 13-1 ■ Commonly Used Herbal Supplements

HERB	USES	POTENTIAL INTERACTIONS
Alfalfa	Cleanses the body; nutritional supplement	Warfarin, contraceptives, estrogens, immunosuppressants, photosensitizing agents
Aloe	For antihistamine effects, decreases pain from burns and skin irritations; also has laxative effects	Digoxin, antidiabetes agents, various oral medications, sevoflurane, stimulant laxatives, warfarin, diuretics
Astragalus	Increases energy; promotes tissue regeneration; increases metabolism; strengthens the body; for upper respiratory infections	Cyclophosphamide, lithium, immunosuppressants
Bilberry (only to be used for a short period of time)	Treats diarrhea, menstrual cramps, vision problems, varicose veins, and circulatory problems	Anticoagulants, antiplatelet agents, aspirin, insulin, iron, NSAIDs, oral antidiabetic agents
Black cohosh (not to be used in pregnancy, lactation, or by women with estrogen-dependent tumors)	Relieves menopausal symptoms and headaches	Antihypertensives, hormone replacement therapies, oral contraceptives, and sedatives/hypnotics
Cayenne	Boosts energy, improve digestion, increase circulation, and stimulate the heart	Cocaine, anticoagulants, antiplatelet agents, theophylline, ACE inhibitors
Chamomile (allergic reactions are common)	Anti-inflammatory, antispasmodic, and anxiolytic; also for mild sedation	Warfarin, ardeparin, dalteparin, danaparoid, enoxaparin, heparin, other blood thinners
Cranberry	For urinary tract infections	Warfarin, cytochrome P450 2C9 (CYP2C9) substrates
Dong quai	For gynecological conditions such as premenstrual syndrome	Anticoagulants, antiplatelet agents, warfarin

HERB	USES	POTENTIAL INTERACTIONS
Echinacea (use cautiously during pregnancy and lactation; may have spermicidal activity)	Enhances the immune system; anti-inflammatory agent; for upper respiratory infections	Amiodarone, anabolic steroids, ketoconazole, methotrexate, immunosuppressants
Evening primrose (oil)	Source of essential fatty acids; relieves premenstrual or menopausal symptoms; relieves rheumatoid arthritis and other inflammatory conditions	Phenothiazines such as chlorpromazine
Feverfew (may alter clotting times)	Blocks inflammatory substances in the blood; for headaches	Many different cytochrome P450 substrates, anticoagulants, antiplatelet agents
Garlic	Reduces blood cholesterol and blood pressure; anticoagulant	Aspirin and other NSAIDs, warfarin, insulin, oral hypoglycemic agents, antiplatelet agents
Ginger	Treats gastrointestinal GI problems such as nausea; for menstrual cramps; anti-inflammatory agent	Aspirin and other NSAIDs, heparin, warfarin, antiplatelet agents
Ginkgo (avoid during pregnancy and lactation)	Improves memory and reduces dizziness	Anticonvulsants, aspirin and NSAIDs, heparin, warfarin, TCAs
Ginseng (Panax ginseng and Siberian ginseng cause a variety of dangerous adverse effects and should be avoided)	Relieves stress; decreases fatigue; enhances the immune system and memory	CNS depressants, digoxin, diuretics, insulin, oral hypoglycemic agents, warfarin, antidepressants, mood stabilizers, antiestrogens, anxiolytics, antihypertensives
Golden seal (avoid during pregnancy or in young children)	Dries secretions; aids in digestion; reduces inflammation; acts as a mild antimicrobial	Cyclosporine, digoxin, various cytochrome P450 substrates, P-glycoprotein substrates
Grape seed extract (avoid during pregnancy, lactation, and in children)	Source of essential fatty acids; antioxidant; restores microcirculation to body tissues; for allergies	Cytochrome P450 1A2 (CYP1A2) substrates, phenacetin, warfarin
Green tea	Antioxidant; lowers LDL cholesterol; prevents cancer; relieves various GI problems	Antacids, bronchodilators, MAOIs, xanthines, dairy products, ephedra
Horny goat weed	Enhances sexual function	High blood pressure medications, anticoagulants, antiplatelet agents, NSAIDs, thrombolytics, ticlopidine, tirofiban, warfarin
Horse chestnut seed extract	Treats circulatory problems, varicose veins, edema, itching, cramping, and hemorrhoids	Anticoagulants, antidiabetic agents, aspirin and other salicylates, iron salts
Kelp	For thyroid disorders; goiter remedy (due to its high iodine content)	Digoxin, ACE inhibitors, potassium supplements, thyroid hormone, potassium-sparing diuretics

(continued)

Table 13-1 ■ **Commonly Used Herbal Supplements** (continued)

HERB	USES	POTENTIAL INTERACTIONS
Melatonin	Sedative and tranquilizer	CNS depressants, contraceptives, caffeine, fluvoxamine, antidiabetes agents, immunosuppressants, anticoagulants, antiplatelet agents, nifedipine GITS, benzodiazepines, verapamil
Milk thistle	Antitoxin; protects against liver disease	Drugs that are metabolized by the P450 enzyme (such as beta-blockers and certain analgesics)
Parsley	For diuretic, expectorant, and laxative effects	Warfarin, diuretics, aspirin
Red clover	Treats menopausal symptoms and cancer	Anticoagulants and antiplatelet agents
Rose hips	For chest and nasal congestion	Aluminum-containing medications, estrogens, fluphenazine, lithium, warfarin, aspirin, choline magnesium trisalicylate, salsalate
Saw palmetto	Treats benign prostatic hypertrophy	Anticoagulants, antiplatelet agents, hormones such as estrogens, oral contraceptives, and androgens, immunostimulants, and NSAIDs
Soy	Protein, vitamin, and mineral supplementation; for menopausal symptoms; prevents cardiovascular disease; anticancer agent	Thyroid agents (dextrothyroxine, levothyroxine, liothyronine, liotrix, thyroglobulin)
St. John's wort (use cautiously due to a variety of adverse effects)	Reduces depression and anxiety; anti-inflammatory agent	CNS depressants, opioid analgesics, cyclosporine, efavirenz, indinavir, protease inhibitors, SSRIs, TCAs, antidepressants, warfarin
Tee tree oil	For skin disorders such as rashes; for burns	No known interactions
Valerian	Relieves stress and promotes sleep	Barbiturates, benzodiazepines, and other CNS depressants
Yohimbe	Increases male sexual potency; aphrodisiac; for weight loss	ACE inhibitors, antihypertensives, beta-blockers, calcium channel blockers, alpha-adrenergic blockers, CNS stimulants, MAOIs, phenothiazines, SSRIs, sympathomimetics, TCAs, caffeine-containing products, and high-tyramine foods (such as wine, beer, aged cheese, liver)

ACE, angiotensin-converting enzyme; CNS, central nervous system; GI, gastrointestinal; LDL, low-density lipoprotein; MAOI, monoamine oxidase inhibitor; NSAID, nonsteroidal anti-inflammatory drug; SSRI, selective serotonin reuptake inhibitor; TCA, tricyclic antidepressant.

Figure 13-3 ■ Labeling of black cohosh: **(A)** front label with general health claim and **(B)** back label with more health claims and FDA disclaimer.

Focus Point

Herbal Supplements as Potential Poisons

Part of the reason that herbal supplements are often used without being fully understood can be explained by this simple fact: Many herbs listed for use as herbal supplements are also listed on the FDA's Poisonous Plant Database! These include herbs such as aloe, black cohosh, chamomile, feverfew, ginkgo, milk thistle, rose hips, St. John's wort, and valerian.

✳ Apply Your **Knowledge 13.1**

The following questions focus on what you have just learned about herbal supplements.

CRITICAL THINKING

1. What are herbal supplements?
2. Which laws regulate herbal supplements?
3. Why was the Dietary Supplement and Nonprescription Drug Consumer Protection Act passed?

Nonherbal Supplements

Nonherbal supplements are specialty supplements that may be obtained from a variety of different animal or plant sources. They are usually more specific in their actions than herbal products and should be used only for very specific conditions. Substances such as chondroitin and glucosamine are natural body substances necessary for healthy cartilage and may be taken in supplement form. Chondroitin is a protein that helps cartilage to remain elastic, and glucosamine has been shown to aid in cartilage formation and repair. Vitamins, minerals, amino acids, flaxseed, and fish oils with omega fatty acids are other examples of specialty supplements. Vitamins and minerals were discussed in Chapter 12. Table 13-2 ■ lists examples of nonherbal supplements.

Table 13-2 ■ Nonherbal Supplements

SUPPLEMENT	USES	POTENTIAL INTERACTIONS
Chondroitin	For osteoarthritis and other arthritic conditions	Warfarin
Chromium	Increases athletic performance; for non-insulin-dependent diabetes	Insulin or other diabetes medications, antacids, acid reflux drugs, corticosteroids, beta-blockers, and NSAIDs
Glucosamine (must be used with caution by diabetic patients)	For osteoarthritis and other arthritic conditions	Warfarin, antimitotic chemotherapeutics, acetaminophen, diabetes medications
S-adenosyl-L-methionine (SAM-e) (must be used with caution in patients with bipolar or movement disorders who are taking serotonin-enhancing drugs)	For depression and osteoarthritis; less studied uses include liver disease, fibromyalgia, Alzheimer's disease, pain, migraine, and bursitis	Antidepressants, MAOIs, dextromethorphan, levodopa, meperidine, pentazocine, tramadol

Focus Point

Nonherbal Supplements

Nonherbal supplements definitely require further study. Examples of these supplements that have been linked to potentially serious adverse effects are many. The nonherbal supplement 5-hydroxytrytophan, along with the similar agent tryptophan, may contain contaminants linked to eosinophilia-myalgia syndrome. Creatine has been sometimes linked to kidney failure.

Alternative Therapies

Complementary and alternative medicine therapies are those that are "outside" of mainstream health care. They focus on treating each person individually, considering the health of the whole person. CAM emphasizes the integration of mind and body, promoting disease prevention, self-care, and self-healing. It also recognizes spirituality as part of health and healing.

Research continues to determine if CAM therapies are totally or partially effective, or not at all effective. Most likely, some CAM therapies have merit, but others do not. CAM therapies include specific diets, homeopathy, chiropractic, acupuncture, massage, yoga and other types of exercise, meditation and other relaxation techniques, hypnotherapy, biofeedback, prayer, counseling, and detoxification therapies, among others. The value of CAM therapies realistically lies in their ability to reduce the need for medications. When drug doses are reduced, this leads to fewer potential adverse effects. The popularity of CAM is growing continually. Examples of CAM are listed in Table 13-3 ■.

Health care professionals should be sensitive to patients' beliefs about CAM therapies. Advantages and limitations of these therapies should be explained to patients so that they can make accurate choices about their health care treatments. Often, alternative therapies can work together with pharmacotherapy to achieve the proper treatment and healing of patients. In many cultures, home remedies and folk remedies are used alongside pharmacotherapy.

In the United States, the majority of cultural groups use their own preferred home or folk remedies. Native Americans continue to use plants and herbs that are "blessed" as part of their healing techniques. Even today, various groups in the United States have become more open to specific dietary changes, acupuncture, massage, and yoga as alternative therapies. Healers in African and Latin American countries use herbs, oils, and roots, along with religious rituals and implements. In Latin American countries, certain foods are heated or cooled to specific temperatures, at which they are believed to have healing properties. Asian medical practitioners believe in keeping the *yin and yang* (balance) of the body constant in order to maintain good health. They use herbs, specific diets, acupuncture, meditation, exercise, and spiritualists in this practice.

Table 13-4 ■ lists a variety of alternative therapies classified as *home remedies* or *folk remedies*.

Table 13-3 ■ Examples of Complementary and Alternative Medicine Therapies

TYPE OF THERAPY	EXAMPLES
Alternative systems	Chinese traditional medicine, including acupuncture and herbs
	Chiropractic
	Homeopathy
	Native American medicine, including medicine wheels, sweat lodges
	Naturopathy
Biologic therapies	Herbs
	Nutritional supplements
	Specially designed diets
Manual therapies	Hand-mediated biofield techniques
	Massage
	Physical therapy
	Pressure-point techniques
Mind–body techniques	Biofeedback
	Guided imagery
	Hypnotherapy
	Meditation
	Movement therapies such as dance and music
	Yoga
Spiritual therapies	Faith, prayer
	Shamans
Other therapies	Animal assistance
	Bioelectromagnetics
	Detoxification

Table 13-4 ■ Home and Folk Remedies as Alternative Therapies

REMEDY	ADMINISTRATION	INDICATION
Apple (and other crunchy fruits or vegetables)	Oral	Tooth whitening
Baking soda in water	Oral	Urinary tract infections
Bay leaf	Oral or topical (chest)	Bronchitis
Chewing gum (cinnamon or peppermint)	Oral	Stress relief
Chicken soup, hot	Oral	Cold, fever, flu

(continued)

Table 13-4 ■ Home and Folk Remedies as Alternative Therapies (continued)

REMEDY	ADMINISTRATION	INDICATION
Clove	Topical	Cuts in the skin
Dandelion tea	Oral	Urinary tract infections
Epsom salt	Topical (bath)	Acute or chronic bronchitis
Eucalyptus oil	Oral or topical	Mucus reduction, sore throat, improved respiratory function
Garlic	Oral	Antibiotic, antitumor agent, blood cholesterol (to decrease), coronary heart disease, hypertension
	Oral or topical	Antiseptic
Gelatin	Oral	Diarrhea
Ginger	Oral	Anti-inflammatory agent, strengthens immunity
Honey	Oral	Antiviral and antibacterial agent, strengthens immunity, also used for sore throat
Lemon balm tea	Topical	Cold sores
Lemon	Oral	Nausea
Lemon in water	Oral	Cold, congestion
Licorice with petroleum jelly (paste)	Topical	Calluses and corns
Mouthwash	Topical	Skin blisters
Mustard	Topical (chest)	Bronchitis
Olive	Oral	Nausea
Olive oil	Topical	Eczema
Onion	Inhaled	Congestion
	Oral	Blood-clotting disorders, cold, heart disease, stomach or intestinal problems
	Topical (hot packs)	Earache
	Topical (to feet)	Fever, headache
	Topical (to neck)	Headache
Orange juice and gelatin	Oral	Arthritis
Oregano oil	Oral	Reduces soreness from bronchitis, relieves deep coughing, reduces uneasy breathing
Papaya (mixed with oatmeal)	Topical	Smooths and softens the skin
Potato juice	Oral	Arthritis
Salt water	Oral (gargle only)	Mucus reduction, sore throat
Savory (herb)	Oral	Mucus reduction, bronchitis
Sesame seed	Oral	Bronchitis, chest pain

REMEDY	ADMINISTRATION	INDICATION
Spinach	Oral	Bronchitis
Sugar	Oral	Hiccups
Thyme	Oral or topical (chest)	Mucus reduction, respiratory function, antibacterial agent, bronchitis
Turmeric	Oral	Relieves cough, anti-inflammatory agent, mucus reduction
Vegetable oil	Topical	Dry fingernails
Vinegar	Gargled	Sore throat
	Oral	Chronic fatigue syndrome
	Topical	Contact dermatitis, pruritus, sunburned skin
Vodka	Topical	Foot odor
Water	Oral	Bronchitis and many other conditions that dehydrate the body
Yogurt	Oral	Halitosis (bad breath)

Focus Point

Apple Cider Vinegar

Apple cider vinegar is effective for treating many different conditions and is often used along with organic honey. It is used for osteoporosis, leg pain and cramps, nausea, sore throat, weight loss, hypertension, sinus congestion, arthritis, hypercholesterolemia, detoxification, improving cognition, fighting infection, treating skin conditions, reducing pain of sunburn and shingles, vaginal infections, and for diabetes mellitus.

✱ Apply Your **Knowledge 13.2**

The following questions focus on what you have just learned about herbal supplements.

CRITICAL THINKING

1. Why should CAM therapies be explained to patients?
2. How is the use of alternative therapies changing in the United States?
3. What home or folk remedies are used for urinary tract infections?

PRACTICAL SCENARIO 1

Though an herbal supplement may be described as "natural," it may not always be totally safe to use. They are not regulated by the FDA, and people must realize that they take them at their own risk. For example, an 80-year-old patient went to her physician for a routine check-up. She was regularly taking warfarin and captopril because of hypertension, atrial fibrillation, coronary artery disease, and a stroke that occurred 3 years previously. During the check-up, she complained of fatigue, swollen ankles, redness of the face, and headaches. She admitted to having added herbal supplements to her daily regimen of medications.

Courtesy of the author

Critical Thinking Questions

1. If this patient was taking garlic, gingko biloba, ginseng, and St. John's wort, could any of these herbal supplements have interacted with her medications?

2. If the physician instructed this patient to immediately stop taking the herbal supplements, what would be the likely outcome in relation to her prescribed medications and their effects?

PRACTICAL SCENARIO 2

Homeopathy is defined as a therapeutic method that uses highly diluted preparations of substances that have effects, when given to a healthy person, correspond to the manifestation of a specific disorder. The idea behind homeopathy is that this administration will trigger the body's natural ability to fight infection. This often does *not* occur, however. For example, a 9-month-old baby who had severe eczema was treated with homeopathic substances by her parents because they feared traditional medicine. The baby became severely malnourished and developed skin and eye infections. She died three days later of sepsis, which caused bleeding in her lungs and airways.

Aldegonde/Shutterstock

Critical Thinking Questions

1. Discuss the controversy over the lack of regulation of homeopathics.

2. In this case, what is the likelihood that the baby's eczema could have been successfully treated with traditional medicines without any severe adverse effects?

Chapter Capsule

This section repeats the objectives from the beginning of the chapter and then provides a summary of the most important concepts for that objective. Use this section as a quick review and to check your knowledge.

Objective 1: Describe the use of herbal supplements.

- Herbal (as well as nonherbal) supplements are used by millions of Americans and can be purchased OTC without any prescription being required. However, they can interact with a variety of other commonly used substances. Consumers who use them often state that they believe they contain more concentrated healing agents than are found in synthetically created medications. Another factor in their popularity is overall lower cost. About 80% of the population of the world uses herbal remedies as their primary form of health care. The use of herbal substances is often aimed at restoring normal balance to the body. They are often used to supplement traditional medical therapies. Patients must consult their physicians when using herbal supplements.

Objective 2: Explain why the Dietary Supplement Health and Education Act was established.

■ This act attempted to regulate herbal supplements as part of its overall description of dietary supplements. These supplements include botanicals, vitamins, minerals, and other extracts or metabolites not already approved as drugs by the FDA. The DSHEA was established because of supplements that posed risks to the public, or that were not clearly labeled as dietary supplements.

Objective 3: Discuss the lack of controls in the dietary supplement industry.

■ There is still no real standardization in the dietary supplement industry. Manufacturers do not have to demonstrate the effectiveness of these products before they can be sold. They also do not have to prove the safety of these supplements. Though labeling must state that these products are not intended to diagnose, treat, cure, or prevent any disease, their labels can still make other claims. Manufacturers can state that supplements may promote healthy immune systems, reduce anxiety and stress, help maintain cardiovascular function, and reduce pain and inflammation. Labels may say that products contain certain substances, but this claim may or may not be correct, and included amounts of ingredients may or may not be factual. Just because a supplement is described as "natural," this is no guarantee of its safety.

Objective 4: Identify herbal supplements that must be avoided during pregnancy.

■ Herbal supplements that must be avoided during pregnancy are labeled "Class 2b." Examples include black cohosh, ginkgo, golden seal, and grape seed extract.

Objective 5: Differentiate between herbal and nonherbal supplements.

■ An herbal supplement is any mixture of ingredients based on plant sources that is designed for the improvement of health or treatment of certain conditions. They are not considered by the FDA to be drugs but, rather, food products. Herbal supplements are available in many different forms, including capsules, liquids, and powders. They may contain a variety of active ingredients, in widely varying quantities and strengths. Nonherbal supplements are specialty supplements that may be obtained from a variety of different animal or plant sources. They are usually more specific in their actions than herbal products and should be used only for very specific conditions. Other examples of specialty supplements include vitamins, minerals, amino acids, flaxseed, and fish oils with omega fatty acids.

Objective 6: List over-the-counter supplements and how they may interact with prescription medications.

■ Examples of OTC supplements that carry significant interactions with prescription medications include alfalfa, aloe, bilberry, black cohosh, cayenne, cranberry, dong quai, Echinacea, and many others. The use of OTC supplements to supplement traditional medical therapies has led to undesired medical outcomes, interactions with drugs, and toxicity. There are many differences between herbal supplements and prescription or OTC drugs. Most modern drugs contain only one active ingredient that is standardized and measured with accuracy, whereas many supplements contain a variety of active ingredients. It is quite possible that the large amounts of active chemicals may not work well together for a controlled effect.

Objective 7: Define various alternative therapies.

■ Complementary and alternative medicine (CAM) therapies are those that are outside of mainstream health care. They focus on treating each person individually, considering the health of the whole person. CAM therapies include specific diets, homeopathy, chiropractic, acupuncture, massage, yoga and other types of exercise, meditation and other relaxation techniques, hypnotherapy, biofeedback, prayer, counseling, and detoxification therapies, among others.

Objective 8: Explain how certain cultures have differing views on the use of supplements and alternative therapies.

■ In many cultures, home remedies and folk remedies are used alongside pharmac-otherapy. In the United States, the majority of cultural groups use their own preferred home or folk remedies. Native Americans continue to use plants and herbs that are "blessed" as part of their healing techniques. Healers in African and Latin American countries use herbs, oils, and roots, along with religious rituals and implements. In Latin American countries, certain foods are heated or cooled to specific temperatures, at which they are believed to have healing properties. Asian medical practitioners use herbs, specific diets, acupuncture, meditation, exercise, and spiritualists to keep the body in balance, to maintain good health.

Objective 9: Identify "home remedies" used for alternative therapies.

■ Alternative therapies classified as home (or folk) remedies include apples, baking soda, bay leaf, chewing gum, chicken soup, clove, dandelion tea, Epsom salt, eucalyptus oil, garlic, gelatin, ginger, honey, lemon, licorice, mouthwash, mustard, olive, onion, orange juice, oregano oil, papaya with oatmeal, potato juice, salt water, savory, sesame seed, spinach, sugar, thyme, turmeric, vegetable oil, vinegar, vodka, water, and yogurt.

Objective 10: Which supplements are known to have antitumor or cancer-fighting properties?

■ Supplements with antitumor or cancer-fighting properties include garlic, green tea, red clover, and soy.

Internet Sites of Interest

■ For general information and resources regarding dietary supplements, search the Food and Nutrition Information Center of the U.S. Department of Agriculture: **www.nal.usda.gov**

■ The Office of Dietary Supplements of the NIH National Institutes of Health offers information on dietary supplement decision making, claims and labeling, research, consumer safety, and nutritional recommendations: **http://ods.od.nih.gov/ Health_Information/Health_Information.aspx**

- A thorough guide to herbal supplements: **www.herbal-supplements-guide.com**
- Information about drug interactions with nutritional supplements: **www.supplements-and-health.com/facts-about-dietary-supplements.html**
- A list of common alternative therapies: **www.nlm.nih.gov/medlineplus/complementaryandalternativetherapies.html**
- The American Herbal Pharmacopoeia: **www.herbal-ahp.org**
- The United States Pharmacopoeia lists a "dietary supplements" section on its website: **www.usp.org**
- The American Herbal Products Association is the only national trade association that is focused primarily on herbs, botanicals, and herbal products: **http://ahpa.org**

Chapter 14

Toxicology

Chapter Objectives

After completing this chapter, you should be able to:

1. Explain the importance of poisons and antidotes.
2. Describe the detection of poisons.
3. List the most common poisonings seen today in the United States.
4. Explain important factors that are related to risks of poisoning.
5. Describe poison prevention programs.
6. Explain how the most common poisonings occur.
7. Compare lead poisoning and mercury poisoning.
8. Name the antidotes for cyanide, methanol, opiates, and organophosphates.
9. Describe arsenic, atropine, and cyanide poisonings.
10. Differentiate between digitalis toxicity and lithium toxicity.

Key Terms

acetaminophen (p. 203)
acids (p. 204)
alkalies (p. 204)
antihistamines (p. 204)
arsenic (p. 204)
atropine (p. 205)
benzene (p. 205)
carbon monoxide (CO) (p. 205)
chelation therapy (p. 205)
cyanide (p. 206)
detergents (p. 206)
diaphoresis (p. 203)
dysphasia (p. 205)

esophagoscopy (p. 204)
ethylene glycol (p. 203)
euphoria (p. 205)
fluorides (p. 206)
formaldehyde (p. 203)
formic acid (p. 203)
gastrotomy (p. 205)
iodine (p. 207)
isopropyl alcohol (p. 207)
lavage (p. 203)
lead (p. 202)
magnesium sulfate (p. 207)
mercury (p. 203)

methyl alcohol (p. 203)
miscible (p. 207)
opioids (p. 207)
petroleum distillates (p. 208)
phenol (p. 208)
phosphorus (p. 209)
preeclampsia (p. 207)
psychotropic (p. 206)
salicylism (p. 204)
soaps (p. 206)
stupor (p. 204)
toluene (p. 205)

Introduction

Identifying cases of poisoning and correctly assessing the potential toxicity of the poison in each case are essential in preserving life. Poisons should always be considered in young children, especially when their symptoms are not specific for any disease. Children commonly eat or drink substances found in the home that may be dangerous. Other high-risk individuals include older adults, hospitalized patients, workers on the job, and people exposed to environmental pollutants. A thorough drug history should be obtained if the patient is conscious. Blood and urine samples should be collected as quickly as possible because the type and speed of onset of symptoms will substantiate whether the patient's condition is due to poison. Poison control centers keep a wealth of information that may be accessed when poisoning is suspected.

Poisoning

A *poison* is defined as any agent that (in relatively small amounts) can cause death or serious bodily harm. All drugs are potential poisons when used improperly or in dosages that are greater than normal. Accidental poisoning by chemicals causes more than 30,000 deaths each year in the United States. In comparison, suicides by using chemicals number more than 6,600 annually. However, a much greater number of persons are made seriously ill by chemical agents than are actually killed by them. Unfortunately, some of these people are left with permanent adverse effects. In 2014, the total number of reported exposures to poisons in the United States was more than 2.2 million.

Accidental poisonings occur far more often at home than through industrial exposure, and the effects are usually acute. Industrial intoxication is more often the result of chronic exposure. Accidental poisoning usually results from the ingestion of toxic substances, with the majority of occurrences involving children. In most instances, accidental poisonings should be preventable. This is especially true in accidental poisonings of young children via drugs and chemicals found in the home. Pharmacists can play a key role in preventing accidental poisonings, especially those caused by drugs.

Focus Point

Accidental Childhood Poisonings

Accidental poisonings in the home occur most commonly in children younger than age 5 years. Widespread use of child-resistant containers with safety caps has reduced poisoning deaths in this age group.

DETECTION OF POISONS

Optimal treatment of poisoned patients requires correct diagnosis. Although some chemical substances have very characteristic toxic effects, most adverse effects from poisonings can simulate other diseases. Poisoning is often included in the diagnoses of coma, convulsions, acute psychosis, acute hepatic or renal insufficiency, and bone marrow depression. Poisoning is usually not considered when the major manifestation is a mild psychiatric disturbance or neurologic disorder, abdominal pain, bleeding, fever, hypotension, pulmonary congestion, or skin eruption. Furthermore, patients may be unaware that they have been exposed to a poison, as seen in cases of chronic intoxication or after attempted suicide or abortion. If they are aware, they may be unwilling to admit it.

In every poisoning case, identification of the toxic agent should be attempted. Specific antidotal therapy is obviously impossible without the poison being correctly identified. Some poisons can produce clinical features that are characteristic enough to strongly suggest the diagnosis. Careful examination may reveal the unmistakable odor of cyanide; a cherry-colored flushing of carboxyhemoglobin in skin and mucous membranes; or the pupillary constriction, salivation, and gastrointestinal (GI) hyperactivity produced by insecticides. Chemical analysis of body fluids provides the most accurate identification of the intoxicating agent. Some common poisons, such as aspirin and barbiturates, can be identified and their amounts ascertained by relatively simple laboratory procedures. Others require more complex toxicologic tests. Chemical analyses of body fluids or tissues are of high importance in the diagnosis and evaluation of chronic intoxications.

INFLUENTIAL FACTORS

Factors that are important in the consideration of poisoning risk and prevention include:

✻ **Age:** Most poisonings occur in children and are accidental. When poisonings occur in teenagers and adults, they may be suicide related or often caused by overdosage or ingestion of various substances concurrently that are contraindicated for such use. Patients should be educated about carefully reading prescription labels and following the prescriber's guidelines exactly as written.

✱ **Location:** Most children experience poisonings in the home, including areas such as the garage, where many dangerous substances may be stored. Also, products actually kept inside cars and other vehicles are usually capable of causing poisonings.

✱ **Access:** Locked medicine cabinets, cupboards, and other areas where poisonous substances are kept offer good protection against children gaining access. At the very least, medications and chemicals should not be stored within reach of children. In the majority of accidental childhood poisonings, poisonous materials are left in easy reach of children (Figure 14-1 ■).

✱ **Containers:** By storing chemicals and medications in their original containers, labeling is usually effective in helping to reduce the risk of poisoning. Dangerous substances should never be stored in containers, such as used soft drink bottles. A child might understandably assume that what is inside is still soda. Drinking glasses, dishes, and bowls should never be used to measure or transfer dangerous substances into other containers.

✱ **Supervision:** The best way to ensure that children do not accidentally poison themselves is to keep them in sight.

Allowing children to play without adult supervision in areas where substances are stored accounts for the majority of at-home poisonings. When substances are being discarded, they should never be left out in sight, especially near areas where children play.

Cathy Melloan/PhotoEdit

Figure 14-1 ■ In the majority of accidental childhood poisonings, poisonous materials are left in easy reach of children.

✸ Apply Your **Knowledge 14.1**

The following questions focus on what you have just learned about accidental poisonings.

CRITICAL THINKING

1. Explain why accidental poisonings occur more often at home.
2. Discuss how pharmacists can play a key role in preventing accidental poisonings.
3. Identify the most important signs and symptoms of cyanide poisoning.
4. List influential factors of poisoning risks.
5. Explain how poisons can be detected.
6. Identify approximately how many reported poisonings occur annually in the United States.
7. Discuss how child-resistant packaging can reduce accidental poisonings.
8. Explain why identification of toxic agents should always be attempted.

Common Poisons

The most common poisonings seen today involve nonprescription drugs, household products, solvents, pesticides, and poisonous plants. The following sections discuss specific poisons and their actions as well as clinical poisonings.

LEAD

Lead poisoning can occur where there is old paint or lead pipes. Vegetable gardens can also be sources of lead. In adults, lead poisoning is rare. However, it

is one of the most common yet preventable childhood health problems today. Children may ingest flakes of old paint containing lead, mistaking it for "candy" because of their attractive colors. Lead can also contaminate water flowing through older lead pipes, slowly poisoning those who drink it. Lead poisoning causes severe damage to the brain, nerves, red blood cells, and digestive system.

Symptoms of acute poisoning include a metallic taste in the mouth, abdominal pain, vomiting, diarrhea, collapse, and coma. Large amounts affect the nervous system directly and cause headache, convulsions, coma, and death. Treatment usually includes the administration of chelating agents to help the body rid itself of lead by binding to lead so it can be excreted. For mild poisoning, the chelating agent penicillamine may be used alone. For chronic poisoning, penicillamine may be used in combination with edetate calcium disodium and dimercaprol. For acute poisoning, gastric **lavage** is performed.

MERCURY

Acute **mercury** poisoning often occurs by the ingestion of inorganic mercuric salts or the inhalation of metallic mercury vapor. Ingestion of mercuric salts causes a metallic taste, salivation, thirst, burning in the throat, discoloration and edema of oral mucous membranes, abdominal pain, vomiting, bloody diarrhea, and shock. Direct nephrotoxicity causes acute renal failure. Acute

chemical pneumonia may be caused by the inhalation of high concentrations of metallic mercury vapor. There is no effective specific treatment for mercury vapor pneumonitis. Ingested mercuric salts can be removed by lavage, with activated charcoal also administered.

For acute ingestion of mercuric salts, dimercaprol can be given unless the patient has severe gastroenteritis. In treating chronic poisoning, the person must be removed from exposure. Neurologic toxicity is not reversible by using chelation. With the advent of many alternate types of thermometers made for home use, the use of mercury thermometers should cease. Mercury in all its forms is toxic and can result in permanent brain and kidney damage. A broken thermometer easily releases the toxic substance. For reference purposes, it takes only 1 g of mercury to contaminate all the fish in a 20-acre lake.

Focus Point

Mercury

Since 2011, the manufacture of mercury thermometers and other medical devices containing mercury was discontinued in the United States. Previously, the average home thermometer contained approximately 0.7 g of mercury, an amount that was highly toxic to anyone exposed to this substance. Today, electronic (digital) thermometers have almost entirely replaced mercury thermometers.

ACETAMINOPHEN

Acetaminophen is a popular alternative to salicylates as an analgesic and antipyretic and a common cause of poisoning. Although toxic and lethal doses of acetaminophen may vary from patient to patient, hepatic damage will most likely occur if an adult has taken more than 8 g as a single dose. Clinical signs of acetaminophen poisoning are nonspecific. In the first few hours after ingestion, lethargy, nausea and vomiting, and **diaphoresis** may occur. Hepatic damage is the most important manifestation of acetaminophen toxicity and becomes evident 1–2 days after ingestion. Treatment should begin with the induction of emesis or gastric lavage, followed by the administration of activated charcoal. Treatment with acetylcysteine is most effective if started within 10 hours after ingestion.

METHYL ALCOHOL AND ETHYLENE GLYCOL

Methyl alcohol is also called *wood alcohol* or *methanol*. Ingestion of methanol and **ethylene glycol** results in the production of metabolic acids and causes metabolic acidosis. A dose as small as 30 mL can be fatal. Ingestion of only 15 mL of methanol has caused permanent blindness by producing severe optic nerve and central nervous system (CNS) toxicity. Symptoms of methanol poisoning usually

do not appear until 12–24 hours after ingestion, when toxic metabolites have accumulated in sufficient quantities. Methanol is converted to **formaldehyde** and **formic acid**. Manifestations include headache, dizziness, nausea and vomiting, CNS depression, and respiratory failure. In the treatment of patients with methyl alcohol intoxication, emesis and gastric lavage are of use only within the first 2 hours after ingestion. Intravenous (IV) administration of large amounts of sodium bicarbonate combats acidosis. Intravenous ethanol therapy should be used.

Ethylene glycol is a solvent found in products ranging from antifreeze and de-icing solutions to carpet and fabric cleaners. It has a sweet taste and is intoxicating—factors that contribute to its abuse potential. A lethal dose is approximately 100 mL. Gastric lavage with syrup of ipecac is ineffective because the syrup is rapidly absorbed by the intestine. Acidosis occurs as ethylene glycol is converted to oxalic and lactic acid. Toxicity manifests in three stages: neurologic symptoms (ranging from drunkenness to coma), which appear within 12 hours; cardiorespiratory disorders (such as tachycardia and pulmonary edema); and flank pain and renal failure (caused by the plugging of the tubules with oxalate crystals).

The enzyme known as *alcohol dehydrogenase* metabolizes methanol and ethylene glycol into toxic metabolites. This enzyme is also used in the metabolism of ethanol. Because alcohol dehydrogenase has an affinity for ethanol that is 10 times greater than its affinity for methanol or ethylene glycol, intravenous or oral ethanol is used as an antidote for methanol and ethylene glycol poisoning.

FORMALDEHYDE

Formaldehyde is a gas available as a 40% solution (formalin), which is used as a disinfectant, fumigant, or deodorant. Poisoning may be diagnosed by the characteristic odor of formaldehyde. This agent reacts chemically with cellular components and depresses cellular functions, with a fatal dose of formalin being about 60 mL. Ingestion of formalin immediately causes severe abdominal pain, nausea and vomiting, and diarrhea. This may be followed by collapse, coma, severe metabolic acidosis, and anuria. Death is usually caused by circulatory failure. Because any organic material can inactivate formaldehyde, milk, bread, and soup should be administered immediately unless activated charcoal is available.

SALICYLATES

Each year, more than 40 million pounds of aspirin are consumed in the United States, and salicylates can be found in most American households. Aspirin is found as an ingredient in many compound analgesic tablets. The ingestion of 10–30 g of aspirin or sodium salicylates may be fatal to adults. Salicylate intoxication may result from the cumulative effect of therapeutic administration of high doses. In adults, toxic symptoms may begin at dosages of 3 g/day. Therapeutic salicylate intoxication is usually mild and is called **salicylism**. The earliest symptoms are vertigo and impairment of hearing.

Further overdosage causes nausea and vomiting, sweating, diarrhea, fever, drowsiness, and headache. Effects on the CNS may progress to hallucinations, convulsions, coma, cardiovascular collapse, pulmonary edema, hyperthermia, and death. Treatment of patients with salicylate poisoning consists of first inducing emesis or using gastric lavage, after which activated charcoal and then an osmotic cathartic are administered. Respiratory depression may require artificial ventilation with oxygen. Convulsions may be treated with diazepam or phenobarbital. Peritoneal dialysis and hemodialysis are also highly effective in removing salicylates from patients with serious poisoning.

Focus Point

Absorption of Methanol

Methanol can be absorbed through the skin or GI tract or inhaled through the lungs. Since it is a central nervous system depressant, in large quantities, it is poisonous and potentially fatal.

ACIDS

Corrosive **acids** are used in many types of industry and laboratories. They are almost always ingested with suicidal intent. Their toxic effects are attributable to direct chemical action. Ingestion of acids may cause irritation; bleeding; severe pain; and severe burns in the mouth, esophagus, and stomach. Profound shock often develops, which may be fatal. Ingested acid should be immediately diluted with large amounts of water or milk. The emesis or gastric lavage is contraindicated because of the danger of perforation. Diagnostic **esophagoscopy**, if performed, should be done within the first 24 hours after ingestion.

ALKALIES

Strong **alkalies** are used throughout various industries as well as in cleansers and drain cleaners. They include ammonium hydroxide, potassium hydroxide (potash), potassium carbonate, sodium hydroxide (lye), and sodium carbonate (washing soda). The toxic effects of alkalies are attributable to irritation and destruction of local tissues. After ingesting any of these agents, the patient will experience severe pain in the mouth, pharynx, chest, and abdomen. Vomiting of blood and diarrhea

is common. The esophagus or stomach may become perforated immediately or after several days. Treatment consists of immediate administration of large amounts of water or milk. Esophagoscopy should be done within the first 24 hours. Steroids are usually administered for about 3 weeks to decrease the incidence of stricture formation.

ANTIHISTAMINES

There is a wide variation among patient tolerance to **antihistamines** and in the symptoms of poisoning. When poisoned by antihistamines, patients may experience CNS excitement or depression. In adults, drowsiness, **stupor**, and coma may occur. Treatment is supportive, focused on the removal of the unabsorbed drug and the maintenance of vital functions. Convulsions may be controlled with phenobarbital or diazepam.

ARSENIC

Arsenic is a cellular toxin that is readily absorbed through the GI tract and lungs. It has a metallic taste and garlic-like odor, causing extreme GI irritation. Signs and symptoms include nausea and vomiting, hemorrhagic gastroenteritis, cardiogenic shock, ventricular tachyarrhythmias, pulmonary edema, pancytopenia, hemolytic anemia, convulsions, coma, polyneuropathy, renal dysfunction, skin lesions, and others. Arsenic poisoning is treated with advanced life support, endotracheal intubation, fluid therapy, gastric lavage, **gastrotomy**, **chelation therapy**, hemodialysis, and blood transfusions. Arsenic poisoning may cause neurotoxic effects and multisystem organ failure.

Focus Point

Arsenic Poisoning

Arsenic is a natural element that is present in water and soil and is easily absorbed by the roots of rice plants. Rice and rice-related products may have dangerous levels of arsenic. Inorganic arsenic is also sprayed onto rice crops as part of pesticides. In children, arsenic toxicity can harm normal development and cause brain damage. Parents must be especially cautious concerning how much rice is consumed by their children, since it is popular childhood food. There are no FDA standards for arsenic levels in food, though there are standards related to its presence in water. Brown rice is healthier, but has more arsenic, due to its shell, than white rice. Washing rice a few times, boiling it in hot water, and then cooking it helps to remove arsenic from rice. Inorganic arsenic may cause lung, bladder, and skin cancer in adults.

ATROPINE

Atropine is a widely prescribed drug. Young children are very susceptible to poisoning with this agent. Older persons appear to be more sensitive to the CNS effects of atropine. The most characteristic symptoms of atropine poisoning are dryness of mouth, thirst, **dysphasia**, hoarseness, dilated pupils, blurred vision, flushing, tachycardia, hypertension, and urinary retention. Treatment includes emesis or gastric lavage, followed by the administration of activated charcoal. Physostigmine salicylate should be given intravenously if symptoms are severe.

BENZENE AND TOLUENE

Benzene and **toluene** are solvents used in paint removers, dry-cleaning solutions, and rubber and plastic cements. Benzene is also present in most types of gasoline. Poisoning may result from ingestion or from breathing the concentrated vapors of these agents. Toluene is an ingredient present in some types of glue that is "sniffed" or "huffed" as a recreational drug. Acute poisoning with these compounds causes CNS manifestations. Restlessness, excitement, **euphoria**, and dizziness, progressing to coma, convulsions, and respiratory failure, are common. The treatment of acute and chronic poisoning with benzene or toluene is symptomatic.

Focus Point

Gastric Lavage Tubing

Gastric lavage should be performed with the largest tube appropriate for the patient.

BENZODIAZEPINES

Benzodiazepines are easily absorbed, exhibiting 85–99% of protein binding the plasma. They are lipid-soluble, weak acids. Benzodiazepines are mainly eliminated by the liver. CNS depressant effects materialize within 30 minutes of acute overdose. Respiratory depression and coma can occur with ultra-short-acting agents and when benzodiazepines are combined with other CNS depressants. Early in the course of poisoning, excitation may occur. Benzodiazepines are absorbed by activated charcoal, which is the method of choice for GI decontamination. Respiratory support should be provided as necessary.

BLEACHES

Whereas industrial-strength bleaches contain 10% or more sodium hypochlorite, household products (e.g., Clorox, Purex, and Sanichlor) contain 3–6%. For reference, the solution used for chlorinating swimming pools contains 20%. The corrosive action of bleaches in the mouth, pharynx, and esophagus is similar to that of sodium hydroxide. Treatment consists of dilution of the ingested bleach with water or milk.

CARBON MONOXIDE

Carbon monoxide (CO) is a colorless, odorless, tasteless, and nonirritating gas present in the exhaust of internal combustion engines in concentrations of 3–7%. Carbon monoxide is responsible for more than 2,500 accidental deaths and suicides every year in the United States. The toxic effects of CO are the result of tissue hypoxia. The most characteristic sign of severe CO poisoning is a cherry color of the skin and mucous membranes. Treatment requires effective ventilation in the presence of high oxygen concentrations and the absence of CO. If necessary, ventilation should be supported artificially. Pure oxygen should be administered. Cerebral edema should be treated with diuretics and steroids.

COCAINE

Cocaine is a colorless crystalline alkaloid derived from coca leaves. Although used as a local analgesic for a century, cocaine is highly toxic, with moderate vasoconstrictor activity as well as significant **psychotropic** effects. Cocaine is rapidly metabolized by the liver, and its effects are seen quickly—in less than 5 minutes. Peak response occurs in 8–12 minutes, lasting for approximately 30 minutes. Signs and symptoms of acute cocaine poisoning include nervous excitement, incoherent speech, restlessness, fever, hypertension, stroke, and cardiac arrhythmias, leading to convulsions, collapse, respiratory arrest, and death. Treatment involves benzodiazepines, oxygen therapy, dextrose, thiamine, barbiturates, fluid replacement, activated charcoal, and advanced life support. Severe cocaine abuse often results in long-term cardiovascular complications, cerebrovascular accidents, and other conditions.

CYANIDE

Cyanide is an exceedingly potent and rapid-acting poison but one for which specific and effective antidotal therapy is available. Cyanide poisoning may result from the inhalation of hydrocyanic acid or from the ingestion of soluble inorganic cyanide salts. Parts of many plants also contain substances such as amygdaline, which release cyanide when they are digested. Cyanide poisoning is characterized by drowsiness, tachycardia, headache, seizures, apnea, and cardiac arrest. It may cause death within 1 to 15 minutes.

Cyanide poisoning is a true medical emergency; however, treatment is highly effective if given rapidly. Chemical antidotes should be immediately available wherever emergency medical care is dispensed. Diagnosis is made by the characteristic "bitter almond" odor on the breath of the victim. Treatment involves the administration of nitrite, which produces methemoglobin in the body. Supportive measures, especially artificial respiration with 100% oxygen, should be instituted as soon as possible.

DETERGENTS AND SOAPS

Detergents and soaps fall into three groups: anionic, nonionic, and cationic. The first group contains common **soaps** and household **detergents**. They may cause vomiting and diarrhea, but have no serious effects, and no treatment is required. However, some laundry compounds contain phosphate water softeners. If ingested, these agents may cause hypocalcemia, but the ingestion of nonionic detergents also does not require treatment.

Cationic detergents are commonly used for bactericidal purposes in hospitals and homes. These compounds are well absorbed in the GI tract and interfere with cellular functions. The fatal oral dose is approximately 3 g. Ingestion produces nausea and vomiting, shock, coma, and convulsions. It may cause death within a few hours. The treatment consists of minimizing GI absorption by emesis and gastric lavage with ordinary soap solution, which rapidly inactivates cationic detergents. Activated charcoal should also be administered.

DIGITALIS

Digitalis contains *digoxin*, which is used for the treatment of heart failure and atrial fibrillation. Toxicity may result from cumulative effects of the drug, or from hypokalemia. Increased digoxin levels may also result from concomitant therapy with such drugs as amiodarone, erythromycin, quinidine, tetracycline, and other drugs. Signs and symptoms of digitalis poisoning include cardiac arrhythmias, tachycardia, nausea and vomiting, seizures, visual abnormalities, dizziness, altered serum potassium levels, and others. The treatment includes activated charcoal, atropine, antiarrhythmics, electrical cardioversion, fragment antigen-binding (Fab fragment) therapy, and advanced life support. Digitalis poisoning may result in multiple-organ failure and recurrence of toxicity after treatment has ended.

FLUORIDES

Fluorides are used in insecticides. The gas called "fluorine" is used in industry. Sodium fluoroacetate is a powerful rodent poison. Methyl fluoroacetate is too toxic to be used as a pesticide. Fluorine and fluorides are cellular poisons. Fluorides also interact with calcium to cause hypocalcemia. Ingestion of 1–2 g of sodium fluoride may be fatal. Inhalation of fluorine or hydrogen fluoride produces coughing and choking. After 1 or 2 days, fever, cough, cyanosis, and pulmonary edema may develop. The ingestion of fluoride salts is followed by nausea and vomiting, diarrhea, and abdominal pain.

Fluoride compounds can also be used safely. They are introduced into drinking water or applied directly to the teeth to prevent tooth decay. The federal safe standard for the ingestion of fluoride is 4 parts per million (ppm) per day. However, each recommended dose of most brands of toothpaste contains 500–1,500 ppm. Toothpaste should never be swallowed for this reason. The fluoride content of fluoridated water is lower—usually only 0.1 ppm (per serving). With a fluoride overdose, death results from bronchospasm, laryngospasm, pulmonary edema, or circulatory collapse. The treatment for acute fluoride poisoning consists of immediate administration of milk, limewater (calcium hydroxide solution), or calcium lactate solution. Gastric lavage or emesis can be used and charcoal can be given.

IODINE

The traditional antiseptic **iodine** tincture is an alcoholic solution of 2% iodine and 2% sodium iodide. A strong iodine solution (Lugol's Solution) is an aqueous solution of 5% iodine and 10% potassium iodide. The fatal dose of tincture of iodine is approximately 2 g. Iodides are less toxic, with no reported fatalities. The diagnosis of iodine poisoning is indicated by a brown discoloration of the oral mucous membranes. Iodine has corrosive effects on the GI tract. Burning abdominal pain, nausea and vomiting, and bloody diarrhea may occur soon after ingestion. Fever, delirium, stupor, laryngeal edema, nephritis, and circulatory collapse have also been observed. The treatment consists of the immediate administration of milk, starch, bread, or activated charcoal.

ISOPROPYL ALCOHOL AND ACETONE

Isopropyl alcohol is a clear, colorless, bitter aromatic liquid that is **miscible** with water, ether, chloroform, and ethyl alcohol. A solution of approximately 70% isopropyl alcohol in water is used as a rubbing compound. Ingestion produces gastric irritation and raises the danger of vomiting with aspiration. The systemic effects of isopropyl alcohol are similar to those of ethyl alcohol, but isopropyl alcohol is twice as potent. Emesis should be induced or gastric lavage should be performed. Acetone is used in cleaners, nail polish removers, and solvents. Isopropyl is actually metabolized to acetone in the liver via the enzyme alcohol dehydrogenase. Acetone is excreted in the kidneys and lungs, and both of these agents are CNS depressants. Hemodialysis is effective for removing isopropyl alcohol and acetone. It should be considered in patients with high serum levels who do not respond to conservative therapy.

Focus Point

Treatment of Simple Goiter

The administration of 1 drop per week of saturated solution of iodine and potassium iodide (Lugol's Solution) is enough for early treatment of simple goiter.

LITHIUM

Lithium is primarily used for bipolar and unipolar depression. It is absorbed, distributed, and eliminated slowly. Acute toxicity usually causes initial GI symptoms followed by CNS complications. Signs and symptoms include nausea and vomiting, memory impairment, delirium, hypertension, tachycardia, tremors, seizures, coma, and hypothermia. The treatment includes advanced life support, fluid therapy, benzodiazepines, whole-bowel irrigation, hemodialysis, amiloride, and other treatments. Complications of lithium poisoning may include permanent encephalopathy, nystagmus, ataxia, and choreoathetosis (the occurrence of involuntary movements).

MAGNESIUM SULFATE

Magnesium sulfate is used intravenously to prevent seizures, especially in **preeclampsia**, as well as for children with acute nephritis. It is also administered orally to treat constipation and heartburn. Magnesium is a profound depressant of the CNS. With normal renal function, poisoning after oral or rectal administration is unlikely. In the presence of impaired renal

function, an oral dose of 30 g may be fatal. Oral ingestion of magnesium sulfate may cause GI irritation. Systemic poisoning can cause paralysis, hypotension, hypothermia, coma, and respiratory failure. The treatment of patients with magnesium poisoning includes an IV administration of 10 mL of a 10% solution of calcium gluconate.

OPIOIDS

Opioids are natural or synthetic chemicals that have opium-like effects similar to morphine, heroin, and codeine. These drugs have widely varying potencies and durations of action. All these agents decrease CNS and sympathetic nervous activity. Mild intoxication is characterized by euphoria, drowsiness, and constricted pupils. More severe intoxication may cause hypotension, bradycardia, hypothermia, coma, and respiratory arrest. Death is usually caused by apnea or pulmonary aspiration of gastric contents. If the patient arrives for medical care shortly after ingestion, the stomach should be emptied by emesis or gastric lavage and activated charcoal should be administered. Naloxone (Narcan) is an opioid antagonist that can rapidly reverse signs of narcotic intoxication.

Focus Point

The Effect of Opioids on the Body

Respiratory depression increases progressively as doses of opioids are increased. It often manifests as a decrease in respiratory rate, with the cough reflex also being depressed.

ORGANOPHOSPHATE

Organophosphate insecticides are compounds that irreversibly inhibit acetylcholinesterase and are absorbed through the skin, lungs, and GI tract. They become widely distributed throughout the tissues and are only slowly eliminated by the liver. Symptoms of organophosphate insecticide poisoning include nausea, vomiting, abdominal cramping, headache, blurred vision, and excessive salivation. Toxicity may be achieved between 30 minutes and 2 hours after absorption. The treatment of patients with organophosphate poisoning includes removing contaminated clothing, washing the skin with soap and water, and using activated charcoal to decontaminate the GI tract. Additional treatment may involve oxygen administration, ventilatory assistance, and treatment of seizures.

PETROLEUM DISTILLATES

Diesel oil, gasoline, kerosene, and paint thinner are all liquid **petroleum distillates**. Kerosene is widely used as a fuel and as a component of cleaning agents, furniture polishes,

insecticides, and paint thinners. Petroleum distillates are CNS depressants; they damage cells by dissolving cellular lipids. Pulmonary damage manifested by pulmonary edema or pneumonitis is a common and serious complication.

Inhalation of gasoline or kerosene vapors induces symptoms that resemble those of alcoholic intoxication. Headache, nausea, and a burning sensation in the chest may be present. Oral ingestion of petroleum distillates causes irritation of the mucous membranes of the upper part of the intestinal tract. During treatment, extreme care must be used to prevent aspiration. When large amounts have been ingested, gastric emptying is indicated. Emesis may be induced if the patient is alert. Oxygen therapy should also be given.

PHENOL

Phenol and related compounds (creosote, cresols, hexachlorophene, Lysol, and tannic acid) are used as antiseptics, caustics, and preservatives. The approximate fatal oral dose ranges from 2 mL for phenol and cresols to 20 mL for tannic acid. Ingestion of these agents

✳ Apply Your Knowledge 14.2

The following questions focus on what you have just learned about common poisons.

CRITICAL THINKING

1. Describe the treatment for acetaminophen poisoning.
2. Differentiate the signs and symptoms of corrosive acid poisonings from alkali poisonings.
3. Discuss the treatment for carbon monoxide poisoning.
4. Define *ethylene glycol* and describe the antidote in cases of poisoning with this agent.
5. Identify the signs and symptoms of the ingestion of formalin.
6. Describe Lugol's Solution.
7. Explain the complications of lead poisoning,
8. Discuss systemic poisoning with magnesium sulfate.
9. Identify three methods used to remove ingested substances.
10. Describe the most common sources of poisons affecting the general population.
11. Explain the effect of alcohol on the CNS.
12. Discuss the type of alcohol that can cause blindness.
13. Describe the signs of poisoning by digoxin.
14. Identify the treatment for ingested bleach.

produces the erosion of mucosa from the mouth to the stomach. Vomiting of blood as well as bloody diarrhea may occur. Other adverse effects include hyperpnea, pulmonary edema, stupor, coma, convulsions, and shock. Emesis and lavage are indicated for treatment when there is no significant corrosive injury to the esophagus. Activated charcoal should be administered.

PHOSPHORUS

Phosphorus occurs in two forms: a red, nonpoisonous form and a yellow, fat-soluble, highly toxic form. The yellow form of phosphorus is used in rodent and insect poisons and in fireworks. Yellow phosphorus causes fatty degeneration and necrosis of tissues, particularly of the liver. The lethal ingested dose of yellow phosphorus is approximately 50 mg. The ingestion of yellow phosphorus may cause stomach pain, vomiting, diarrhea, and a garlic odor of the breath. Patients may also develop hepatomegaly, jaundice, hypocalcemia, hypotension, and oliguria. The treatment includes emesis or gastric lavage and the administration of activated charcoal and an osmotic cathartic.

Antidotes

Antidotes are drugs or other substances that oppose the action of a poison. An antidote may be mechanical, such as activated charcoal, which absorbs poisons in the GI tract and prevents their absorption. It may also be chemical, having actions that neutralize the toxin, as well as physiologic, in which its actions oppose the actions of the poison. Specific antidotal therapy is available for only a few poisons. Some systemic antidotes exert their therapeutic effect by reducing the concentration of the toxic substance. They may do this by combining with the poison or by increasing its rate of excretion.

Other systemic antidotes compete with the poison for its receptor site. Specific antidotes are listed in Table 14-1 ■.

Table 14-1 ■ Poisons and Antidotes

POISON	ANTIDOTES
Acetaminophen	*N*-Acetylcysteine
Benzodiazepines	Flumazenil (e.g., Romazicon)
Carbon monoxide	Oxygen
Cyanide	Amyl nitrate
Iron	Deferoxamine
Methanol	Ethanol
Opiates	Naloxone (e.g., Narcan)
Organophosphates	Atropine (Atropen) or pralidoxime

CYANIDE ANTIDOTE KIT

Most cyanide antidote kits consist of the following:

✳ Two ampules of sodium nitrate injection (USP 300 mg in 10 mL of sterile water)

✳ One vial of sodium thiosulfate injection (intraperitoneal; 25 g in 50 mL of sterile water)

✳ Twelve gauze-covered ampules of amyl nitrate inhalant (0.3 mL)

✳ One sterile 10-mL plastic disposable syringe with a 22-gauge needle

✳ One sterile 50-mL plastic disposable syringe with a 22-gauge needle

✳ One stomach tube

✳ One nonsterile 50-mL syringe

✳ One set of instructions for the treatment of cyanide poisoning

Sodium nitrite reacts with hemoglobin to form methemoglobin, which removes cyanide ions from various tissues and couples with them to become cyanmethemoglobin, which has a relatively low toxicity. Sodium thiosulfate converts cyanide to thiocyanate. The combination of sodium nitrite and sodium thiosulfate is the best therapy against cyanide and hydrocyanic acid poisoning. The two substances are injected IV—one after the other (the nitrite followed by the thiosulfate). They are capable of detoxifying approximately 20 lethal doses of sodium cyanide and are effective even after respiration has stopped. As long as the heart is still beating, the chances of recovery after using this method are very good.

Prevention

Quality, in-depth education about poisons and poisonings is the best method to address the problem. Directions and steps for poison prevention should be clear and determinate. Accurate lists of all potential poisons should be supplied. Often, parents are unaware that a specific product is actually poisonous. Naming actual locations to store specific products in the household does far more than generalizing about how many children are poisoned at home each year. Person-to-person counseling about specific medications and other substances, detailing their poisoning potential, is invaluable. The use of safety containers and child-resistant packaging must be stressed to parents and family members (Figure 14-2 ■). Certain medications sold over the counter are not currently required to have child-resistant packaging even though, if taken in large quantities, they could cause severe harm and even death.

Figure 14-2 ■ Child-resistant packaging.

Poison Control Centers

A network consisting of more than 600 poison control centers exists in the United States. Poison treatment information is available free of charge 24 hours a day. The first poison control center was established in Chicago, led by the Illinois chapter of the American Academy of Pediatrics. Shortly afterward, the Duke University Poison Control Center was established in North Carolina. The idea of poison control centers then spread across the country.

In 1957, the FDA established the National Clearinghouse for Poison Control Centers to coordinate activities at poison control centers across the United States. This clearinghouse collected and standardized product toxicology data, reproduced this information on large file cards, and distributed them nationwide to poison control centers.

✳ Apply Your Knowledge 14.3

The following questions focus on what you have just learned about antidotes, cyanide poisoning, and poison control centers.

CRITICAL THINKING

1. Identify the antidotes for methanol poisoning, opiate overdose, and benzodiazepine overdose.
2. Explain why the administration of nitrite is preferred to treat cyanide poisoning.
3. Discuss the functions of poison control centers.

PRACTICAL SCENARIO 1

A 76-year-old grandmother with a history of angina pectoris and heart attacks went to Florida to visit her daughter and granddaughter. She had medications in her purse that did not have childproof lids because she lived alone and there was no danger of a child being poisoned. A few hours after she arrived at her daughter's house, her granddaughter wouldn't awaken from her nap and had a nosebleed. The child's mother called 911, and the child was taken to the emergency room in an ambulance. It was soon discovered that she had swallowed half of the bottle of one of her grandmother's medications, presumably taking them from her grandmother's purse while she was taking a shower and the child's mother was cooking.

Critical Thinking Questions

1. What could have been done to prevent this type of accident?
2. If the medication the child consumed was aspirin, what treatments would be indicated?

PRACTICAL SCENARIO 2

On a cold winter evening, a family lit its fireplace to help warm up the house. One of the family's children was using his laptop near the fire. A while later, as his father was working in his office, he noticed that the air in the house smelled of smoke. He entered the family room and noticed that his son was asleep. He tried to get him to go to bed, but he was unresponsive. He quickly opened all the house's windows and got his children and wife, who was in the back bedroom, outside. He then went back in and found that the chimney flue had not been opened.

Michael Macsuga/Shutterstock

Critical Thinking Questions

1. What gas had most likely overcome the family?
2. Why did the father open the windows and take the family outside?

Chapter Capsule

This section repeats the objectives from the beginning of the chapter and then provides a summary of the most important concepts for that objective. Use this section as a quick review and to check your knowledge.

Objective 1: Explain the importance of poisons and antidotes.

- A poison is any agent that in relatively small amounts can cause death or serious bodily harm. All drugs are potential poisons when used improperly or in dosages that are greater than normal.

- Specific antidotal therapy is available for only a few poisons. Some systemic antidotes exert their therapeutic effect by reducing the concentration of the toxic substance. They may do this by combining with the poison or by increasing its rate of excretion. Other systemic antidotes compete with the poison for its receptor site.

Objective 2: Describe the detection of poisons.

- The optimal treatment of poisoned patients requires correct diagnosis. Most adverse effects from poisonings can simulate other diseases. In every poisoning case, the identification of the toxic agent should be attempted. Specific antidotal therapy is obviously impossible without the poison being correctly identified. Some poisons can produce clinical features that are characteristic enough to strongly suggest the diagnosis. Chemical analysis of body fluids provides the most accurate identification of the intoxicating agent.

Objective 3: List the most common poisonings seen today in the United States.

- The most common poisonings in the United States involve lead, mercury, acetaminophen, methyl alcohol, ethylene glycol, formaldehyde, salicylates, acids, alkalies, antihistamines, arsenic, atropine, benzene, toluene, benzodiazepines, bleaches, carbon monoxide, cocaine, cyanide, detergents, soaps, digitalis, fluorides, iodine, isopropyl alcohol, acetone, lithium, magnesium sulfate, opioids, organophosphate and carbamate insecticides, petroleum distillates, phenol, and phosphorus.

Objective 4: Explain important factors that are related to risks of poisoning.

■ Factors that are important in the consideration of poisoning risk and prevention include age (most poisonings occur in children and are accidental), location (usually at home), access (locked medicine cabinets, cupboards, and other areas are helpful in protecting against poisonings), containers (using original containers with proper labeling), and supervision (keeping children in sight at all times).

Objective 5: Describe poison prevention programs.

■ The best method of poison prevention is quality, in-depth education. All directions and steps should be clear and determinate, and accurate lists of all potential poisons should be supplied. Naming actual locations to store specific products in the household does far more than generalizing about how many children are poisoned at home each year. Person-to-person counseling about specific medications and other substances, detailing their poisoning potential, is invaluable. The use of safety containers and child-resistant packaging must be stressed to parents and family members. Lack of the use of child-resistant packaging can lead to severe harm and even death.

Objective 6: Explain how the most common poisonings occur.

■ Most common poisonings occur at home, with acute effects. These mostly accidental poisonings usually result from the ingestion of toxic substances—most often by children. These examples are usually preventable if proper measures are taken. Common cases of poisoning are usually caused by unlocked storage areas, repackaging poisons into containers that do not bear warning labels or other accurate labeling, and the lack of proper supervision of children.

Objective 7: Compare lead poisoning and mercury poisoning.

■ Lead poisoning usually affects children and may involve old paint containing lead, pipes made of lead, and vegetable gardens. Lead poisoning causes severe damage to the brain, nerves, red blood cells, and digestive system. Symptoms include a metallic taste, abdominal pain, vomiting, diarrhea, collapse, coma, headache, convulsions, and death. Treatment usually involves such chelating agents as penicillamine, edetate calcium disodium, and dimercaprol. Gastric lavage may also be indicated.

■ Mercury poisoning often occurs by the ingestion of inorganic mercuric salts or the inhalation of metallic mercury vapor. Symptoms include a metallic taste, salivation, thirst, burning in the throat, discoloration and edema of oral mucous membranes, abdominal pain, vomiting, bloody diarrhea, shock, acute renal failure, and acute chemical pneumonia. There is no specific treatment for mercury vapor pneumonitis. Ingested mercuric salts can be removed by lavage, with activated charcoal also administered. Dimercaprol can be given, and if poisoning is chronic, the patient must be removed from exposure to mercury.

Objective 8: Name the antidotes for cyanide, methanol, opiates, and organophosphates.

■ Cyanide—antidote: amyl nitrate

■ Methanol—antidote: ethanol

■ Opiates—antidote: naloxone

■ Organophosphates—antidote: atropine or pralidoxime

Objective 9: Describe arsenic, atropine, and cyanide poisonings.

■ *Arsenic poisoning:* Arsenic is a cellular toxin readily absorbed through the GI tract and lungs; it has a metallic taste and garlic-like odor, and it causes extreme GI irritation. Signs and symptoms include nausea and vomiting, hemorrhagic gastroenteritis, cardiogenic shock, ventricular tachyarrhythmias, pulmonary edema, pancytopenia, hemolytic anemia, convulsions, coma, polyneuropathy, renal dysfunction, and skin lesions. Patients are treated with advanced life support, endotracheal intubation, fluid therapy, gastric lavage, gastrotomy, chelation therapy, hemodialysis, and blood transfusions.

■ *Atropine poisoning:* Although young children are very susceptible to atropine poisoning, older persons appear to be more sensitive to its CNS effects; symptoms include dryness of the mouth, thirst, dysphasia, hoarseness, dilated pupils, blurred vision, flushing, tachycardia, hypertension, and urinary retention. The treatment includes emesis, gastric lavage, activated charcoal, and physostigmine salicylate.

■ *Cyanide poisoning:* A potent, rapid-acting poison, cyanide may exert its effects via the inhalation of hydrocyanic acid or from the ingestion of soluble inorganic cyanide salts. Many plants also release cyanide when they are digested. In a true medical emergency, patients with cyanide poisoning respond to rapid treatment. Chemical antidotes should be readily available at emergency care facilities. A distinct "bitter almond" odor will be present on the breath of the victim, and the treatment involves the administration of nitrite. Supportive measures include artificial respiration with 100% oxygen.

Objective 10: Differentiate between digitalis toxicity and lithium toxicity.

■ Digitalis toxicity: Digitalis poisoning may result in multiple-organ failure and recurrence of toxicity after treatment with activated charcoal, atropine, antiarrhythmics, electrical cardioversion, fragment antigen-binding therapy, and advanced life support.

■ Lithium toxicity: Acute lithium toxicity causes initial GI symptoms, followed by CNS complications. It is absorbed, distributed, and eliminated slowly.

 Internet Sites of Interest

■ Symptoms of mercury poisoning, mercury prognosis, and detoxification guide: **http://heartspring.net/mercury_poison_symptoms.html**

■ American Association of Poison Control Centers: **www.aapcc.org**

■ Alcohol poisoning symptoms: **www.md-health.com/Alcohol-Poisoning-Symptoms.html**

■ Poisoning causes, symptoms, diagnosis, and treatment: **www.emedicinehealth .com/poisoning/article_em.htm**

■ Lead poisoning: **www.mayoclinic.com/diseases-conditions/lead-poisoning/ basics/definition/con-20035487**

■ Aspirin and other salicylate poisoning: **www.emedicinehealth.com/ aspirin_poisoning/article_em.htm**

■ Common poisons at home and at work: **www.ncpoisoncenter.org/body.cfm?id=87**

■ Household poisons: **www.poison.org/common-and-dangerous-poisons**

Chapter 15

Substance Abuse and Misuse

Chapter Objectives

After completing this chapter, you should be able to:

1. Define *addiction* and list several factors on which it may be based.
2. Identify the most commonly abused drugs in the United States.
3. List five substances that cause relaxation or sedation.
4. Explain opioid addiction and its withdrawal.
5. Discuss cannabinoids and their effects on the central nervous system.
6. Compare hallucinogens and opioid drugs.
7. Explain the effects of substance abuse.
8. Describe withdrawal from nicotine.
9. Explain the psychological and physical effects of alcoholism.
10. Discuss signs and symptoms of withdrawal from alcohol.

Key Terms

additive effect (p. 215)
benzodiazepines (p. 216)
cannabinoids (p. 217)
delirium tremens (DT) (p. 223)
detoxification (p. 221)

hallucinogens (p. 218)
polysubstance abuse (p. 216)
psychological treatment (p. 221)
sedatives (p. 216)
substance abuse (p. 215)

substance-dependent (p. 215)
tetrahydrocannabinol (THC) (p. 217)
tobacco dependence (p. 221)
withdrawal (p. 216)

Introduction

Substance abuse is a major issue in today's society. Throughout history, natural and prescription drugs have been used to increase physical or mental performance. These substances cause a relaxed feeling and a change in psychological state. The most commonly abused substances include alcohol, prescription medications, over-the-counter (OTC) medications, and illegal drugs. Addiction is very prevalent and refers to any physical or psychological dependence on any substance. It is a psychological and biological problem. Many people who take drugs use more than one drug, which is referred to as *polysubstance abuse*. Drug abuse is generally associated with anxiety and depression. The most common addiction today does not involve any of the previously mentioned substances; rather, the most common addiction is to nicotine, as found in cigarettes and other tobacco products.

Substance Abuse

Substance abuse may affect every level of a person's life. People are described as having a substance abuse problem when they experience significant distress in their lives and when any four of the following things occur:

1. Failure to fulfill parenting, school, or work obligations
2. Hazardous behavior, such as driving under the influence
3. Recurrent legal problems related to hazardous behaviors
4. Continued use of substances despite continuing social or interpersonal problems

People are termed to be **substance-dependent** when they exhibit any three of the following signs:

1. Tolerance
2. Withdrawal
3. Increasing consumption
4. Desire to quit
5. Excessive time spent on abuse
6. Fewer occupational, recreational, or social activities
7. Continued use while understanding the physiologic and psychological effects

A *substance abuse disorder* is one that includes both substance abuse and dependence. Addiction is defined as progressive, chronic abuse of a substance that causes a person to use the substance repeatedly despite serious health and social consequences. It depends on varying factors based on the drug or drugs used. These include cost, availability, dose, and method of administration. Other factors that may influence addiction include experience with drugs, risk-taking behaviors, certain diseases that require scheduled drugs to be taken, educational opportunities, and peer influences.

Sedatives and hypnotics are used to promote relaxation in small doses but can induce sleep and confusion when used in higher doses. Very high doses can induce coma and even death. Any combination of these agents can be lethal, known as the **additive effect**.

Substance Misuse

Substance misuse is defined as the use of drugs or other agents for other than their indications. It is common in patients in primary care settings, and it is often difficult to identify. Patients should be screened for determination of hazardous use of substances, actual substance abuse, and substance dependence. Substance use disorders often accompany mental illness and domestic violence. Prescription opioids are examples of drugs that are often misused.

When a patient is screened for substance misuse and the result is negative, it is important to reinforce healthy behavior. However, when the result is positive, there are many steps to be taken. The first is to assess substance use and comorbidities to determine whether there is hazardous use, substance abuse, or substance dependence. If there is hazardous use, treatment includes brief counseling and ongoing assessment. If there is substance abuse, treatment includes brief counseling, negotiating a plan, close follow-up; if abuse continues, more intensive treatment is recommended. If there is substance dependence, treatment includes brief counseling, referral for treatment, consideration of pharmacotherapy, and finally ongoing assessment and support.

Addictive Drugs

The majority of drugs of abuse are addictive. Addiction is chronic and characterized by compulsive drug seeking and use despite negative consequences and long-lasting brain changes. Strong cravings for a drug make it difficult to stop, and addiction often results in poor and dangerous choices to be made concerning behavior. According to the Drug Enforcement Agency (DEA), the most commonly abused substances include alcohol, tobacco, marijuana, cocaine, club drugs, hallucinogens, heroin, inhalants, methamphetamine, prescription opioids, prescription sedatives, prescription stimulants, synthetic cannabinoids, and anabolic steroids.

Addictive drugs include cannabinoids (e.g., hashish and marijuana), depressants (e.g., barbiturates and benzodiazepines), dissociative anesthetics (e.g., ketamine and phenylcyclohexylpiperidine [PCP]), hallucinogens (e.g., lysergic acid diethylamide [LSD] and mescaline), opioids and morphine derivatives (e.g., codeine and morphine), stimulants (e.g., amphetamine and cocaine), and other compounds such as anabolic steroids and dextromethorphan. Misuse of prescription drugs exceeds the combined use of *all* street drugs except marijuana. Currently, about 8% of Americans age 12 or older are dependent on drugs or alcohol. Use of two or more different substances of abuse is referred to as **polysubstance abuse**.

Recent studies have shown the following percentages and numbers of users of abused drugs:

✳ Marijuana: 4.9% of Americans or 15.2 million people

✳ Opioids: 3.6% of Americans or 11 million people

✳ Sedatives: 2.9% of Americans or 8.9 million people

✳ Hallucinogens: 0.36% of Americans or 1.1 million people

✳ Cocaine: 0.33% of Americans or 1 million people

✳ Methamphetamines: 0.17% of Americans or 529,000 people

Out of all substance abusers, only 4.8% on average believe they need treatment. Drug addiction can start early. Of people older than age 18 who first tried marijuana before age 14, a total of 13% are now substance abusers. Apparently, the earlier in life the person begins using drugs, the higher the chance he or she will have a long-term substance use disorder.

Focus Point

Withdrawal Syndrome

Withdrawal syndrome is defined as the unpleasant symptoms that are experienced when a client with physical dependence discontinues the use of an abused drug.

Central Nervous System Depressants

Central nervous system (CNS) depressants cause relaxation or sedation and include barbiturates, nonbarbiturate sedative–hypnotics, benzodiazepines, opioids, and gamma hydroxybutyrate. The CNS depressants allowed for medical use are controlled because of their abuse potential. The following paragraphs explain these agents in detail. Alcohol and alcoholism are explained later in this chapter.

BARBITURATES AND NONBARBITURATE SEDATIVE–HYPNOTICS

There are two major types of **sedatives** (tranquilizers): barbiturates and nonbarbiturate sedative–hypnotics. They are used for sleep disorders and certain forms of epilepsy. These agents have similar actions to each other and may cause physical or psychologic dependence as well as tolerance when taken at high doses or for extended periods. Sedatives are often combined with alcohol and other CNS stimulants. Those who become addicted often vary between these drugs and amphetamines in an attempt to control their wakefulness and sleep patterns.

Some sedatives last for as long as an entire day, with higher doses causing similar effects to those of alcohol intoxication. Commonly abused barbiturates include amobarbital (Amytal), secobarbital (Seconal Sodium), pentobarbital (Nembutal), and the combination of amobarbital and secobarbital (known as Tuinal). Medical use of these agents has decreased greatly since the 1970s. Overdoses of these agents are very dangerous, potentially causing respiratory arrest, coma, and death. Barbiturates were responsible for the deaths of entertainers such as Marilyn Monroe and Judy Garland.

BENZODIAZEPINES

Benzodiazepines are CNS depressants that are widely prescribed, largely replacing barbiturates for various conditions. They are usually used to treat anxiety but also for muscle relaxation and the prevention of seizures. Commonly used benzodiazepines include alprazolam (Xanax), diazepam (Valium), midazolam (Versed), temazepam (Restoril), and triazolam (Halcion). Flunitrazepam (Rohypnol) began being abused in the early 1990s in the United States, even though it has no approved medical use in this country and its importation is banned.

Frequently abused, benzodiazepines may cause patients to appear remote from others, lightheaded, disoriented, or sleepy. Although these agents seldom cause death because of overdose, users frequently combine them with alcohol and illegal drugs to increase their effects. In these cases, the outcome may be fatal. **Withdrawal** from benzodiazepines is not as severe compared with withdrawal from alcohol or barbiturates. However, drug levels of benzodiazepines, remain higher in the body for several weeks, making abuse of these agents extremely dangerous.

OPIOIDS

Opioids (narcotic analgesics) are used for severe pain, diarrhea, and persistent cough. This class of drugs includes natural substances derived from unripe poppy seeds (codeine, morphine, and opium). Synthetic forms of these agents are available, including fentanyl (Sublimaze), meperidine (Demerol HCl), methadone (Dolophine), oxycodone (OxyCONTIN), and the illegal drug heroin. Orally administered opioids take effect within 30 minutes and can last for more than a day. Parenteral forms, including heroin, cause a euphoric rush, intense sedation, and abnormally slow body functions. Signs of use include constricted pupils, respiratory depression, and the ability to tolerate increased amounts of pain. Overdose is extremely dangerous and potentially fatal. Famous deaths from heroin have included singer Janis Joplin; actor Philip Seymour Hoffman died from a toxic mixture of heroin, cocaine, amphetamines, and benzodiazepines. Approximately 42,000 people die every year in the United States from opioid overdoses.

Opioid addiction may develop rapidly and withdrawal is very unpleasant (although not life-threatening compared with barbiturate withdrawal). Methadone is often used to treat patients with addiction to other opioids because it does not produce the same degree of euphoria and has longer-lasting effects. It may also be addictive—but to a lesser degree—and helps those who are addicted to heroin to withdraw from that drug without unpleasant withdrawal symptoms. Methadone is an orally administered opioid, which helps to remove further risks (via parenteral injection) of contact with such diseases as AIDS and hepatitis. Methadone may be used throughout a patient's lifetime (in certain cases), with withdrawal taking longer than that of heroin or morphine but with less intense symptoms.

GAMMA HYDROXYBUTYRATE

Gamma hydroxybutyrate, also called GHB or Xyrem, is a CNS depressant first approved for narcolepsy, but as a metabolite of the neurotransmitter gamma-aminobutyric acid (GABA), it is finding popularity as a club or party drug of abuse. In these situations, GHB is often put into someone's alcoholic beverage. Negative effects may include sweating, loss of consciousness, nausea, hallucinations, amnesia, and coma. The prescription form, Xyrem, was approved by the FDA in 2002 to treat narcolepsy, is a Schedule III controlled substance, and requires patient enrollment in a restricted access program. GHB is available in odorless, colorless, and tasteless liquid or powder forms. It also has anabolic effects, aiding in fat reduction and muscle building.

✳ Apply Your Knowledge 15.1

The following questions focus on what you have just learned about substance abuse and addictive drugs.

CRITICAL THINKING

1. Describe the effects of substance abuse on an individual.
2. Explain polysubstance abuse.
3. Give six examples of CNS system depressants.
4. Identify the indications of benzodiazepines.
5. Describe the indications of opioids for various conditions.

Cannabinoids

Cannabinoids are obtained from the hemp plant (*Cannabis sativa*) and are usually smoked to obtain their effects. Cannabinoids include marijuana, hashish, and hash oil, with the most psychoactive agent being delta-9-**tetrahydrocannabinol (THC)**.

MARIJUANA

Marijuana is a natural substance that is the most commonly used illicit drug in the United States. It is regularly referred to as "dope," "grass," "pot," "reefer," or "weed." The effects of marijuana include decreased coordination and motor activity, confusion, paranoia, euphoria, increased thirst and hunger, and bloodshot eyes. Effects occur within a few minutes and last for up to 24 hours. Marijuana smoke is generally inhaled more deeply than cigarette smoke, introducing four times the particulates of tar into the lungs. Daily use increases the risks of lung cancer and respiratory conditions and leads to a lack of motivation.

However, marijuana produces very little physical dependence or tolerance, with withdrawal symptoms being nearly nonexistent. Because THC metabolites remain in the body for many months (or years depending on usage), tests can easily show that a person has been using marijuana or has quit before the tests. THC is detectable in the urine for several days after using marijuana. As of November 2016, medical marijuana usage laws have been established in 28 states, yet the drug is still federally classified as a Schedule I drug. Its medical value is still controversial, but legalized use of the drug is growing. Recently, in California, marijuana extract has been approved for sale as an additive to ice cream for patients who are approved to use medical marijuana. Other recent studies have included the testing of Epidiolex, which is a purified oil-based extract of cannabidiol, to treat children with types of epilepsy that did not respond to currently available treatments. Marijuana has also been tested in

monkeys with AIDS and has shown an ability to stimulate appetite, prevent weight loss, and decrease damaged immune tissue in the stomach, which is a common spot for the infection to occur.

Focus Point

The Use and Legalization of Marijuana

Marijuana is currently allowed for medical use in 28 states and also in the District of Columbia, Puerto Rico, and Guam. State penalties for use, possession, and cultivation of marijuana have been decriminalized for patients who have written documentation from a physician that their health might benefit from its medical use. Another important point to consider about marijuana is that the amount of THC it contains may widely vary, based on the type harvested and the methods that were used. In general, marijuana is more potent today than in earlier decades.

Hallucinogens

Hallucinogens are quite diverse but produce similar effects, including altered consciousness that may appear "dreamlike." They are all Schedule I drugs with no approved medical use. The prototype hallucinogen is LSD.

LSD

Hallucinogens such as LSD have widely variable effects that are based on the user's mood, expectations, and environment. Repeated use may bring about entirely different effects. However, common effects include laughter, hallucinations or "visions," deep personal insight, *afterimages* (trailing images of other people as they move), or religious "revelations." Users often mention that colors, lights, sounds, and other sensations are greatly intensified. However, hallucinogens also have the potential to bring about terrifying experiences, which may include anxiety, confusion, panic attacks, paranoia, and severe depression.

Commonly referred to as "acid," LSD was originally derived from a fungus growing on the grain known as rye and can also be obtained from fungal growths on other grains. It is usually administered orally as a liquid, capsule, or tablet. LSD is often placed, in droplet form, onto paper that contains cartoon images related to the drug culture. After drying, the user may ingest a piece of the paper to experience the drug's effects. LSD is immediately distributed through the body, with effects usually beginning within 1 hour. These effects may last for up to 12 hours, increasing blood pressure and heart rate, raising body temperature, and dilating the pupils. Repeated use can lead to impaired memory and reasoning ability as well as psychoses. Flashbacks occur in some users, wherein the drug's effects reoccur without further administration. Tolerance to LSD may occur, but little or no dependence has been seen.

OTHER HALLUCINOGENS

Other hallucinogens with similar effects to LSD include:

✳ Ketamine (also known as "special coke" or the "date rape drug"): legally used as a dissociative anesthetic, but also produces unconsciousness and amnesia; this drug is primarily used legally by veterinarians, but abuse rates are increasing in club or party situations; addicts only consume about 10–25% of the therapeutic dose needed to induce anesthesia, but fatalities have occurred when ketamine is combined with other CNS depressants (including alcohol and benzodiazepines) or with other illicit drugs.

✳ MDMA (3,4-methylenedioxymethamphetamine; also known as "Ecstasy," "XTC," or more recently as "Molly"): an amphetamine originally used for research but has become very popular among young adults and teenagers for recreational use; it is actually classified as a psychostimulant that in extreme cases can cause *serotonin syndrome*, a rapid increase in body temperature, heart rate, and blood pressure, which can lead to hyperthermia and death. MDMA is a Schedule I drug with no medical use and a high potential for abuse.

✳ Flakka, a new party drug that can be as potent as crystal meth, bath salts, or cocaine; it causes erratic, uncontrollable, and dangerous behaviors and can be injected, snorted, smoked, or swallowed; body temperature may reach 105°F, and the individual becomes psychotic and violent, often removing all clothing, with their strength intensified; this drug is usually made from the chemical alpha-PVP, a synthetic version of the stimulant cathinone, which is grouped with bath salts.

✳ Mephedrone (also known as "bath salts," "Ivory Wave," "White Lightning," and "Hurricane Charlie"): a white, powdery drug that can be swallowed, snorted, or injected; while having the effects of methamphetamine, it is currently legal to sell since it is listed as "not for human consumption"; mephedrone is a synthetic drug that causes intense cravings, hallucinations, paranoia, and rapid heart rate, and may cause seizures, suicidal thoughts, coma and death, especially if taken with alcohol.

✳ Mepherone (also 4-methylmethcathinone, 4-MMC, or 4-methylephedrone): a synthetic stimulant grouped along with amphetamine and cathinone; its street names include "drone," "M-CAT," "White Magic," and "meow meow"; the drug is available in tablet or powder forms that can be swallowed, snorted, or injected.

✳ MDA (3,4-methylenedioxyamphetamine; also known as the "love drug," tenamfetamine, "INN," "Sally," "Sass," "Sass-a-frass," or the "Mellow Drug of America"): believed to increase sexual desire; it is in the same chemical family as mescaline and is closely related to the more widely used MDMA; it is a Schedule I drug that users report has more stimulant and psychedelic qualities with less *enactogenic* (empathy or sympathy with others) effects than MDMA.

✳ DOM or STP (2,5 dimethoxy-4-methylamphetamine): a synthetic hallucinogen often used at "rave" parties recreationally; it is illegal and causes effects that are similar to LSD or "magic mushrooms," including hallucinations, euphoria, distorted perceptions and thoughts, and delusions.

✳ Mescaline: found in the peyote cactus of Mexico and Central America and used by Native Americans as part of traditional religious ceremonies; as a party drug, it is used to produce hallucinations and altered consciousness, but may also cause anxiety, tachycardia, dizziness, diarrhea, vomiting, and headache; it is not physically addictive.

✳ PCP (also known as "Angel Dust," phencyclidine, and "Ozone"): produces a long, trancelike state that can cause severe brain damage; it has a distinctive bitter taste and is available in many formulations, including tablets, capsules, and colored powders, which are taken orally or snorted; a liquid form is also available, which is highly flammable; deaths linked to PCP have involved accidental drowning, leaping from tall buildings, vehicular accidents, self-mutilation, suicides, and homicides.

Central Nervous System Stimulants

CNS stimulants increase the activity of the CNS and are legally available (by prescription) to treat narcolepsy, attention-deficit/hyperactivity disorder (ADHD), and obesity. These drugs produce improved mental and physical performance, a sense of exhilaration, prolonged wakefulness, and are often used illegally to "get high." CNS stimulants have similar effects to norepinephrine by activating neurons in the reticular formation of the brain. Most of them affect cardiovascular and respiratory activity to increase blood pressure and respiration, dilate the pupils, and cause sweating and tremors. Overdoses of certain CNS stimulants may cause seizures and cardiac arrest. Stimulants include amphetamines, methylphenidate, cocaine, and caffeine.

AMPHETAMINES

In high doses and short-term use, amphetamines cause feelings of euphoria, self-confidence, alertness, and empowerment. Long-term use usually results in feelings of anxiety, restlessness, and rage (especially when "coming down" from the ultimate effects of the drug). After years of prescribing amphetamines and dextroamphetamines, it became understood that their risks outweighed their medical uses. Newer agents that are much safer have replaced these agents except for certain conditions. However, illegally produced amphetamines continue to be popular drugs in substance abuse.

Dextroamphetamine (Dexedrine) is used for short-term weight loss after other methods have failed and for narcolepsy. Methamphetamine (commonly known as "ice") is a common recreational drug administered in powdered or crystallized form that gives users a "rush." It may also be smoked and is a Schedule II drug (marketed as Desoxyn). Most abusers obtain methamphetamine from illegal "meth" laboratories. Another variant, methcathinone (known as "cat"), is a Schedule I agent that is illegally made for injection, inhalation, or oral administration.

METHYLPHENIDATE

Methylphenidate (Ritalin) is a CNS stimulant used for children diagnosed with ADHD. For those who are hyperactive or inattentive, Ritalin has a calming effect, helping the patient to focus on specific tasks for longer periods of time than he or she normally can. When taken by adults, Ritalin usually causes the opposite effects. It is a Schedule II drug with similar effects to amphetamines and cocaine. Illegally, the drug is administered by inhalation or injection—sometimes being mixed with heroin (known as a "speedball").

COCAINE

Cocaine is obtained from the leaves of the South American coca plant and has been used since 2500 B.C. Users who chew coca leaves or make teas from them only receive slow absorption of the drug, and only tiny amounts of cocaine are present in the leaves. However, in the United States, cocaine is a Schedule II drug that is used entirely differently. It produces rapid and intense effects that are similar to but greater than the effects of amphetamines. It is usually inhaled, smoked, or injected to produce intense euphoria, analgesia, decreased hunger, increased sensory perception, and illusions of physical strength. Large doses heighten these effects and also cause rapid heartbeat, pupil dilation, elevated body temperature, and sweating. When the euphoric feelings diminish, the user experiences insomnia, irritability, depression, and extreme distrust of others. A "crawling" skin sensation may occur, and chronic use (by inhalation) results in many nasal problems. These include continual running of the nose, a reddened "crusting" around the nostrils, and nasal cartilage deterioration.

Overdose may lead to convulsions, dysrhythmias, stroke, and death from respiratory arrest. Withdrawal from amphetamines and cocaine is usually less intense than from barbiturates or alcohol. Celebrity deaths that have been linked to cocaine use have included musician John Entwistle and singer Whitney Houston.

Focus Point

Cocaine

Cocaine is a Schedule II drug that produces actions similar to those of amphetamines. However, its effects are usually more rapid and intense. It is the second-most commonly abused illegal drug in the United States.

CAFFEINE

Caffeine occurs naturally in the seeds, fruits, or leaves of more than 63 different plants. Coffee, chocolate, ice cream, soft drinks, and tea contain significant amounts of caffeine. It increases the effectiveness of OTC pain relievers and is commonly added to their formulations. Two or three cups of coffee per day, with the caffeine it contains, are good for the heart. The body metabolizes caffeine after several hours, and the drug causes pronounced diuresis. It produces increased mental alertness, restlessness, irritability, nervousness, and insomnia. Physical effects include bronchodilation, increased blood pressure and production of stomach acid, and alterations in blood glucose level. Repeated use results in physical dependence and tolerance. Withdrawal from caffeine produces fatigue, headaches, depression, and impaired physical and mental performance.

Effects of Substance Abuse

The mental states that often encourage drug abuse include anxiety and depression. Abuse often prevents users from seeking proper treatment for the reason they chose to abuse drugs in the first place. Anxiety, panic disorder, and insomnia are all increased by the use of stimulants. Although depression is numbed by alcohol, opioids, and sedatives initially, they cause depression over longer periods of time. Psychoses can be precipitated by hallucinogens and stimulants. Results of drug abuse include imprisonment, unemployment, cognitive dysfunction, family disharmony, financial loss, poor decisions, and sexual relationships that otherwise would not have occurred.

The physical effects of substance abuse may include sexually transmitted infections. These may include hepatitis B and C and human immunodeficiency virus (HIV). Drug use is more prevalent in victims of sexual assault, and intravenous drug abuse may be associated with hepatitis, HIV, and *Staphylococcal endocarditis*. Smoking and alcohol have been linked to more serious drug abuse. Heart attacks and strokes are commonly linked to the use of cocaine. Drug overdoses can lead to respiratory depression, seizures, confusion, pneumonia, coma, and death. Drugs can also cause motor vehicle accidents, fetal impairment, suicide, and violence.

✳ Apply Your Knowledge 15.2

The following questions focus on what you have just learned about cannabinoids, hallucinogens, and CNS stimulants.

CRITICAL THINKING

1. Describe the substance that is the most commonly used illicit drug in the United States.
2. Explain the adverse effects of repeated use of LSD on the CNS.
3. Identify the most commonly used CNS stimulants.
4. Discuss the adverse effects of cocaine overdose.
5. Explain the symptoms of withdrawal from caffeine.

Prevention and Treatment

Schools can receive grants for drug testing and education of parents, students, and teachers through the Office of National Drug Control Policy (ONDCP). More than 4,000 schools across the United States used random student drug testing programs to provide early intervention for those students labeled "at risk." Risk factors for drug abuse include:

✳ Absent or permissive parents

✳ Substance-abusing peers or parents

✳ Access to prescriptions

✳ Student absenteeism

✳ Aggressive behavior in adolescents

✳ Poor social skills

✳ Poor academic performance

✳ Transition periods in adolescent life

✳ Early drug use

✳ Method of drug administration

Yellow Dog Productions/The Image Bank/Getty Images

Figure 15-1 ■ Alcoholics Anonymous is one of the most popular treatment programs available for substance abusers.

When treating patients with addiction, **detoxification** must first take place. Withdrawal may cause physical and psychological symptoms and can require hospitalization or other inpatient treatment. Detoxification is the period of getting over physical withdrawal when an addict stops taking a drug, and medical management may be required to prevent serious health problems. Medications used for ongoing management of withdrawal include methadone or Suboxone. However, most treatment is psychological in nature.

Psychological treatment uses motivational interviewing. The most popular treatment programs are Narcotics Anonymous (NA) and Alcoholics Anonymous (AA) (Figure 15-1 ■). Often, members attend both programs' meetings because of their combined use of narcotics and alcohol. These programs use group therapy with addicts, family members, and peers. Additional individual psychotherapy and drug counseling may be used. Continuous urine tests are used to prevent the addict from relapsing, and recovering addicts are sometimes given financial or other incentives to stay clean.

Pharmacologic treatment involves substances that are used in lieu of the addictive substances, although this type of treatment is not used for hallucinogen or stimulant addicts. Methadone eliminates the physical cravings for heroin; Suboxone does the same but also makes the user ill if he or she tries to use heroin. Again, frequent urine toxicology screens are used to find if the addict is occasionally using his or her addictive substances.

✳ Apply Your Knowledge 15.3

The following questions focus on what you have just learned about the prevention and treatment of substance abuse.

CRITICAL THINKING

1. Identify the risk factors for drug abuse.

2. Discuss the drug of choice to treat heroin addiction.

3. Describe the role of schools regarding the prevention of addiction to substances.

Cigarette Smoking

The single-largest cause of preventable death and illness in the United States is smoking. It is the most common addiction of all, and nicotine is highly addictive (Figure 15-2 ■). Continued consumption of tobacco despite significant physical, economic, or social side effects is termed **tobacco dependence**. The physical adverse effects of smoking are usually serious later in life and include cancer, emphysema, and heart attacks. Smoking-related cancers often attack certain people in their early 30s and often result in death. Nearly 20% of

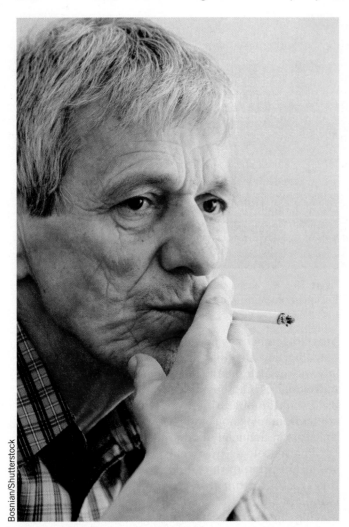

Bosnian/Shutterstock

Figure 15-2 ■ Smoking is the single largest preventable cause of death and illness in the United States.

Americans smoke. Because it is legal, smoking is not perceived to be an addiction by many. It has been linked to the deaths of celebrities such as singer Nat "King" Cole, actor Patrick Swayze, and musician George Harrison.

Nicotine is sometimes considered to be a CNS stimulant, but it is unique because of its legality, high potential for addiction, and carcinogenic effects. It affects most body systems, increasing alertness, ability to focus, and relaxation and causing lightheadedness. Directly stimulating the CNS, nicotine accelerates the heart rate and increases blood pressure and may result in muscular tremors in certain people. It also increases the basal metabolic rate, leading to weight loss and appetite reduction. Physical and psychologic dependence occur relatively quickly.

Withdrawal from nicotine causes anxiety, cravings, impaired attention, insomnia, continual thoughts about smoking, gastrointestinal disturbances, and headaches. Nicotine has been proven to be a psychoactive substance. The adverse effects of nicotine are caused by carbon monoxide levels, its addictive properties, irritants in the tar found in tobacco, and passive smoke inhalation.

Approximately 480,000 people die annually in the United States from various effects of smoking. Half of all Americans who continue to smoke will die from a smoking-related disease. Tobacco smoking affects all body systems but primarily the respiratory, cardiovascular, and nervous systems. Smoking is the major cause of lung cancer deaths. For example, in males, lung cancer risk is 23 times greater than in lifelong nonsmokers. Cancers throughout the body are much greater in occurrence as a result of smoking.

Those who do not die from smoking-related illnesses experience pneumonia, being chronically short of breath and sometimes having to be on a respirator for much of their lives. Chronic smoking leads to heart disease and chronic obstructive pulmonary disorder. Statistically, one cigarette shortens a smoker's life by 5–11 minutes. Stopping smoking has many long-term health benefits. Because every body system is affected (in varying degrees) by the use of tobacco products, morbidity and mortality are greatly affected by the cessation of smoking.

Passive smoking involves *side-stream smoke* (from the end of the cigarette) and *mainstream smoke* (that which has been exhaled by the smoker). Passive smoking can affect a fetus via the mother's respiratory system, causing low birth weight, which can lead to neonatal death, stillbirth, and intellectual disabilities. Children of smokers have a higher incidence of bronchitis, pneumonia, asthma, middle ear problems, growth retardation, and sudden infant death syndrome.

On average, smoking reduces life expectancy by 10–14 years. For an average individual, smoking adds $2,555 to the budget per year. Approximately 70% of smokers say they would like to quit. A further reason to quit is that insurance premiums of all types are lower for nonsmokers. The following reasons help to convince a person to quit:

✳ Those with a familial history of cancers may have a higher risk level for contracting the disease themselves.

✳ Heart disease is greatly increased by smoking.

✳ Chronic lung disease will shorten a smoker's life.

✳ Lower back pain is greatly increased by smoking.

✳ Smoking repels many potential dates, girlfriends or boyfriends, wives or husbands, and so on.

✳ Smoking increases wrinkling and premature aging.

Smoking cessation techniques include:

✳ Smoking cessation clinics

✳ Literature about quitting techniques

✳ Nicotine replacements

✳ The drugs bupropion and varenicline (Chantix)

✳ Drug counseling

✳ Hypnotherapy

✳ Acupuncture

✳ Progressive filters

✳ Employer-offered financial incentives

Focus Point

Cigarette Smoking

Tobacco smoke contains about 4,000 chemical agents, including more than 60 carcinogens (agents that cause cancer).

✳ Apply Your Knowledge 15.4

The following questions focus on what you have just learned about cigarette smoking.

CRITICAL THINKING

1. Explain the serious complications of cigarette smoking later in life.
2. Describe the effects of nicotine on the cardiovascular system.
3. Identify the symptoms of withdrawal from nicotine.
4. Discuss techniques that are used for smoking cessation.
5. Explain the benefits of stopping cigarette smoking.

Alcoholism

Ethyl alcohol is a widely abused drug that is legal and readily available. Alcohol has enormous economic, health, and social consequences. In small quantities, alcohol has been shown to reduce the risk of heart attack and stroke, but long-term abuse can have devastating effects. Alcohol use has been linked to the deaths of celebrities such as singer Amy Winehouse, actor Oliver Reed, and athlete Mickey Mantle.

Alcohol is a CNS depressant that easily crosses the blood–brain barrier to cause effects within 5 to 30 minutes. Effects are based on the amount consumed and include relaxation, memory impairment, sedation, loss of coordination, decreased inhibition, and reduced judgment. Alcohol affects the breath of the user and increases blood flow to the face and cheeks as well as other parts of the body. It mimics the effects of many antidepressants, antianxiety agents, and sedatives, and health care personnel should verify which drugs a patient has consumed before any treatment. Also, mouthwashes containing alcohol can make the patient's breath smell from the drug—similar to the effects of drinking.

Alcohol is absorbed more slowly when there is food in the stomach. Detoxification of alcohol by the liver (metabolism) occurs slowly at a constant rate of about 15 mL per hour. This is essentially the same as one serving of alcohol per hour, which is based on the following:

✳ 12 fl oz of regular beer (about 5% alcohol)

✳ 8–9 fl oz of malt liquor (about 7% alcohol)

✳ 5 fl oz of wine (about 12% alcohol)

✳ 3–4 fl oz of fortified wine (sherry or port) (about 17% alcohol)

✳ 2–3 fl oz of an aperitif, cordial, or liqueur (about 24% alcohol)

✳ 1.5 fl oz of brandy or "hard liquor" (about 40% alcohol or more)

PSYCHOLOGICAL AND PHYSICAL EFFECTS OF ALCOHOLISM

Acute overdoses of alcohol cause vomiting, severe hypotension, respiratory failure, and coma. Almost 88,000 Americans die every year due to alcohol use and related behaviors. High rates of alcohol consumption produce increased depressant effects on the brain. Alcohol should never be combined with other CNS depressants because effects are cumulative, resulting in profound sedation or coma. Withdrawal from alcohol is severe and potentially life-threatening, causing anxiety, insomnia, or seizures. Long-term alcoholics may experience **delirium tremens (DT)**, commonly referred to as "the DTs." Symptoms include confusion, disorientation, agitation, hallucinations, anxiety, panic, a "crawling" sensation of the skin, and paranoia.

The liver is the most affected organ when chronic alcohol abuse occurs. *Cirrhosis* is the debilitating and potentially fatal failure of the liver to function normally. When the liver becomes impaired, blood clotting and nutritional states are affected. Liver impairment makes the organ more sensitive to all substances that it metabolizes. Patients should be honest with their physicians and nurses about their use of alcohol because dosage levels must be determined based on this information. When a patient does not admit his or her alcohol consumption correctly, dosage levels of medications may be too high to be processed and may harm the patient.

TREATMENT OF ALCOHOLISM

Patients with acute alcohol withdrawal are treated with such benzodiazepines as Valium or Librium as well as antiseizure medications. Additional treatments for

alcohol abuse include behavioral counseling, self-help groups (such as AA), and the drug disulfiram (Antabuse), which discourages relapses of alcohol use. Antabuse works by stopping the metabolism of alcohol, bringing about headache and nausea and vomiting within 5 to 10 minutes after alcohol is consumed. After it is discontinued, the patient will be sensitive to alcohol consumption for an additional 2 weeks. Other agents used to treat patients with alcoholism include acamprosate calcium (Campral) and naltrexone (ReVia).

Focus Point

Consumption of Alcohol

Consuming more than one alcoholic drink per hour will usually result in blood alcohol levels above the legal limit for operating a vehicle.

✸ Apply Your Knowledge 15.5

The following questions focus on what you have just learned about alcoholism.

CRITICAL THINKING

1. What are the effects of alcohol in small quantities?
2. What are the effects of acute overdoses of alcohol, and how do high rates of alcohol consumption affect the brain?
3. Why should alcohol never be combined with other CNS depressants?
4. Which organ is most affected by chronic alcohol abuse?
5. What are the treatments for acute alcohol withdrawal?

PRACTICAL SCENARIO 1

A 17-year-old female student begins to demonstrate signs of depression and irritability. She begins to spend more and more time alone in her room. She continually comes home later than she is supposed to. Several weeks later, her mother receives a phone call from the school when her daughter is found having convulsions on the restroom floor. The mother is instructed to go to the local hospital, where her daughter has been transported by ambulance. After several tests and verifying that the patient has had no history of epilepsy, the physician acknowledges that the girl has been using cocaine.

Mita Stock Images/Shutterstock

Critical Thinking Questions

1. Why is substance abuse common among teenagers?
2. What are the common symptoms of an overdose of cocaine?

PRACTICAL SCENARIO 2

Suzanne was hired as a medical assistant at a family practice office. At the time she was hired, the office manager told her that the facility conducted random drug screening tests, and Suzanne signed an agreement indicating her compliance. After being employed for a few months, the physician noticed that Suzanne was occasionally behaving suspiciously while at work. She was sometimes late or did not show up to work without calling to let the office know. One day, she asked her physician if he could order a urine test for her because she suspected she was pregnant. He ordered the pregnancy test, and because he was suspicious of her recent behavior, also ordered tests

AVAVA/Shutterstock

for the presence of any drugs in her system. After 48 hours, the results came back. Suzanne was indeed pregnant, and the physician noticed that the drug test indicated the presence of nicotine and cocaine.

Critical Thinking Questions

1. What do you think were the consequences of these events?
2. What are the adverse effects of nicotine and cocaine on a developing fetus?

Chapter Capsule

Objective 1: Define *addiction* and list several factors on which it may be based.

- Addiction is defined as a progressive and chronic abuse of a substance that causes a person to use it repeatedly despite serious health and social consequences.

- Addiction may be based on the cost, availability, dose, and method of administration as well as risk-taking behavior, prior drug experience, certain diseases requiring the use of scheduled drugs, educational opportunities, and peer influences.

Objective 2: Identify the most commonly abused drugs in the United States.

- The most commonly abused drugs in the United States include alcohol, marijuana, sedatives, opioids, cocaine, hallucinogens, and methamphetamine.

Objective 3: List five substances that cause relaxation or sedation.

- Five substances that cause relaxation or sedation are barbiturates, nonbarbiturate sedative–hypnotics, benzodiazepines, opioids, and alcohol.

Objective 4: Explain opioid addiction and its withdrawal.

- Opioid addiction may develop rapidly. Methadone is often used to treat an addiction to other opioids because it does not produce the same degree of euphoria and has longer-lasting effects.

- Opioid withdrawal is very unpleasant (although not life-threatening compared with barbiturate withdrawal). Methadone is used, in part, to help heroin addicts withdraw with less unpleasant symptoms. Withdrawal from methadone itself—if a person becomes addicted—takes longer than that from heroin or morphine but with less intense symptoms.

Objective 5: Discuss cannabinoids and their effects on the central nervous system.

- Cannabinoids are obtained from the hemp plant (*Cannabis sativa*) and are usually smoked to obtain their effects. They include marijuana, hashish, and hash oil, with the most psychoactive agent being delta-9-tetrahydrocannabinol (THC).

■ The effects of cannabinoids on the central nervous system include decreased coordination and motor activity, confusion, paranoia, and euphoria. Effects occur within a few minutes and last for up to 24 hours. The most commonly used cannabinoid—marijuana—produces very little physical dependence or tolerance, with withdrawal symptoms being nearly nonexistent.

Objective 6: Compare hallucinogens and opioid drugs.

■ Hallucinogens produce altered, "dreamlike" consciousness and are all Schedule I drugs with no approved medical use. The prototype hallucinogen is LSD. Common effects include laughter, hallucinations or "visions," deep personal insight, afterimages, and religious "revelations." Other common effects include greatly intensified colors, lights, sounds, and other sensations.

■ Opioid drugs are used for severe pain, diarrhea, and persistent cough. They are derived from unripe poppy seeds and include codeine, morphine, opium, and heroin. Oral opioids take effect within 30 minutes and can last for more than a day. Signs of use include a euphoric rush, intense sedation, abnormally slow body functions, constricted pupils, respiratory depression, and the ability to tolerate increased amounts of pain.

Objective 7: Explain the effects of substance abuse.

■ Substance abuse may affect every level of a person's life. It is signified by a failure to fulfill parenting, school, or work obligations; hazardous behavior, such as driving under the influence; recurrent legal problems related to hazardous behaviors; and continued use of substances despite continuing social or interpersonal problems.

■ A person is "substance dependent" when he or she exhibits any three of these signs: tolerance; withdrawal; increasing consumption; desire to quit; excessive time spent on abuse; fewer occupational, recreational, or social activities; and continued use while understanding the physiologic and psychologic effects.

Objective 8: Describe withdrawal from nicotine.

■ Withdrawal from nicotine causes anxiety, cravings, impaired attention, insomnia, continual thoughts about smoking, gastrointestinal disturbances, and headaches.

Objective 9: Explain the psychological and physical effects of alcoholism.

■ Psychological effects of alcoholism include increased depressant effects on the brain, sedation, confusion, disorientation, agitation, hallucinations, anxiety, panic, and paranoia.

■ Physical effects of alcoholism include vomiting, severe hypotension, respiratory failure, potential coma, severe withdrawal symptoms, insomnia, seizures, delirium tremens, a crawling sensation of the skin, liver cirrhosis and liver failure, impaired blood clotting, and an impaired nutritional state.

Objective 10: Discuss signs and symptoms of withdrawal from alcohol.

■ Withdrawal from alcohol is severe and potentially life-threatening, causing anxiety, insomnia, or seizures. Long-term alcoholics may experience "the DTs" (delirium tremens), which causes confusion, disorientation, agitation, hallucinations, anxiety, panic, crawling of the skin, and paranoia.

Internet Sites of Interest

- The DEA's multimedia library of abused drugs: **www.dea.gov/pr/multimedia-library/publications/drug_of_abuse.pdf#page=68**
- Hallucinogens: **http://emedicine.medscape.com/article/293752-overview**
- Cigarette smoking: **www.cancer.org/Cancer/CancerCauses/TobaccoCancer/CigaretteSmoking/cigarette-smoking-toc**
- Marijuana Infofacts: **www.drugabuse.gov/publications/drugfacts/marijuana**
- A list of the most addictive drugs: **www.michaelshouse.com/drug-addiction/most-addictive-drugs-world/**
- Substance abuse: **www.emedicinehealth.com/substance_abuse/article_em.htm**
- CNS stimulants: **www.drugs.com/drug-class/cns-stimulants.html**
- Prescription drug abuse and addiction: **www.drugabuse.gov/publications/research-reports/prescription-drugs/director**
- Alcoholism: **www.mayoclinic.org/diseases-conditions/alcoholism/basics/definition/con-20020866**
- The Substance Abuse and Mental Health Services Administration: **www.samhsa.gov**

Chapter 16

Antibacterial Agents

Chapter Objectives

After completing this chapter, you should be able to:

1. Identify the major types of antibiotics by drug class.
2. Describe the mechanism of action of the sulfonamides.
3. Outline the five classes of penicillins.
4. Describe the principal mechanisms of action of cephalosporins, vancomycin, and isoniazid.
5. Explain the classifications of cephalosporins.
6. Outline the main adverse effects of macrolides, aminoglycosides, and chloramphenicol.
7. Contrast bactericidal and bacteriostatic actions.
8. Discuss the contraindications, precautions, and interactions of the penicillins and tetracyclines.
9. Describe the indications of vancomycin.
10. List the first-line antituberculosis agents and two characteristic adverse effects of each drug.

Key Terms

Introduction

Infection is the most common cause of death for many people afflicted with a chronic or critical illness, with the very young and the very old being particularly susceptible. Infections are caused by microorganisms that gain entry into the body. After a microorganism invades the human body, the signs and symptoms generally associated with infection are generated, including fever and an elevated white blood cell (WBC) count. The microorganisms that cause infection and disease are called *pathogens*, and the major types of microorganisms that can cause infection include bacteria, viruses, fungi, and parasites.

Different pathogens inhabit various environments, such as hospitals, the food supply, water, and animals or humans. Globalization of the world's population and faster air travel to nearly every spot on Earth have major implications for the worldwide spread of infectious agents. Rapidly spreading infections may be particularly dangerous to populations when infected individuals are asymptomatic for long periods or the infection itself is difficult to identify for other reasons.

Infection with **pathogenic** microorganisms has become a tool of war and terrorism throughout the world. Weapons of mass destruction may be nuclear, chemical, or biological in nature. Whether the situation involves anthrax spores sent through the mail or the threat of smallpox being introduced to a nonimmunized population, the various methods of preventing infections have key roles in the defense of humanity. Healthcare professionals play a vital part in the prevention, early detection, and management of infections.

Transmission of Infection

Transmission of disease requires a chain of events that must occur unbroken to allow one human to infect another. The pathogenic organism must live and reproduce in a reservoir (Figure 16-1 ■). The reservoir may be a human being, an animal, or soil.

The pathogen must have a portal of exit, with a mode of transmission from the reservoir to a susceptible victim. For example, *Neisseria gonorrhoeae*—the organism that is responsible for gonorrhea—usually resides in the urethra of the male and the vaginal canal of the female. The microorganism is transmitted by sexual contact.

Control of infectious disease occurrence depends on breaking this chain of transmission in one or more places (Figure 16-2 ■). A pathogen can be vulnerable in one or more links of the transmission chain. Some **bacteria** are susceptible to direct attack with antibiotics. Antibiotics are designed to kill the bacteria directly or hold it in check so the body's defenses can eradicate it.

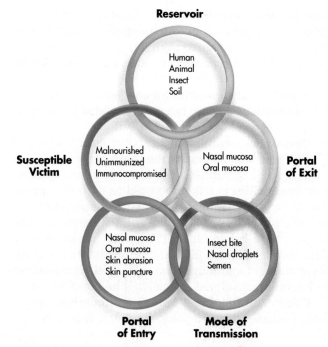

Figure 16-1 ■ Chain of transmission of microorganisms from host to victim.

Figure 16-2 ■ Breaking the chain of transmission of microorganisms from host to victim.

Some bacteria have developed resistance to **antibiotics** (substances produced by microorganisms that in low concentrations are able to inhibit or kill other microorganisms) through repeated exposure to **subtherapeutic doses** (doses that are below the level used to treat diseases) and use of antibiotics for nonbacterial infections. This antibiotic resistance is a major threat to the success of the management of bacterial infections.

Destroying nonhuman reservoirs and vectors of the pathogen can also break the chain of transmission. For example, controlling the number of mosquitoes with insecticides is a method used to curb the spread of malaria (see Chapter 19). Blocking the portal of exit can also block transmission of the pathogen. Having patients with tuberculosis (TB) wear masks as they move through the hospital and implementing respiratory isolation techniques to stop droplet transmission are interventions aimed at blocking the portal of exit.

Finally, host susceptibility is an important aspect of the transmission of a pathogen. Such factors as age, gender, ethnic group, and genetic makeup affect the susceptibility of the host. Although these factors cannot be changed, improving the host's immune system by improving his or her nutritional status, decreasing stress, and limiting fatigue can decrease the host's susceptibility to infection. Immunization of the host also has a key role in blocking the transmission of infection and provides active immunity, thus allowing the creation of host antibodies to help prevent future infections. In contrast, immunoglobulin given to the host can provide passive immunity to some infections, allowing for short-term prevention of disease transmission or infection.

Antibiotic use has had a tremendous impact on the way microorganisms respond to various agents. Using subtherapeutic doses of or overusing antibiotics can affect the resistance that microorganisms have to them. Resistance may be altered because of *mutation* (a change in gene chemistry that continues in subsequent cell divisions) or by the continuous exposure of a microbe to an antibiotic.

Focus Point

Handwashing Reduces Transmission

Frequent handwashing with soap, friction, and warm running water is one of the most effective ways to reduce pathogenic transmission.

Types of Microorganisms

The four basic types of microorganisms that can be helpful or pathogenic to the host are:

1. **Bacteria:** single-celled organisms with a cell wall and cellular organelles that allow them to live independently in the environment

2. **Viruses:** tiny genetic parasites that require the host cell to replicate and spread (see Chapter 17)
3. **Fungi:** nonphotosynthetic, eukaryotic single- or multicellular organisms that are found throughout the environment; fungi have a cell wall containing sterol (see Chapter 18)
4. **Parasites:** protozoa, roundworms, flatworms, and arthropods (see Chapter 19)

✳ Apply Your Knowledge 16.1

The following questions test your understanding of the transmission of infection and the types of microorganisms.

CRITICAL THINKING

1. Explain how infectious disease can be controlled.
2. Identify "weapons of mass destruction."
3. Describe the chain of transmission of infectious diseases.
4. Define *subtherapeutic doses.*
5. Describe the structure of bacteria.

Antibacterial Agents

Little distinction exists today between the terms *antibiotic* and **antimicrobial** (referring to an agent that tends to destroy microbes, prevent their multiplication or growth, or prevent their pathogenic action). The most common sources of natural antibiotics are molds and bacteria. Antibiotics are produced by one microorganism and inhibit the growth of others. However, many antibiotics are now partially or wholly synthesized in commercial laboratories. Included in this group are the penicillins, cephalosporins, aminoglycosides, tetracyclines, and macrolides. Important synthetic antibacterial agents, including nitrofurantoin and the quinolones, are also used clinically.

Antibiotics inhibit the growth of or kill microorganisms when given in sufficient concentrations—ideally, low enough to exert their effect but remain harmless to the host. Systemic antibacterial agents can be **bactericidal** or **bacteriostatic** but also rely on host defenses to aid in eliminating bacterial pathogens.

Antibiotics were discovered in 1928 when Sir Alexander Fleming was performing research on influenza. One year later, he found penicillin by culturing the mold *Penicillium notatum*. In 1938, British researchers studied the effects of natural penicillins on infectious disease. In 1941, natural penicillins were used clinically for the treatment of infections.

Factors to consider when selecting antibiotics for therapy in patients should include identification of:

✳ Likely or specific microorganisms
✳ Antimicrobial susceptibility
✳ Bactericidal versus bacteriostatic properties
✳ Host status, such as allergy history, age, pharmacokinetic factors, renal and hepatic function, pregnancy status, anatomic site of infection, and host defenses

Focus Point

Resistance to Antibiotics

All antibiotics are able to cause drug-resistant microorganisms to develop, but some antibiotics cause this to a greater degree. Because broad-spectrum antibiotics destroy more microorganisms than narrow-spectrum antibiotics, they also cause more resistant microorganisms to emerge. In fact, the greater the use of antibiotics, the quicker that drug-resistant microorganisms develop. Antibiotics also promote overgrowth of normal flora, which may also increase resistance.

Focus On

Sulfonamides

Sulfanilamides (sulfa drugs) are antibacterial agents that were first synthesized in 1908, but it was many years before their therapeutic value was discovered. In 1937, researchers in England synthesized sulfapyridine, which was the first sulfonamide used with great success in combating pneumonia. After that, a large number of other sulfonamides, such as sulfathiazole and sulfadiazine, were synthesized. Today, sulfamethoxazole is still commonly used, usually combined with trimethoprim and abbreviated SMZ/TMP.

The sulfonamides and trimethoprim act by inhibiting the folic acid synthesis that most bacteria require. Although humans rely on dietary sources for the folic acid they need, most bacteria must synthesize it on their own. Sulfonamides were the first antimicrobial agents, but their clinical use has been greatly restricted as a result of the development of resistant bacteria, their significant side effects, and the availability of other drugs. Although the sulfonamides are no longer preferred for the treatment of urinary tract infections (UTIs), they are still important and effective for other infections. This is particularly true for new sulfa drugs. Table 16-1 ■ lists the various sulfa drugs.

How do they work?

The mechanism of the antimicrobial action of the sulfonamides has been analyzed extensively. These agents block a specific step in the biosynthetic pathway of folic acid. They are primarily bacteriostatic, meaning that they slow the multiplication of bacteria. Bacteria cannot absorb folic acid; therefore, it is made from precursors, specifically para-aminobenzoic acid (PABA). The sulfonamides interfere with PABA and folic acid formation, thereby destroying the bacteria. The efficacy of sulfonamides is generally enhanced when the drugs are used in combination with trimethoprim, which inhibits the conversion of dihydrofolate to folinic acid.

(continued)

Focus On (*continued*)

. . . .

How are they used?

Sulfonamide therapy alone has a minor place in the treatment of patients with infectious diseases. Major advantages of sulfonamides are their low cost and ease of administration. The combination of trimethoprim with sulfamethoxazole is the treatment of choice for most UTIs, otitis media (especially in children), sinusitis, some lower respiratory infections, and ulcerative colitis.

What are the adverse effects?

Major disadvantages of sulfonamides are their untoward effects (blood dyscrasias, crystalluria, hematuria, and life-threatening hepatitis). However, the new sulfa drugs in use today cause fewer allergic reactions than do the older drugs. Sulfonamides may cause several adverse effects, such as aplastic anemia, leukopenia, thrombocytopenia, and even agranulocytosis. Loss of appetite is a common mild adverse effect, with nausea and vomiting, diarrhea, fever, *stomatitis* (inflammation of the mouth), and photosensitivity also being seen. Crystalluria may occur during use of older sulfonamides but may be reduced by increasing fluid intake in patients receiving these agents.

What are the contraindications and interactions?

Sulfonamides must be avoided in patients with known hypersensitivity, during lactation, and in children younger than 2 years of age. These drugs are contraindicated near the end of pregnancy.

Sulfonamides may interact with oral anticoagulants and cause increased anticoagulant effects. Sulfonamides accompanied by methotrexate may increase the risk of bone marrow suppression. These agents may prevent the metabolism of oral hypoglycemic drugs, resulting in an increase of hypoglycemic reaction. When a sulfonamide is administered with a hydantoin, the serum hydantoin level may be increased.

What are the important points patients should know?

Instruct patients to take sulfonamide drugs on an empty stomach either 1 hour before or 2 hours after a meal with a full glass of water. (*Note:* At least eight to ten 8-oz glasses of water should normally be consumed every day.) Instruct patients to complete the full course of therapy and avoid prolonged exposure to sunlight, which may result in a skin reaction that is similar to severe sunburn.

Table 16-1 ■ Various Sulfa Drugs

GENERIC NAME	TRADE NAME	AVERAGE ADULT DOSAGE	ROUTE OF ADMINISTRATION
mafenide	Sulfamylon	Apply to burned area 1–2 times/d	Topical
silver sulfadiazine	Silvadene, Thermazene, SSD (cream)	Apply to burned area 1–2 times/d	Topical
sulfadiazine	(Generic only)	Loading dose: 2–4 g; maintenance dose: 2–4 g/d in 4–6 divided doses	PO
sulfamethizole	Thiosulfil Forte	0.5–1 g tid–qid	PO
sulfamethoxazole	Gantanol	Initial dose: 2 g; maintenance dose: 1 g bid–tid	PO
sulfasalazine	Azulfidine	Initial dose: 1–4 g/d in divided doses; maintenance dose: 2 g/d in evenly spaced doses of 500 mg qid	PO
sulfisoxazole	Gantrisin	Loading dose: 2–4 g; maintenance dose: 4–8 g/d in 4–6 divided doses	PO
trimethoprim (TMP) and sulfamethoxazole (SMZ)	Bactrim, Septra	160 mg TMP/800 mg SMZ q12h	PO
		8–10 mg/kg/d (based on TMP) in 2–4 divided doses	IV

IV, intravenous; PO, oral; qid, four times a day; tid, three times a day.

Focus Point

Sulfonamides

Special considerations are needed for patients who are taking sulfonamides. They must avoid direct sunlight or use sunscreen when exposed, and drink plenty of water to prevent crystallization in the urine.

Focus On

Penicillins

The name *penicillin* now designates a number of antibiotic substances produced by the growth of various types of *Penicillium* or by other means. Penicillins are some of the most valuable antibiotics used in primary care. They are bactericidal, very well distributed, and highly effective against susceptible organisms. Development of synthetic penicillins has broadened the spectrum of activity and enhanced their effectiveness. Occasionally, resistant bacterial strains may develop. Therefore, this has limited the usefulness of penicillins in recent years. Penicillins still remain the drugs of choice for many mild, local soft tissue infections. They are particularly important in specific situations during pregnancy. In some cases, penicillins may still be used even if there is a history of penicillin allergy. The penicillins are listed in Table 16-2 ■.

How do they work?

Penicillin interferes with the synthesis of peptidoglycans—important building blocks of bacterial cell walls. The penicillins are bactericidal. There are five classes of penicillins: (1) natural penicillins; (2) semisynthetic, penicillinase-resistant penicillins; (3) amino penicillins; (4) extended-spectrum or carboxy penicillins; and (5) ureido penicillins. The natural penicillins are effective against most **Gram-positive** bacteria and anaerobes and certain **Gram-negative** bacteria and spirochetes. The semisynthetic, penicillinase-resistant penicillins are effective against Gram-positive bacteria. The amino penicillins are effective against a variety of Gram-positive and Gram-negative cocci, as well as some Gram-negative rods, but have a limited spectrum due to sensitivity to most beta-lactamases. The extended-spectrum or carboxy penicillins are more effective in high doses. The ureido penicillins act similarly to the extended-spectrum penicillins.

How are they used?

Although penicillin G is the original penicillin, it remains the drug of choice for the treatment of almost all infections caused by nonpenicillinase-producing and non-methicillin-resistant Gram-positive bacteria. These bacteria have the ability to resist decolorization with alcohol after being treated with Gram's crystal violet stain, which imparts a violet color to the bacterium when viewed by microscope. Penicillin is the drug of choice against infections by Gram-positive, nonpenicillinase-producing *cocci*, such as *Staphylococcus aureus*, *Staphylococcus epidermidis*, and *Streptococcus* group B. Therefore, penicillins can be used for UTIs, gonorrhea, syphilis, septicemia, meningitis, pneumonia, and other respiratory infections. Because of penicillinase-producing organisms, many skin and other types of infections must be treated with an extended-spectrum (carboxy) penicillin—sometimes along with another drug.

Penicillin V is primarily used to treat mixed aerobic–anaerobic infections such as dental abscesses and other head or neck infections. It also prevents recurrent rheumatic fever and recurrent streptococcal cellulitis in patients who have lymphedema. Penicillin G is used for certain pneumococcus and *S. pyogenes* bacteria, some *Neisseria* species, Gram-positive *Clostridium* rods, most anaerobes, syphilis, and *Leptospira*.

The semisynthetic, penicillinase-resistant penicillins are used mostly for skin and soft tissue infections or methicillin-sensitive *S. aureus* infections. The amino penicillins are used for *Neisseria gonorrhoeae*, *Haemophilus influenzae*, invasive enterococcal infections, *Listeria* meningitis, uncomplicated ear/nose/throat infections, in the prevention of endocarditis during dental procedures, and as part of combination therapy for *Helicobacter pylori* infection. Both ampicillin and amoxicillin have broadened effects when administered with beta-lactamase inhibitors. The extended-spectrum or carboxy penicillins are used against *Enterobacter* and *Pseudomonas* infections; the ureido penicillins are used for similar infections as well as enterococci and *Klebsiella*.

(continued)

Focus On (*continued*)

What are the adverse effects?

Penicillin is a very safe drug in most cases, with low toxicity. However, hypersensitivity reactions may occur in a low percentage of patients. The most common manifestation of this allergic response is a raised, itchy skin rash, **serum sickness** (a reaction to a foreign serum), angioedema and difficulty breathing, and nephropathy. Penicillin G, in high doses, can also cause seizures. All types of penicillins can cause acute interstitial nephritis.

Side effects of oral administration of penicillins are nausea and vomiting, diarrhea, and a black "hairy" tongue, which is due to a temporary overgrowth of harmless bacteria or yeast in the mouth. A nonallergic and harmless rash may also occur during amoxicillin therapy and is differentiated from a true hypersensitivity reaction based on the absence of a raised or itchy rash. Very high concentrations of penicillin are neurotoxic, and nerve damage has resulted from intramuscular (IM) administration. Oral antistaphylococcal penicillins may also cause *Clostridium difficile* colitis. Intravenous nafcillin may cause phlebitis at the injection site, agranulocytosis, and acute interstitial nephritis. Oxacillin is linked to hepatotoxicity, which may be reversed if the drug is discontinued.

What are the contraindications and interactions?

Penicillins are contraindicated in patients with a history of hypersensitivity to penicillin or the cephalosporins. The drugs should be used cautiously in patients with renal disease or during pregnancy and lactation. Some penicillins, such as penicillin V and ampicillin, may interfere with the effectiveness of birth control pills that contain estrogen. Penicillins can potentiate the anticoagulant effects of warfarin.

The effectiveness of penicillin decreases when it is used with the tetracyclines because penicillin is bactericidal and requires actively producing bacteria for full effect (whereas the tetracyclines are bacteriostatic). Absorption of most penicillins is affected by food. They should be given 1 hour before or 2 hours after meals.

What are the important points patients should know?

Advise patients to take penicillin on an empty stomach (1 hour before or 2 hours after meals), with water, to facilitate absorption. Note that amoxicillin may be taken with meals to decrease gastric upsets. Hypersensitivity may occur after oral administration of penicillin, so advise the patient to discontinue the medication and immediately contact his or her physician.

Table 16-2 ■ Penicillins

GENERIC NAME	TRADE NAME	AVERAGE ADULT DOSAGE	ROUTE OF ADMINISTRATION
Natural (Classic) Penicillins			
penicillin G potassium	Pfizerpen	≤ 20–30 million units/d; dosage may also be based on weight	IV or IM
penicillin G benzathine	Bicillin L-A	≤ 2.4 million units/d	IM
procaine penicillin	Wycillin	600,000–2.4 million units/d	IM
penicillin V potassium	Pen-Vee-K	125–500 mg q6h or q8h	PO
Semisynthetic, Penicillinase-Resistant Penicillins			
cloxacillin	Cloxapen, Tegopen	250–500 mg q6h	PO
dicloxacillin	Dynapen, Dycill, Pathocil	125–250 mg q6h	PO
methicillin	Staphcillin	1,000 mg q4-6h	IM, IV
nafcillin	Unipen, Nallpen	250 mg–1,250 mg/d	PO
		500 mg q4–6h	IM
		3–6 g/d for 24–48h only	IV

GENERIC NAME	TRADE NAME	AVERAGE ADULT DOSAGE	ROUTE OF ADMINISTRATION
oxacillin	Bactocill	500 mg–1 g q4–6h	PO
		250 mg–1 g q4–6h	IM, IV
Amino Penicillins			
amoxicillin	Amoxil, Trimox, Wymox	250–500 mg q8h or 875 mg bid	PO
amoxicillin and clavula-nate potassium	Augmentin	250–500 mg q8h or 875 mg q12h	PO
ampicillin (oral)	Omnipen, Principen	250–500 mg q6h	PO
ampicillin (parenteral)	Omnipen-N	1–12 g/d in divided doses q4–6h	IM, IV
ampicillin and sulbactam	Unasyn	0.5–1 g sulbactam with 1–2 g ampicillin q6–8h	IM, IV
bacampicillin	Spectrobid	400–800 mg q12h; dosage may also be based on weight	PO
Extended-Spectrum, Carboxy Penicillins			
carbenicillin indanyl sodium	Geocillin	1–2 tablets (382 mg each) qid	PO
ticarcillin	Ticar	150–300 mg/kg/d q3h, q4h, or q6h; 24 g/d	IM
		150–300 mg/kg/d q3h, q4h, or q6h; maximum dosage, 2 g/d	IV
ticarcillin and clavulanate	Timentin	3.1 g q4–6h or 200–300 mg/kg/d in divided doses q4–6h	IV
Ureido Penicillins			
mezlocillin	Mezlin	200–300 mg/kg/d in 4–6 divided doses; ≤ 350 mg/kg/d	IM, IV
piperacillin	Pipracil	3–4 g q4–6h; maximum dosage, 25 g/d	IM, IV
piperacillin and tazobactam	Zosyn	12 mg/1.5 g given as 3.375 g q6h	IV

bid, twice a day; IM, intramuscular; IV, intravenous; PO, oral.

Focus Point

Methicillin

Methicillin is another example of the semisynthetic, penicillinase-resistant penicillins, but is only used rarely today because so many bacteria have become resistant to its effects. It has widely been replaced with vancomycin (Vancocin). Methicillin is also known as staphcillin. The condition known as MRSA stands for "methicillin-resistant *Staphylococcus aureus.*" When MRSA is discovered in a hospitalized patient, special precautions are used to prevent its spread, and treatment usually involves vancomycin.

Focus On

Cephalosporins

The cephalosporins are a group of antibiotics closely related to the penicillins. Currently, they are classified into four generations based on their Gram-negative spectrum and stability in the presence of beta-lactamases (agents that retard the actions of enzymes). Gram-negative bacteria cannot resist decolorization with alcohol after being treated with Gram's crystal violet. After decolorization, they can be readily counterstained with safranin, which gives them a pink or red color when viewed under a microscope. However, this classification scheme is becoming less reliable because newer agents have led to more exceptions and less precise criteria for differences in the **antibacterial spectrum** (the range of bacteria against which an agent is effective). Whereas those with a broad spectrum are effective against many different kinds of bacteria, those with a narrow spectrum may be effective against only a single type or a few (Table 16-3 ■).

The different generations of cephalosporins are:

✳ *First generation:* Exhibit highest activity against Gram-positive bacteria and lowest activity against Gram-negative bacteria

✳ *Second generation:* Are more active against Gram-negative bacteria and less active against Gram-positive bacteria than first-generation cephalosporins

✳ *Third generation:* Are considerably less active than first-generation agents against Gram-positive bacteria (especially staphylococci), have a much expanded spectrum of activity against Gram-negative organisms, and are more resistant to Gram-negative beta-lactamases

✳ *Fourth generation:* Have improved Gram-positive spectrum and expanded Gram-negative activity of third-generation cephalosporins

How do they work?

The cephalosporins have a mechanism of action that is very similar to that of the penicillins. They affect the bacterial cell wall and are bactericidal, resulting in the destruction of bacteria.

How are they used?

The cephalosporins are effective against a wide variety of infections because they have a broad spectrum. The first- and second-generation cephalosporins are used frequently for prophylaxis during certain surgical procedures to reduce the risk of postoperative wound infections. Cefazolin is preferred because it has a higher serum concentration and longer elimination half-life. A number of second- and third-generation cephalosporins are effective alternatives as prophylactic agents for various surgical procedures. Cephalosporins are generally not the first drugs of choice for any bacterial infections because equally effective and less expensive alternatives are available. Overall, cephalosporins are used for dental work, heart and pacemaker procedures, orthopedic surgery, pneumonia, upper respiratory infections (URIs), and sinus infections.

What are the adverse effects?

Hypersensitivity occurs in about 5–10% of patients taking cephalosporins; manifestations include drug fever, skin rash, urticaria (hives), serum sickness, anaphylaxis, neutropenia, and nephritis. Other adverse effects of cephalosporins include pain, sterile abscess, nausea and vomiting, glossitis, diarrhea, and abdominal pain. Cephalosporins have a 5–10% cross-sensitivity with penicillins.

What are the contraindications and interactions?

Cephalosporins should not be used in combination with other antibiotics that cause nephrotoxicity or ototoxicity. Diuretics such as furosemide and ethacrynic acid also enhance nephrotoxicity and make certain cephalosporins ototoxic. Estrogen-containing oral contraceptives and cephalosporins taken concurrently may result in therapeutic failure.

What are the important points patients should know?

Instruct patients to take cephalosporins on an empty stomach. If gastric irritation occurs, patients may take these drugs with food.

Focus Point

Penicillin Allergy

Allergic reaction to penicillin is an immediate life-threatening systemic reaction that typically occurs after exposure to penicillin injection. The patient must be closely observed for this reaction after injection. The usual treatment is one or more injections of epinephrine and, in some cases, intravenous antihistamines and corticosteroids, as well as oxygen therapy.

Table 16-3 ■ Cephalosporins

GENERIC NAME	TRADE NAME	AVERAGE ADULT DOSAGE	ROUTE OF ADMINISTRATION
First Generation			
cefadroxil	Duricef	500 mg–1 g/d	PO
cefazolin	Ancef, Kefzol	250 mg–1 g/d	IM or IV
cephalexin	Keflex	25 mg–1 g/d	PO
cephapirin	Cefadyl	25 mg–4 g/d	PO
cephradine	Velosef	250 mg/d	PO, IM, or IV
Second Generation			
cefaclor	Ceclor	125–500 mg/d	PO
cefonicid	Monocid	50 mg–12 g/d	IM or IV
cefoxitin	Mefoxin	2 g/d	IV
cefuroxime	Ceftin	125–500 mg/d	PO
Third Generation			
cefixime	Suprax	100–400 mg/d	PO
cefoperazone	Cefobid	1–6 g/d	IM or IV
cefotaxime moxalactam	Claforan	75 mg–4 g/d	IV
cefprozil	Cefzil	250–500 mg/d	PO
ceftazidime	Ceptaz, Fortaz	1 gram q8-12h	IM or IV
ceftriaxone	Rocephin	1–2 g/d	IV
Fourth Generation			
cefepime	Maxipime	500 mg–2 g/d	IM or IV
Combination Agent			
ceftazidime/avibactam*	Avycaz	2.5 grams (2 g/0.5 g) q8h infused over 2h for 5–14 days	IV

IM, intramuscular; IV, intravenous; PO, oral.

*Note: Avibactam is the first non-beta-lactam beta-lactamase inhibitor (BLI).

Focus On

Ceftazidime/avibactam

Ceftazidime/avibactam (Avycaz) is a new combination drug that contains a third-generation cephalosporin with the *first available* non-beta-lactam beta-lactamase inhibitor.

How does it work?

Ceftazidime/avibactam works in several ways. The ceftazidime component binds to essential penicillin-binding proteins, inhibiting enzymes responsible for cell-wall synthesis. The avibactam component improves the in vitro activity of ceftazidime against various bacteria.

How is it used?

Ceftazidime/avibactam is used to treat complicated intra-abdominal infections and complicated urinary tract infections, including pyelonephritis.

(continued)

Focus On (*continued*)

What are the adverse effects?

Ceftazidime/avibactam may cause severe diarrhea, nausea and vomiting, constipation, and anxiety. There are no other significant adverse effects.

What are the contraindications and interactions?

Ceftazidime/avibactam is contraindicated in patients with known serious hypersensitivity to this drug, its components, or other cephalosporins. There are no known drug interactions.

What are the important points patients should know?

The patient should be instructed not to take this drug if there are kidney abnormalities and should understand that this medication must be stopped if an allergic reaction occurs. The physician must be contacted in this situation, as well as if diarrhea develops.

❋ Apply Your Knowledge 16.2

The following questions focus on what you have just learned about sulfonamides, penicillins, and cephalosporins.

CRITICAL THINKING

1. Define the terms *bacteriostatic* and *bactericidal*.
2. Explain the mechanism of action of the sulfonamides.
3. Identify the characteristics of Gram-positive bacteria.
4. Discuss the characteristics of the four generations of cephalosporins.

SUPERINFECTIONS

Superinfections may be caused by a disruption of the nonpathogenic microorganisms within the human body (also known as *normal flora*) that is often attributed to the use of antibiotics. When antibiotics destroy large numbers of normal flora, the chemical environment of the body is altered and a new infection is "superimposed" on an original infection (hence the term *superinfection*). The altered chemical environment allows for the uncontrolled growth of microorganisms (fungal or bacterial) that are not affected by the antibiotic in use.

Superinfections may occur with any antibiotic, most often when antibiotics are used for long periods or over repeated therapy courses.

Superinfections can develop rapidly and become very serious or even life-threatening. Oral penicillins and cephalosporins often cause bacterial superinfections in the bowel, characterized by diarrhea (or bloody diarrhea), abdominal cramping, fever, and rectal bleeding. A common bacterial superinfection is *pseudomembranous colitis*. Penicillins and cephalosporins are commonly associated with vaginal yeast infections.

Focus on Geriatrics

The Risk of Superinfection Among Elderly Patients

Older patients taking penicillin over a long period and those who are chronically ill or debilitated are more likely to contract a superinfection such as pseudomembranous colitis. This condition is potentially life-threatening and produces a toxin that affects the lining of the colon. Signs and symptoms include abdominal cramping and severe diarrhea that contains visible blood and mucus. Use of antibiotics should be discontinued, and severe cases may require treatment with intravenous (IV) fluids and electrolytes, oral vancomycin, and protein supplements.

Focus On

Aminoglycosides

Aminoglycosides have been very important antibiotics for the treatment of infections caused by Gram-negative bacilli. They are **broad-spectrum** antibiotics (effective against a wide range of organisms). The clinically important aminoglycosides are amikacin (Amikin), gentamicin (generic only), kanamycin (Kantrex), neomycin (Mycifradin), netilmicin (Netromycin), paromomycin (Humatin), streptomycin (the first aminoglycoside ever discovered), tobramycin (Tobrex), and vancomycin (Vancocin). Because of lower toxicity and broader effectiveness against various microorganisms, amikacin, gentamicin, and tobramycin are most widely used. Kanamycin is an older aminoglycoside to which many bacteria are resistant. Table 16-4 ■ lists various aminoglycosides.

How do they work?

The aminoglycosides combine with bacterial (not human) ribosomes to arrest protein synthesis, but their complete mechanism of action is not fully understood. They prevent cell reproduction, resulting in death of the bacteria. Aminoglycosides are bactericidal, which is different than other protein synthesis inhibitors. Aminoglycosides also act synergistically with beta-lactams and other agents that inhibit cell wall synthesis. As a result, aminoglycosides are often used along with beta-lactams and similar agents.

How are they used?

Aminoglycosides are used for the treatment of life-threatening infections, sepsis, and immunocompromised patients. Large doses of aminoglycosides are given orally before abdominal surgery to reduce the number of intestinal bacteria. Since these agents are charged molecules that are not bioavailable via the oral route, they are administered parenterally. The usual route of administration for systemic effects is either IM or IV. Aminoglycosides are also commonly administered via the ophthalmic or otic route in the form of eyedrops or eardrops to treat localized infections.

What are the adverse effects?

The serious adverse effects of aminoglycosides include ototoxicity, nephrotoxicity, and neuromuscular blockade. Ototoxicity manifests as auditory or vestibular damage, and it is the most important factor that restricts the use of these agents. Nephrotoxicity depends on the renal function of the patient, his or her age, and the drug dose. These agents can cause acute renal failure, probably because of their accumulation in the proximal tubular cells. The biochemistry of aminoglycosides in these situations is not fully understood, but mitochondrial poisoning and abnormal effects upon the plasma membrane are believed to occur.

What are the contraindications and interactions?

Aminoglycosides should not be used during pregnancy because they may cause fetal harm, particularly hearing loss and deafness in newborn babies. When aminoglycosides are used concurrently with penicillins, their desired effects may be greatly decreased. Still, these drugs are often used in combination, especially in the treatment of bacterial endocarditis. These drugs should be given several hours apart. The drug action of warfarin (an oral anticoagulant) can increase if taken simultaneously with aminoglycosides. The risk of ototoxicity increases when ethacrynic acid and aminoglycosides are given.

What are the important points patients should know?

Instruct patients to increase fluid intake while taking aminoglycosides. This measure assists in preventing renal failure from nephrotoxicity. To minimize toxicity problems, short treatment periods (7–10 days) and once-daily administration should be used. Once-per-day dosage has the tendency to reduce toxicity; however, monitoring is still required.

Aminoglycoside Toxicity

Careful drug dosing is very important with younger and older patients. Prolonged use of aminoglycosides may cause a superinfection. Toxicity from aminoglycosides may result in hypersensitivity reactions and drug-induced fever. Tobramycin may also cause *C. difficile*-related diarrhea. Neomycin is the most ototoxic and nephrotoxic aminoglycoside. Therefore, it is used topically for eye, ear, and skin infections. It is also used orally before intestinal surgery to suppress normal flora. However, oral administration may cause superinfection of the bowel along with intestinal malabsorption syndrome.

Table 16-4 ■ Aminoglycosides

GENERIC NAME	TRADE NAME	AVERAGE ADULT DOSAGE	ROUTE OF ADMINISTRATION
amikacin	Amikin	15 mg/kg/d in 2–3 divided doses	IV or IM
gentamicin	(Generic only)	3–5 mg/kg/d (standard dose)	IM
		6–7 mg/kg/d (once daily)	IV or PO
kanamycin	Kantrex	15 mg/kg/d q8–12h	PO, IM, or IV
neomycin	Mycifradin	50–100 mg/kg/d	PO
		10–15 mg/d	Topical
netilmicin	Netromycin	3–6 mg/kg/d	IV or IM
paromomycin	Humatin	25–35 mg/kg/d, in 3 doses with meals, for 5–10 days	PO
streptomycin	Streptomycin	0.5–1 g q12–24h	IM
tobramycin	Tobrex	3–5 mg/kg/d (standard dose)	IV, IM, or ophthalmic
vancomycin	Vancocin	6–7 mg/kg/d (once daily)	PO or IV

IM, intramuscular; IV, intravenous; PO, oral.

Focus On

Macrolides

The term *macrolide* refers to the large chemical ring structure characteristic of these antibiotics. One or more deoxy sugars are attached to these rings. The macrolides include erythromycin (e.g., E-mycin), azithromycin (Zithromax), clarithromycin (Biaxin), troleandomycin (Tao), and dirithromycin (Dynabac). Erythromycin is produced by *Streptomyces erythreus*. Macrolides are broad-spectrum agents that are bacteriostatic at normal doses and bactericidal at higher doses. They are also commonly used as alternative drugs in patients who are allergic to penicillin because they are effective against many of the same organisms. Table 16-5 ■ lists common macrolides. The macrolides are active against Gram-positive and Gram-negative aerobic bacteria and atypical organisms, including chlamydiae, mycoplasmae, legionellae, rickettsia, and spirochetes. Erythromycin is the oldest known macrolide, with new agents such as azithromycin and clarithromycin being derivatives of erythromycin.

How do they work?

The mechanism of action of the macrolides is inhibition of bacterial protein synthesis by binding to the bacterial ribosome, which stops bacterial growth. Macrolides bind equally to ribosomes from Gram-positive and Gram-negative bacteria. Erythromycin is one of the safest antibiotics of all, is usually bacteriostatic, but can be bactericidal against highly susceptible microorganisms. It is selectively toxic to bacteria since ribosomes in cytoplasm do not bind the drug. The antibacterial spectrum of erythromycin is similar to that of penicillin.

How are they used?

Macrolides are indicated for treatment of bacterial-related exacerbations of chronic obstructive pulmonary disease, skin structure infections, pharyngitis, tonsillitis, sinusitis, bronchitis, other respiratory tract infections, pneumonia, acute otitis media, duodenal ulcers, pelvic inflammatory disease, intestinal amebiasis, rheumatic fever, soft tissue infections, urethritis, syphilis, Legionnaires' disease, UTIs, and rectal infections. Because of broader spectrums of effects and their ability to be better tolerated by most patients, azithromycin and clarithromycin are increasing in popularity. Erythromycin is a preferred treatment for pneumonia caused by *Legionella pneumophila*. It is the drug of first choice for *Bordetella pertussis*, which causes **whooping cough**. Erythromycin is also the treatment of choice for acute diphtheria and is one of the most effective agents for chlamydial urethritis or cervicitis, as well as for ***Mycoplasma pneumoniae***.

What are the adverse effects?

In general, the macrolides are considered safe agents. Gastrointestinal (GI) effects, such as abdominal pain and nausea and vomiting, are the most common adverse effects. The newer macrolides cause fewer GI side effects. Hepatotoxicity related to the use of the macrolides is rare but may be serious. Extremely high doses of IV erythromycin and oral clarithromycin have been associated with ototoxicity. Phlebitis may occur with IV administration of the macrolides. Though extremely safe overall, the most common adverse effects of erythromycin include diarrhea, epigastric pain, and nausea and vomiting. Rarely, when it is combined with drugs that can raise its plasma level (class IA or class III antidysrhythmic drugs, verapamil, diltiazem, ketoconazole, itraconazole, ritonavir, saquinivir, or nefazodone), it has resulted in fatal ventricular dysrhythmias. It can also promote superinfection of the intestines or **thrombophlebitis**.

What are the contraindications and interactions?

Macrolides are contraindicated in patients with hypersensitivity to them. They must be avoided in individuals who have a history of erythromycin-associated hepatitis or liver dysfunction. Erythromycin inhibits the hepatic metabolism of theophylline. It may interfere with the metabolism of digoxin, carbamazepine, warfarin, chloramphenicol, clindamycin, corticosteroids, and cyclosporine. In fact, drug interaction between macrolides and cyclosporine and the resulting toxicity has led to the removal of several drugs from the market in the United States. Erythromycin should not be used with drugs that inhibit its metabolism such as verapamil, diltiazem, azole antifungals, and HIV protease inhibitors.

What are the important points patients should know?

Instruct patients to take oral macrolides with a full glass of water and food to get the maximum effect. Clarithromycin may leave a metallic taste in the mouth.

Table 16-5 ■ Commonly Used Macrolides

GENERIC NAME	TRADE NAME	AVERAGE ADULT DOSAGE	ROUTE OF ADMINISTRATION
azithromycin	Zithromax	500–2,000 mg	PO
clarithromycin	Biaxin	500 mg	PO
dirithromycin	Dynabac	250 mg	PO
erythromycin base	Eryc, E-mycin	250 mg	PO
erythromycin estolate	Ilosone	125 mg or 250 mg per 5 mL of oral suspension	PO
erythromycin stearate	Erythrocin	500–1,000 mg	IV or PO
troleandomycin	Tao	125–500 mg	PO

IM, intramuscular; IV, intravenous; PO, oral.

✳ Apply Your Knowledge 16.3

The following questions focus on aminoglycosides and macrolides.

CRITICAL THINKING

1. Describe how aminoglycosides work.
2. Give the trade names of kanamycin, netilmicin, and tobramycin.
3. Explain the mechanisms of action of the macrolides.
4. Give the generic names of Biaxin, Ilosone, and Zithromax.
5. Identify the important points that patients should know about macrolides.

Focus On

Fluoroquinolones

The antibacterial drugs known as quinolones have been in use since 1964, when nalidixic acid was released. Since 1990, the fluoroquinolones have become a dominant class of bactericidal antimicrobial agents.

In general, the fluoroquinolones possess activity against Gram-positive, Gram-negative, and atypical organisms. The older fluoroquinolones (ciprofloxacin [Cipro], norfloxacin [Noroxin], and ofloxacin [Floxin]) are highly active against Gram-negative pathogens, but their activity against Gram-positive pathogens is limited. The newer fluoroquinolones have enhanced activity against the Gram-positive pathogens while maintaining similar Gram-negative activity (Table 16-6 ■).

How do they work?

The fluoroquinolones exert their bactericidal effect by interfering with an enzyme (DNA gyrase) that is required by bacteria for the synthesis of DNA. This action inhibits cell reproduction, resulting in the death of the bacteria.

How are they used?

The fluoroquinolones have a broad spectrum of antimicrobial activity. They are used for prophylactic purposes before dental procedures and also to treat UTIs, prostatitis, gonorrhea, anthrax, pneumonia and other respiratory tract infections, and infections of the bones and joints.

What are the adverse effects?

Adverse effects are usually mild and transient. They include nausea and vomiting, diarrhea, flatulence, abdominal discomfort, skin rashes, photosensitivity (especially severe with sparfloxacin), and some nephrotoxicity. Rare but severe reactions that have also been reported include neuropsychiatric effects, cardiac abnormalities, and liver dysfunction. In children, fluoroquinolones may damage developing cartilage.

What are the contraindications and interactions?

Fluoroquinolones should be avoided in children younger than 18 years, patients older than 60 years of age, and in pregnant or lactating women. When used with caffeine, such symptoms as insomnia and hyperactivity may occur. Antacids decrease the absorption of the drug and should not be given for 2 hours after the administration of the antibiotic.

What are the important points patients should know?

Advise patients that fluoroquinolones should not be taken with milk or other dairy products, antacids, magnesium laxatives, or iron supplements. Advise patients to drink adequate fluids to maintain a high urine output, thereby preventing crystalluria. Instruct patients to report visual disturbances, dizziness, lightheadedness, or depression that may indicate potential early central nervous system (CNS) toxicity. If these manifestations occur, advise patients to avoid driving and operating heavy machinery and to report the effects immediately. Alcohol may worsen these effects and should be avoided. Ciprofloxacin and ofloxacin injections should be protected from light.

Table 16-6 ■ Fluoroquinolones

GENERIC NAME	TRADE NAME	AVERAGE ADULT DOSAGE	ROUTE OF ADMINISTRATION
Classical Fluoroquinolones			
ciprofloxacin	Cipro	500–750 mg q12h (PO) 400 mg q12h (IV)	PO, IV
enoxacin	Penetrex	200–400 mg q12h for 1–2 wk	PO
levofloxacin	Levaquin	PO: 250–500 mg/d; IV: 25 mg/mL	PO, IV
lomefloxacin	Maxaquin	400 mg/d for 2 wk	PO
nalidixic acid	NegGram	500 mg (tablet form) and 300 mg/5 mL (suspension form)*	PO
norfloxacin	Noroxin	400 mg q12h for 3 d	PO
ofloxacin	Floxin	200–400 mg q12h	PO

GENERIC NAME	TRADE NAME	AVERAGE ADULT DOSAGE	ROUTE OF ADMINISTRATION
Newest Fluoroquinolones			
gatifloxacin	Tequin	PO: 400 mg/d for 7–14 d; IV: 400 mg/40 mL	PO, IV
moxifloxacin	Avelox	400 mg/d for 5–10 d	PO
sparfloxacin	Zagam	Loading dose: 400 mg on day 1; then 200 mg/d for 10 d	PO
trovafloxacin	Trovan	100 mg	PO

*Most antibiotic suspensions such as this example should be refrigerated after constitution.

IM, intramuscular; IV, intravenous; PO, oral.

Focus on Pediatrics

Avoid Fluoroquinolones in Children

Fluoroquinolones should be avoided in children because studies in young animals have documented the erosion of cartilage. However, these agents have been used safely in children with cystic fibrosis without harm.

Focus On

Tetracyclines

The tetracyclines are all very much alike with respect to their antimicrobial spectra and the untoward effects they elicit. They differ mainly in their absorption, duration of action, and suitability for parenteral administration (Table 16-7 ■). The tetracyclines available in the United States include chlortetracycline, demeclocycline, doxycycline, minocycline, oxytetracycline, and tetracycline.

How do they work?

The tetracyclines are broad-spectrum antibiotics and are mainly bacteriostatic. They bind to the bacterial ribosomes and prevent protein synthesis. The tetracyclines have activities against Gram-positive and Gram-negative bacteria, mycobacteria, rickettsia, and chlamydiae.

How are they used?

The tetracyclines are used in the treatment of infections caused by a wide range of microorganisms. They are effective against certain types of *Rickettsia* (Rocky Mountain spotted fever and typhus fever). These drugs are also indicated for therapy of chlamydial infections, cholera, brucellosis, tularemia, and amebiasis. Tetracyclines are prescribed as an alternative to penicillin for the treatment of gonorrhea, syphilis, Lyme disease, anthrax, and *Haemophilus influenzae* respiratory infections. Doxycycline hyclate is highly effective in the prophylaxis of "traveler's diarrhea."

What are the adverse effects?

The tetracyclines cause a large number of different adverse effects. GI toxicity is common with oral use; it is probably caused by the combined effect of local irritation and alteration of the intestinal flora. Manifestations are heartburn, nausea and vomiting, and diarrhea. They are also associated with photosensitivity reactions, predisposing patients to severe sunburn. Kidney toxicity is also a significant adverse effect. Doxycycline is safest in this regard because less of this drug is eliminated via the kidneys. It also does not alter intestinal flora as much as the other tetracyclines. Expired tetracyclines can result in severe kidney damage and even death.

(continued)

Focus On (*continued*)

The broad-spectrum antibacterial activity of the tetracyclines may cause superinfections in the manner of penicillins, cephalosporins, and sulfa drugs. This occurs most commonly in the bowel, but it may also readily occur in the mouth, lungs, and vagina. The most common superinfection is **candidiasis**, which is an infection or disease caused by certain types of *Candida*, especially *Candida albicans*—usually resulting from debilitation, physiologic change, prolonged administration of antibiotics, and barrier breakage. Overgrowth from staphylococci may also occur. Staphylococcal enteric superinfections are frequently fatal.

Various hypersensitivity reactions or hepatotoxicity may occur. Tetracyclines may cause a darker pigment (graying) in developing teeth in children younger than 8 years old and may impair bone growth.

What are the contraindications and interactions?

The tetracyclines should be avoided in patients with hypersensitivity and renal or liver diseases. They should not be used in children younger than 8 years old. These drugs are also contraindicated in pregnant and lactating women.

Certain foods (such as dairy products) and drugs (such as laxatives, antacids that contain aluminum and calcium, and iron preparations) may reduce the absorption of tetracyclines. Therefore, it is recommended that tetracyclines be taken on an empty stomach. Phenytoin and barbiturates can decrease the effectiveness of tetracyclines.

What are the important points patients should know?

Instruct patients that tetracyclines should be taken on an empty stomach (1 hour before or 2 hours after meals) to facilitate absorption. The absorption of tetracyclines is strongly influenced by the presence of food and other drugs. Advise patients that because tetracyclines can cause photosensitivity reactions, they should avoid the sun during the warmest time of day (10:00 A.M. to 2:00 P.M.), use a sunblock, and wear a hat as well as protective clothing. Tetracyclines should be stored away from light and extreme heat because their effects cause tetracyclines to decompose and produce toxic breakdown products. Expired tetracyclines should be disposed of immediately.

Table 16-7 ■ Tetracyclines

GENERIC NAME	TRADE NAME	AVERAGE ADULT DOSAGE	ROUTE OF ADMINISTRATION
chlortetracycline	Aureomycin	250–500 mg q6h	PO
demeclocycline	Declomycin	150 mg q6h	PO
doxycycline hyclate	Vibramycin	100–200 mg initially; then 100 mg bid	PO
doxycycline monohydrate	Monodox	100 mg/d	PO
minocycline	Minocin	200 mg initially; then 100 mg bid (both)	PO, IV
oxytetracycline	Terramycin	250 mg/d	PO
tetracycline	Achromycin, Sumycin, Panmycin	250–500 mg q6h; 100 mg bid–tid	PO, IM

bid, twice a day; IM, intramuscular; IV, intravenous; PO, oral; tid, three times a day.

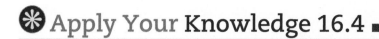

Apply Your Knowledge 16.4

The following questions focus on what you have just learned about fluoroquinolones and tetracyclines.

CRITICAL THINKING

1. Describe the mechanism of action of the fluoroquinolones.
2. Identify the contraindications of fluoroquinolones.
3. Explain the main indications of tetracyclines.
4. Discuss why tetracyclines are contraindicated in pregnant women and in children younger than 8 years of age.
5. Give the trade names of minocycline, doxycycline, and chlortetracycline.

MISCELLANEOUS ANTIBACTERIAL AGENTS

These antibacterial agents are principally second-line drugs because of emerging resistance, concerns with toxicity, or special activity against selected organisms (Table 16-8 ■). Discussion of chloramphenicol, clindamycin, vancomycin, and other miscellaneous antibacterial agents follows (in several of the following tables).

Table 16-8 ■ Miscellaneous Antibacterial Agents

GENERIC NAME	TRADE NAME	AVERAGE ADULT DOSAGE	ROUTE OF ADMINISTRATION
chloramphenicol	e.g., Chloromycetin	12.5 mg/kg qid	IV infusion
clindamycin	Cleocin	600–1,200 mg/d in 3–4 divided doses, bid to qid	IV infusion, IM
		150–300 mg q6h	PO
		100 mg into vagina daily	Vaginal cream
linezolid	Zyvox	600 mg bid	PO
spectinomycin	Trobicin	2 g as single dose	IM
vancomycin	Vancocin	125–500 qid	PO
		30 mg/kg daily divided bid	IV infusion

bid, twice a day; IM, intramuscular; IV, intravenous; PO, oral; qid, four times a day.

Focus On

Chloramphenicol

Chloramphenicol (e.g., Chloromycetin) is highly effective against rickettsial diseases (such as Rocky Mountain spotted fever), chlamydial diseases, and many bacterial infections.

How does it work?

Chloramphenicol is primarily bacteriostatic and a secondary bactericidal medication against a few bacterial strains. This agent interferes with protein synthesis. It is active against both Gram-positive and Gram-negative microorganisms.

How is it used?

Because of serious toxic reactions, the systemic use of chloramphenicol should be limited only to very serious infections that cannot be managed by other drugs.

(continued)

Focus On (continued)

Chloramphenicol is very effective against *Haemophilus influenzae*, *Neisseria meningitides*, and certain *Bacteroides* strains. It is used occasionally for typhoid fever, bacterial meningitis, and rickettsial diseases when safer alternatives are not available or because of drug allergy or resistance.

What are the adverse effects?

Chloramphenicol is extremely toxic, and bone marrow injury is its major toxic effect. Thrombocytopenia, granulocytopenia, and aplastic anemia are the most serious blood cell formation disturbances observed and have resulted in a number of fatalities. In neonates, its use may cause gray-baby syndrome. Chloramphenicol, in high doses, may cause fatal aplastic anemia.

What are the contraindications and interactions?

Chloramphenicol must be avoided in patients with known hypersensitivity to the drug. It must be used cautiously in patients with severe liver or kidney disease, in elderly patients, and during pregnancy and lactation.

Chloramphenicol may inhibit the metabolism of dicumarol, tolbutamide, warfarin, and phenytoin, leading to prolonged action and increased effects of these drugs. Phenobarbital can reduce the effect of chloramphenicol levels and may cause toxicity.

What are the important points patients should know?

Advise patients to take oral chloramphenicol with a full glass of water on an empty stomach and to avoid driving or operating heavy machinery if confusion or visual disturbances occur. Instruct patients to report any manifestation of blood dyscrasias, such as sore throat, weakness, unexplained bruising or bleeding, and fever, to their physician promptly.

Focus on Pediatrics

Gray-Baby Syndrome

Gray-baby syndrome is a fatal cyanosis. Its symptoms include vomiting; abdominal distension; and loose green stools. It results from the inability of infants to metabolize the drug.

Focus On

Clindamycin

Clindamycin (Cleocin) is an antibacterial agent used as an alternate drug for treating infections caused by penicillin-resistant *S. aureus*. It is classified as a lincosamide, along with lincomycin.

How does it work?

Clindamycin is bacteriostatic and inhibits bacterial protein synthesis. This agent is active against most Gram-positive and many anaerobic organisms.

How is it used?

Clindamycin is the drug of choice for the treatment of GI infections caused by *Bacteroides fragilis*. It is perhaps the best drug for the topical treatment of acne vulgaris. Clindamycin is also used for serious respiratory tract infections, serious skin and soft tissue infections, septicemia, intra-abdominal infections, infections of the female pelvis and genital tract, and for bone and joint infections.

What are the adverse effects?

Clindamycin may cause abdominal pain, nausea and vomiting, mucosal ulcerations, fever, and bloody diarrhea. It may also result in antibiotic-associated (pseudomembranous) colitis.

What are the contraindications and interactions?

The contraindications include previous hypersensitivity to clindamycin, as well as impaired liver function. Clindamycin must be used cautiously in patients with impaired kidney function, a history of GI disease (particularly colitis) or liver disease, or asthma. It may potentiate the effects of neuromuscular blocking agents.

What are the important points patients should know?

Clindamycin should be taken with a full glass of water in order to avoid throat irritation. The patient should not take clindamycin if he or she is allergic to it, or to lincomycin. Clindamycin should not be taken with erythromycin. Clindamycin must be taken for the full prescribed length of time, and doses must not be skipped. The patient should stop taking clindamycin if watery or bloody diarrhea develops and should inform the physician immediately. Regular blood tests should be performed to assess for harmful adverse effects, and kidney or liver function may also need to be tested.

Spectinomycin

Spectinomycin (Trobicin) is an antibiotic produced by *Streptomyces spectabilis.* This agent is bacteriostatic and not bactericidal. It has variable activity against a wide variety of Gram-negative and Gram-positive organisms.

How does it work?

Spectinomycin suppresses protein synthesis in Gram-negative bacteria, especially *Neisseria gonorrhoeae.*

How is it used?

Spectinomycin is used only for the treatment of uncomplicated gonorrhea in patients sensitized or resistant to penicillin.

What are the adverse effects?

The common adverse effects of spectinomycin include headache, dizziness, chills, fever, insomnia, nervousness, and nausea and vomiting. It also causes pain and soreness at the injection site.

What are the contraindications and interactions?

The safety of spectinomycin during pregnancy, lactation, and in infants or children is not established. This drug is also contraindicated in known cases of hypersensitivity to spectinomycin. No significant drug or food interactions for this agent are known.

What are the important points patients should know?

Advise patients to use condoms to prevent transmission of gonorrheal infection. It may be necessary to treat patients' partners to prevent reinfection. Instruct patients to avoid driving or operating heavy machinery if dizziness occurs after administration.

Vancomycin

Vancomycin (Vancocin) is the drug of choice for severe infections caused by drug-resistant *Staphylococcus* and *Clostridium* infections. It is the most widely used antibiotic in hospitals in the United States. Vancomycin is active only against Gram-positive bacteria.

How does it work?

Vancomycin suppresses cell wall synthesis and is bactericidal. This drug is eliminated unchanged by the kidneys. This drug, unlike most antibiotics, does not contain a beta-lactam ring.

How is it used?

Vancomycin is usually reserved for serious infections such as *S. aureus* and *S. epidermidis.* It is especially effective against infections caused by methicillin-resistant staphylococci. It is useful in patients who are allergic to penicillin or cephalosporins. Typical uses include osteomyelitis, endocarditis, and staphylococcal pneumonia. When given orally, vancomycin is useful in the treatment of pseudomembranous colitis. However, because it is poorly absorbed from the GI tract, vancomycin is usually given by slow intravenous infusion. It is the drug of choice for severe *C. difficile* infection, but not for mild cases of this infection.

What are the adverse effects?

The most serious side effects of vancomycin are dose-related nephrotoxicity (resulting in renal failure) and, less commonly, ototoxicity. Additional adverse effects include chills, fever, nausea, flushing, skin rashes, pruritus, urticaria, tachycardia, and hypotension. Local pain and thrombophlebitis at the site of IV injection have been reported, as well as a flushing sensation that can occur if the agent is infused too rapidly. Most adverse effects are avoided if vancomycin is infused over 60 minutes or more.

What are the contraindications and interactions?

Vancomycin must be avoided in patients with known hypersensitivity to this drug. It is also contraindicated in patients with previous hearing loss. Vancomycin should

(continued)

Focus On (continued)

. . . .

be administered with caution in neonates, children, older adults, pregnant women, and patients with impaired kidney function or renal failure. Vancomycin increases the neuromuscular blockade of the muscle relaxants atracurium, pancuronium, tubocurarine, and vecuronium. Vancomycin should not be administered concurrently with aminoglycosides, cyclosporine, NSAIDs, and other nephrotoxic drugs.

What are the important points patients should know?

Advise patients to notify their health care providers if they experience ringing in the ears while taking this medicine.

Focus Point

Red-Man Syndrome and Vancomycin

Vancomycin may cause *red-man syndrome*, a condition that is manifested by facial flushing and hypotension caused by very rapid infusion of the drug. Other symptoms include rash, pruritus, urticaria, and tachycardia. A 1-g dose should be infused over at least 60 minutes.

Focus On

Linezolid

Linezolid is one of the oxazolidinones, a class of totally synthetic antibiotics first investigated in the late 1980s as antidepressant drugs. Later, these agents were discovered to have excellent antibacterial activity. The main reason for their development has been the increased resistance of Gram-positive pathogens. The Food and Drug Administration approved linezolid (Zyvox), the first oxazolidinone, in April 2000. The only other commercially available oxazolidinone in the United States is tedizolid (Sivextro).

How does it work?

Linezolid is a protein synthesis–inhibiting compound that usually produces a bacteriostatic effect. The principal activity is against Gram-positive aerobic organisms, including staphylococci, streptococci, and enterococci.

How is it used?

Linezolid is used for Gram-positive drug-resistant microorganisms that are highly virulent. These include MRSA, penicillin-resistant streptococcus, and vancomycin-resistant enterococcus.

What are the adverse effects?

In general, linezolid is well tolerated. The most common adverse effects are nausea and vomiting, diarrhea, and leukopenia.

What are the contraindications and interactions?

Linezolid is contraindicated in patients who are hypersensitive to the drug or its components. The use of linezolid with such adrenergic drugs as dopamine, epinephrine, or pseudoephedrine may cause hypertension. Blood pressure and heart rate should be monitored. Other items that may cause interactions include serotoninergic drugs and foods and beverages high in tyramine (including aged cheeses, air-dried meats, chocolate, fish, sauerkraut, red wines, tap beers, and soy sauce).

What are the important points patients should know?

Advise patients to avoid foods that contain tyramine or over-the-counter cold remedies while taking linezolid. The patient must notify his or her physician if severe diarrhea develops during or up to 2 months after linezolid therapy. The patient must report vision changes or pain, numbness, or tingling of the limbs. Since the teeth can become discolored by linezolid, the patient should be instructed about professional dental cleaning to restore normal tooth color. If the patient is diabetic, he or she should be instructed to monitor blood glucose closely and be prepared to treat hypoglycemia if it occurs.

Streptogramins

Streptogramins are protein synthesis inhibitors, of which the first drug, Synercid , was approved in 1999. It is a combination of dalfopristin (a group A streptogramin) and quinupristin (a group B streptogramin). This combination agent was approved for life-threatening vancomycin-resistant *Enterococcus faecium* or *Streptococcus pyogenes* infections. The streptogramins bind similarly to the macrolides and are believed to also block peptide emergence from ribosomes. These agents are bactericidal against many, but not all, susceptible bacterial species.

Pleuromutilins

The first pleuromutilin, called *retapamulin*, was approved in 2007. It is used topically for bacterial skin infections and has similar binding to that of linezolid and the group A streptogramins. These agents inhibit peptide bond formation.

Cyclic Lipopeptides

Cyclic lipopeptides are natural products with promising antibiotic properties. They are amphiphilic molecules, meaning they have a polar, water-soluble group attached to a nonpolar, water-insoluble hydrocarbon chain. Cyclic lipopeptides have a fatty acid tail linked to a short oligopeptide, forming a macrocyclic ring structure.

How do they work?

Cyclic lipopeptides bind to bacterial membranes and cause the cell membrane to depolarize. This results in an inhibition of DNA and RNA synthesis.

How are they used?

Cyclic lipopeptides are indicated for the treatment of life-threatening infections, sepsis, and immunocompromised patients.

What are the adverse effects?

Cyclic lipopeptides may cause nephrotoxicity, ototoxicity, tinnitus, and permanent deafness.

What are the contraindications and interactions?

Cyclic lipopeptides should be avoided in patients with kidney impairment. They need to be adjusted for each patient after the first dose and closely monitored. Once-per-day dosage has the tendency to reduce toxicity. However, monitoring is still required.

What are the important points patients should know?

If using a cyclic lipopetide at home, the patient should administer it the same time every day. The exact prescribed amount must be used. The patient should finish the prescription, even if symptoms improve while taking the medication. Doses must not be skipped or doubled up if a previous dose is missed. The patient must report any of the following symptoms to his or her physician immediately: diarrhea, constipation, nausea and vomiting, stomach pain, difficulty falling asleep or staying asleep, headache, increased sweating, injection site reactions, unusual weight gain, sore throat, increased urge to urinate, or a burning sensation when urinating.

✳ Apply Your Knowledge 16.5

The following questions focus on what you have just learned about the miscellaneous antibacterial agents.

CRITICAL THINKING

1. Describe the indications of chloramphenicol and discuss its toxicity.
2. Identify the mechanism of action of spectinomycin.
3. Briefly explain how vancomycin works.
4. Identify the drug of choice for the treatment of GI infections caused by *Bacteroides fragilis*?
5. Point out the most serious side effects of vancomycin.

Antituberculosis Agents

Tuberculosis is a slow, progressive respiratory disease. It occurs worldwide and is caused by *Mycobacterium tuberculosis*, an acid-fast aerobic bacillus. Worldwide, approximately 1.5 million people die of TB each year. An estimated 10–15 million people in the United States have latent TB, of which 10% will develop active tuberculosis in the future. Ninety percent of cases involve the reactivation of prior infection; the remainder of cases are new infections. The majority of new cases occur in malnourished individuals, those living in overcrowded conditions, immunosuppressed individuals, incarcerated persons, immigrants, and older adults.

The twentieth century was characterized by a decline in the incidence of TB in most developed countries. This was largely because of antibiotic drugs, active immunization, screening of people and livestock, and better living conditions. More recently, a disturbing increase in occurrence of this infection has been seen. This increase appears to be attributable to immigration patterns, drug-resistant strains of TB, and a prevalence of conditions that impair immunity (e.g., HIV/AIDS and organ transplant therapy).

As many as four different drug combinations may be required to treat TB. These combinations are divided into the first- and second-line antituberculotics on the basis of their efficacy, activity, and adverse effects. Therapy is usually started with ethambutol (Myambutol), isoniazid (INH), rifampin (Rifadin, Rimactane), and pyrazinamide (PZA) for the first 2 months, followed by isoniazid and rifampin for a further minimum of 4 months. This regimen is suitable if bacteriology shows fully sensitive acid-fast bacilli (which may include *Mycobacteria* or *Nocardia* species) on culture (Table 16-9 ■).

Table 16-9 ■ Most Commonly Used Antituberculotics

GENERIC NAME	BRAND NAME	AVERAGE ADULT DOSAGE	ROUTE OF ADMINISTRATION
capreomycin	Capastat	1 g/d	IM
ciprofloxacin	Cipro	100–750 mg q12h	PO
		200–400 mg 8–q12h	IV
cycloserine	Seromycin	500–750 mg q12h	PO
ethambutol	Myambutol	15–25 mg/kg/d	PO
ethionamide	Trecator-SC	500–750 mg/d	PO
isoniazid (INH)	Laniazid, Nydrazid	5–10 mg/kg/d (≤ 300 mg/d)	PO, IM
isoniazid-pyrazinamide-rifampin	Rifater	300 mg/d	PO, IV
ofloxacin	Floxin	200–400 mg q12h	PO
pyrazinamide	(Generic only)	15–35 mg/kg/d in 3–4 divided doses (≤ 2 g/d)	PO
rifampin	Rifadin, Rimactane	600 mg/d with other antitubercular agents	PO, IV
rifapentine	Priftin	600 mg twice weekly for 2 months; then 600 mg/wk for 4 months	PO
streptomycin	Streptomycin	15 mg/kg (≤ 1 g) as a single dose	IM, IV

IM, intramuscular; IV, intravenous; PO, oral.

Focus On

Isoniazid

Isoniazid or INH is the most potent and selective of the known tuberculostatic antibacterial agents. It is tuberculocidal to growing bacteria and the most effective agent in the therapy of TB. The drug is never used alone because of the rapid emergence of resistance.

How does it work?

INH acts by interfering with the biosynthesis of bacterial proteins, nucleic acid, and lipids.

How is it used?

INH is used in the treatment of all forms of active TB caused by susceptible organisms and as a preventive agent in high-risk persons, such as household members and persons with positive tuberculin skin test reactions.

What are the adverse effects?

The common adverse effects include restlessness, insomnia, convulsions, optic neuritis, and psychoses. The drug also may cause nausea and vomiting, aplastic anemia, fever, and skin rashes.

What are the contraindications and interactions?

History of INH-associated hypersensitivity reactions, liver damage, and pregnancy are contraindications for its use. This drug should be used cautiously in patients with chronic liver disease, renal dysfunction, history of convulsive disorders, and chronic alcoholism.

What are the important points patients should know?

Advise patients that INH is better absorbed on an empty stomach. Instruct patients to avoid driving or operating heavy machinery if dizziness or drowsiness occurs and to contact their physicians if *tinnitus* (ringing in the ears), visual changes, dizziness, or *ataxia* (an inability to coordinate muscle activity) occurs. Patients must notify their physicians if symptoms of hepatotoxicity occur, including fever, liver tenderness, loss of appetite, malaise, or jaundice.

Focus on Geriatrics

Risk of Fatal Hepatitis with Isoniazid Therapy

Older patients taking INH are very susceptible to a potentially fatal hepatitis, especially if they regularly drink alcohol. Careful monitoring for signs of liver impairment is necessary. Good patient observation alerts the caregiver to the warning signs, which include increased serum alanine transferase and increased serum aspartate transaminase (liver enzymes), increased serum *bilirubin* (a substance released into the blood when red blood cells break down), and jaundice. Liver dysfunction in older adults may also be caused by the antitubercular drugs PZA and rifampin.

Focus On

Ethambutol

Ethambutol is a tuberculostatic drug that is effective against tubercle bacilli that are resistant to INH or streptomycin.

How does it work?

The mechanism of action of ethambutol is not completely understood, but it appears to inhibit RNA synthesis and arrest multiplication of tubercle bacilli. The emergence of resistant TB strains is delayed by administering ethambutol in combination with other antituberculosis drugs.

How is it used?

Ethambutol can be used in conjunction with at least one other antituberculotic in the treatment of pulmonary TB.

What are the adverse effects?

Ethambutol occasionally causes optic neuritis, with blurred vision and diminished visual acuity to green light. Although these effects disappear on discontinuation, the drug should be discontinued at the first indication of a loss

(continued)

Focus On (continued)

in visual acuity. Eye tests should be made before and at monthly intervals after the onset of therapy.

Other adverse effects include pruritus, anorexia, nausea and vomiting, abdominal pain, headache, vertigo, fever, hallucinations, and abnormal liver function.

What are the contraindications and interactions?

Ethambutol is contraindicated in patients with optic neuritis or a history of hypersensitivity to the drug. It is also contraindicated in children younger than 6 years. Ethambutol should be used cautiously in patients with renal impairment, hepatic disease, gout, cataracts, or diabetic retinopathy and in those who are pregnant or lactating. Ethambutol absorption is decreased with aluminum salts.

What are the important points patients should know?

Instruct patients about the importance of regular eye examinations while taking ethambutol. If the patient experiences problems with vision, the drug should be stopped immediately.

Advise patients to take ethambutol with meals to lessen gastric irritation and to avoid driving or operating heavy machinery if drowsiness or dizziness occurs.

Rifampin

Rifampin (Rifadin, Rimactane) is a broad-spectrum antibiotic that is effective against most Gram-positive bacteria and variably active against Gram-negative organisms. *M. tuberculosis* is very susceptible to this drug.

How does it work?

Rifampin inhibits the activity of DNA-dependent RNA polymerase (an enzyme responsible for creating different RNA molecules) in susceptible bacterial cells, thereby suppressing RNA synthesis.

How is it used?

Rifampin is used primarily with other antituberculosis agents for the initial treatment and retreatment of clinical TB and as short-term therapy to eliminate meningococci from the nasopharynx of an asymptomatic carrier of *Neisseria meningitides* when the risk of meningococcal meningitis is high.

What are the adverse effects?

Fatigue, drowsiness, headache, confusion, dizziness, nausea and vomiting, heartburn, skin rashes, and renal insufficiency may be observed with rifampin administration. This drug may also cause a reddish-orange discoloration of such body fluids as tears, urine, sweat, and saliva.

What are the contraindications and interactions?

Rifampin must be avoided in patients with a history of hypersensitivity to the drug. It should be used with caution in patients with hepatic disease or a history of alcoholism and in those who are pregnant or lactating.

Rifampin decreases concentrations of alfentanil (Alfenta, an opioid analgesic), alosetron (Lotronex, which is used to treat irritable bowel syndrome), barbiturates, benzodiazepines, and many other drugs. The use of rifampin with oral anticoagulants or oral hypoglycemics may decrease the effects of these drugs.

What are the important points patients should know?

Inform patients that rifampin may cause urine, feces, saliva, sputum, sweat, and tears to develop a red-orange appearance. This effect is harmless. Advise patients not to wear soft contact lenses because they may become permanently stained. Instruct patients to take rifampin on an empty stomach and to avoid driving or operating heavy machinery if drowsiness or dizziness occurs. Instruct patients to notify their physicians if manifestations of hepatotoxicity—including fever, loss of appetite, liver tenderness, malaise, or jaundice—occur.

Pyrazinamide

Pyrazinamide is an antituberculosis drug used for initial treatment in combination with INH and rifampin. It is generally administered with INH, which it potentiates. However, it is quite toxic and should be held in reserve until other therapies fail.

How does it work?

Pyrazinamide is bacteriostatic against *M. tuberculosis*. When used alone, resistance may develop in 6–7 weeks. Therefore, administration with other effective agents is recommended.

How is it used?

Pyrazinamide is used for short-term therapy of advanced TB before surgery and to treat patients unresponsive to such primary agents as INH and streptomycin.

What are the adverse effects?

Hepatotoxicity is the principal adverse effect reported with pyrazinamide use. Other adverse effects include nausea and vomiting, diarrhea, skin rashes, and myalgia.

What are the contraindications and interactions?

Pyrazinamide should be avoided in patients with a history of hypersensitivity to the drug. It is contraindicated in patients who have severe liver damage and patients who are pregnant or lactating. Pyrazinamide must be used cautiously in patients with gout or diabetes mellitus, a history of peptic ulcer, and impaired kidney function. This drug decreases the effects of allopurinol, colchicine, and probenecid. It increases liver toxicity when used with rifampin.

What are the important points patients should know?

Instruct patients to notify their physician if manifestations of hepatotoxicity—including fever, liver tenderness, loss of appetite, malaise, or jaundice—occur.

✳ Apply Your Knowledge 16.6

The following questions focus on what you have just learned about the antituberculosis agents.

CRITICAL THINKING

1. Explain the characteristics of *Mycobacterium tuberculosis*.
2. Identify the first-line antituberculotics.
3. Discuss the most effective agent in the therapy of tuberculosis.
4. Detail the adverse effects of rifampin.
5. Explain how pyrazinamide is used in the treatment of tuberculosis.

Factors of Antibacterial Effectiveness

Resistance to antibacterial drugs is a major problem in health care today. Bacteria routinely respond to various agents by evolving new strains that are resistant to them. The spread of resistance genes is another factor concerning antibacterial effectiveness. These genes can be transferred into other bacteria by bacteriophages and various components of DNA. The selection of resistant forms can happen during or after treatment with antibacterial agents. Since many of these agents remain present long after treatment ends, alteration of bacteria is highly likely. This means that both resistant and susceptible bacteria can be altered, as well as which of these can survive when an agent is used or used more than one time. An important factor of antibacterial effectiveness is the reintroduction of normal flora to help reverse antibiotic resistance. The emergence of multidrug resistance is another factor, and is related to the amounts of antibacterials being used, as well as how they are actually used. In addition, the development of opportunistic bacteria that are resistant to a variety of drugs is complicating the situation. Opportunistic pathogens include enterococci, coagulase-negative staphylococci, *Pseudomonas aeruginosa*, and *Acinetobacter baumanii*.

PRACTICAL SCENARIO 1

A physician orders penicillin for a 15-year-old patient without closely checking the patient's chart. While the medical assistant prepares to explain to the patient and her mother how she should take the medication, he notices that the chart indicates that the patient has an allergy to penicillin.

Brian Warling/PH College

Critical Thinking Questions

1. What is the first thing the medical assistant should do?
2. How might the medical assistant ensure that the physician sees information about drug allergies in a patient's chart?
3. When taking a patient history, what important question should always be asked each time the patient is seen in the office or clinic?

PRACTICAL SCENARIO 2

Kasey, a 34-year-old woman who tested positive for Lyme disease, went to a family practice office. The physician ordered tetracycline, which is the drug of choice for Lyme disease. After 2 weeks of taking antibiotics, at a routine gynecologic examination, the nurse practitioner asked Kasey if she knew she was pregnant. Kasey was surprised, and as they discussed her health, the nurse practitioner asked if she was on any medication. Kasey told her about the Lyme disease and the prescription for tetracycline.

Lana K/Shutterstock

Critical Thinking Questions

1. What are the contraindications of tetracycline related to pregnant women?
2. Does Lyme disease cause any harm to a developing fetus?

Chapter Capsule

This section repeats the objectives from the beginning of the chapter and then provides a summary of the most important concepts for that objective. Use this section as a quick review and to check your knowledge.

Objective 1: Identify the major types of antibiotics by drug class.

- Sulfa drugs, penicillins, cephalosporins, aminoglycosides, tetracyclines, macrolides, synthetic antibacterial agents (such as nitrofurantoin and the quinolones)

Objective 2: Describe the mechanism of action of the sulfonamides.

- The mechanism of the antimicrobial action of the sulfonamides has been analyzed extensively. These agents block a specific step in the biosynthetic pathway of folic acid. They are primarily bacteriostatic, meaning that they slow the multiplication of bacteria. Bacteria cannot absorb folic acid; therefore, it is made from precursors, specifically para-aminobenzoic acid (PABA). The sulfonamides interfere with PABA and folic acid formation, thereby destroying the bacteria. The efficacy of sulfonamides is generally enhanced when the drugs are used in combination with trimethoprim, which inhibits the conversion of dihydrofolate to folinic acid.

Objective 3: Outline the five classes of penicillins.

- Natural penicillins: effective against Gram-positive and Gram-negative bacteria, most anaerobes, and certain spirochetes.
- Semisynthetic, penicillinase-resistant penicillins: effective against Gram-positive bacteria.
- Amino penicillins: effective against a variety of Gram-positive and Gram-negative cocci, as well as some Gram-negative rods, but have a limited spectrum due to sensitivity to most beta-lactamases.
- Extended-spectrum or carboxy penicillins: more effective in high doses
- Ureido penicillins: act similarly to the extended-spectrum penicillins.

Objective 4: Describe the principal mechanisms of action of cephalosporins, vancomycin, and isoniazid.

- Cephalosporins: bactericidal, affecting the bacterial cell wall
- Vancomycin: bactericidal, suppressing cell-wall synthesis
- Isoniazid: interfering with biosynthesis of bacterial proteins, nucleic acid, and lipids

Objective 5: Explain the classifications of cephalosporins.

- First generation: highest activity against Gram-positive bacteria and lowest activity against Gram-negative bacteria
- Second generation: more active against Gram-negative bacteria and less active against Gram-positive bacteria than the first-generation cephalosporins
- Third generation: considerably less active than first-generation agents against Gram-positive bacteria; much expanded spectrum of activity against Gram-negative organisms
- Fourth generation: improved Gram-positive spectrum of activity; expanded Gram-negative activity of third-generation cephalosporins

Objective 6: Outline the main adverse effects of macrolides, aminoglycosides, and chloramphenicol.

- Macrolides: abdominal pain and nausea and vomiting
- Aminoglycosides: ototoxicity and nephrotoxicity
- Chloramphenicol: bone marrow injury, blood cell formation disturbances, and gray-baby syndrome

Objective 7: Contrast bactericidal and bacteriostatic actions.

- Bactericidal: kills bacteria
- Bacteriostatic: inhibits growth of bacteria

Objective 8: Discuss the contraindications, precautions, and interactions of the penicillins and tetracyclines.

- Penicillins—contraindications: hypersensitivity, renal disease, pregnancy, lactation; precautions: give 1 hour before or 2 hours after meals; interactions: estrogen-containing birth control pills, tetracyclines

■ Tetracyclines—contraindications: hypersensitivity, liver diseases, children younger than 8 years, pregnancy, lactation; precautions: take tetracyclines on an empty stomach; interactions: dairy products, laxatives, antacids containing aluminum and calcium, iron preparations, phenytoin, barbiturates

Objective 9: Describe the indications of vancomycin.

■ Vancomycin is usually reserved for serious infections such as *S. aureus* and *S. epidermidis*. It is especially effective against infections caused by methicillin-resistant staphylococci. It is useful in patients who are allergic to penicillin or cephalosporins. Typical uses include osteomyelitis, endocarditis, and staphylococcal pneumonia. When given orally, vancomycin is useful in the treatment of pseudomembranous colitis. However, because it is poorly absorbed from the GI tract, vancomycin is usually given by slow intravenous infusion. It is the drug of choice for severe *Clostridium difficile* infection, but not for mild cases.

Objective 10: List the first-line antituberculosis agents and two characteristic adverse effects of each drug.

■ Isoniazid: restlessness, insomnia
■ Ethambutol: optic neuritis, blurred vision
■ Rifampin: fatigue, drowsiness
■ Pyrazinamide: hepatotoxicity, nausea

 Internet Sites of Interest

■ A wealth of information on treatments for infectious diseases is available at the website of the National Foundation for Infectious Diseases: **www.nfid.org/ publications**

■ The appropriate use of antibiotics is a topic of great concern for the public and health care providers. For consumer and professional information: **http://emerald.tufts.edu/med/apua**

■ A list of the various classes of antibiotics: **http://antibioticsfor.com/antibiotic-classes.phtml**

■ For treating infections, a comparison of bactericidal versus bacteriostatic drugs: **www.news-medical.net/news/2004/10/21/5741.aspx**

■ Common bacterial infections: **www.livestrong.com/article/128682-common-bacterial-infections/**

Chapter 17

Antiviral Agents

Chapter Objectives

After completing the chapter, you should be able to:

1. Describe the structures of viruses.

2. Explain CD4 cells.

3. Describe the pathophysiology of the human immunodeficiency virus.

4. Explain how HIV is transmitted.

5. List three antiviral drugs for HIV- and AIDS-related secondary viral infections and explain their mechanisms of action.

6. List the trade names of nucleoside reverse transcriptase inhibitors.

7. Identify common adverse effects for lamivudine and stavudine.

8. Describe the indications of zidovudine and darunavir.

9. Identify the actions, indications, and contraindications of ganciclovir.

10. Compare and contrast influenza A and influenza B.

Key Terms

capsid (p. 261)
CD4 T-lymphocytes (p. 261)
cirrhosis (p. 287)
erythema multiforme (p. 272)
fulminant hepatitis (p. 286)
gingivostomatitis (p. 284)
helper T-lymphocytes (p. 261)

herpes keratitis (p. 284)
herpes labialis (p. 284)
immunocompromised (p. 284)
lipoatrophy (p. 269)
macrophages (p. 261)
microglial cells (p. 261)
nucleoside (p. 264)

physiochemical (p. 259)
polyneuropathy (p. 269)
reverse transcriptase (p. 260)
symptomatology (p. 259)
toxic epidermal necrolysis (p. 272)
virions (p. 259)

Introduction

There are many different viral infections, caused by a variety of viruses, but far less antiviral agents available to combat them. This chapter focuses on antiviral agents used against HIV/AIDS and related opportunistic infections, as well as herpes simplex, varicella-zoster, cytomegalovirus, hepatitis, influenza, and respiratory syncytial virus. With the human immunodeficiency virus or HIV, CD4 T-lymphocytes are killed, which means that affected patients are more likely to develop opportunistic infections and certain types of cancer. The development of effective antiviral drugs has generally been much less successful than the development of effective antibacterial drugs. This is partially because of the fact that viruses are intracellular microorganisms that reproduce by using the biochemical processes of host cells. It is very difficult to stop viral replication without causing great harm to host cells. Antiviral drugs work by suppressing the cell processes that are unique to viral reproduction. However, increased knowledge of these processes is helping to develop more effective antiviral drugs.

Virus Characteristics

A minute microorganism that is much smaller than a bacterium is called a *virus*. This type of agent has no independent metabolic activity, and may replicate only within a cell of a living plant or animal host. Viruses are able to live only inside cells and are the smallest of all microorganisms. They are unable to derive nourishment or reproduce outside of cells. They are not considered to be "cellular" and are much simpler in structure than bacteria. Viruses contain cores of nucleic acid (deoxyribonucleic acid or ribonucleic acid) that are abbreviated DNA and RNA. These cores are surrounded by protein coatings. Certain viruses are able to create an additional coating called an *envelope*, which protects the virus from attack by the immune system. A virus damages the cell containing it by blocking normal protein synthesis, as well as by utilizing the cell's metabolic mechanisms to reproduce. Viruses are classified in several ways, which include:

✳ **Physiochemical** characteristics of **virions**
✳ Mode of transmission
✳ Range of the host cells
✳ **Symptomatology**

A particular viral infection is able to cause different symptoms between various people. While some viruses are latent for many years, causing no symptoms for a long time, others immediately trigger disease responses.

Focus On

Viral Detection

As of 2015, there is a new blood test that can identify approximately 1,000 viruses that have reached a person's bloodstream in their lifetime. It is called VirScan, and it uses just one drop of blood. The test is able to identify how acquired viruses can affect immune system responses and possibly add to future occurrence of cancer and chronic diseases. It may also aid in research regarding the patterns of disease development. VirScan searches for imprint "memories" of viruses that have been previously contracted. It may be available in the near future.

Antiviral Agents

Viruses cause much of the morbidity and mortality in populations worldwide, but the number of drugs available to treat such viruses is still quite low. Antiviral drug development has become very active in the past decade, especially with the challenges of the AIDS epidemic.

Relatively few antiviral drugs have been successfully used in the United States. However, several viral diseases, including measles, mumps, rubella, polio, chickenpox, smallpox, and rabies, are prevented by vaccines. The antiviral agents reviewed here are acyclovir (Zovirax), amantadine (Symmetrel), didanosine (Videx), ribavirin (Virazole), zanamivir (Relenza), ganciclovir (Cytovene), and zidovudine (Retrovir). Table 17-1 ■ lists examples of antiviral agents successfully used in the United States.

HIV Infections

Human immunodeficiency virus (HIV), which results in *acquired immunodeficiency syndrome* (AIDS), is caused mainly by two viruses, HIV-1 and HIV-2. HIV-1 is found worldwide; HIV-2 infections are most common in parts of Africa and India. The antiviral drugs used to suppress HIV are effective mostly against the HIV-1 strain. The

Table 17-1 ■ Examples of Effective Antiviral Agents

GENERIC NAME	TRADE NAME	AVERAGE ADULT DOSAGE	ROUTE OF ADMINISTRATION
acyclovir	Zovirax	IV: 5–15 mg/kg q8h for 7–21 days; PO: 20–400 mg (800 mg max) 4–5 times/d for 5–14 days; Topical: 5% cream 5 times/d for 4 days	IV, PO, topical
amantadine	Symmetrel	Two 100 mg tablets/d or 4 teaspoons of syrup/d; may be split into 1 tablet bid or 2 teaspoons of syrup bid	PO (tablets and syrup)
didanosine	Videx, Videx EC	EC Capsules: 400 mg once/d (or 250 mg once/d with tenofovir); Oral solution: 200 mg bid	PO (enteric-coated capsules or oral solution) (take 30 minutes before meals or 2 hours after)
ganciclovir	Cytovene, Vitrasert, Zirgan	IV infusion: 5 mg/kg over 1 hour q12h for 14–21 days; Oral: 1000 mg tid with food; Ocular implant: inserted surgically and replaced q5–8m; Ocular 0.15% gel: 1 drop in affected eye 5 times/d prn, followed by 1 drop tid for 7 days	IV, PO, ocular implant, ocular gel
ribavirin	Virazole	20 mg/mL as starting solution in SPAG-2 unit with continuous aerosol administration for 12–18 hours/d for 3–7 days (this concentration = 190 micrograms/liter of air)	Inhalation (powder for solution)
zanamivir	Relenza	10 mg, provided in 2 inhalations using Diskhaler	Inhalation (powder for PO inhalation)
zidovudine	Retrovir	200 mg tid or 300 mg bid	PO

IV, intravenous; PO, oral; bid, twice a day; tid, three times a day.

virus infects a group of helper T lymphocytes, which are called *CD4 cells*. This results in the individual with AIDS becoming more susceptible to other infections, such as bacteria, fungi, protozoans, and other viruses. Most AIDS patients die from these secondary infections. It is important to remember that not all individuals infected with HIV develop AIDS, but they continue to be carriers of the virus. AIDS develops years after the HIV infection is acquired. It is defined as when an HIV-positive individual has one of the following:

✳ An AIDS-defining illness such as cytomegalovirus retinitis, disseminated histoplasmosis, Kaposi's sarcoma, *Pneumocystis* pneumonia, or tuberculosis

✳ CD4 T-lymphocyte count below 200 cells/mL

AIDS was first identified in 1981, and it became a worldwide epidemic that has killed more than 22 million people; more than 58 million people worldwide have contracted the HIV virus since 1981. In the

United States alone, more than 1.2 million people are living with HIV infection, with nearly one in seven being unaware of their HIV status. While the annual number of new HIV infections has remained relatively the same, the number of people living with HIV has increased. There are about 50,000 new HIV infections per year. Homosexual or bisexual men have the highest rates of HIV infection, with most of these being young black males. In the United States, more than 658,000 people have died from AIDS since it was first identified.

HIV PATHOPHYSIOLOGY

Retroviruses such as HIV have genetic material that consists of positive-sense, single-stranded RNA. They must transcribe their RNA into DNA in order to replicate. This requires the enzyme RNA-dependent DNA polymerase, which is also called **reverse transcriptase**. In fact, the term *retrovirus* is derived from "reverse transcriptase."

Because of differences between HIV-1 and HIV-2, not all drugs are effective against both. HIV mostly attacks **CD4 T-lymphocytes**, which are also called **helper T-lymphocytes**. The immune system becomes progressively weaker and opportunistic infections become more prevalent. HIV is able to attach to CD4 proteins on the surface of the helper T-lymphocytes. The cells then die within approximately 30 hours. Only a small percentage of this type of cells circulate in the blood, and most are found in the lymphoid tissues, including the lymph nodes. HIV also infects **macrophages** and **microglial cells**, which carry CD4 proteins. These cells are resistant to HIV and are not killed, but instead act as HIV reservoirs.

The structure of HIV is simplistic (see Figure 17-1 ■). The HIV virion is made up of RNA (nucleic acid), surrounded by core proteins, which are then surrounded by a protein shell (**capsid**). The capsid is then surrounded by a lipid bilayer envelope created from the host cell's membrane. Two identical yet separate strands of RNA make up the central core. Each has its own reverse transcriptase molecule attached. The RNA helps DNA to be synthesized. The outer HIV envelope contains glycoproteins that are used to attach to host cells. A small subunit called gp41 of each glycoprotein embeds in the viral envelope's lipid bilayer, while remaining attached to a larger subunit called gp120.

The replication cycle of HIV is shown in Figure 17-2 ■. The steps involved in this cycle, as it progresses toward becoming AIDS, are:

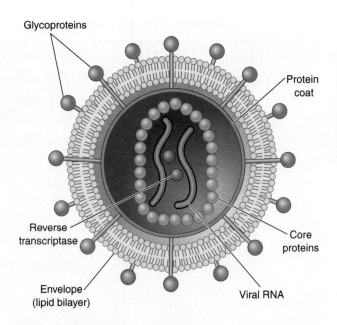

Figure 17-1 ■ Simple structure of HIV.

Source: Adams, Michael Patrick; Holland, Leland; Urban, Carol, *Pharmacology for Nurses: A Pathophysiologic Approach, 4th Ed.,* ©2014. Reprinted and Electronically reproduced by permission of Pearson Education, Inc., New York, NY

1. The HIV virus attaches to CD4 receptors on T4-helper lymphocytes. Structural proteins on the HIV viral cell surfaces fuse with CD4 receptors.

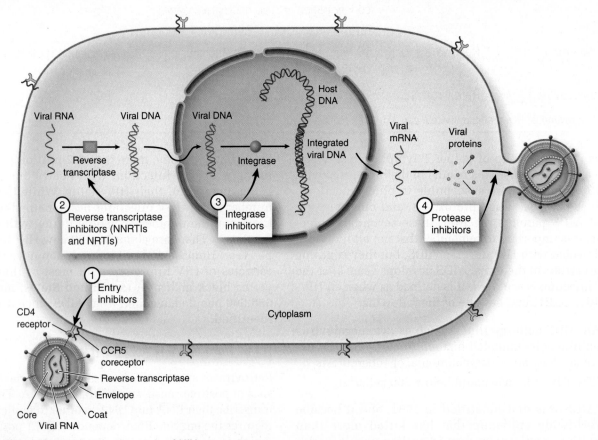

Figure 17-2 ■ Replication cycle of HIV.

Source: Adams, Michael Patrick; Holland, Leland; Urban, Carol, *Pharmacology for Nurses: A Pathophysiologic Approach, 4th Ed.,* ©2014. Reprinted and Electronically reproduced by permission of Pearson Education, Inc., New York, NY

2. The HIV virus becomes uncoated, and its genetic material (single-stranded RNA) enters host cells.

3. The RNA strands are converted to double-stranded DNA via the actions of reverse transcriptase, a viral enzyme. This DNA eventually enters T4 lymphocyte nuclei and is incorporated into the chromosomes of the host. This occurs via HIV integrase, an enzyme that is unique to HIV.

4. Over years, the viral DNA becomes activated and produces more viral particles that eventually "bud" from host cells and enter the bloodstream. These virions are not yet infectious.

5. Protease, another viral enzyme, cleaves certain proteins associated with the HIV DNA. This enables the virion to infect other T4 lymphocytes.

6. Budding of viral particles triggers the immune system to recognize infected cells, and T4 lymphocytes are killed as a result. However, by this time, the patient may be producing up to 10 billion new virions per day. The immune system is overcome and cannot remove all of them.

7. HIV progresses to AIDS as the immune system is gradually destroyed. This is signified by declining numbers of CD4 T-lymphocytes. Once this count has reduced below a certain amount, the patient develops opportunistic bacterial, fungal, and viral infections, as well as various malignancies.

8. Once the immune system no longer has any ability to defend itself, the patient will die.

Focus Point

Mechanism of Action of HIV Medications

It is important to understand how specific drugs used against HIV actually work, in relation to the steps listed above. The drug called maraviroc affects Step 1, blocking HIV entry by binding to the CCR4 co-receptor. The drug called enfuvirtide blocks the fusion process of Step 2. Twelve different antiretroviral drugs inhibit the reverse transcriptase enzyme's effects in Step 3. The drug called raltegravir inhibits the integrase enzyme and its effects in Step 5. Several drugs target HIV protease and its effects in Step 10.

During all stages of HIV infection, the virus replicates very quickly, but particularly during the initial stage. This is because the amount of CD4 cells is still very large, and the host has not developed an immune response against the virus. Therefore, plasma levels of HIV can initially exceed 10 million virions per mL. Patients often experience acute retroviral syndrome as a result. In the next few months, HIV plasma levels decline sharply but eventually level off to between 1,000 and 100,000 virions per mL. This is not what it seems, since the HIV plasma half-life is 6 hours, meaning that one-half of HIV virions in plasma are lost every 6 hours. Therefore, to remain a relatively steady level when infection is chronic, replication occurs at between 1 and 10 billion virions per day. Even so, the patient is usually asymptomatic for approximately 10 years. After this period, advanced signs and symptoms appear.

HIV mutates very quickly due to errors in reverse transcriptase. Up to 10 incorrect base pairs may be incorporated into HIV DNA with each replication. Therefore, HIV can easily develop a drug-resistant form even though it was previously in a drug-sensitive form. The chance of HIV becoming resistant to drugs is related to the total viral load. There is more chance of at least one virion becoming resistant with increased amounts of total virions. Therefore, patients are treated with combination antiretroviral agents.

Focus Point

Acute Retroviral Syndrome

Acute retroviral syndrome is signified by a variety of signs and symptoms, which include fever, lymphadenopathy, pharyngitis rash and mucocutaneous ulceration (face, trunk, extremities including palms and soles, mouth, esophagus, genitals), arthralgia or myalgia, diarrhea, headache, nausea and vomiting, hepatosplenomegaly, weight loss, thrush, and neurologic symptoms (brachial neuritis, cognitive impairment or psychosis, facial palsy, Guillain-Barré neuritis, meningoencephalitis or aseptic meningitis, and peripheral neuropathy or radiculopathy).

HIV TRANSMISSION AND PREVENTION

The HIV virus may be present in all body fluids of infected patients. It can be transmitted through intimate contact with blood, semen, or vaginal secretions. Methods of transmission also include sharing intravenous needles, blood transfusions, accidental needlesticks, and transmission from an infected mother to her fetus. When HIV was first recognized, it mostly affected homosexual males, people who injected drugs, and hemophiliacs, but it is now found in nearly every segment of the population. Methods to reduce sexual transmission of HIV include using condoms, limiting sexual partners, male circumcision, and total sexual abstinence. The prevention of HIV being transmitted can also be accomplished with certain drugs.

Antiretroviral drugs can greatly reduce risks of HIV transmission through sexual, mother-to-infant, and accidental exposure. Immediate treatment of HIV-positive individuals significantly reduces the risk of it being transmitted to their sexual partners. In one test, these drugs stopped all transmission of HIV between sexual partners, except for 1 out of 886 test couples. When use of antiretroviral drugs was delayed in another test group, 27 out of 877 couples transmitted HIV between partners.

Pre-exposure prophylaxis means using antiretroviral drugs to prevent HIV infection instead of treating it. Recent studies have shown that certain orally administered agents can protect high-risk homosexual men from acquiring HIV. Another study concerned use of topical pre-exposure prophylaxis, applied vaginally. This offered less effectiveness, though was more effective when applied immediately before and after intercourse.

Though a single exposure to HIV carries only a small risk of infection, it is still quite possible to result in another person becoming HIV-positive. Unprotected vaginal or anal intercourse, receptive oral intercourse, sharing contaminated needles, accidental needlesticks, and contact with blood or other body fluids all carry the potential to transfer HIV, even through a single exposure. The risk is higher with exposure to a large amount of infected blood or blood that contains a high virus titer, as well as after deep percutaneous needle penetration when that needle was recently removed from an infected person's vein.

However, prophylactic antiretroviral drugs can reduce the risk of developing HIV after a single exposure. It should be administered as quickly as possible, within 1–2 hours, and no longer than 72 hours after exposure. These drugs must be continued for 28 days. Each patient must be tested for antibodies against HIV at the time of exposure, if possible, and then again 6 weeks, 12 weeks, and 6 months after. For nonoccupational postexposure prophylaxis, the following drug regimens are used:

* Non-nucleoside reverse transcriptase inhibitor (NNRTI)–based treatment: efavirenz plus lamivudine or emtricitabine, plus zidovudine or tenofovir
* Protease inhibitor (PI)–based treatment: lopinavir/ritonavir plus lamivudine or emtricitabine, plus zidovudine

For occupational postexposure prophylaxis, a determination is made based on the nature of the exposure, its severity, and the HIV status of the exposure source. As a result, any of the following may be initiated:

* No postexposure prophylaxis needed
* Two NRTIs, such as emtricitabine plus tenofovir
* PI-based treatment such as lopinavir/ritonavir plus emtricitabine plus tenofovir

For preventing perinatal HIV transmission, which accounts for nearly all new HIV infections in American children, antiretroviral drugs are given to the mother during gestation and labor. They are also given to the infant for 6 weeks after birth. Cesarean section delivery is recommended if the mother has a viral load above 1,000 copies per mL. The drug of choice is zidovudine, regardless of whether antiretroviral therapy was used during gestation. It is administered intravenously to the mother during labor and delivery, then by IV or orally to the infant. The rate of HIV transmission is nearly zero when this regimen is used. Neonatal dosage is based on gestational age.

HIV Infection Development Process

There are three phases in which HIV develops (see Table 17-2 ■). These include the massive replication phase that triggers acute retroviral syndrome, the clinical latency phase, and the final phase in which AIDS occurs. After the initial phase, the immune system combats the condition to cause HIV levels to fall and the acute retroviral syndrome symptoms to reduce. In many cases, the acute retroviral syndrome is mistaken for influenza. During the clinical latency phase, HIV levels are lower and patients are usually asymptomatic. Even so, HIV does continue to replicate as CD4 T-lymphocytes progressively decline. This period averages about 10 years in duration. In the final phase, the CD4 T-lymphocytes drop below 200 cells per mL and the patient becomes susceptible to opportunistic infections and certain types of cancer. Peripheral and central nervous complications often develop. The neurological symptoms may be directly caused by HIV or may develop because of an opportunistic infection.

Table 17-2 ■ The Three Phases of HIV

PHASE	CHARACTERISTICS
Initial	Massive replication of HIV
	Extremely high blood levels of HIV
	Between 50 and 90% of patients develop flu-like acute retroviral syndrome
	After this, immune system combats HIV; levels fall and symptoms subside
Middle	Prolonged clinical latency with low blood levels of HIV
	Most patients are asymptomatic
	HIV does continue to replicate as CD4 T-lymphocytes decline
	This period averages 10 years
Late	CD4 T-lymphocytes drop below 200 cells per mL
	Opportunistic infections and certain cancers (such as Kaposi's sarcoma) occur
	AIDS occurs
	Neurologic complications may occur (20–40% of patients develop peripheral neuropathies, which can actually develop in any phase of HIV); central nervous system complications usually occur in the late phase, including decreased cognition, memory loss, reduced concentration, mental slowness, and motor abnormalities such as ataxia or tremors
	Neuronal injury may be caused by HIV or by an opportunistic infection in the CNS

Antiretroviral Drugs

Antivirals known as *antiretroviral drugs* are used alone or in combinations for the treatment of HIV infection. Highly active antiretroviral therapy (HAART) has been shown to reduce viral load, increase CD4 lymphocyte counts in individuals infected with HIV, delay the onset of AIDS, and prolong survival of patients with AIDS. Both the incidence of and mortality from AIDS have declined substantially since 1996 because of HAART. The benefits of HAART, which involves the combination of three to four drugs effective against HIV, have been widely publicized. Two distinct categories of drugs are combined: **nucleoside** analogues (derived from nucleic acid) and protease inhibitors.

The use of HAART presents formidable challenges, including harsh side effects and the potential for rapid development of drug resistance. Protease inhibitors do not work as well with a third category of HIV drugs, the non-nucleoside analogues. Therefore, the non-nucleoside analogues should not be taken alone. Presently, because of the limited number of HAART medications available in the United States, only a few drug combinations are possible. HAART regimens can also fail because of lack of *viral load response* (the body's reaction to antiviral agents) or the patient's poor adherence to treatment. Missing a

single dose of HAART even twice a week can cause the development of drug-resistant HIV. This is a real danger because adherence to the drug regimen is difficult. The simplification of HIV antiretroviral therapy regimens has been shown to improve adherence. One combination antiviral agent approved for the treatment of HIV infection and AIDS is 2'-3'-dideoxycytidine (ddC; also called zalcitabine), which is to be used only with the popular drug zidovudine (Retrovir).

NUCLEOSIDE REVERSE TRANSCRIPTASE INHIBITORS

There are six classifications of antiretroviral drugs: nucleoside reverse transcriptase inhibitors, nonnucleoside reverse transcriptase inhibitors, protease inhibitors, integrase strand transfer inhibitors, fusion inhibitors, and chemokine receptor 5 antagonists. Nucleoside reverse transcriptase inhibitors (NRTIs) inhibit synthesis of viral DNA by reverse transcriptase. These are structural analogs of nucleosides or nucleotides, the basics of DNA. They are administered orally, except for zidovudine, which may also be administered intravenously. These were the first drugs used against HIV and are the mainstays of therapy. They remain the core drugs in all treatment regimens, and must undergo intracellular conversion to their active triphosphate forms. There are few drug interactions. Most NRTIs can be taken with or without meals. In rare cases, NRTIs may cause a potentially fatal syndrome (lactic acidosis, hepatomegaly with steatosis). Pregnant women who take two NRTIs may be at increased risk for this syndrome. The seven currently available NRTIs (see Table 17-3 ■) are abacavir, didanosine, emtricitabine, lamivudine, stavudine, tenofovir disoproxil fumarate, and zidovudine. NRTIs are also available as components of fixed-dose combinations.

Table 17-3 ■ Nucleoside Reverse Transcriptase Inhibitors

GENERIC NAME	TRADE NAME	AVERAGE ADULT DOSAGE	ROUTE OF ADMINISTRATION
abacavir (ABC)	Ziagen	Tablet: 300 mg bid Oral solution (20 mg/mL): 600 mg once/d	PO
didanosine (ddI)	Videx, Videx EC	Videx (oral solution): 200–400 mg, based on body weight and if taken with TDF, 1/2 hour before or 2 hours after a meal, split into 2 doses per day Videx EC (capsules): 200–400 mg, with same restrictions, but taken once/d	PO
emtricitabine (FTC)	Emtriva	Capsule: 200 mg once/d Oral solution: 240 mg (24 mL) once/d	PO
lamivudine (3TC)	Epivir, Epivir HBV	Tablet: 150 mg bid or 300 mg once/d Oral solution (10 mg/mL): same dosage	PO
stavudine (d4T)	Zerit	Capsule: 30–40 mg bid Oral solution (1 mg/mL): same dosage	PO
tenofovir disoproxil fumarate (TDF)	Viread	Tablet: 300 mg once/d Oral powder (40 mg/g): 7.5 level scoops once/d mixed into 2–4 ounces of a soft food such as applesauce or yogurt	PO
zidovudine (AZT or ZDV)	Retrovir	Capsule, tablet (generic version only), or oral solution (10 mg/mL): 300 mg bid or 200 mg tid IV (10 mg/mL): same dosage	PO IV
Combination Formulations			
abacavir-lamivudine	Epzicom	1 tablet (600 mg abacavir/300 mg lamivudine) once/d	PO
emtricitabine-tenofovir	Truvada	1 tablet (200 mg emtricitabine/300 mg tenofovir) once/d	PO
zidovudine-lamivudine (CBV)	Combivir	1 tablet (300 mg zidovudine/150 mg lamivudine) bid	PO
zidovudine-lamivudine-abacavir (TRZ)	Trizivir	1 tablet (300 mg zidovudine/150 mg lamivudine/300 mg abacavir) bid	PO

bid, twice a day; PO, oral; tid, three times a day; IV, intravenous.

Focus On

Abacavir

Abacavir (Ziagen) is also referred to as ABC. It is an analog of the naturally occurring pyrimidine known as guanine. Abacavir is approved only for HIV-1 infection and should always be combined with other antiretroviral drugs. It offers 83% bioavailability and penetrates the cerebrospinal fluid well. Abacavir has a plasma half-life of 1.5 hours and an intracellular half-life of 12–36 hours.

How does it work?

After being taken up by host cells, abacavir is converted to its active form, which is called carbovir triphosphate. This is an analog of deoxyguanosine triphosphate. Viral replication is suppressed when carbovir triphosphate causes early termination of growing DNA strands and also by competing with natural nucleoside triphosphates for binding to reverse transcriptase. Abacavir is converted to inactive metabolites by alcohol dehydrogenase.

How is it used?

Abacavir is administered orally and absorption is unaffected by food. Its metabolites are excreted in the urine.

What are the adverse effects?

The adverse effects of abacavir include headache, nausea and vomiting, diarrhea, hypersensitivity reactions, and extremely rarely, myocardial infarction. Abacavir may also (rarely) cause potentially fatal lactic acidosis with hepatic steatosis. In pregnant women, it should not be combined with other NRTIs. Hypersensitivity reactions usually occur during the first 6 weeks of use, with the potential to be severe or even fatal. Symptoms include fever, myalgia, rashes, arthralgia, and GI disturbances. When severe, hypersensitivity may lead to liver or renal failure, anaphylaxis, and death. The drug should be withdrawn and never administered again. Often, hypersensitivity begins as respiratory symptoms and must be assessed quickly due to rapid progression.

What are the contraindications and interactions?

Abacavir is contraindicated in previously demonstrated hypersensitivity and in moderate or severe hepatic impairment. It may compete with alcohol for metabolism by alcohol dehydrogenase, causing abacavir levels to increase by approximately 40%. Alcohol consumption should therefore be minimized. No other significant drug interactions have been reported.

What are the important points patients should know?

The patient should be instructed to stop using abacavir and contact his or her physician if there are any signs of hypersensitivity. There is a warning card that accompanies the medication, and patients must carry it at all times in order to be aware of the various hypersensitivity reactions. Also, if there are any signs of lactic acidosis, the patient must be aware that he or she needs to get emergency help immediately. Patients must also be instructed about symptoms of liver damage from this drug. They should also be told not to allow the medication to run out completely before getting a refill, and that dosage instructions must be followed exactly.

Didanosine

Didanosine (Videx, Videx EC) is an antiretroviral and nucleoside reverse transcriptase inhibitor. It is also known as dideoxyinosine or ddI. This drug is an analog of inosine, which is a natural nucleoside. It is approved only for HIV-1 infection and must be used along with other antiretroviral drugs due to resistance against it if used alone. This drug is administered orally, but its absorption is greatly reduced by food as well as gastric acidity. It does not cross the blood–brain barrier well and between 35 and 60% is excreted in the urine without being changed. Its plasma half-life is 1.5 hours in patients with normal renal function but up to three times longer in those with renal failure; its intracellular half-life is more than 20 hours.

How does it work?

Didanosine can inhibit the replication of the HIV virus that has become resistant to zidovudine. Its mechanism of action is similar to that of zidovudine, being taken up by host cells and converted to its active form, which is called dideoxyadenosine triphosphate or ddATP. It then suppresses viral replication mostly via terminating growing

(continued)

Focus On (*continued*)

DNA strands. It also competes with natural nucleoside triphosphates for binding to reverse transcriptase, which suppresses DNA synthesis even more. It has been clinically shown to increase CD4 T-lymphocytes, decrease viremia, and reduce symptoms in patients who have developed AIDS.

How is it used?

Didanosine is used in advanced HIV infection in patients who are intolerant to zidovudine or who demonstrate significant clinical or immunologic deterioration during zidovudine therapy.

What are the adverse effects?

The major adverse effects of didanosine are peripheral neuropathies and pancreatitis, which may be fatal. These effects are more likely in high doses of the drug. This drug is minimally toxic to bone marrow. Common adverse effects include headache, dizziness, insomnia, seizures, abdominal pain, nausea and vomiting, diarrhea, constipation, and dry mouth. Didanosine may also cause lactic acidosis with hepatic steatosis that can be fatal. In pregnancy, this has occurred when combined with stavudine and other NRTIs.

What are the contraindications and interactions?

Contraindications for didanosine include hypersensitivity to the drug and pregnancy or lactation. It must be administered cautiously to individuals with peripheral vascular disease, history of neuropathy, chronic pancreatitis, renal impairment, or liver disease.

Aluminum and magnesium-containing antacids may increase the aluminum- and magnesium-associated adverse effects. The effectiveness of dapsone may be reduced by didanosine. Absorption of didanosine is significantly decreased by food.

What are the important points patients should know?

Instruct patients to maintain an adequate fluid intake to increase urine output, thereby preventing renal problems.

Emtricitabine

Emtricitabine (Emtriva) is derived from lamivudine and is active against HIV-1 and the hepatitis B virus (HBV). It has a long intracellular half-life, so it can be taken once per day. The plasma half-life is 10 hours, and the intracellular half-life is longer than 20 hours.

How does it work?

Emtricitabine is taken up by host cells and then converted to the active form, called emtricitabine triphosphate. This inhibits the synthesis of viral DNA in two ways. The first is by competing with natural substrates regarding binding to reverse transcriptase. The second is by causing early termination of growing DNA strands. Emtricitabine weakly inhibits nuclear and mitochondrial DNA polymerases.

How is it used?

Emtricitabine is quickly and nearly completely absorbed with or without food. After each dose, plasma levels reach their peak within 1 to 2 hours. Protein binding in blood and hepatic metabolism is low. The drug is generally eliminated with little change in the urine.

What are the adverse effects?

This mostly well-tolerated drug may cause headache, diarrhea, nausea, and rashes. Rarely, hyperpigmentation of the palms and soles develops. Predominately in women, emtricitabine carries a risk of lactic acidosis and severe hepatomegaly with steatosis. It should be withdrawn in these cases. This drug can suppress HBV, and patients who also have HBV may have severely worsened hepatitis symptoms when the drug is discontinued.

What are the contraindications and interactions?

Emtricitabine is contraindicated with previously demonstrated hypersensitivity to any of its components. It is unlikely to interact with other drugs since it does not affect cytochrome P450. There are no significant drug interactions.

What are the important points patients should know?

Patients should be made aware of the possibility of this drug causing lactic acidosis and its related symptoms, as well as the possibility of liver damage. The patient must understand that a physician should be contacted immediately in these cases. Patients should understand that this drug will not keep them from passing HIV to other individuals and follow all physician instructions.

Lamivudine

Lamivudine (Epivir) is an analog of the naturally occurring nucleoside called cytidine. It is also known as dideoxy-3'-thiacytidine or 3TC. It is effective against HIV-1 and HBV. Lamivudine has 86% bioavailability. It has a plasma half-life of 5–7 hours, and its intracellular half-life is 18–22 hours.

How does it work?

After being taken up by host cells, lamivudine is converted to the active form called lamivudine triphosphate. This suppresses the replication of HIV in two ways. The first is by causing early termination of growing DNA strands, and the second is by competing with natural nucleoside triphosphates in their binding to reverse transcriptase. It must be combined with at least one other antiretroviral drug in order to decrease possibilities of resistance.

How is it used?

Lamivudine is given orally, and its rate of absorption is reduced by food. It is eliminated intact in the urine. Lamivudine is the best tolerated of all NRTIs.

What are the adverse effects?

Lamivudine has only minimal adverse effects, including insomnia and headache, which usually subside within a few weeks. It does carry a slight risk of potentially fatal lactic acidosis, and it should not be combined with another NRTI in pregnant women. If a patient also has HBV, its withdrawal may cause severe acute worsening of hepatitis symptoms.

What are the contraindications and interactions?

Lamivudine is contraindicated with previously demonstrated, clinically significant hypersensitivity to any of its components. This drug may interact with interferon- and ribavirin-based antiretroviral therapies, with zalcitabine, and with trimethoprim/sulfamethoxazole.

What are the important points patients should know?

Patients with symptoms of hypersensitivity to lamuvidine should be instructed not to use it with any HIV combination medicine containing this same drug or emtricitabine, and not to use it if there is kidney or liver disease, history of pancreatitis, or if a similar medication has been used in the past. The patient must understand to seek emergency help if symptoms of lactic acidosis develop. If liver or pancreatic abnormalities develop during or after use of this medication, the patient must notify his or her physician.

Stavudine

Stavudine (Zerit) is an analog of the natural nucleoside called thymidine. It is also known as didehydrodeoxythymidine or d4T. Stavudine is effective only against HIV-1 and should be combined with other antiretroviral drugs to decreased chances of resistance. Its bioavailability is 86% and penetration to the CNS is good. It is eliminated by both hepatic metabolism and renal excretion. Its plasma half-life is 1 hour, and its intracellular half-life is 7.5 hours.

How does it work?

After being taken up by cells, it is converted to stavudine triphosphate, its active form. This suppresses HIV replication in two ways. The first is by causing early termination of growing DNA strands, and the second is by competing with natural nucleoside triphosphates in binding to reverse transcriptase.

How is it used?

Stavudine is administered orally, with or without food. It is used to treat HIV, but may also be used for other purposes. It is not a cure for HIV or AIDS. This drug must be taken at regular intervals to keep a steady amount of the drug present at all times, and it is usually administered once every 12 hours. Because stavudine doses are based on body weight, each patient must inform his or her physician if there are any changes in weight.

What are the adverse effects?

Stavudine may cause peripheral neuropathy, which may resolve if it is withdrawn. If this occurs, treatment at a lower dose may be attempted. Stavudine may also cause pancreatitis, which has been fatal in 1% of cases. The patient must be monitored for symptoms of pancreatitis

(continued)

Focus On (continued)

and, if present, the drug must be withdrawn. This drug is more likely than other NRTIs to cause lactic acidosis with hepatic steatosis. Pregnant women should not be given this drug with didanosine due to higher incidence of fatal lactic acidosis. It is probably wise to avoid combining stavudine with any other NRTI during pregnancy. This drug has sometimes caused ascending demyelinating **polyneuropathy** that results in neuromuscular weakness beginning in a few months, but increasing quickly. Serious motor weakness then occurs within days to weeks, possibly requiring mechanical ventilation due to respiratory paralysis. If this occurs, all antiretroviral drugs should be stopped. Recovery is slow, over several months, and may never be total. Other adverse effects include hyperlipidemia, insulin resistance/diabetes, and **lipoatrophy**.

What are the contraindications and interactions?

Stavudine is contraindicated in patients with clinically significant hypersensitivity to any of its components. It should not be used with didanosine since both drugs can cause peripheral neuropathy. It should also be avoided with zidovudine. Due to lack of sufficient data, stavudine should be used with caution with doxorubicin and ribavirin.

What are the important points patients should know?

Patients must be told about early symptoms of neuropathy such as numbness, pain, or tingling in the hands or feet. They must inform their physician of these symptoms immediately. Patients must be instructed about symptoms of lactic acidosis and the need to request emergency care if these develop. They should also be told about liver or pancreatic abnormalities and to contact their physician immediately if they develop. Every patient must tell his or her physician about kidney or liver disease, history of pancreatitis, or use of any medicine similar to stavudine.

Tenofovir Disoproxil Fumarate

Tenofovir disoproxil fumarate (Viread) is a nucleotide reverse transcriptase inhibitor, instead of a nucleoside reverse transcriptase inhibitor. It is also known as TDF. A nucleotide is actually a nucleoside that has an added phosphate group, and it has similar effects. Its blood levels peak approximately 1 hour after administration and binding to plasma proteins is low. Tenofovir is eliminated mostly by the kidneys via glomerular filtration and active tubular secretion. It has a prolonged half-life of 17 hours in plasma and 60-plus hours inside cells, so it can be administered one time per day.

How does it work?

Inside host cells, it is converted to tenofovir, then to its active form known as tenofovir diphosphate. This drug inhibits viral DNA by competing with deoxyadenosine triphosphate for binding to reverse transcriptase and after it is incorporated into the growing DNA chain, to prematurely terminate the chain. Partially from inhibiting mitochondrial DNA polymerase, toxicity occurs.

How is it used?

Tenofovir is now approved for both HIV-1 and HBV, though previously it was only approved for HIV-1. It should always be used with other antiretroviral agents to prevent resistance. It is administered orally, with 39% bioavailability when taken with food and 25% when taken without food.

What are the adverse effects?

It is possible for tenofovir to accumulate to dangerous levels with impaired kidney function, but this is relatively rare. Adverse effects are not significant and include nausea and vomiting, diarrhea, asthenia, headache, and flatulence. It can suppress HBV, so if it is withdrawn in a patient who also has HBV, severe exacerbation of hepatitis symptoms may occur. This drug is able to reduce bone mineral density, increasing risk of osteoporotic hip, vertebrae, or wrist fractures. There is also a small risk of possibly fatal lactic acidosis with hepatic steatosis. In pregnant women, it should not be combined with NRTIs.

What are the contraindications and interactions?

There are no significant contraindications to tenofovir disoproxil fumarate. Regarding interactions, combining this drug with another that undergoes active tubular secretion may lead to accumulation of either drug, or both. Tenofovir can raise plasma levels of didanosine. Therefore, patients receiving these two drugs must be monitored for long-term toxicity.

What are the important points patients should know?

Patients should be instructed not to take this drug with adefovir or with combination medicines that also contain tenofovir. This drug should not be used in HIV-positive children under 2 years of age or to treat HBV in anyone younger than 18 years of age. Patients should be instructed to monitor for symptoms of lactic acidosis and request emergency care. They should also be told to contact a physician if severe or life-threatening effects upon the liver develop. For patients with HBV, liver function tests may be required over several months.

Zidovudine

Zidovudine (Retrovir) is often known by its original abbreviation AZT, which stands for azidothymidine (its simplified chemical name). It is also known by its newer abbreviation, ZDV. Zidovudine was the first NRTI available. After it is absorbed, some ZDV is converted to its active form, which is known as ZTP. The remainder is quickly converted to an inactive metabolite by the liver, then eliminated by the kidneys. Its plasma half-life is 1.1 hours, and its intracellular half-life is 7 hours.

How does it work?

Zidovudine is a major nucleoside in DNA. On entering host cells, this drug is converted to a triphosphate by *endogenous* (grown from within) cellular enzymes. It appears to act by being incorporated into growing DNA chains by viral reverse transcriptase, thereby terminating viral replication. When used with other antiretrovirals, it decreases viral load, increases CD4 T-lymphocyte counts, delays onset of symptoms, and reduces severity of symptoms.

How is it used?

Zidovudine is used for patients who have asymptomatic HIV-1 infection and early or late symptomatic HIV disease. It is the drug of choice for prevention of perinatal transfer of HIV during pregnancy. Zidovudine is always combined with other antiretroviral agents because monotherapy with any antiretroviral drug can quickly lead to resistance. It is used for relieving cognitive symptoms because of its ability to better penetrate the CNS.

What are the adverse effects?

Common adverse effects of zidovudine include fever, dyspnea, malaise, weakness, myalgia, and myopathy. In some patients, headache, insomnia, dizziness, anxiety, or bone marrow depression may be seen. The main dose-limiting toxicities are neutropenia and severe anemia. Multiple transfusions may be required. Hematologic status must be continually monitored. In rare cases, lactic acidosis with hepatic steatosis occurs, which also involves severe hepatomegaly. This syndrome can be fatal if not treated. During pregnancy, combining this drug with other NRTIs may increase the risk of lactic acidosis.

What are the contraindications and interactions?

Acetaminophen (Tylenol), ganciclovir (Cytoven), and pegylated interferon α-2A (Roferon-A) may enhance bone marrow suppression. Interaction of aspirin, dapsone (DDS or Aczone), indomethacin (Indocin), methadone (Dolophine), vincristine (Oncovin), and valproic acid (Depakote) may increase the risk of zidovudine toxicity.

Zidovudine is contraindicated in patients who are hypersensitive to the drug; in severe bone marrow depression, hepatomegaly, hepatitis, or other liver disease risk factors; and in those with renal insufficiency. It interacts with a wide variety of drugs, including atovaquone (Mepron), fluconazole (Diflucan), probenecid (Probalan), doxorubicin (Adriamycin), ribavirin (Virazole), stavudine (Zerit), and phenytoin (Dilantin).

What are the important points patients should know?

Advise patients to avoid taking nonsteroidal anti-inflammatory drugs such as aspirin or indomethacin (Indocin) or paracetamol (which is also known as acetaminophen or the trade name Tylenol) while taking zidovudine. These drugs may inhibit the metabolism of zidovudine, therefore increasing the possibility of toxicity.

Non-Nucleoside Reverse Transcriptase Inhibitors

The non-nucleoside reverse transcriptase inhibitors (NNRTIs) inhibit enzymes needed for HIV replication. They are structurally different from naturally occurring nucleosides and work differently. The NNRTIs bind to active reverse transcriptase centers, directly inhibiting them. These agents are active as administered. They are administered orally. Currently, there are five NNRTIs available, which include delavirdine (Rescriptor), efavirenz (Sustiva), etravirine (Intelence), nevirapine (Viramune, Viramune XR), and rilpivirine (Edurant). These agents all may cause rashes, which can be severe. The NNRTIs are listed in Table 17-4 ■.

Table 17-4 ■ Non-Nucleoside Reverse Transcriptase Inhibitors

GENERIC NAME	TRADE NAME	AVERAGE ADULT DOSAGE	ROUTE OF ADMINISTRATION
delavirdine (DLV)	Rescriptor	Tablets: 400 mg tid, with or without food; can also be mixed with at least 3 ounces of water and swallowed as a suspension. Otherwise, tablets should swallowed whole. If patient has a lack of stomach acid, tablets should be taken with acidic beverages such as juices.	PO
efavirenz (EFZ)	Sustiva	Tablets or capsules: 600 mg once/d on an empty stomach, preferably at bedtime	PO
etravirine	Intelence	Tablets: 200 mg bid, following meals	PO
nevirapine (NVP)	Viramune, Viramune XR	Immediate-release tablets or oral suspension: start with 200 mg once/d for 14 days, then may increase to 200 mg bid. Extended-release tablets (for adults only): start with 200 mg once/d for 14 days, then may increase to 400 mg once/d	PO
rilpivirine	Edurant	Tablets: 25 mg once/d with food. This drug is also available in a combination tablet (along with emtric-itabine and tenofovir)	PO

tid, three times a day; PO, oral; bid, twice a day.

Focus On

Delavirdine

Delavirdine (Rescriptor) is used to treat HIV and has similar actions to efavirenz. It must be used in combination with at least two other anti-HIV medications. Delavirdine is a NNRTI that blocks the growth of HIV.

How does it work?

Delavirdine acts directly to inhibit reverse transcriptase, suppressing HIV replication. Due to resistance, it must always be combined with other antiretroviral drugs.

How is it used?

Delavirdine is only effective against HIV-1. It is not a cure for HIV or AIDS. This drug may also be used for other purposes. This drug must not be taken in larger or smaller amounts, or for longer than recommended. It may be taken with or without food. If the patient has a condition of decreased stomach acid, it may need to be taken with an acidic beverage, such as orange or cranberry juice. Delavirdine tablets may be dissolved in water to make swallowing easier. The patient should place 4 tablets into at least 3 ounces of water, which is just below one-third cup. The liquid should be left to stand for a few minutes, then stirred to disperse the tablets evenly. The patient should drink this mixture right away. Then, a little more water should be added to the same glass, swirled, and swallowed so that any residue from the pills is also administered.

What are the adverse effects?

Delavirdine causes potentially serious rashes and other hypersensitivity reactions. Approximately half of patients develop rashes, though serious forms such as erythema multiforme and Stevens-Johnson syndrome are rare. When they do develop, the drug must be withdrawn. Other adverse effects may include fatigue, headache, diarrhea, nausea and vomiting, or elevated liver enzymes.

What are the contraindications and interactions?

Delavirdine is contraindicated with known hypersensitivity to any of its components. It should not be administered concurrently with ergot derivatives (dihydroergotamine, ergonovine, ergotamine, methylergonovine), the gastrointestinal motility agent cisapride, the neuroleptic pimozide, and certain sedative/hypnotics (alprazolam, midazolam, triazolam). Delavirdine is different from efavirenz and nevirapine in that it inhibits cytochrome P450, meaning that certain concurrent drug levels may increase. These drugs include cisapride, lovastatin, simvastatin, indinavir, saquinavir, clarithromycin, dapsone, warfarin, quinidine, sildenafil, and the dihydropyridine-type calcium channel blockers. Also, levels of delavirdine can be decreased by St. John's wort, rifampin, rifabutin, phenytoin, phenobarbital, and carbamazepine. Drugs that can decrease the absorption of delavirdine include antacids, histamine$_2$ receptor antagonists, proton pump inhibitors, and buffered didanosine formulations.

What are the important points patients should know?

Patients must be informed about the many drugs that can cause serious or life-threatening outcomes if used with delavirdine. Any new medications should not be started while using delavirdine without telling your physician. Patients should be instructed that use of delavirdine will not prevent them from passing HIV to others.

Efavirenz

Efavirenz (Sustiva) is considered a preferred agent against HIV, making it unique among the other NNRTIs. It can be given once per day due to its long half-life, but does cause teratogenicity and transient adverse effects to the central nervous system. Plasma levels peak 3–5 hours after administration, and this drug is over 99% protein bound in the blood. It has a long serum half-life of between 40 and 55 hours, so it can be taken once per day.

How does it work?

Efavirenz binds directly to HIV reverse transcriptase, disrupting its active center and suppressing its activity. It is only effective against HIV-1. It does not inhibit human DNA polymerases. Efavirenz crosses the blood–brain barrier and can reduce HIV levels in the CNS. It is metabolized by CYP3A4 and CYP2B6, then excreted in the urine and feces.

How is it used?

Efavirenz is the only NNRTI considered first-line therapy against HIV and is highly effective. When combined with the NRTIs called zidovudine and lamivudine, its effects and ability to be tolerated are better than when the protease inhibitor called indinavir is combined with the same two NRTIs. Efavirenz must be combined with other anti-retroviral agents due to resistance. It is administered orally on an empty stomach because meals (especially high-fat meals) increase plasma levels significantly.

What are the adverse effects?

Efavirenz causes CNS symptoms in more than half of patients, which include dizziness, impaired consciousness, insomnia, drowsiness, nightmares, and vivid dreams. Other effects such as delusions, hallucinations, and severe acute depression can occur, but these are mostly in patients with histories of drug abuse or mental illness. The drug should be discontinued in these cases. Most CNS symptoms resolve within 2 to 4 weeks of beginning treatment. Rashes may also occur, which can range from mild to severe. Severe rashes are signified by moist desquamation, ulceration, and vesiculation. Rarely, these may evolve into potentially fatal **erythema multiforme**, Stevens-Johnson syndrome, or **toxic epidermal necrolysis**, and the drug should be withdrawn immediately. Efavirenz has been shown to cause fetal malformation in animal studies, so women must avoid pregnancy while taking this drug. It is listed as FDA Pregnancy Risk Category D.

(*continued*)

Focus On (continued)

This drug may also cause liver damage, so liver enzymes must be monitored, especially in patients with HBV or HCV.

What are the contraindications and interactions?

Efavirenz is contraindicated in patients who have had serious hypersensitivities such as erythema multiforme, Stevens-Johnson syndrome, or toxic skin eruptions. It is also contraindicated in any hypersensitivity to its components. Efavirenz competes with other drugs for metabolism by cytochrome P450, resulting in possibly dangerous accumulations. It should not be combined, therefore, with alprazolam, cisapride, midazolam, triazolam, dihydroergotamine, or ergotamine. Because of efavirenz inducing P450, there may be increased metabolism of indinavir and saquinavir. Efavirenz can also decrease effects of oral contraceptives, the etonogestrel contraceptive implant, and other hormonal contraceptives. Contraceptive failure may result, leading to teratogenicity. Efavirenz should not be combined with ritonavir because of possibilities of toxicity. It should also not be combined with the herbal supplement St. John's wort due to accelerated metabolism.

What are the important points patients should know?

Patients must be informed that efavirenz should not be taken while trying to become pregnant or if pregnant. If sexual activity is occurring, two forms of birth control should be used, with one of these being a barrier form such as a condom or diaphragm with spermicide gel. The same procedures must be continued for at least 12 weeks after treatment with efavirenz ends. The physician must be informed if pregnancy occurs during treatment with this drug. Patients must also be informed about severe psychiatric symptoms that this drug can cause and to tell their physician if any occur. Patients must be aware of the many contraindicated drugs as well as the contraindicated use of St. John's wort. It should also be discussed with patients that efavirenz will not prevent passage of HIV to others.

Etravirine

Etravirine (Intelence) is a newer NNRTI with similar features. It has a serum half-life of 41 hours and is excreted in the urine and feces.

How does it work?

Etravirine binds to and inhibits reverse transcriptase, to suppress HIV replication. In the blood, this drug is 99% protein bound, mostly to albumin. It is metabolized by cytochrome P450 isozymes.

How is it used?

Etravirine is effective only against HIV-1 and does not inhibit human DNA polymerases. It is indicated for HIV strains that are resistant to other NNRTIs as well as other antiretroviral drugs, including protease inhibitors. Therefore, etravirine must always be combined with other effective agents. Etravirine is administered orally, following a meal because food increases its absorption by 50%.

What are the adverse effects?

Though mostly well tolerated, etravirine can also cause rashes and other hypersensitivity reactions, which may be fatal. Severe skin reactions are very rare, and the drug should be discontinued should they occur. Other adverse effects may include diarrhea, nausea and vomiting, fatigue, abdominal pain, peripheral neuropathy, hypertension, and headache. This drug is classified in FDA Pregnancy Risk Category B.

What are the contraindications and interactions?

There are no significant contraindications to etravirine. However, it has many drug interactions, which include drugs that inhibit or induce cytochrome P450 and related substrates. These drugs include efavirenz, nevirapine, delavirdine, rilpivirine, ritonavir, maraviroc, digoxin, carbamazepine, phenobarbital, phenytoin, fluconazole, voriconazole, itraconazole, ketoconazole, posaconazole, clarithromycin, rifampin, rifapentine, rifabutin, dexamethasone, telaprevir, St. John's wort, atorvastatin, fluvastatin, lovastatin, pitavastatin, pravastatin, rosuvastatin, simvastatin, buprenorphine, and methadone.

What are the important points patients should know?

Patients must be instructed about a rare condition in which etravirine causes a breakdown of skeletal muscle tissue, leading to kidney failure. The patient must contact his or her physician if symptoms of this condition develop. Patients must inform their physicians about all medications, vitamins, or herbal products that they take, and also avoid starting anything new while on etravirine therapy. Patients must understand that etravirine will not prevent them from passing HIV to others.

Nevirapine

Nevirapine (Viramune, Viramune XR) is active against HIV-1 and is available as oral tablets or as a suspension. The Viramune brand is approved for adults and children, whereas Viramune XR is approved only for adults. Nevirapine is eliminated mostly in the urine (80%) but also in the feces.

How does it work?

Nevirapine binds directly to HIV reverse transcriptase to cause noncompetitive inhibition of this enzyme. It is effective for HIV-1 only, does not affect HIV-2, and does not inhibit human DNA polymerase. Nevirapine is more than 90% absorbed, with or without food, and can cross the placenta and blood–brain barrier as well as enter the breast milk. Its concentrations in the cerebrospinal fluid are approximately 45% of those in the plasma.

How is it used?

Nevirapine is approved for HIV-1 and resistance develops quickly if it is used alone; therefore, it must be combined with other antiretroviral drugs.

What are the adverse effects?

Nevirapine predominantly causes rashes early in therapy, which can become life-threatening. The drug should be withdrawn if fever, blisters, conjunctivitis, oral lesions, and muscle or joint pain occur. To protect against such developments, nevirapine is usually begun in low doses and then increased if no rashes occur. It can also cause severe and potentially fatal hepatotoxicity, especially during the first 12 weeks of therapy. This is increased if the patient has a history of chronic HBV or HCV. Liver function tests are required on an as-needed basis. If liver damage is present, the drug must be withdrawn.

What are the contraindications and interactions?

Nevirapine is contraindicated in patients with moderate or severe hepatic impairment. It is also contraindicated for use as part of occupational and nonoccupational postexposure prophylaxis regimens. Nevirapine induces cytochrome P450 and can result in declining levels of drugs that include hormonal contraceptives, methadone, and protease inhibitors. Since rifampin can also induce P450, it should not be combined with nevirapine. Nevirapine should also not be used with St. John's wort.

What are the important points patients should know?

Patients must be informed about the hepatotoxic effects of nevirapine and the symptoms that they should report to their physician. They must also understand and report severe skin reactions, which are considered medical emergencies. No new medicines, vitamins, or herbal products should be started while taking nevirapine unless approved by a physician. Patients must also understand that taking nevirapine will not prevent them from passing HIV to others.

Rilpivirine

Rilpivirine (Edurant) is the newest NNRTI, and has similar actions and uses to the others. It is more than 99.7% protein-bound in the blood, mostly to albumin. Rilpivirine is mostly metabolized by the liver, then excreted mostly in the feces but also in the urine.

How does it work?

Rilpivirine binds to and inhibits reverse transcriptase to suppress HIV replication. It is active only against HIV-1. Its serum half-life is approximately 50 hours.

How is it used?

Rilpivirine is indicated, along with other antiretroviral agents, for HIV-1. It is as effective as efavirenz and may be better tolerated, but with other risk factors. It is administered orally with food because its absorption is increased by 50% when taken in this manner.

What are the adverse effects?

Rilpivirine has a greater risk than efavirenz of resistance and virologic failure, especially when a patient's viral load exceeds 100,000 virions per mL. Overall, rilpivirine is well tolerated. Adverse effects include depression, insomnia, headache, and mild to moderate rash. Rilpivirine can prolong the QT interval. Based on studies in animals, this drug is classified in FDA Pregnancy Risk Category B.

What are the contraindications and interactions?

Rilpivirine should not be administered with certain anticonvulsants (carbamazepine, oxcarbazepine,

(continued)

Focus On (continued)

phenobarbital, phenytoin), certain antimycobacterials (rifampin, rifapentine), certain proton pump inhibitors (esomeprazole, lansoprazole, omeprazole, pantoprazole, rabeprazole), the glucocorticoid systemic dexamethasone (in more than one dose), and the supplement St. John's wort. Rilpivirine may interact with all of these drugs, which inhibit or induce cytochrome P450, and those that elevate gastric pH. Drugs that should be used with caution along with rilpivirine include antacids, histamine$_2$-receptor blockers, azole antifungal drugs, and macrolides.

What are the important points patients should know?

Rilpivirine should not be used if breastfeeding due to possible toxicity. Because of potential drug interactions,

the patient must tell his or her physician about any medications currently being used, or any medications that are started or stopped while taking rilpivirine. Patients must discuss with physicians if they have liver or kidney disease, a history of depression or mental illness, or if any HIV medication has been taken previously. This drug must be used in combination with other HIV medications. The physician must be contacted if the patient experiences anxiety, mood changes, feelings of hopelessness, severe depression, or thoughts about suicide or self-harm. Taking this medication will not prevent passing HIV to others.

Protease Inhibitors

Protease inhibitors (PIs) restrain enzymes needed for HIV replication. They are some of the most effective antiretroviral drugs used today. They are able to reduce viral loads to undetectable levels when used along with NRTIs. Widespread use of PIs has demonstrated a variety of adverse effects beyond the originally discovered gastrointestinal disturbances. These include abnormal fat distribution, diabetes and hyperglycemia, increased bleeding (in hemophiliacs), reduced bone mineral density, and elevated levels of triglycerides and transaminases.

PIs inhibit cytochrome P450 enzymes, possibly increasing levels of certain drugs and leading to widely different drug interactions. HIV resistance to PIs is also significant. Since PIs do not work the same way as many other drugs used against HIV, cross-resistance between them and the other classifications does not occur. Therefore, PIs are always used in combination with at least one reverse transcriptase inhibitor, or ideally, at least two of these agents. These agents, of which there are nine currently available, are administered orally. Due to lack of available data, choosing which PIs to use is based on adverse effects, interactions, and how acceptable they are to individual patients. The protease inhibitors are listed in Table 17-5 ■.

Table 17-5 ■ Protease Inhibitors

GENERIC NAME	TRADE NAME	AVERAGE ADULT DOSAGE	ROUTE OF ADMINISTRATION
atazanavir	Reyataz	Capsule: 300 mg once/d	PO
darunavir	Prezista	Tablet or oral suspension: 800 mg once/d with ritonavir 100 mg once/d with food	PO
fosamprenavir	Lexiva	Tablet or oral suspension: 1400 mg bid without ritonavir; or 1400 mg once/d with ritonavir 200 mg; or 1400 mg once/d with 100 mg ritonavir; or 700 mg bid with 100 mg ritonavir; in PI-experienced patients: 700 mg bid with 100 mg ritonavir	PO
indinavir	Crixivan	Capsule: 800 mg (usually two 400-mg capsules) q8h, without food, but with water 1 hour before or 2 hours after a meal	PO

GENERIC NAME	TRADE NAME	AVERAGE ADULT DOSAGE	ROUTE OF ADMINISTRATION
lopinavir/ritonavir (lopinavir is only available in combination with ritonavir)	Kaletra, Aluvia	Tablet or oral liquid: 400 mg lopinavir/100 mg ritonavir bid (if less than 3 lopinavir resistance-associated substitutions, may use lopinavir 800 mg/ritonavir 200 mg bid); with concomitant efavirenz, nelfinavir, or nevirapine therapy: tablets—lopinavir 500 mg/ritonavir 125 mg bid or pinavir 533 mg/ritonavir 133 mg bid	PO
nelfinavir	Viracept	Tablet or oral powder: 1250 mg (five 250 mg or two 625 mg tablets) bid or 750 mg (three 250 mg tablets) tid, taken with food. If unable to swallow the tablets, they may be dissolved in a small amount of water. Oral powder should be mixed with a small amount of water, milk, or dietary supplements	PO
ritonavir	Norvir	Capsule: 600 mg bid (may need to be started at 300 mg bid, increased at 2- to 3-day intervals by 100 mg bid)	PO
saquinavir	Invirase	Tablet or capsule: 1000 mg bid (five 200 mg capsules or two 500 mg tablets) in combination with ritonavir 100 mg bid, within 2 hours after a meal	PO
tipranavir	Aptivus	Capsule or oral solution: 500 mg (two 250 mg capsules or 5 mL oral solution), in combination with 200 mg ritonavir bid	PO

PO, oral; bid, twice a day; tid, three times a day.

Focus On

Atazanavir

Atazanavir (Reyataz) is an HIV-1 protease inhibitor. It is most commonly used with ritonavir.

How does it work?

Atazanavir disrupts normal functions of HIV protease, interrupting replication of the HIV virus.

How is it used?

Atazanavir is used in combination with other antiretrovirals for HIV-1 infection in patients older than 3 months of age. It is not used in infants younger than this due to risk of kernicterus. Its use in treatment-experienced patients must be based on how many baseline primary PI resistance substitutions have been made.

What are the adverse effects?

Atazanavir may cause cardiac conduction abnormalities, rashes, hyperbilirubinemia, nephrolithiasis, and cholelithiasis. Other adverse effects include nausea and jaundice.

What are the contraindications and interactions?

Atazanavir is contraindicated with previously demonstrated clinically significant hypersensitivity to any of its components. Contraindications include alfuzosin, rifampin, irinotecan, triazolam, orally administered midazolam, ergot derivatives, cisapride, lovastatin, simvastatin, pimozide, sildenafil, indinavir, nevirapine, and the herbal supplement St. John's wort. If atazanavir is used without ritonavir, it may interact with paclitaxel or repaglinide. In general, atazanavir may interact with proton pump inhibitors, antacids, buffered medications, or H_2-receptor antagonists.

What are the important points patients should know?

Patients must be instructed not to take atazanavir if they are allergic to any of its components. The physician must tell the patient about the many drugs that cannot be taken along with atazanavir. The patient must inform the physician about all other medications

(continued)

Focus On (continued)

being taken and should not start any new medication without discussing this with the physician. Patients must discuss previous use of PIs and whether they have any liver disease, kidney disease, diabetes, bleeding disorders, high cholesterol, or heart problems.

Darunavir

Darunavir (Prezista) is a second-generation PI that is boosted with ritonavir, then combined with other antiretroviral drugs. It is 95% protein-bound in the blood. Combined with ritonavir, darunavir has a half-life of 15 hours.

How does it work?

Darunavir is mostly metabolized by CYP3A whereas ritonavir inhibits this drug. Therefore, plasma concentrations of darunavir are increased. Studies have shown that ritonavir increases levels of darunavir by 14 times.

How is it used?

Darunavir is used for HIV-1 strains that are resistant to other PIs. However, any strain that resists darunavir is usually also resistant to the other PIs, except for tipranavir. Darunavir is indicated for HIV-1 infection in adults and children. Darunavir with ritonavir as a booster is very effective in patients who have been previously under treatment for strains of HIV resistance to one or more PIs. It is administered orally and its absorption is increased with food. If taken alone, it is quickly inactivated in the liver.

What are the adverse effects?

Darunavir primarily causes diarrhea, nausea, rash, and headache. Less common adverse effects include elevated serum lipids and activity of aminotransferase. Darunavir differs from other PIs in that it has not been shown to cause newly developing diabetes, worsening of existing diabetes, or hyperglycemia.

What are the contraindications and interactions?

Darunavir is contraindicated with ergonovine, ergotamine, dihydroergotamine, methylergonovine, midazolam, triazolam, cisapride, and pimozide. Darunavir must be used cautiously in patients allergic to sulfonamides because it has a sulfonamide component.

What are the important points patients should know?

Patients must be instructed not to take darunavir if allergic to any of its components, the components of ritonavir, or if they have severe liver disease. Patients must follow the darunavir–ritonavir dosage regimen exactly. They should be informed about potentially life-threatening adverse effects if darunavir is taken with a large variety of other drugs and substances. Patients should provide their physician with a list of all other medications, vitamins, and herbal supplements that they take.

Fosamprenavir

Fosamprenavir (Lexiva) is a prodrug that is quickly converted to its active form, known as amprenavir. Fosamprenavir is better tolerated than amprenavir itself, and in fact replaced a previously marketed product known as amprenavir (Agenerase). The withdrawal of amprenavir was based on high incidence of nausea and vomiting, and rashes that it caused. Amprenavir is chemically related to the sulfonamide antibiotics. Fosamprenavir has a half-life that is long enough to enable dosing to occur twice per day. It is metabolized by cytochrome P450 in the liver, then excreted in the feces (75%) and urine (14%).

How does it work?

Fosamprenavir inhibits HIV protease to prevent maturation of the HIV virus. It is quickly converted to amprenavir by gastrointestinal enzymes.

How is it used?

Fosamprenavir is used along with other antiretrovirals to treat HIV infection in adults and children.

What are the adverse effects?

The most common adverse effects of fosamprenavir include nausea and vomiting, diarrhea, headache, and mild to moderate rashes. There is the less common chance that serious rashes may develop, including Stevens-Johnson syndrome, which can be fatal. Fosamprenavir may also cause hyperglycemia, newly occurring diabetes, worsening of existing diabetes, fat maldistribution, bone loss, hyperlipidemia, elevated transaminase, and increased bleeding (in hemophiliacs). In rare cases, kidney stones (nephrolithiasis) may develop.

What are the contraindications and interactions?

Fosamprenavir is contraindicated with cisapride, alprazolam, triazolam, midazolam, bepridil, ergot alkaloids, simvastatin, lovastatin, rifampin, and the herbal supplement St. John's wort. It may also interact with oral contraceptives, so alternate forms of contraception should be used while taking fosamprenavir.

What are the important points patients should know?

Patients must be informed that fosamprenavir may cause abdominal or back pain, as well as pain in the groin or testicles. They should report these symptoms to their physician, and the drug should be temporarily or permanently discontinued.

Indinavir

Indinavir (Crixivan) is administered on an empty stomach, with which it has 65% bioavailability. It must not be administered with meals high in calories, fats, or proteins due to significantly decreased absorption. Indinavir is excreted mostly in the feces and to a lesser degree in the urine. Its plasma half-life is 1.5–2 hours; however, this may be prolonged in patients with liver dysfunction.

How does it work?

Indinavir inhibits HIV protease, preventing cleavage of large HIV polyproteins into smaller functional forms. The particles then remain immature and noninfectious. Indinavir is metabolized by hepatic cytochrome P450.

How is it used?

Indinavir is used only for HIV infections, usually combined with two NRTIs. This indication is based on clinical trials that have demonstrated a reduced risk of AIDS-defining illnesses or death, as well as a prolonged suppression of HIV RNA.

What are the adverse effects?

Though generally well tolerated, the major adverse effect of indinavir is kidney stones or nephrolithiasis, which causes flank pain, and may cause hematuria. This usually does not affect kidney function and resolves with

hydration and withdrawal of the drug for 1–3 days. Patients can reduce risk of kidney stones by consuming at least 48 ounces of water daily. Additional adverse effects include newly developing diabetes, hyperglycemia, worsening of existing diabetes, fat maldistribution, bone loss, hyperlipidemia, elevated transaminase levels, and increased bleeding in hemophiliacs. Less common effects include GI problems, headache, weakness, blurred vision, dizziness, metallic taste, rash, indirect hyperbilirubinemia, and thrombocytopenia.

What are the contraindications and interactions?

Indinavir is contraindicated in hypersensitivity to any of its components, and the drugs alfuzosin, amiodarone, dihydroergotamine, ergonovine, ergotamine, methylergonovine, cisapride, lovastatin, simvastatin, pimozide, sildenafil, oral midazolam, triazolam, and alprazolam. Drug interactions with indinavir may occur with buffered didanosine, rifampin, rifabutin, ketoconazole, and the herbal supplement St. John's wort.

What are the important points patients should know?

Patients must be instructed about the many medications that can cause life-threatening adverse effects if taken with indinavir. They must tell their physician about all medications they are using concurrently and not to change doses or medication schedule without notifying their physician. Indinavir will not prevent them from passing HIV to others.

Lopinavir/Ritonavir

This fixed-dose combination, marketed as Kaletra and Aluvia, is approved for adults and children over 6 months old. Lopinavir is the active retroviral; ritonavir is included to increase its effects by inhibiting cytochrome P450. The lower levels of ritonavir mean that this component is insufficient to have significant antiretroviral effects. Lopinavir is mostly excreted in the feces and somewhat in the urine. It has a half-life of 5–6 hours.

How does it work?

While the actions of ropinavir are explained in detail under its section below, lopinavir is absorbed better when taken with food. It is 99% bound to plasma proteins in the blood and undergoes extensive metabolism by CYP3A4. In this combination drug, lopinavir achieves much higher concentrations than ritonavir, yet is effective at much lower concentrations.

(continued)

Focus On (continued)

How is it used?

Lopinavir/ritonavir is used for many HIV strains and has been effective against certain strains that resist other PIs. This combination is preferred in multidrug antiretroviral treatment regimens.

What are the adverse effects?

Lopinavir/ritonavir is extremely well tolerated, with the most common adverse effects being diarrhea and nausea. The other adverse effects include tiredness or weakness and headache. There are risks for new-onset diabetes, hyperglycemia, worsening of existing diabetes, fat mal-distribution, bone loss, hyperlipidemia, elevated transaminases, and increased bleeding in hemophiliacs. Children may experience rashes as a result of this combination drug. This drug also prolongs the PR and QT intervals. In relation to the PR interval, this may be linked to increased risk of atrioventricular block. Therefore, it must be used cautiously in patients taking other drugs that prolong the PR interval. In relation to the QT interval, there is increased risk of severe dysrhythmias. Additionally, the oral solution formulation of this combination drug has caused serious cardiac, renal, and respiratory problems in newborns, leading to fatalities. It should be avoided in full-term infants for the first 14 days following birth and in preterm infants until 14 days after their predicted due date.

What are the contraindications and interactions?

Lopinavir/ritonavir must be avoided with congenital long QT syndrome and if other drugs that prolong the QT interval are being taken. Other contraindications include structural heart disorders, ischemic heart disease, myocardial disease with enlargement, heart block, torsades de pointes, dysrhythmias, chronic HBV or HBC, liver diseases, pancreatitis, hyperbilirubinemia, hyperglycemia, abnormal liver function tests, during lactation, with diabetes, with hypertriglyceridemia, high blood cholesterol, hypomagnesemia, hypokalemia, with hemophilia A, and with blood clotting disorder due to clotting factor IX. Drug interactions with lopinavir/ritonavir include clarithromycin, ketoconazole, itraconazole, rifabutin, sildenafil and similar erectile dysfunction drugs, cisapride, flecainide, propafenone, dihydroergotamine, ergonovine, ergotamine, methylergonovine, pimozide, midazolam, triazolam, lovastatin, and simvastatin. Additional interactions may include methadone, ethinyl estradiol, rifampin, efavirenz, nevirapine, phenobarbital, phenytoin, carbamazepine, disulfiram, metronidazole, and the herbal supplement St. John's wort.

What are the important points patients should know?

Patients must be aware of hypersensitivity reactions to this combination drug, as well as the medications to avoid taking during therapy.

Nelfinavir

Nelfinavir (Viracept) prevents HIV maturation by inhibiting HIV protease. More than 98% of this drug is protein-bound in the blood. It is extensively metabolized in the liver and 99% is excreted in the feces, with the remainder in the urine. Its plasma half-life is 3.5–5 hours.

How does it work?

Nelfinavir works by blocking the HIV protease enzyme, which prevents HIV from replicating, lowering the amount of HIV in the blood.

How is it used?

Nelfinavir is approved for HIV in adults and in children 2 years of age or older. It must be combined with at least one reverse transcriptase inhibitor. Nelfinavir is administered orally, and its absorption is doubled or tripled when taken with food.

What are the adverse effects?

Nelfinavir may cause diarrhea in patients, which is dose-limited. This is also successfully treated with loperamide, available OTC. This drug may also cause hyperglycemia, newly occurring diabetes, worsening of existing diabetes, fat maldistribution, bone loss, hyperlipidemia, elevated transaminase, and increased bleeding (in hemophiliacs).

What are the contraindications and interactions?

Nelfinavir is contraindicated with cisapride, midazolam, and ergot alkaloids. It may also interact with ethinyl estradiol, norethindrone, rifampin, rifabutin, and the herbal supplement St. John's wort.

What are the important points patients should know?

Patients must be instructed about life-threatening adverse effects that may occur if nelfinavir is taken with many other drugs. They must tell their physician about all medications they use, including vitamins and herbal products. It is important not to start any new medication without discussing this with their physician. Nelfinavir will not prevent the patient from passing HIV to others.

Ritonavir

Ritonavir (Norvir) prevents the multiplication of HIV cells and is an effective "booster" of antiretroviral actions when used in combination with lopinavir. Nearly 33% of HIV patients take ritonavir. This agent is excreted mostly in the feces, with lesser excretion in the urine. Its plasma half-life is 3–5 hours.

How does it work?

Ritonavir inhibits HIV protease, preventing maturation of HIV. It is well absorbed when administered orally. Ritonavir is metabolized by cytochrome P450 enzymes.

How is it used?

Ritonavir is used to treat HIV-1 and HIV-2 in adults and children. It must be combined with at least one reverse transcriptase inhibitor in order to reduce possibility of resistance. Due to the poor taste of ritonavir, its oral solution formulation is often taken with chocolate milk, nutritional drinks, or other flavored liquids.

What are the adverse effects?

The adverse effects of ritonavir happen most often during the first weeks of therapy. The most common adverse effects include nausea and vomiting, diarrhea, muscle weakness, altered taste sensations, and, in lesser amounts, tingling or numbness around the mouth or in the extremities. Adverse effects are reduced by beginning therapy at lower dosages and titrating them upward to the maintenance dosage. There are also risks of hyperglycemia, newly developing diabetes, fat maldistribution, worsening of existing diabetes, bone loss, hyperlipidemia, elevated transaminases, and in hemophiliacs, increased bleeding.

What are the contraindications and interactions?

Ritonavir is contraindicated with many different drugs, including amiodarone, bepridil, bupropion, clorazepate, clozapine, diazepam, encainide, estazolam, flecainide, flurazepam, meperidine, piroxicam, propoxyphene, propafenone, quinidine, and zolpidem. Drug interactions with ritonavir include ethinyl estradiol, rifabutin, ketoconazole, clarithromycin, desipramine, didanosine, and the supplement St. John's wort.

What are the important points patients should know?

Patients must be alerted that life-threatening adverse effects may occur if ritonavir is taken with a large variety of medications. They must tell their physician about all other medications or supplements being taken. Patients must also be instructed not to change doses or medication schedules without physician approval. They must understand that ritonavir will not prevent them from passing HIV to others.

Saquinavir

Saquinavir (Invirase) was the first protease inhibitor approved by the FDA. It appears to be more potent than the other PIs. Both the tablet and hard-gelatin capsule formulations are sold under the same trade name. This drug's effectiveness is boosted by administration along with ritonavir. It is excreted in the feces and has a plasma half-life of 1–2 hours.

How does it work?

Saquinavir inhibits HIV protease, preventing cleavage of larger HIV polyproteins into smaller, functional forms, with these remaining immature and noninfectious. It is metabolized by cytochrome P450.

How is it used?

Saquinavir is used only for HIV infection, in combination with at least one reverse transcriptase inhibitor. It is administered orally and food does not affect its blood levels if given with ritonavir.

What are the adverse effects?

Generally well tolerated, saquinavir may cause nausea, diarrhea, dyspepsia, and abdominal pain. Like other PIs, it is also linked to newly occurring diabetes, hyperglycemia, worsening of existing diabetes, fat maldistribution, bone loss, hyperlipidemia, elevated transaminase levels, and increased bleeding in hemophiliacs. It also prolongs PR and QT intervals, with similar outcomes to those of lopinavir/ritonavir.

(continued)

Focus On (continued)

. . . .

What are the contraindications and interactions?

Saquinavir must be avoided with congenital long QT syndrome, refractory hypokalemia or hypomagnesemia, and with drugs that both increase its concentrations while prolonging the QT interval. It is also contraindicated with complete AV block without implanted pacemakers, or if patients are at high risk of complete AV block, in those with clinically significant hypersensitivity to its components, and if the patient has severe hepatic impairment. It is contraindicated with drugs that are CYP3A substrates. Drug interactions with saquinavir include ketoconazole, clarithromycin, rifampin, rifabutin, phenobarbital, cisapride, alprazolam, triazolam, midazolam, bepridil, ergot alkaloids, simvastatin, and lovastatin. Other substances that may interact with saquinavir include grapefruit juice and St. John's wort.

What are the important points patients should know?

Patients must be instructed not to take saquinavir if they are allergic to its components or those of ritonavir. They must tell their physician if they have liver disease, diabetes, hemophilia, high cholesterol, heart disease including dysrhythmias, or history of long QT syndrome. Physicians must educate patients about the potential life-threatening adverse effects if saquinavir is taken with many other drugs. Patients must inform their physician about all medications used and must not start any new medication without first discussing this with their physician. Doses must remain as prescribed. Saquinavir will not prevent the patient from passing HIV to others.

. . . .

Tipranavir

Tipranavir (Aptivus) is used along with ritonavir, which boosts its actions, along with other antiretrovirals. It is better absorbed when taken with a high-fat meal. Tipranavir is more than 99.9% bound to proteins in the blood and is a substrate for CYP3A4. When given with ritonavir, its conversion to metabolites is insignificant; therefore, it is excreted mostly unchanged in the feces. Its plasma half-life is 6 hours.

How does it work?

Tipranavir prevents maturation of the HIV virus by inhibiting HIV protease. Differently from the other PIs, it is a flexible nonpeptide that adapts to changes in HIV protease. These changes make the enzyme able to resist the other PIs. Therefore, tipranavir is able to suppress strains that have been resistant to other PIs.

How is it used?

Tipranavir is indicated for HIV infection in adults who have continuing viral replication, if they have been taking antiretrovirals for a long time, or if they are infected with strains of HIV that resist a variety of PIs. Tipranavir is not used without being boosted by ritonavir.

What are the adverse effects?

The most significant adverse effect of tipranavir is liver damage. It may cause potentially fatal hepatitis as well. Therefore, liver function must be assessed before use and continually monitored. This is especially true for patients with HBV or HCV. Cases of potentially fatal intracranial hemorrhage have also been reported. Other adverse effects include nausea and vomiting, diarrhea, fatigue, and headache. This drug may also cause hyperglycemia, newly occurring diabetes, worsening of existing diabetes, fat maldistribution, and increased bleeding (in hemophiliacs). Compared to other PIs, tipranavir causes the largest increases in plasma triglycerides and cholesterol.

What are the contraindications and interactions?

Contraindications include amiodarone, flecainide, pimozide, midazolam, triazolam, simvastatin, lovastatin, and ergot alkaloids. Tipranavir should be used cautiously in patients allergic to sulfonamides because it contains a sulfonamide group. Tipranavir may require reductions of other substrates for CYP3A or CYP2D6. It also interacts with fosamprenavir, lopinavir, saquinavir, ethinyl estradiol (resulting in use of different contraceptives while taking tipranavir), rifampin, and the herbal supplement St. John's wort.

What are the important points patients should know?

The patient must be instructed to contact his or her physician immediately if symptoms of bleeding in the brain occur, which include confusion, vision or speech problems, or one-sided weakness. The patient must also contact his or her physician if symptoms of liver problems develop, which include jaundice, dark urine, pale stools, stomach pain or tenderness, severe or persistent nausea or tiredness, or loss of appetite.

Integrase Strand Transfer Inhibitors

The integrase strand transfer inhibitors (INSTIs) inhibit enzymes needed for HIV replication. These are also called simply *integrase inhibitors (IIs)*. Administered orally, there are three INSTIs available: raltegravir (Isentress), dolutegravir (Tivicay), and elvitegravir (Vitekta).

Fusion Inhibitors

The fusion inhibitors (FIs) block fusion of the viral membrane with the bilipid layer of the plasma membrane. This is very different than the actions of other antivirals, and patients who do not respond to other antivirals usually do respond to fusion inhibitors. They are used in the treatment of HIV. Administered subcutaneously, there is actually only one fusion inhibitor currently available, which is enfuvirtide (Fuzeon). It is a highly expensive drug to manufacture. They are contraindicated in patients with pulmonary diseases such as pneumonia, since they may increase severity of these conditions. Serious adverse effects include hypersensitivity, nephrotoxicity, neutropenia, and thrombocytopenia. Common but less severe adverse reactions to enfuvirtide include bruising, cysts, skin nodules, itching, abscesses, cellulitis, severe pain, redness, nausea, diarrhea, and fatigue. This drug has a Pregnancy Category B Rating.

Chemokine Receptor 5 Antagonists

The chemokine receptor 5 antagonists (CRAs) block viral entry into cells. These are also known as CCR5 antagonists. Administered orally, there is actually only one CRA available: maraviroc (Selzentry). It is used in the treatment of HIV infection, and is also classified as an entry inhibitor. Its actions involve blocking the HIV protein from its receptors, making it unable to enter the cells. Studies have shown maraviroc to be safe for use in HIV patients.

✱ Apply Your Knowledge 17.1

The following questions focus on what you have just learned about antiviral agents and HIV infections.

CRITICAL THINKING

1. Differentiate between HIV and AIDS.
2. Give the trade names of acyclovir, ganciclovir, and zidovudine.
3. Identify the indications of amantadine (Symmetrel).
4. Explain the mechanism of action of acyclovir.
5. Discuss why patients with AIDS become more susceptible to other infections.
6. Differentiate between NRTIs and NNRTIs.

Other Antiviral Agents

Besides the antivirals used for HIV, there are other classes of antiviral agents available. They are used for conditions such as cytomegalovirus, herpes zoster, herpes simplex, influenza, and hepatitis, which are discussed next.

CYTOMEGALOVIRUS

Cytomegalovirus (CMV) is also known as *human herpes virus type 5*. It is transmitted through blood, body fluids, or transplanted organs. It can also pass through the placenta to affect a fetus. Prevalence is increased with age, and between 60 and 90% of adults have had CMV infection. It is also more prevalent in lower socioeconomic groups. Congenital CMV may be asymptomatic, but can cause abortion, stillbirth, or postnatal death. Complications include extensive hepatic or CNS damage. There are several antivirals used to treat CMV, which include ganciclovir, valganciclovir, foscarnet, and cidofovir. Here we focus on ganciclovir and valganciclovir, which are most commonly used for the treatment of cytomegalovirus.

Focus On

Ganciclovir

Ganciclovir (Cytovene) is a synthetic purine (crystalline, organic base) nucleoside analogue that is approved for the treatment of cytomegalovirus infections but not for HIV itself.

How does it work?

After conversion to ganciclovir triphosphate, ganciclovir is incorporated into viral DNA and inhibits viral DNA polymerase. By this action, it can terminate viral replication.

How is it used?

Ganciclovir is used for prophylaxis and treatment of systemic CMV infections in immunocompromised patients, including those who are HIV-positive or have a transplant. It is also prescribed for CMV retinitis.

What are the adverse effects?

Black box warnings for ganciclovir include increased potential for dose-limited neutropenia, thrombocytopenia, and anemia. Other adverse effects are fever, headache, disorientation, ataxia, confusion, tremor, edema, and phlebitis.

What are the contraindications and interactions?

Ganciclovir is contraindicated in patients with hypersensitivity to the drug or to acyclovir (Zovirax). It must be avoided in lactating women. Ganciclovir should be used cautiously in patients with renal impairment, older adults, and pregnant women. Its safety and efficacy in children are not established. No specific drug interactions have been identified.

What are the important points patients should know?

Instruct patients to report adverse effects of therapy, including CNS changes such as confusion, depression, ataxia, and tremor.

Valganciclovir

Valganciclovir hydrochloride (Valcyte) is a salt of ganciclovir that prevents viral cells from multiplying that is predominantly used for cytomegalovirus infections.

How does it work?

After oral administration, valganciclovir is quickly converted to ganciclovir by intestinal and hepatic esterases. It then works by inhibiting replication of CMV in vitro and in vivo.

How is it used?

Valganciclovir is indicated for CMV retinitis in patients with AIDS, for the prevention of CMV disease in kidney, heart, and kidney-pancreas transplant patients who are at high risk, and to prevent CMV in pediatric patients.

What are the adverse effects?

The most common adverse effects caused by valganciclovir include diarrhea, nausea and vomiting, abdominal pain, fever, headache, insomnia, peripheral neuropathy, paresthesias, and retinal detachment. There are potentially serious adverse effects, including liver toxicity and acute renal failure.

What are the contraindications and interactions?

Valganciclovir is contraindicated in patients who have had a clinically significant hypersensitivity reaction to this drug, ganciclovir, or any component of these formulations. Since valganciclovir is quickly and extensively converted to ganciclovir, drug–drug interactions associated with ganciclovir should be considered for valganciclovir. These include interactions with zidovudine, probenecid, mycophenolate/mofetil, and didanosine.

What are the important points patients should know?

Valganciclovir tablets may be administered for adults or children, but the oral liquid form is only used for children. Adults should not use the oral solution or the dose may be incorrect. Valganciclovir must never be taken with ganciclovir. Valganciclovir must not be used if the patient is a pregnant female, and birth control must be used during its administration and for at least 30 days after treatment ends. Men taking valganciclovir should use contraception to avoid fathering a child because of the possibility of birth defects. They should continue using contraception for 90 days after stopping treatment with valganciclovir. Tablets should never be broken or crushed, and contact between tablets and the eyes or skin must be prevented. Regular blood testing is required during treatment because valganciclovir lowers the body's ability to fight infections.

HERPES ZOSTER

Herpes zoster is also referred to as *shingles*, an infection caused by the varicella-zoster virus. This virus is the same one that causes chickenpox. When a person has previously had chickenpox, the virus remains in their nervous systems for life, specifically in the dorsal root ganglia. Later, it can emerge because of physical stress or immune system impairment. Reactivation of the varicella-zoster virus causes inflammation of the nerves in the skin of the abdomen and trunk. This manifests as blisters and severe pain. There may be flu-like symptoms, headache, and a low-grade fever. Complications of shingles include repeated outbreaks, blindness, deafness, encephalitis, or sepsis. For prevention of herpes zoster, the zoster vaccine is available. For treatment, antiviral medications such as acyclovir, valacyclovir, and famciclovir are used, as well as analgesics to relieve the pain. The antivirals used for shingles will shorten the length and severity of the illness, but must be started as soon as possible after the rash appears in order to be effective.

HERPES SIMPLEX

The herpes simplex viruses, HSV-1 and HSV-2, often cause recurrent infection that affects the skin, mouth, lips, eyes, and genitals. Most commonly, HSV-1 causes **gingivostomatitis**, **herpes keratitis**, and **herpes labialis**. Genital lesions are usually caused by HSV-2. The transmission of HSV results from close contact with another individual who has an actively shedding virus. This viral shedding occurs from lesions, but can occur even when there are no visible ones. After an initial infection, HSV stays dormant in the nerve ganglia. Symptoms occur when it periodically emerges. Eruptions of herpes are triggered by fevers, overexposure to the sun, immunosuppression, physical or emotional stress, and from unknown factors. Usually, recurrent eruptions of herpes are less severe and occur less often over time. The most common medications used to treat herpes simplex include acyclovir, valacyclovir, and famciclovir. In this chapter, we focus on acyclovir.

Focus On

Acyclovir

Acyclovir (Zovirax) is an antiviral agent used for initial and recurrent mucosal and cutaneous herpes simplex virus types 1 and 2. It is also used for herpes zoster infections in **immunocompromised** patients, which are those with weakened immune systems. Valacyclovir (Valtrex), which is a chemically modified version of acyclovir, is used for the suppression and treatment of mucosal herpes infections. It is also used to treat shingles.

How does it work?

Acyclovir interferes with DNA synthesis and inhibits viral multiplication.

How is it used?

Acyclovir is also used to treat herpes simplex, herpes simplex encephalitis in patients older than 6 months, acute herpes zoster (shingles), and chickenpox.

What are the adverse effects?

Adverse effects of acyclovir include vertigo, headache, tremors, depression, hair loss, and phlebitis at injection sites. It may also cause nausea and vomiting, anorexia, and diarrhea.

What are the contraindications and interactions?

Acyclovir is contraindicated in patients who are allergic to this agent. It should not be used in patients with renal disease or seizures or during lactation.

What are the important points patients should know?

Instruct patients to report adverse effects of therapy, including decreased urination, CNS changes (such as confusion, anxiety, or depression), and gastric irritation.

INFLUENZA

Influenza is an extremely infectious viral illness. The influenza virus is classified as an orthomyxovirus; it is single-stranded, with its RNA shaped like a helix that has a curved, cyclical appearance. The basic antigen types are labeled A, B, and C, which are determined by varying types of nuclear material. The three types are further explained as follows:

✳ **Influenza A:** affects humans, pigs, birds, and other animals; causes moderate to severe illness in all ages. An example is the H1N1 influenza or "swine flu," which was named a pandemic virus by the World

Health Organization in June 2009. Otherwise, this form of influenza is not common in the United States.

✳ **Influenza B:** affects only humans, mostly children; usually causes less severe illness than Influenza A, is more stable, has less antigenic shift and more immunological stability. Seasonal influenza B is highly common in the United States, and its vaccine became available in 2009.

✳ **Influenza C:** rarely linked to disease in humans; most cases are subclinical, and this type has not been associated with epidemics. It mostly affects the upper respiratory tract.

The incubation period for influenza ranges between 1 and 5 days, with 2 days being most common. An individual's previous immunology in regard to antigenically related variants of the virus determines the severity of illness. The "classic" symptoms of influenza include abrupt onset of fever, myalgia, nonproductive cough, and sore throat. The disease is spread through aerosolized or droplet transmission from the respiratory tract of other infected people.

The most common complication of influenza is bacterial pneumonia. Primary influenza viral pneumonia is rare, yet has a high fatality rate. Risks for complications and hospitalizations are higher in people age 65 or older, in very young children, or in any age if there are certain underlying medical conditions. Other complications may include:

✳ *Reye syndrome:* most common in children taking aspirin, mostly associated with influenza B or varicella zoster; symptoms include severe vomiting, confusion, and brain swelling that may progress to coma; therefore, aspirin should be avoided in infants, children, or teenagers with influenza. Patients usually recover quickly or may have depression and lack of strength or energy for several weeks.

✳ *Myocarditis:* inflammation of the myocardium (heart muscle) along with worsening chronic bronchitis or other chronic pulmonary diseases.

✳ *Death:* of the 200,000 Americans hospitalized every year for influenza, between 3,000 and 49,000 die; this range is based on changing viral strains, which vary in severity.

Influenza occurs most often in temperate climates between late December and early March of each year. The inactivated influenza vaccine that is available in the United States is discussed in detail in Chapter 20.

Focus On

Amantadine

Amantadine (Symmetrel) is used to prevent or treat symptoms of influenza A viral infections (also known as the *flu* or *grippe*) as well as respiratory tract illnesses.

How does it work?

Amantadine inhibits replication of the influenza A virus by interfering with viral attachment and by the *uncoating* (disassembly or disintegration) of the virus.

How is it used?

Amantadine is used to treat a wide variety of patients of all ages who have symptoms of influenza, but it may also be used to treat some patients with parkinsonism.

What are the adverse effects?

The most pronounced adverse effects of amantadine are insomnia, nightmares, confusion, *ataxia* (loss of muscular control), headache, dizziness, dyspnea, hypotension, edema, urine retention, constipation, nausea, and dry mouth.

What are the contraindications and interactions?

Amantadine is contraindicated in patients with hypersensitivity to the drug and should be used cautiously in elderly patients and patients with seizure disorders, peripheral edema, heart failure, hepatic disease, eczema-type rash, mental illness, orthostatic hypotension, renal impairment, and cardiovascular disease. Amantadine interacts with anticholinergics and CNS stimulants. It also should not be used with the herb known as jimsonweed or with alcohol.

What are the important points patients should know?

Advise patients to report adverse effects of therapy, including CNS changes (such as confusion, insomnia, nightmares) and urine retention. Instruct patients to rise slowly from sitting and lying positions to avoid experiencing dizziness caused by postural hypotension.

Ribavirin

Ribavirin (Virazole) is a synthetic nucleoside analogue with broad-spectrum antiviral activity against both DNA and RNA viruses.

How does it work?

Its exact mechanism of action is not fully understood, but it is believed to involve multiple mechanisms, including selective interference with viral ribonucleic protein synthesis.

How is it used?

Ribavirin given by aerosol into an infant oxygen hood has been effective for the treatment of respiratory syncytial virus pneumonia.

What are the adverse effects?

The adverse effects of ribavirin include abdominal cramps, jaundice, anemia, and hypotension.

What are the contraindications and interactions?

Ribavirin is contraindicated in patients with severe cardiovascular disease, congestive heart failure, angina, pancreatitis, and hepatitis. It is also contraindicated in patients with renal failure, sickle-cell disease, pregnancy, and lactation. No specific drug interactions have been identified, but clinical experience with the systemic administration of ribavirin is limited.

What are the important points patients should know?

Advise patients to report adverse effects of hepatotoxicity, including fever, liver tenderness, loss of appetite, and jaundice.

HEPATITIS

Hepatitis is defined as inflammation of the liver and may be nonviral or viral. *Nonviral hepatitis* is usually caused by exposure to certain drugs or chemicals and protozoa. The majority of patients recover from nonviral hepatitis, though a small amount develop sudden and severe **fulminant hepatitis**, which is also called **cirrhosis**. Another outcome of hepatitis is liver failure.

Viral hepatitis is a common liver infection that causes destruction of liver cells and necrosis. Fortunately, in some cases, the liver is able to repair itself with little or no damage, depending on the types of viral hepatitis. All forms of viral hepatitis are highly communicable. There are six major forms of viral hepatitis, which include hepatitis A, B, C, D, E, and G (see Table 17-6 ■).

Table 17-6 ■ Six Major Forms of Viral Hepatitis

FORM	MODE OF TRANSMISSION	COMMENTS
HAV	Usually spread via the fecal–oral route by ingestion of fecal contaminants.	Most common among male homosexuals and individuals with human immunodeficiency virus (HIV) infection. Symptoms develop slowly.
HBV	Usually spread by drug users via sharing of needles and contact with blood, semen, or vaginal secretions. Also spread from mothers to their fetuses during birth.	Most common in HIV-positive individuals. Routine screening of blood donors has reduced posttransfusion cases.
HCV	Spread through contact with blood products, IV drug use, and donations of blood, organs, semen, or tissue.	Accounts for most posttransfusion cases of hepatitis. Also accounts for approximately 20% of all viral hepatitis cases.
HDV	Only develops after individuals have contracted hepatitis B. In the U.S., only occurs in individuals frequently exposed to blood products, including IV drug users and hemophiliacs.	Has a high mortality rate and is responsible for nearly 50% of all cases of fulminant hepatitis.

(continued)

Table 17-6 ■ Six Major Forms of Viral Hepatitis (*continued*)

FORM	MODE OF TRANSMISSION	COMMENTS
HEV	Mostly transmitted through fecal–oral route, via contaminated drinking water. Less commonly, it is transmitted through contaminated food, blood transfusions, and during pregnancy.	More common in young adults and those visiting endemic areas (Africa, Asia, Central America, India). More severe when contracted by pregnant women.
HGV	Transmitted by infected blood or blood products. It may be transmitted by sharing personal items that are contaminated, sharing needles, via vertical transmission from mother to newborn at birth, or through sexual activity.	High-risk individuals include recipients of infected blood or blood products, hemodialysis patients, and injection drug users.

ANTIVIRALS FOR HEPATITIS

Though hepatitis A and B are preventable through available vaccines, there is also a variety of drugs used once viral hepatitis has developed in a patient.

✻ Hepatitis A may be treated with intramuscular immunoglobulins.

✻ Hepatitis B may be treated with NRTIs and antiviral interferons

✻ Hepatitis C may be treated with combinations of antivirals, miscellaneous antivirals, protease inhibitors, inhaled anti-infectives/purine nucleosides, antineoplastic interferons, and antiviral interferons. A vaccine is being developed, but is not currently available in the United States. Interferon reduces production of translation inhibitory protein (TIP) in noninfected cells. TIP blocks translation of viral RNA, giving other cells protection against the original virus and other viruses.

✻ Hepatitis D is not greatly affected by antiviral medications, so large doses of interferon may be administered for up to 12 months, which can cause the disease to go into remission. For some patients, a liver transplant will be required.

✻ Hepatitis E usually resolves on its own without medication, and there are no approved hepatitis D or E vaccines available in the United States.

Table 17-7 ■ lists the drugs used in the treatment of the various forms of viral hepatitis. The hepatitis A and B vaccines are further discussed in Chapter 20.

Table 17-7 ■ Drugs Used to Treat Viral Hepatitis

GENERIC NAME	TRADE NAME	AVERAGE ADULT DOSAGE	ROUTE OF ADMINISTRATION
Immunoglobulins			
immunoglobulin (human)	BayGam, Biogam, GamaSTAN S/D	0.01 mL/lb (0.02 mL/kg)	IM
Nucleoside Reverse Transcriptase Inhibitors			
adefovir	Hepsera	10 mg/day	PO
entecavir	Baraclude	0.5 mg/day (taken 2 hours before or after food)	PO
lamivudine	Epivir, Epivir-HBV	100 mg/day	PO
telbivudine	Tyzeka	600 mg/day	PO
tenofovir	Viread	300 mg/day	PO

GENERIC NAME	TRADE NAME	AVERAGE ADULT DOSAGE	ROUTE OF ADMINISTRATION
Antiviral or Antineoplastic Interferons			
interferon alfacon-1	Infergen	9 mcg 3×/week for 24 weeks	SC
interferon alfa-2a	Roferon-A	3 million IU/m², 3×/week for 12 mo.	SC
interferon alfa-2b	Intron A	10 million IU/m², 3×/week for up to 6 mo.	IM or SC
peginterferon alfa-2a	Pegasys	180 mcg/week for 48 weeks	SC
peginterferon alfa-2b	PegIntron	1.5 mcg/kg/week	SC
Combination Antivirals			
dasabuvir/ombitasvir/ paritaprevir/ritonavir	Viekira Pak	2 pink tablets plus 1 beige tablet same time q A.M. with food; 1 beige tablet same time q P.M. with food	PO
interferon alfa-2b/ ribavirin	Rebetron	Interferon alfa-2b 3 million IU 3×/week; ribavirin (either 400 mg a.m. and 600 mg p.m. per day OR 600 mg bid)	SC/PO combination
ledipasvir/sofosbuvir	Harvoni	90 mg ledipasvir; 400 mg sofosbuvir per day	PO
Miscellaneous Antivirals			
sofosbuvir	Solvadi	400 mg per day	PO
Protease Inhibitors			
boceprevir	Victrelis	Four 200-mg capsules tid, with food	PO
simeprevir	Olysio	150 mg per day, with food	PO
telaprevir	Incivek	Three 375-mg tablets bid with food	PO
Anti-infectives/Purine Nucleosides			
ribavirin	Copegus, Rebetol, RibaPak, Ribasphere, RibaTab	800–1200 mg in two doses (based on individual genotype of patient) for 24–48 weeks	PO

IM, intramuscular; PO, oral; SC, subcutaneous; bid, twice a day; tid, three times a day.

✳ Apply Your Knowledge 17.2

The following questions focus on what you have just learned about other antiviral agents, such as those used for cyto-megalovirus, herpes zoster, herpes simplex, influenza, and hepatitis.

CRITICAL THINKING

1. Explain the groups in which cytomegalovirus (CMV) is most prevalent.
2. Identify the symptoms of shingles.
3. Differentiate between the effects of herpes simplex viruses HSV-1 and HSV-2.
4. Identify the most common complication of influenza, and discuss its other complications.
5. Point out the types of viral hepatitis that are most common in HIV patients.

PRACTICAL SCENARIO 1

A 52-year-old woman is diagnosed with hepatitis C. She has worked as a registered nurse for 25 years. The patient has no physical complaints, does not drink alcohol, and does not have an infection with either HIV or hepatitis B. A blood test reveals that her serum transaminases are mildly elevated. An ultrasound of her liver shows no evidence of liver cancer, but a biopsy of her liver revealed moderate fibrosis. Her physician prescribes interferon and three different antivirals. Eight weeks after her therapy begins, she complains of profound fatigue, nausea, and extreme depression.

AZP Worldwide/Shutterstock

Critical Thinking Questions

1. What is the role of interferon in treating hepatitis C?
2. Name antivirals that are used as combination agents to treat hepatitis C.

PRACTICAL SCENARIO 2

A 64-year-old man went to his physician's office complaining of a slight fever, headache, flu-like symptoms, and a burning pain on his neck and chest. Upon examination, a blistering rash was discovered. His physician diagnosed the patient with shingles.

CLS Design/Shutterstock

Critical Thinking Questions

1. What is the cause of shingles?
2. What is the treatment for shingles?
3. What are the complications of shingles?

Chapter Capsule

This section repeats the objectives from the beginning of the chapter and then provides a summary of the most important concepts for that objective. Use this section as a quick review and to check your knowledge.

Objective 1: Describe the structures of viruses.

- Viruses are much smaller than bacteria and contain cores of nucleic acid (deoxyribonucleic acid or ribonucleic acid) that are abbreviated DNA and RNA.
- These cores are surrounded by protein coatings.
- Certain viruses are able to create an additional coating called an envelope, which protects the virus from attack by the immune system.

Objective 2: Explain CD4 cells.

- CD4 cells are a group of helper T-lymphocytes. These cells are affected by, for example, the HIV virus. In fact, when the CD4 T-lymphocyte count falls below 200 cells per milliliter, the HIV-positive individual is classified as having developed AIDS.

Objective 3: Describe the pathophysiology of the human immunodeficiency virus.

- The pathophysiology of HIV requires that the virus must transcribe its RNA into DNA in order to replicate. The enzyme RNA-dependent DNA polymerase (or reverse transcriptase) is needed.
- HIV mostly attacks CD4 T-lymphocytes (helper T-lymphocytes).
- The immune system becomes progressively weaker, and opportunistic infections become more prevalent.
- Once HIV attaches to CD4 proteins on helper T-lymphocyte surfaces, the cells die within about 30 hours. HIV also infects macrophages and microglial cells, which are resistant to HIV, but then act as HIV reservoirs instead of being killed.
- The RNA helps the DNA to be synthesized, and the outer HIV envelope contains glycoproteins that attach to host cells. A small subunit (gp41) then embeds in the viral envelope's lipid bilayer, while remaining attached to a larger subunit (gp120).
- The virus replicates most quickly during the initial stage because no immune response has yet developed.
- Acute retroviral syndrome often results, and HIV plasma levels decline sharply in the next few months, remaining relatively steady when the infection is chronic.
- The patients are often asymptomatic for about 10 years, but then advanced signs and symptoms appear.

Objective 4: Explain how HIV is transmitted.

- The HIV virus is present in all body fluids of infected patients and is transmitted sexually as well as by other methods. It can be transmitted through intimate contact with blood, semen, or vaginal secretions.
- Methods of transmission also include sharing intravenous needles, blood transfusions, accidental needlesticks, and transmission from an infected mother to her fetus, usually in the perinatal period.

Objective 5: List three antiviral drugs for HIV- or AIDS-related secondary viral infections and explain their mechanisms of action.

- Didanosine—enters host cells and is incorporated into growing DNA chains by viral reverse transcriptase, thereby terminating viral replication
- Ganciclovir—after conversion to ganciclovir triphosphate, incorporated into viral DNA, inhibiting viral DNA polymerase and then terminating viral replication
- Zidovudine—mechanism of action similar to didanosine

Objective 6: List the trade names of nucleoside reverse transcriptase inhibitors.

- The trade names of NRTIs include Ziagen, Videx, Videx EC, Emtriva, Epivir, Epivir HBV, Zerit, Viread, and Retrovir.

Objective 7: Identify common adverse effects for lamivudine and stavudine.

- Lamivudine has only minimal adverse effects, including insomnia and headache, which usually subside within a few weeks. It does carry a slight risk of potentially fatal lactic acidosis. If a patient also has HBV, its withdrawal may cause severe acute worsening of hepatitis symptoms.
- Stavudine may cause peripheral neuropathy, which may resolve if it is withdrawn. If this occurs, treatment at a lower dose may be attempted. This drug may also cause pancreatitis, which has been fatal in 1% of cases. The patient also must be monitored for symptoms of pancreatitis and, if present, the drug must be withdrawn. This drug is more likely than other NRTIs to cause lactic acidosis with hepatic steatosis. It has sometimes caused ascending demyelinating polyneuropathy that results in neuromuscular weakness beginning in a few months, but increasing quickly. Serious motor weakness then occurs within days to weeks, possibly requiring mechanical ventilation due to respiratory paralysis. Other adverse effects include hyperlipidemia, insulin resistance/diabetes, and lipoatrophy.

Objective 8: Describe the indications of zidovudine and darunavir.

- Zidovudine is used for patients who have asymptomatic HIV-1 infection and early or late symptomatic HIV disease. It is the drug of choice for prevention of perinatal transfer of HIV during pregnancy. It is used for relieving cognitive symptoms because of its ability to better penetrate to the CNS.
- Darunavir is used for HIV-1 strains that are resistant to other protease inhibitors. It is indicated for HIV-1 infection in adults and children. Darunavir with ritonavir as a booster is very effective in patients who have been previously under treatment for strains of HIV resistance to one or more protease inhibitors.

Objective 9: Identify the actions, indications, and contraindications of ganciclovir.

- After conversion to ganciclovir triphosphate, ganciclovir is incorporated into viral DNA and inhibits viral DNA polymerase. By this action, it can terminate viral replication.
- Ganciclovir is used for prophylaxis and treatment of systemic CMV infections in immunocompromised patients, including HIV-positive and transplant patients. It is also prescribed for CMV retinitis.
- Ganciclovir is contraindicated in patients with hypersensitivity to the drug or to acyclovir (Zovirax). It must be avoided in lactating women. Ganciclovir should be used cautiously in patients with renal impairment, older adults, and pregnant women. Its safety and efficacy in children are not established.

Objective 10: Compare and contrast influenza A and influenza B.

- Influenza A affects humans, pigs, birds, and other animals. It causes moderate to severe illness in all ages. An example is the H1N1 influenza or "swine flu," which was named a pandemic virus in 2009. Otherwise, this form of influenza is not common in the United States.

- Influenza B affects only humans, mostly children. It usually causes less severe illness than Influenza A, is more stable, has less antigenic shift and more immunological stability. Seasonal influenza B is highly common in the United States and its vaccine became available in 2009.

Internet Sites of Interest

- AIDSLINE contains abstracts on AIDS topics compiled by the U.S. National Library of Medicine, arranged by year: **https://aidsinfo.nih.gov/news/311/aidsline**

- Reports and news articles on HIV/AIDS in children around the world is available on the UNICEF website: **www.unicef.org/aids**

- Immunocompromised patients are more prone to infections than other people. For information: **www.cdc.gov/parasites/crypto/gen_info/infect_ic.html**

- The latest news about viral diseases in humans and animals: **www.livescience.com/topics/virus/**

- Basic information about HAART therapy: **www.who.int/topics/antiretroviral_therapy/en/**

- For Antiviral agents go to: **www.aids.gov/hiv-aids-basics/hiv-aids-101/global-statistics/**

- Additional HIV infection statistics: **www.cdc.gov/hiv/statistics/overview/ataglance.html**

Chapter 18

Antifungal Agents

Chapter Objectives

After completing this chapter, you should be able to:

1. Distinguish between superficial and systemic fungal infections.
2. Explain how fungi may gain access to a human host.
3. Describe an opportunistic fungal infection.
4. Identify the risk factors that will most likely cause patients to acquire systemic and serious fungal infections.
5. Distinguish the classifications of antifungal agents.
6. Distinguish the trade names of topical antifungal agents.
7. Describe the adverse effects of amphotericin B.
8. Describe the contraindications of griseofulvin and micafungin.
9. Explain the mechanism of action and indications for ketoconazole.
10. Describe the mechanism of action for sulconazole and terbinafine.

Key Terms

Introduction

Fungi were originally believed to have been primitive plants that lacked chlorophyll. However, today it is understood that fungi are unique spore-producing organisms that include yeasts and molds. They obtain their food by absorbing dissolved organic materials and are composed of one or more cells that contain visible nuclei and organelles. Most healthy human beings are resistant to fungal infections but may become infected when overwhelming numbers of fungi infiltrate their systems. Fungi may enter the body in routes that include the skin, mucous membranes, and respiratory tract. Because of the common use of antibiotics and drugs, such as oral contraceptives, more and more patients are at risk for fungal infections.

Fungal Characteristics

The characteristics of fungi are extremely unique, though like bacteria, they are able to break down complex organic substances. **Fungi** are essential to the recycling of elements such as carbon. They are used as food for other organisms and also in the **fermentation** process of medical substances, industrial substances, and alcohol. Examples of medical substances for which fungi are used include antibiotics and antitoxins. Fungi cause the majority of diseases that affect plants, yet cause very few human diseases. Most cases of fungal diseases in humans occur in immunologically impaired patients.

Fungi grow in single cells (such as **yeasts**) or in colonies (such as **molds**). Fungal infections may affect the skin, nails, hair, and mucous membranes. They may be superficial or life-threatening systemic infections. Systemic fungal infections are serious infections that occur when fungi involve the interior body organs such as the lungs, brain, or gastrointestinal tract. Fungi may be identified by Gram staining. Also, culture and sensitivity tests that follow Gram staining help to determine if specific antibiotics should be prescribed to treat a fungal infection.

Fungal Infections

A *fungus* is a one-celled plant that lacks both color and chlorophyll. The various fungi that can cause human diseases are either mold-like or yeast-like. Molds and yeasts are so widely distributed in air, dust, contaminated objects, and normal flora that humans are constantly being exposed to them. More than 1 million species of fungi have been identified. Only about 20 of these are associated with systemic infections and cause opportunistic infections. Normal healthy individuals are resistant to most fungal infections, called **mycoses** or *mycrotic infections*, and are infected only when faced with overwhelming numbers of the fungi. In other cases, opportunistic pathogens may invade an individual whose natural resistance is low because of other illnesses or even some medications. A mycrotic infection may be superficial, such as when the skin is infected, or life-threatening if it becomes systemic. Superficial fungal infections occur on the skin or nail surfaces or just below them. When fungi are able to enter the interior of the body, a serious systemic infection can develop. This type of infection often affects the brain, gastrointestinal tract, or lungs, and requires lengthy and difficult modes of treatment.

Mycoses involve complex interactions among the portal of entry into the human body, the number of infecting organisms generally required to cause disease, the **virulence** of the fungus, and the host's resistance. Fungi enter the body mainly via respiratory, mucous, and cutaneous routes. In general, the agents of primary mycoses have a respiratory portal (spores inhaled from the air). Subcutaneous agents enter through compromised skin and cutaneous and superficial agents enter through contamination of the skin surface. Spores and yeasts can all be infectious, but spores are most often involved because of their durability and abundance.

The human body is extremely resistant to fungi. Among its numerous antifungal defenses are the normal integrity of the skin, mucous membranes, and respiratory cilia, but the most important defenses are cell-mediated immunity, *phagocytosis* (a process in which cells, called *phagocytes*, consume foreign material), and the inflammatory reaction.

A common opportunistic infection is *candidiasis* (also called *moniliasis* or *thrush*). **Thrush** is a yeast infection in the mouth caused by ***Candida albicans***, a normal resident of the gastrointestinal tract and vagina (Figure 18-1 ■). Thrush can occur during the use of broad-spectrum antibiotics or by the alteration of the environmental conditions in the female reproductive system because of pregnancy or oral contraceptive use. This disease usually results from debilitation (immunosuppression, especially AIDS). Candidiasis also may affect the vulvovaginal area in women, and the mouth, perineum, or all body systems in immunocompromised

Kirkpatrick Charles H Entremed Inc.

Figure 18-1 ■ Oral *Candida albicans*.

patients who have chronic conditions. Those at highest risk for candidal infections include diabetics, pregnant women, females taking oral contraceptives, and patients taking antibiotics or corticosteroids, including postsurgical or posttransplant patients.

The incidence of human fungal infections has increased in recent years because more patients are now at risk for these pathogens. Causes include increased exposure resulting from more frequent surgeries, use of broad-spectrum antimicrobials, immunosuppressive drug therapy for cancer and organ transplantation patients, and HIV.

Antifungal Agents

Antifungal drugs are called *fungicidal* (destroying fungi) or *fungistatic* (slowing fungal multiplication). Many antifungal agents—including amphotericin B, nystatin, voriconazole, micafungin, and ketoconazole—affect the cell membranes of fungi and act in relation to their concentration in body tissues. Fluconazole has fungistatic actions that are believed to deplete *sterols*, which are

substances in fungal cells that are similar to fats. Griseofulvin works by being deposited in keratin precursor cells. As these cells are lost during normal skin shedding, they are then replaced by new cells that are not infected. Flucytosine inhibits DNA and RNA synthesis in fungi.

Antifungal drugs are classified into three categories:

1. Drugs for systemic mycoses (see Table 18-1 ■)
2. Oral drugs for **mucocutaneous** infections
3. Topical drugs for mucocutaneous infections (see Table 18-2 ■)

SYSTEMIC ANTIFUNGALS

The major drugs for systemic mycoses include amphotericin B (Amphocin), caspofungin (Cancidas), fluconazole (Diflucan), flucytosine (Ancobon), griseofulvin (Grifulvin V), itraconazole (Sporanox), ketoconazole (Nizoral), micafungin (Mycamine), nystatin (Nilstat, Nystex), posaconazole (Noxafil), terbinafine (Lamisil), and voriconazole (Vfend).

Table 18-1 ■ Systemic Antifungal Agents

GENERIC NAME	TRADE NAME	AVERAGE ADULT DOSAGE	ROUTE OF ADMINISTRATION
amphotericin B	Amphocin	0.25–1.5 mg/kg/d	IV
caspofungin	Cancidas	70 mg on day 1; then 50 mg/d; infuse doses over 1 h	IV
fluconazole	Diflucan	100–200 mg/d	PO, IV
flucytosine	Ancobon	12.5–37.5 mg/kg q6h	PO
griseofulvin	Grifulvin V	500 mg/d	PO
itraconazole	Sporanox	200 mg/d	PO
ketoconazole	Nizoral	200–400 mg/d	PO
micafungin	Mycamine	10–60 mg/d divided into 2 or 3 doses (highly individualized), 30–45 minutes before meals, taken with at least 8 ounces of water or another fluid	PO
nystatin	Nilstat, Nystex	400,000–600,000 mg qid	PO
posaconazole	Noxafil	IV (initial): 300 mg bid; delayed-release tablet (initial): 300 mg bid; oral suspension (initial): 100 mg (2.5 mL) to 400 mg (10 mL) bid-tid	IV (slow infusion) or PO
terbinafine	Lamisil	250 mg/d for 6–12 weeks	PO
voriconazole	Vfend	IV: 3 mg/kg/hr over 1–2 hours; tablets or suspension: 200 mg q12h	IV (slow infusion) or PO

bid, twice a day; IV, intravenous; PO, oral; qid, four times a day; tid, three times a day.

Focus On

Amphotericin B

Amphotericin B has the widest spectrum of antifungal activity of any systemic antifungal drug.

How does it work?

Most antifungal drugs act by interfering with the synthesis of ergosterol, a chemical found in fungal cell membranes. This results in a change in the permeability of the fungal cell membrane and either slowed growth or destruction of the fungal organism.

How is it used?

Administration of amphotericin B by the intravenous (IV) route is extremely useful for therapy of systemic fungus diseases such as *Candida albicans*. It is also used by nasal spray in the prophylaxis of aspergillosis in immunocompromised patients and orally for treatment of oral candidiasis. This drug is also available in a generic form for topical use.

What are the adverse effects?

Amphotericin B may induce chills and fever, nausea and vomiting, diarrhea, abdominal cramps, dyspepsia, headache, vertigo, thrombophlebitis, anemia, cardiac arrest, and skin rashes. The most serious adverse effect of amphotericin B is renal damage. This drug is also able to cause blood dyscrasias and loss of hearing.

What are the contraindications and interactions?

Amphotericin B is contraindicated in patients hypersensitive to the drug and should be used cautiously in patients with impaired renal function. It interacts with many other drugs, including antineoplastics, cardiac glycosides, corticosteroids, nephrotoxic drugs (including antibiotics and pentamidine), thiazides, and flucytosine (Ancobon); it should not be used with leukocyte transfusions.

What are the important points patients should know?

Inform patients that when given IV, this drug may cause fever, chills, headache, and nausea in the first few hours of therapy, but these adverse reactions usually decrease as therapy continues. Advise patients to notify their physicians if improvement does not occur within 1 to 2 weeks and to report loss of hearing, dizziness, cloudy or pink urine, or greatly increased urination. The treatment of cutaneous infections, such as nail infections, usually requires several months or longer of therapy. Advise patients to wash towels and clothing that were in contact with affected areas after each treatment. Topical cream discolors the skin slightly when rubbed in, and nail lesions may be stained. Instruct patients to drink plenty of fluids.

Focus on Geriatrics

Amphotericin B and Kidney Damage

Amphotericin B is a very toxic agent that in most cases should be administered intravenously. Elderly patients who use this drug must be very careful because kidney damage is the most serious toxic effect of amphotericin B. Older adults who have renal impairment must be tested for creatinine clearance.

Focus on Natural Products

Interactions Between Gossypol and Amphotericin B

The herb gossypol, which is derived from cottonseed oil, may be used to treat endometriosis in women. It may also be used by men and women to prevent pregnancy. Gossypol used with amphotericin B may increase the risk of renal toxicity.

Focus On

Caspofungin

Caspofungin is an antifungal medication used to treat a variety of serious internal fungal infections and is often used in patients who cannot use or do not respond to other antifungals. It is administered intravenously via slow infusion, which can take at least 1 hour to complete.

How does it work?

Caspofungin works by stopping the growth of fungi. It inhibits synthesis of essential components of the cell walls.

How is it used?

Caspofungin is used to treat fungal infections of the esophagus, lungs, stomach, and other internal body areas. It is usually administered for at least 14 days.

What are the adverse effects?

Caspofungin may cause rash, facial swelling, itching, sensation of warmth, bronchospasm, and anaphylaxis.

What are the contraindications and interactions?

Caspofungin is contraindicated in patients with hypersensitivity to any component of this drug. It may interact with tacrolimus, cyclosporine, rifampin, and drugs that induce drug clearance, which include efavirenz, nevirapine, phenytoin, dexamethasone, and carbamazepine.

What are the important points patients should know?

The patient taking caspofungin should be instructed to inform the physician about any medical conditions, medications, and allergies. He or she should also be instructed to inform the physician of any severe or unusual adverse effects.

Fluconazole

Fluconazole is used to treat and prevent many fungal and yeast infections. It is an azole antifungal.

How does it work?

Fluconazole works by stopping the growth of certain types of fungi. It interacts with enzymes that are essential fungal cell membrane components, inhibiting their synthesis.

How is it used?

Fluconazole is administered orally, with or without food as directed, usually once per day. Dosage is based on the medical condition and the response to treatment. Fluconazole is indicated for the treatment of vaginal candidiasis, oropharyngeal and esophageal candidiasis, and cryptococcal meningitis. Intravenous injection is used for systemic infection such as cryptococcal meningitis, because it has good central nervous system (CNS) penetration.

What are the adverse effects?

Fluconazole may cause headache, nausea and vomiting, abdominal pain, diarrhea, dyspepsia, dizziness, taste sensation changes, angioedema, anaphylaxis, and skin rash. Rarely, hepatobiliary reactions have occurred, including mild transient elevations in transaminases, hepatitis, cholestasis, and fulminant hepatic failure, which have caused death.

What are the contraindications and interactions?

Fluconazole is contraindicated in hypersensitivity to this drug or its components, coadministration of terfenadine, cisapride, astemizole, erythromycin, pimozide, and quinidine. Many drugs interact with fluconazole, including oral hypoglycemics, coumarin-type anticoagulants, phenytoin, cyclosporine, rifampin, theophylline, rifabutin, voriconazole, tacrolimus, short-acting benzodiazepines, tofacitinib, triazolam, oral contraceptives, hydrochlorothiazide, alfentanil, amitriptyline, nortriptyline, amphotericin B, azithromycin, carbamazepine, calcium channel blockers, celecoxib, cyclophosphamide, fentanyl, halofantrine, HMG-CoA reductase inhibitors, losartan, methadone, NSAIDs, prednisone, saquinavir, sirolimus, vinca alkaloids, vitamin A, and zidovudine.

What are the important points patients should know?

If taking the liquid suspension form of fluconazole, the patient must shake the bottle well before each dose and carefully measure the dose using a special measuring device. Household spoons should never be used for this purpose. It is important to take fluconazole at the same time every day.

Flucytosine

Flucytosine is an antifungal agent used for a wide variety of severe fungal infections.

How does it work?

Flucytosine is converted in the fungus to 5-fluorouracil, which is incorporated into RNA and interferes with normal protein synthesis.

How is it used?

Certain fungal organisms are more sensitive to interference from the drug than are human cells, so flucytosine is useful in the treatment of some fungal infections. It is the drug of choice to treat **chromomycosis** and of second choice to treat systemic candidiasis. It may be combined with amphotericin B for first-choice treatment of **aspergillosis** or **cryptococcosis** (a fungal disease of the lungs), especially in patients with meningitis.

What are the adverse effects?

Flucytosine commonly causes nausea and vomiting, diarrhea, and skin rashes. Bone marrow suppression, manifest by anemia, leukopenia, and thrombocytopenia, has been reported. Sedation, confusion, hallucinations, headache, and vertigo occur infrequently.

What are the contraindications and interactions?

Flucytosine is contraindicated in patients who are hypersensitive to the drug and should be used with extreme caution in patients who have impaired hepatic or renal function or who have bone marrow suppression. It interacts with amphotericin B, causing synergistic effects and increasing toxicity.

What are the important points patients should know?

Instruct patients to report fever, sore mouth or throat, and a tendency for unusual bleeding or bruising to their physicians. They must be aware that the general duration of therapy is 4–6 weeks, but it may need to be continued for several months. Instruct patients not to breastfeed while taking this drug without consulting their physician.

Griseofulvin

Griseofulvin is an effective agent in the treatment of superficial fungal infections.

How does it work?

Griseofulvin is fungistatic and not **fungicidal** (having a killing action on fungi). Its action involves deposition in newly formed skin and nail beds, where it binds to keratin, protecting these sites from new infection.

How is it used?

Griseofulvin is used systemically and is highly effective in the management of **dermatophyte** infections of the skin, hair, and nails. Dermatophytoses require keratin for nutrition and live on the top layer of the epidermis. Because it does not kill, but only arrests reproduction of the organism, it is necessary to continue medication for three months or longer. This allows the entire epidermis to be replaced, thereby removing reinfecting organisms.

What are the adverse effects?

Griseofulvin may cause hypersensitivity, skin rashes, pruritus, serum sickness, severe headache, insomnia, fatigue, mental confusion, psychotic symptoms, and vertigo. This agent also causes heartburn, nausea and vomiting, diarrhea, flatulence, dry mouth, and unpleasant taste sensations. Nephrotoxicity and hepatotoxicity may occur.

What are the contraindications and interactions?

Griseofulvin is contraindicated in patients with **porphyria** or liver disease. Safe use of this drug during pregnancy, lactation, or in children younger than 2 years has not been established.

Griseofulvin with alcohol may cause flushing and tachycardia. Barbiturates may decrease hypoprothrombinemic effects of oral anticoagulants. Griseofulvin may increase estrogen metabolism and decrease contraceptive efficacy of oral contraceptives.

What are the important points patients should know?

Advise patients to continue treatment as prescribed to prevent relapse. Instruct them to avoid exposure to intense natural or artificial sunlight because photosensitivity reactions may occur. Advise women to not breastfeed while taking this drug without consulting their physician.

Focus Point

Onychomycosis

Onychomycosis is a chronic fungal disease of the nails. It is also known as *tinea unguium*. The nails thicken, discolor, disfigure, and split. Without treatment, the nails can become so thick that they press against the insides of gloves or shoes, causing pressure, irritation, and pain. About 50% of all nail disorders are caused by onychomycosis, which is the most common nail disease in adults. Toenails are much more likely to be infected than fingernails, and incidence of onychomycosis has been increasing. This disease is associated with diabetes, a suppressed immune system, warmer climates, and increasing age. Older adults are most commonly affected.

Focus On

Itraconazole

Itraconazole is an azole antifungal that is used for many fungal infections. It carries a black box warning related to potential congestive heart failure, cardiac effects, and drug interactions.

How does it work?

Like other azole antifungals, itraconazole inhibits fungal-mediated synthesis of **ergosterol**. However, it is the only drug in its class that inhibits both the hedgehog signaling pathway and angiogenesis.

How is it used?

Itraconazole has a broader spectrum of activity than fluconazole, but not as broad as posaconazole or voriconazole. It is particularly effective against *Aspergillus* and is used to treat **blastomycosis**, **histoplasmosis**, and **sporotrichosis**, as well as many systemic infections when other antifungals are ineffective or inappropriate.

What are the adverse effects?

Itraconazole may cause elevated alanine aminotransferase levels, congestive heart failure, liver failure that may be potentially fatal, nausea and vomiting, abdominal pain, fatigue, anorexia, jaundice, itching, dark urine, pale stools, and headache.

What are the contraindications and interactions?

Itraconazole is contraindicated with chronic obstructive lung disease; numbness, tingling, or pain in the hands or feet; hearing loss; inadequate blood flow to the heart muscle, heart valve disease, or chronic heart failure; absence of or decreased stomach acid; kidney disease; visible water retention; abnormal liver function tests; and hypersensitivity. The most serious drug interactions with itraconazole include fluticasone, salmeterol, acetaminophen, hydrocodone, guaifenesin, chlorpheniramine, pseudoephedrine, fentanyl, emtricitabine, lopinavir, ritonavir, tenofovir, caffeine, phenylephrine, oxycodone, nifedipine, lovastatin, niacin, and many others.

What are the important points patients should know?

Patients must be instructed not to take itraconazole if they have had heart failure, including congestive heart failure, or if they are taking certain medications. They also must be instructed to tell their physician if they have had lung, liver, kidney, or other serious health problems.

Ketoconazole

Ketoconazole is an antifungal used to treat many varieties of candidiasis infections as well as **coccidioidomycosis**, blastomycosis, histoplasmosis, chromomycosis, paracoccidioidomycosis, and severe cutaneous dermatophyte infections that resist griseofulvin therapy.

How does it work?

Ketoconazole blocks the fungal synthesis of ergosterol, which is essential to the integrity of the cell membranes of nearly all pathogenic fungi.

How is it used?

Ketoconazole has a broad spectrum of antifungal activity. This drug, or amphotericin B, is the drug of choice for the treatment of blastomycosis, coccidioidomycosis, and histoplasmosis. It is an alternative drug for candidiasis. Successful treatment sometimes requires months.

What are the adverse effects?

The most common adverse effects of ketoconazole include nausea and vomiting, diarrhea, pruritus (severe itching), abdominal cramps, headache, **photophobia**, fever, and **impotence**.

What are the contraindications and interactions?

Ketoconazole should not be used in patients with hypersensitivity to this drug or in patients with chronic alcoholism or fungal meningitis. Safety during pregnancy and lactation and in children younger than 2 years has not been established. Ketoconazole should be used cautiously in patients with a history of liver disease or with HIV infection.

Cimetidine inhibits and rifampin induces the metabolism of ketoconazole. Rifampin decreases the biosynthesis of androgens and estrogens.

What are the important points patients should know?

Instruct patients to promptly report the signs and symptoms of hepatotoxicity to their physician. Advise them to avoid over-the-counter drugs for gastric distress (such as Rolaids, Tums, and Alka-Seltzer) and to check with their physicians before taking any other nonprescription medications. Tell patients to not alter the dose or dose interval before consulting their physician.

Micafungin

Micafungin is classified as an **echinocandin**. It treats severe *Candida* fungal infections.

How does it work?

Micafungin stops the growth of fungus. It affects enzymes in the fungal cell wall and causes cellular contents to leak out, resulting in cellular death.

How is it used?

Micafungin is injected intravenously, usually once per day, with slow infusion that takes about 1 hour. Dosage and length of treatment are based on the medical condition and response to treatment.

What are the adverse effects?

Micafungin may cause nausea and vomiting, diarrhea, headache, insomnia, and irritation at the site of injection, as well as less common adverse effects.

What are the contraindications and interactions?

Micafungin is contraindicated in hypersensitivity to the drug or its components, as well as hypersensitivity to other echinocandins. Drug interactions with micafungin include sirolimus, itraconazole, and nifedipine.

What are the important points patients should know?

Patients must not be given micafungin if they have liver or kidney disease or if they may be allergic to any of the components of the drug.

Nystatin

Nystatin is an antifungal that is available for oral and topical administration, with activity against many species of yeast and *Candida albicans*. Nystatin is not absorbed through the stomach and has not been linked to drug-induced liver injury.

How does it work?

Nystatin binds to sterols in the plasma membranes of fungi, causing their contents to leak outward, resulting in cell death.

(*continued*)

Focus On (*continued*)

How is it used?

Nystatin is used orally to treat thrush as well as *Candida* infections of the mouth, skin, nails, vagina, stomach, or intestines.

What are the adverse effects?

Nystatin may cause hypersensitivity reactions and nausea, vomiting, diarrhea, and other less common effects.

What are the contraindications and interactions?

Nystatin is contraindicated with hypersensitivity to the drug or any of its components. It has no reported drug interactions.

What are the important points patients should know?

Patients should be instructed to take all of the prescribed nystatin even if their symptoms begin to improve. The entire drug regimen is necessary to eradicate the fungal infection fully.

Posaconazole

Posaconazole is an azole antifungal agent that is available as a concentrated solution to be diluted before IV administration, as a delayed-release tablet, or as an oral suspension.

How does it work?

Posaconazole blocks synthesis of ergosterol in the fungal cell membrane, weakening its structure and function.

How is it used?

Posaconazole is used to treat invasive *Aspergillus* and *Candida* infections in patients at high risk of developing these infections because of being severely immunocompromised.

What are the adverse effects?

Posaconazole may cause hypersensitivity reactions, arrhythmias, QT interval prolongation, and hepatic toxicity.

What are the contraindications and interactions?

Posaconazole is contraindicated in hypersensitivity to this drug or any of its components and concomitant use of sirolimus, pimozide, quinidine, atorvastatin, lovastatin, simvastatin, ergotamine, and dihydroergotamine. It may also interact with tacrolimus, cyclosporine, alprazolam, triazolam, efavirenz, ritonavir, atazanavir, fosamprenavir, rifabutin, phenytoin, cimetidine, esomeprazole, vincristine, vinblastine, verapamil, diltiazem, nifedipine, nicardipine, felodipine, digoxin, metoclopramide, and glipizide.

What are the important points patients should know?

Patients must be instructed not to use posaconazole if they are allergic to this drug or similar antifungals, including clotrimazole, fluconazole, itraconazole, ketoconazole, miconazole, or voriconazole. They also must be instructed to take posaconazole for the prescribed length of time in order to completely treat the infection. If chronic vomiting or diarrhea occurs, the patient must notify his or her physician.

Terbinafine hydrochloride

Terbinafine hydrochloride is an allylamine antifungal agent that is fungicidal. It is structurally and pharmacologically related to naftifine.

How does it work?

Terbinafine is fungicidal against certain types of fungi. It works by inhibiting biosynthesis of ergosterol, causing cell death.

How is it used?

When used systemically, terbinafine is indicated for the treatment of onychomycosis of the nails due to dermatophytes.

What are the adverse effects?

Terbinafine may cause nasopharyngitis, headache, pyrexia, coughing, nausea and vomiting, upper respiratory tract infection, abdominal pain, diarrhea, influenza, pharyngolaryngeal pain, rash, rhinorrhea, nasal congestion, pruritus, and toothache.

What are the contraindications and interactions?

Terbinafine is contraindicated if there is hypersensitivity, due to risk of anaphylaxis. It may interact with tricyclic antidepressants, selective serotonin reuptake inhibitors, beta-blockers, flecainide, propafenone, monoamine oxidase inhibitors Type B, dextromethorphan, caffeine, cyclosporine, fluconazole, ketoconazole, amiodarone, rifampin, and cimetidine.

What are the important points patients should know?

Patients must tell their physician about liver or kidney disease, or autoimmune disorders, before taking terbinafine. This medication must be taken for the prescribed length of time. If any symptoms of liver damage develop, the patient must call his or her physician immediately. These symptoms include nausea, upper stomach pain, itching, anorexia, dark urine, clay-colored stools, and jaundice. The patient should be informed of the need to have regular blood and liver function tests while taking terbinafine.

- -

Voriconazole

Voriconazole is an azole antifungal that may be administered in a variety of ways. It usually works equally well in patients who do not have other conditions and in patients who are at risk of aspergillosis, such as those with malignant neoplasms of the lymphatic or hematopoietic tissues.

How does it work?

Voriconazole inhibits sterols used for fungal biosynthesis, damaging cell walls and resulting in death of the fungus.

How is it used?

Voriconazole is used for invasive aspergillosis, **candidemia** in non-neutropenic patients, and *Candida* infections of the skin, abdomen, kidneys, bladder, and various types of wounds. It is also used for esophageal Candidiasis.

What are the adverse effects?

Voriconazole may cause visual disturbances, fever, nausea and vomiting, rash, chills, headache, liver function changes, tachycardia, and hallucinations.

What are the contraindications and interactions?

Voriconazole is contraindicated with known hypersensitivity and concurrent use of terfenadine, astemizole, cisapride, pimozide, quinidine, sirolimus, rifampin, carbamazepine, long-acting barbiturates, efavirenz, ritonavir, rifabutin, ergotamine, dihydroergotamine, and St. John's wort. Drug interactions with voriconazole include phenytoin, oral contraceptives containing ethinyl estradiol and norethindrone, fluconazole, HIV protease inhibitors, NNRTIs, cyclosporine, methadone, fentanyl, alfentanil, oxycodone, NSAIDs, tacrolimus, warfarin, omeprazole, HMG-CoA reductase inhibitors, dihydropyridine calcium channel blockers, sulfonylurea oral hypoglycemics, vinca alkaloids, and everolimus.

What are the important points patients should know?

Female patients must not be given voriconazole while pregnant, since this drug has teratogenic effects. The patient must tell his or her physician about all other medications being used, including over-the-counter medications. The patient must discuss any heart rhythm problems, electrolyte imbalances, liver or kidney disease, or a history of allergy to other antifungal medications. The patient must be instructed to take voriconazole for the prescribed length of time, and should also be instructed that use of this drug for more than 28 days may require an eye examination because of potential vision problems.

TOPICAL ANTIFUNGALS

The topical forms of nystatin (e.g., Mycostatin) are used for local *C. albicans* infections of the skin. Overall, the "azole" antifungals are the most commonly prescribed antifungals in the United States. Other commonly used topical antifungals include butenafine (e.g., Mentax), ciclopirox (Loprox, Penlac), clotrimazole (Lotrimin), econazole (Econazole Nitrate Cream), miconazole (e.g., Monistat-Derm), naftifine (Naftin), oxiconazole (Oxistat), sulconazole (Exelderm), terbinafine (Lamisil Topical), terconazole (Terazol), tioconazole (Monistat), and tolnaftate (Tinactin). The topical antifungals are listed in Table 18-2 ■.

Table 18-2 ■ **Topical Antifungal Drugs**

GENERIC NAME	TRADE NAME	USAGE INSTRUCTIONS	TYPE OF TOPICAL AGENT
butenafine	e.g., Mentax	Apply a thin layer to and around the affected area and gently rub in, usually 1–2 times/d	Cream
ciclopirox	Loprox, Penlac	Massage into affected area and surrounding skin in the morning and evening	Lotion, gel/jelly, cream, suspension, shampoo, solution, powder
clotrimazole	Lotrimin	Apply small amount to affected areas in the morning and evening	Lotion, solution, cream
econazole	Econazole Nitrate Cream	Apply sufficient amount to affected areas in the morning and evening	Cream, foam, solution, powder
miconazole	e.g., Monistat-Derm	Apply to affected area, usually twice per day	Lotion, effervescent tablet, cream, ointment, powder, tincture, gel/jelly, spray, vaginal cream, vaginal suppository, tampon
naftifine	Naftin	Apply 1–2 times/d; may use up to 4 wk	Cream, gel/jelly
nystatin	e.g., Mycostatin	100,000 units (1 g) on affected area bid-tid for at least 2 weeks	Cream, ointment, powder
oxiconazole	Oxistat	Apply to affected area once daily in the evening	Lotion, cream
sulconazole	Exelderm	Massage a small amount into affected and surrounding areas 1–2 times/d	Cream, solution
terbinafine	Lamisil Topical	Cream: apply a thin layer on and around affected area, usually 1–2 times/d; Solution: apply enough medication to wet the skin on and around affected area, usually 1–2 times/d	Cream, solution
terconazole	Terazol	Apply once/d at bedtime for 3–7 days per physician instructions	Vaginal cream, vaginal suppository
tioconazole	Monistat	Apply 1–2 times/d as directed for 2–4 weeks	Cream, lotion, spray, powder
tolnaftate	Tinactin	Apply to affected skin, usually 1–2 times/d as directed	Ointment, spray, cream, lotion, gel/jelly, powder, solution

Focus on Pediatrics

Thrush in Babies

In babies, thrush causes difficulty in breastfeeding and chronic diaper rash. Oral thrush (white patches in the mouth or throat) in babies may infect the nipples of the mother, causing drying or cracking.

Focus On

Butenafine

Butenafine is a synthetic antifungal agent and is classified as a benzylamine. It is structurally related to the allylamines.

How does it work?

The mechanism of action of butenafine is not fully understood. It appears to prevent the growth of fungus by affecting the sterols in the fungal membrane, causing damage and cell death.

How is it used?

Butenafine is used for skin infections, which include **tinea versicolor (pityriasis)**, **tinea pedis (athlete's foot)**, **tinea corporis (ringworm)**, and **tinea cruris (jock itch)**.

What are the adverse effects?

Butenafine may cause burning, stinging, itching, and worsening of the fungal infection, but all adverse effects are usually mild. Additional adverse effects may include contact dermatitis, erythema, and irritation.

What are the contraindications and interactions?

Butenafine is contraindicated with hypersensitivity to this drug or any of its components. There has been no systematic evaluation of drug interactions with butenafine.

What are the important points patients should know?

The patient must be instructed to use butenafine for the prescribed amount of time and not to use bandages or dressings that do not allow air to circulate to the affected area. The patient must also be instructed to wear loose-fitting clothing, preferably made of cotton, and to avoid getting the medication in the eyes, nose, or mouth. The patient must not skip doses.

Ciclopirox

Ciclopirox is a synthetic antifungal that is available in a variety of different topical formulations.

How does it work?

Ciclopirox works by *chelation*, which inhibits enzymes responsible for degradation of peroxides within the fungal cell.

How is it used?

Ciclopirox is intended for topical dermatologic use only. It is used to treat superficial dermatophyte infections as well as **seborrheic dermatitis**.

What are the adverse effects?

Ciclopirox may cause burning, contact dermatitis, itching, dry skin, acne, rash, hair loss, pain upon application, eye pain, and facial edema.

What are the contraindications and interactions?

Ciclopirox is contraindicated with hypersensitivity to this drug or its components. There are no known drug interactions with ciclopirox.

What are the important points patients should know?

The patient should be instructed to rinse the eyes, nose, or mouth with water if ciclopirox accidentally gets into these areas. The patient should also be instructed not to use bandages or dressings that do not allow air to circulate and to wear loose-fitting clothing. The patient must use ciclopirox for the prescribed length of time and not skip doses.

(continued)

Focus On (*continued*)

....

Clotrimazole

Clotrimazole is a synthetic antifungal agent with broad-spectrum effects against many skin infections.

How does it work?

Clotrimazole's primary mechanism of action is against fungi that are actively dividing and growing. It has both fungistatic and fungicidal activity and breaks down the fungal cell walls, causing cell death very quickly.

How is it used?

Clotrimazole is indicated for the treatment of candidiasis due to *Candida albicans* and tinea versicolor due to *Malassezia furfur*.

What are the adverse effects?

Clotrimazole may cause erythema, stinging, blistering, peeling, edema, itching, urticaria, burning, and general skin irritation.

What are the contraindications and interactions?

Clotrimazole is contraindicated with hypersensitivity to this drug or its components. There are no known drug interactions.

What are the important points patients should know?

Patients must be instructed to use clotrimazole for the prescribed amount of time, even though symptoms may begin to improve. This will ensure complete healing of the fungal infection.

....

Econazole

Econazole is a topical antifungal that exhibits extremely low systemic absorption. Most of the applied drug remains on the skin surface.

How does it work?

Econazole has broad-spectrum antifungal activity against many fungi, including **Epidermophyton floccosum**, *Microsporum* species, *Trichophyton* species, *Candida* species, and **Malassezia furfur**.

How is it used?

Econazole is used to treat tinea pedis, tinea cruris, tinea corporis, cutaneous candidiasis, and tinea versicolor.

What are the adverse effects?

Econazole may cause burning, itching, stinging, erythema, and an itchy rash. These effects were only seen in less than 5% of clinical trials.

What are the contraindications and interactions?

Econazole is contraindicated with hypersensitivity to this drug or its components. There are no known drug interactions.

What are the important points patients should know?

The patient should be instructed to use econazole for the prescribed amount of time, not to use bandages or dressings that do not allow air to circulate to the affected area, wear loose-fitting clothing (preferably cotton), and avoid getting the medication into the eyes, nose, or mouth.

....

Miconazole

Miconazole is a synthetic azole antifungal that is available in a large variety of different formulations.

How does it work?

Miconazole inhibits the growth of many common dermatophytes, yeast-like fungi, and *Malassezia furfur*, which causes tinea versicolor. It affects the cell walls of the fungi.

How is it used?

Miconazole is used to treat athlete's foot, jock itch, tinea corporis, cutaneous candidiasis (moniliasis), and tinea versicolor.

What are the adverse effects?

Miconazole has only caused isolated cases of irritation, burning, maceration (softening and breaking-down of skin), and allergic contact dermatitis.

What are the contraindications and interactions?

Miconazole has no known contraindications or interactions.

What are the important points patients should know?

The patient should be instructed to use miconazole for the prescribed amount of time in order to fully eradicate the infection. The patient should not use bandages or dressings that do not allow air to circulate and should wear loose-fitting clothing, preferably made of cotton. The patient should also avoid getting miconazole into the eyes, nose, or mouth.

Naftifine

Naftifine is a synthetic allylamine antifungal agent that is available in several different topical formulations.

How does it work?

Naftifine penetrates the stratum corneum of the skin to inhibit the growth of dermatophytes by interfering with sterol biosynthesis and harming fungal cells.

How is it used?

Naftifine is used to treat athlete's foot, whether it is caused by **Trichophyton rubrum**, **Trichophyton mentagrophytes**, or *Epidermophyton floccosum*.

What are the adverse effects?

Naftifine may cause application site reactions, blisters, burning, crusting, dryness, erythema, inflammation, irritation, softening and breakdown of skin, pain, itching, rash, and swelling. Fortunately, all of these adverse effects are usually mild.

What are the contraindications and interactions?

Naftifine has no known contraindications or interactions.

What are the important points patients should know?

The patient should be instructed to use naftifine for the prescribed amount of time, to not use bandages or dressings that do not allow air to circulate to the affected area, and to wear loose-fitting clothing, preferable made of cotton. The patient must avoid getting naftifine into the eyes, nose, or mouth.

Oxiconazole

Oxiconazole is a derivate of imidazole that is active against *Epidermophyton*, *Tricophyton*, and *Malassezia* species.

How does it work?

Oxiconazole works by inhibiting ergosterol biosynthesis and degrading fungal cell membranes, which results in its antifungal properties.

How is it used?

Oxiconazole is used to treat athlete's foot, jock itch, tinea corporis, and tinea versicolor. It is effective against several different causative microorganisms.

What are the adverse effects?

Oxiconazole may cause itching, burning, irritation, allergic contact dermatitis, folliculitis, erythema, papules, fissures, skin softening and degradation, rash, stinging, nodules, scaling, tingling, pain, and **dyshidrotic eczema**.

What are the contraindications and interactions?

Oxiconazole is contraindicated with hypersensitivity to this drug or its components. There has been no systematic evaluation of any drug interactions.

What are the important points patients should know?

The patient should be instructed to use oxiconazole for the prescribed amount of time, to not use bandages or dressings that do not allow air to circulate to the affected area, and to wear loose-fitting clothing, preferably made of cotton. The patient must avoid getting oxiconazole into the eyes, nose, or mouth.

(continued)

Focus On (continued)

Sulconazole

Sulconazole is a broad-spectrum antifungal agent that inhibits growth of many types of fungi.

How does it work?

Sulconazole works by affecting components of fungal cell walls, slowing their activities, and also affects certain Gram-positive bacteria.

How is it used?

Sulconazole is used to treat jock itch and tinea corporis caused by *Trichophyton rubrum*, *Trichophyton mentagrophytes*, *Epidermophyton floccosum*, and *Microsporum canis*. It is also used to treat tinea versicolor. However, it has not been proven effective against athlete's foot.

What are the adverse effects?

Very few adverse effects have been reported with sulconazole. The only reported effects are mild itching, burning, and stinging.

What are the contraindications and interactions?

Sulconazole is contraindicated with hypersensitivity to this drug or its components. There are no known drug interactions.

What are the important points patients should know?

The patient should be instructed to use sulconazole for the prescribed amount of time, to not use bandages or dressings that do not allow air to circulate to the affected area, and to wear loose-fitting clothing, preferably made of cotton. The patient must avoid getting sulconazole into the eyes, nose, or mouth.

Terbinafine

Terbinafine is a synthetic allylamine antifungal agent that also has systemic uses, which were previously discussed in this chapter.

How does it work?

Terbinafine works by inhibiting biosynthesis of ergosterol in the fungal cell membrane, leading to fungal cell death.

How is it used?

Terbinafine is used to treat onychomycosis of the toenails or fingernails that are caused by dermatophytes, also known as *tinea unguium*.

What are the adverse effects?

Terbinafine may cause rash, urticaria, itching, blisters, erythema, skin peeling, skin dryness, and other signs of irritation.

What are the contraindications and interactions?

Terbinafine is contraindicated in patients with a history of allergy. There are no known drug interactions.

What are the important points patients should know?

The patient should be instructed to wash and dry the affected area before applying terbinafine and to use the medication for the entire prescribed amount of time. After applying this drug, the patient must wash the hands carefully and avoid getting it into the eyes, nose, or mouth.

Terconazole

Terconazole is a vaginally applied antifungal that is available in a variety of formulations.

How does it work?

While not fully understood, terconazole appears to break down fungal cell wall permeability, leading to disruption of fungal cell processes.

How is it used?

Terconazole is used only for the local treatment of vulvovaginal candidiasis (moniliasis), once diagnosis is confirmed by smears or cultures.

What are the adverse effects?

Terconazole, based on the type of formulation, may cause headache or other body pain, burning, itching, irritation, fever, chills, and dysmenorrhea.

What are the contraindications and interactions?

Terconazole is contraindicated with hypersensitivity to this drug or its components. There are no significant drug interactions.

What are the important points patients should know?

The patient should be instructed to use terconazole for the prescribed amount of time and not to skip doses. Patients should avoid any tight clothing that does not allow good air flow to the affected area. If terconazole gets into the eyes, nose, or mouth, these areas should be rinsed thoroughly with water.

- -

Tioconazole

Tioconazole is a broad-spectrum antifungal agent that inhibits the growth of pathogenic yeasts. It has fungicidal activity in vitro against *Candida albicans*, other *Candida* species, and against *Torulopsis glabrata*.

How does it work?

Tioconazole works by disrupting normal fungal cell membrane permeability, causing leakage of contents and cell death.

How is it used?

Tioconazole is used for the local treatment of moniliasis after this infection is confirmed by smears or cultures.

What are the adverse effects?

Tioconazole may cause burning, itching, irritation, discharge, vulvar edema and swelling, vaginal pain, dysuria, nocturia, dyspareunia, dryness of vaginal secretions, and skin shedding.

What are the contraindications and interactions?

Tioconazole is contraindicated with hypersensitivity to this drug or other imidazole antifungals, as well as any of the contained components. Tioconazole may interact with progesterone-based agents.

What are the important points patients should know?

Patients must be instructed to use tioconazole for the full amount of time prescribed, to avoid wearing tight-fitting, synthetic clothing that does not allow air circulation, and to instead wear loose-fitting clothing that is made of cotton or other natural fibers. The patient must avoid getting tioconazole into the eyes, nose, or mouth.

- -

Tolnaftate

Tolnaftate is a topical antifungal that is used for a variety of fungal infections, effectively blocking fungal growth.

How does it work?

Tolnaftate is believed to inhibit an enzyme required for biosynthesis of ergosterol in the fungal membrane, causing permeability and ultimately, cell death.

How is it used?

Tolnaftate is indicated for athlete's foot, jock itch, tinea corporis, and tinea versicolor. It is not the preferred drug for tinea versicolor, however.

What are the adverse effects?

Tolnaftate may cause skin irritation and a temporary stinging sensation. In general, these adverse effects are mild.

What are the contraindications and interactions?

Tolnaftate is contraindicated with hypersensitivity to this drug or any of its components. There have been no formal drug interaction studies performed.

What are the important points patients should know?

The patient must be instructed to complete the full course of treatment, contact the physician if improvement does not occur by the end of treatment, and also contact the physician if irritation, blisters, swelling, or oozing occurs. The patient must apply tolnaftate to affected areas as directed and avoid contact with the eyes, nose, mouth, or other body openings.

✳ Apply Your **Knowledge** 18.1

The following exercises focus on what you have just learned about antifungal agents.

CRITICAL THINKING

1. Describe how fungi enter the body and cause infection.
2. Compare molds with yeasts.
3. Explain mycoses and how they may cause disease.
4. Describe moniliasis and describe why it occurs.
5. Identify the classifications of antifungal agents.
6. Give the trade names of amphotericin B, fluconazole, ketoconazole, and clotrimazole.
7. Point out the indications of amphotericin B.
8. Explain the mechanism of action for griseofulvin.

Focus Point

Fungal Superinfections

Usually occurring in the anal and genital areas or in the vagina or mouth, fungal superinfections cause anal or vaginal itching, vaginal discharge, and lesions on the tongue or mouth. A common type of fungal superinfection is known as *candidiasis* or *moniliasis*. This superinfection may occur because of an overgrowth of yeast-like fungi in the vagina. Normally, multiplication of these microorganisms is controlled because of a strain of vaginal bacteria known as *Doderlein bacillus*. Penicillin therapy may destroy these bacteria, causing the fungi to multiply at a rapid rate. Symptoms include vaginal discharge and itching.

PRACTICAL SCENARIO 1

A 62-year-old woman with lung cancer is exhibiting symptoms of an infection. She is admitted to her local hospital and, after testing, her physician diagnoses her as having aspergillosis, a fungal disease of the lungs. He prescribes amphotericin B by intravenous injection.

Michal Heron/Pearson Education/PH College

Critical Thinking Questions

1. The patient asks the nurse what adverse effects she can expect from the drug. What would be the appropriate answer for the nurse to give the patient?
2. Can you think of any adverse reactions the nurse needs to monitor this patient for?
3. What patient education should the nurse provide?

PRACTICAL SCENARIO 2

A 46-year-old woman who lives in Florida visits her dermatologist because her fingernails have become brittle, yellowed, cracked, visibly thickened, and are beginning to pull away from the actual nail beds. The dermatologist takes a sample from under one of her nails, which results in diagnosis of onychomycosis. The dermatologist prescribes griseofulvin tablets for 3 months.

Critical Thinking Questions

1. What is the mechanism of action of griseofulvin?
2. What are the serious adverse effects of griseofulvin?
3. What advice should the nurse give to this patient while she is taking griseofulvin?

Chapter Capsule

This section repeats the objectives from the beginning of the chapter and then provides a summary of the most important concepts for that objective. Use this section as a quick review and to check your knowledge.

Objective 1: Distinguish between superficial and systemic fungal infections.

■ Superficial fungal infections may affect the skin, nails, hair, and mucous membranes.

■ Systemic fungal infections are serious infections that occur when fungi involve the interior body organs such as the lungs, brain, or gastrointestinal tract.

Objective 2: Explain how fungi may gain access to a human host.

■ Respiratory route

■ Mucous membrane route

■ Cutaneous route

Objective 3: Describe an opportunistic fungal infection.

■ Candidiasis is an opportunistic fungal infection that is also called moniliasis or thrush

❑ Thrush is a yeast infection in the mouth caused by *Candida albicans*

❑ It can occur during use of broad-spectrum antibiotics or by alteration of environmental conditions in the female reproductive system

❑ Usually results from debilitation (immunosuppression, especially AIDS)

■ Candidiasis may also affect the vulvovaginal area and the mouth, perineum, or all body systems in immunocompromised patients who have chronic conditions

Objective 4: Identify the risk factors that will most likely cause patients to acquire systemic and serious fungal infections.

■ Constant exposure to systemic-causing infections present in the air, dust, fomites, and even among the normal flora in the environment of humans

- Exposure to overwhelming numbers of fungi
- Immunosuppression (especially HIV and AIDS) and immunosuppressive drug therapies (including those used for cancer and organ transplantation patients)
- Frequent surgeries
- Use of broad-spectrum antimicrobials

Objective 5: Distinguish the classifications of antifungal agents.

- Antifungal agents are classified into three categories:
  - Drugs for systemic mycoses
  - Oral drugs for mucocutaneous infections
  - Topical drugs for mucocutaneous infections

Objective 6: Distinguish the trade names of topical antifungal agents.

- Topical antifungals include Mentax, Loprox, Penlac, Lotrimin, Econazole Nitrate Cream, Monistat-Derm, Naftin, Oxistat, Exelderm, Lamisil Topical, Terazol, Monistat, and Tinactin.

Objective 7: Describe the adverse effects of amphotericin B.

- Chills, fever, nausea and vomiting, diarrhea, abdominal cramps, dyspepsia, headache, vertigo, thrombophlebitis, anemia, cardiac arrest, and skin rashes
- The most serious adverse effect is renal damage.
- This drug is also able to cause blood dyscrasias and loss of hearing.

Objective 8: Describe the contraindications of griseofulvin and micafungin.

- Griseofulvin is contraindicated in patients with porphyria or liver disease. Safe use of this drug during pregnancy, lactation, or in children younger than 2 years has not been established.
- Micafungin is contraindicated in hypersensitivity to the drug or its components, as well as hypersensitivity to other echinocandins.

Objective 9: Explain the mechanism of action and indications for ketoconazole.

- Ketoconazole blocks the fungal synthesis of ergosterol, which is essential to the integrity of the cell membranes of nearly all pathogenic fungi.
- It has a broad spectrum of antifungal activity and is (with amphotericin B) one of the drugs of choice for blastomycosis, coccidioidomycosis, and histoplasmosis. Ketoconazole is an alternative drug for candidiasis, but successful treatment sometimes requires months.

Objective 10: Describe the mechanism of action for sulconazole and terbinafine.

- Sulconazole works by affecting components of fungal cell walls, slowing their activities, and also affects certain Gram-positive bacteria.
- Terbinafine works by inhibiting biosynthesis of ergosterol in the fungal cell membrane, leading to fungal cell death.

Internet Sites of Interest

- For information on nail fungus, including diagnosis and treatments, check out the Mayo Clinic website: **www.mayoclinic.org**. Search for "nail fungus."

- Patients with HIV and those who are immunocompromised are more susceptible to fungal infections than healthy individuals. Information on opportunistic fungal infections in HIV-positive individuals: **www.thebodypro .com/index/treat/candida.html**

- Characteristics of fungi: **www.biology-online.org/articles/fungi/characteristics_ fungi.html**

- Fungal infections: **https://www.nlm.nih.gov/medlineplus/fungalinfections.html**

- Topical and oral antifungals, as well as conditions they are used for, side effects, interactions, and uses: **http://drugs.nmihi.com/antifungal.htm**

- Human fungal infections are described at: **www.cdc.gov/fungal/**

Chapter 19

Antiprotozoal Agents

Chapter Objectives

After completing this chapter, you should be able to:

1. Describe the causes of protozoal infections.
2. Describe the most common cause of malarial infections and the most serious type of infection.
3. Describe the general drug indications of antimalarial agents.
4. Describe the indications of chloroquine and its adverse effects.
5. Explain the indications of doxycycline.
6. Explain amebic dysentery.
7. Explain the drugs that are most frequently used in the treatment of intestinal amebiasis and their contraindications.
8. List three generic and trade names of medications used for giardiasis.
9. Describe the mode of transmission of toxoplasmosis.
10. Briefly explain Chagas disease.

Key Terms

Introduction

Parasitic infections are responsible for significant morbidity and mortality throughout the world. These infections are prevalent in Africa, Asia, Central America, and South America and are much less common in Australia, Canada, Europe, Japan, New Zealand, and the United States. Though most parasitic infections occur in developing areas, they are also present in developed countries among immigrants and travelers who return from endemic regions.

Parasitic infections are often spread through fecal contamination of food or water. They occur most frequently in impoverished areas that have poor hygiene and sanitation. There are a variety of methods by which **parasites** can cause infection. Hookworms can enter the skin during contact with infected dirt; schistosomes are present in contaminated water. Malaria is transmitted through the bites of infected mosquitos.

Parasites can be divided into two primary groups: protozoa and helminths (worms). Protozoa are single-celled organisms that multiply by simple binary fission. Protozoa are able to multiply inside human hosts and increase in number to cause overwhelming infections. This chapter focuses on protozoal infections and their treatment, including malaria, amebiasis, trichomoniasis, giardiasis, toxoplasmosis, and Chagas disease.

Protozoal Infections

Protozoal infections are very common, often restricted geographically to the tropics and subtropics. *Amebiasis* is relatively rare in the United States. Another important protozoal infection is *Trichomonas vaginalis*, which causes a sexually transmitted disease called *trichomoniasis*, which is common in the United States (Figure 19-1 ■).

MALARIA

Malaria is caused by several species of the protozoan **Plasmodium**, of which *Plasmodium vivax* and

Centers for Disease Control and Prevention

Figure 19-1 ■ Vaginal discharge with microorganisms caused by trichomoniasis.

Plasmodium falciparum are the most common. The most serious infections involve *P. falciparum*, which causes a higher incidence of complications and deaths. These protozoans all have complex life cycles involving the anopheles mosquito and the red blood cells of the human host. The infection caused by *P. vivax* is a persisting tissue phase that continues to infect the blood at intervals for many years. Thus, the ideal drug to combat malarial infections should eradicate the *microzoan* from not only the blood but from the tissue as well to effect what is termed a **radical cure**.

For treatment of malaria, several antimalarial agents differ in their points of interruption of the cycle of the parasite and in the type of malaria affected. In addition, parasite resistance (especially that of *P. falciparum*) to these drugs is an important therapeutic problem.

Antimalarial drugs include chloroquine, doxycycline, hydroxychloroquine, primaquine, and quinine. Some agents are used for the actual prevention of malaria. They include mefloquine and folic acid antagonists such as pyrimethamine (Table 19-1 ■).

Table 19-1 ■ Antimalarial Drugs

GENERIC NAME	TRADE NAME	AVERAGE ADULT DOSAGE	ROUTE OF ADMINISTRATION
chloroquine	Aralen	300–700 mg/wk, 2 wk before exposure and for ≤4 wk after leaving endemic area	PO
doxycycline	Vibramycin	100 mg daily 1–2 days before, continuously during, and 4 wk after travel	PO
hydroxychloroquine	Plaquenil	400 mg/wk	PO
mefloquine	Lariam	5 tablets with water as a single oral dose, and then 250 mg/wk and then every other wk	PO
primaquine	Primaquine	15 mg/d for 14 d	PO

GENERIC NAME	TRADE NAME	AVERAGE ADULT DOSAGE	ROUTE OF ADMINISTRATION
pyrimethamine (folic acid antagonist)	Daraprim	25 mg once/wk up to 10 wk	PO
quinine	Qualaquin	648 mg q8h for 7 days	PO
PO, oral.			

Focus On

Chloroquine

Chloroquine is one of the most commonly used drugs for prophylaxis and the treatment of acute malarial attacks that are caused by *P. vivax, Plasmodium malariae, Plasmodium ovale,* and susceptible strains of *P. falciparum.*

How does it work?

Chloroquine is a protozoacidal drug. The agent destroys *Plasmodia* organisms by interfering with their metabolism or inhibiting normal replication of the **protozoan**.

How is it used?

Chloroquine is used for the control of acute attacks of *P. vivax* malaria and for suppression against all plasmodia except chloroquine-resistant *P. falciparum.* The drug is neither a prophylactic nor a radical curative agent in *P. vivax* malaria. In regions where *P. falciparum* is generally sensitive to chloroquine, it is markedly effective in terminating acute attacks of nonresistant *P. falciparum* malaria and usually brings about a complete cure in this type of malaria. Chloroquine is the drug of choice for the oral treatment of all malaria except that caused by resistant *P. falciparum.*

What are the adverse effects?

Adverse effects include pigmentation of the skin and nail beds, pruritus, fatigue, toxic psychosis, and ototoxicity.

Chloroquine may also cause clouding of the corneas of the eyes and retinopathy.

What are the contraindications and interactions?

Chloroquine is contraindicated in patients with liver disease, hypersensitivity to 4-aminoquinolines, psoriasis, porphyria, and renal disease. This drug should also not be used by children or by pregnant or lactating women. Certain antacids and laxatives decrease chloroquine absorption, and chloroquine may interfere with the response to the rabies vaccine.

What are the important points patients should know?

Advise patients to promptly report visual or hearing disturbances, muscle weakness, loss of balance, and symptoms of blood dyscrasia, which include fever, sore mouth or throat, unexplained fatigue, easy bruising, or bleeding. Instruct them to wear dark glasses in sunlight and bright light because of photophobia, to reduce the risk of ocular damage, and to avoid driving or other potentially hazardous activities until a reaction to the drug is known. Inform patients that this drug may cause rusty yellow or brown discoloration of the urine.

Doxycycline

Doxycycline is also known as *doxycycline calcium oral suspension* (syrup), *doxycycline hyclate* (capsules or film-coated tablets), and *doxycycline monohydrate* (for oral suspension). It is active against many different types of bacteria as well as parasites.

How does it work?

Doxycycline inhibits bacterial protein synthesis by binding to ribosomal subunits and is bacteriostatic against a broad range of Gram-positive and Gram-negative bacteria.

How is it used?

Doxycycline should be used only to treat or prevent infections that are proven or strongly suspected to be caused by bacteria, in order to reduce development of drug-resistant bacteria and maintain effectiveness of this and other antibacterial drugs. This drug is primarily indicated for Rickettsial infections such as Rocky Mountain spotted fever and typhus fever and for chlamydia. Doxycycline is used for the prevention of malaria.

What are the adverse effects?

Doxycycline, like all of the tetracyclines, may cause anorexia, nausea and vomiting, diarrhea, glossitis, dysphagia, enterocolitis, inflammatory lesions, toxic epidermal necrolysis, Stevens-Johnson syndrome, erythema multiforme, rashes, increased blood urea nitrogen, hypersensitivity reactions, haemolytic anemia, thrombocytopenia, neutropenia, eosinophilia, and intracranial hypertension.

What are the contraindications and interactions?

Doxycycline is contraindicated with hypersensitivity to any of the tetracyclines. Doxycycline may interact with anticoagulants, penicillin, antacids, bismuth subsalicylate, barbiturates, carbamazepine, phenytoin, methoxyflurane, and oral contraceptives.

What are the important points patients should know?

Patients should be instructed not to use doxycycline if they are pregnant or using a hormone-based method of contraception. The patient must tell his or her physician about liver or kidney disease, asthma, or allergies to sulphites. It is important to drink plenty of liquids while taking this and other tetracyclines. Doxycycline must be taken for the prescribed length of time and doses must not be skipped. This drug should not be used in children.

- -

Hydroxychloroquine

Hydroxychloroquine suppresses malaria attacks that are caused by *P. vivax*, *P. malariae*, *P. ovale*, and susceptible strains of *P. falciparum*.

How does it work?

The mechanism of action of hydroxychloroquine is based on its ability to form complexes with the DNA of parasites, thereby inhibiting replication and transcription to RNA and DNA synthesis of the parasites.

How is it used?

Hydroxychloroquine is a suppressive prophylaxis agent that is also used for the treatment of acute malarial attacks caused by all forms of susceptible malaria. This drug is used adjunctively with primaquine for the eradication of *P. vivax* and *P. malariae*. Hydroxychloroquine is commonly prescribed for the treatment of rheumatoid arthritis and lupus erythematosus.

What are the adverse effects?

Hydroxychloroquine may cause nausea and vomiting, anorexia, diarrhea, abdominal cramps, and weight loss. This agent may also produce fatigue, vertigo, headache, anxiety, retinopathy, blurred vision, and mood changes.

The serious adverse effects, which are rare, include aplastic anemia, agranulocytosis, thrombocytopenia, and alopecia.

What are the contraindications and interactions?

Hydroxychloroquine should be avoided in patients with known hypersensitivity to the drug or in patients with visual field changes associated with quinoline compounds. It is also contraindicated in patients who have psoriasis or porphyria. Safe use of hydroxychloroquine for juvenile arthritis or in lactating women is not established. It must be used cautiously in patients with liver disease, alcoholism, and impaired renal function. Aluminum- and magnesium-containing antacids and laxatives decrease hydroxychloroquine absorption. This agent may interfere with the response to the rabies vaccine.

What are the important points patients should know?

Inform patients about adverse effects and related symptoms when receiving prolonged therapy with this drug. Advise them to follow the drug regimen exactly as prescribed by their physician and to keep this drug out of the reach of children. Instruct women to not breastfeed while taking this drug without first consulting their physicians.

- -

Mefloquine

Mefloquine is an orally administered antimalarial agent that is absorbed significantly better when it is taken with food.

How does it work?

Mefloquine destroys sporozoan parasites in the blood. Its exact mechanism of action is unknown.

(continued)

Focus On (continued)

How is it used?

Mefloquine is indicated for mild to moderate acute malaria caused by *P. falciparum* or *P. vivax*. It is also used for the prophylaxis of malaria caused by these organisms.

What are the adverse effects?

Mefloquine may cause nausea, vomiting, dizziness, syncope, extrasystoles, myalgia, fever, headache, chills, diarrhea, skin rash, abdominal pain, fatigue, anorexia, and tinnitus. Rare but serious adverse effects include cardiopulmonary arrest and encephalopathy.

What are the contraindications and interactions?

Mefloquine is contraindicated with hypersensitivity to this drug or related compounds such as quinine and quinidine, or to its components. It is also contraindicated with depression, generalized anxiety disorder, psychosis, schizophrenia, and other major psychiatric disorders or a history of convulsions. Mefloquine may interact with propranolol, halofantrine, similar drugs (quinine, quinidine, chloroquine), antiseizure medications, and the oral live typhoid vaccine.

What are the important points patients should know?

Patients must tell their physician about liver or kidney disease, severe complications from infection with malaria, or uncontrolled vomiting or diarrhea. After beginning mefloquine, the patient must call the physician if vomiting is chronic. The patient must begin taking this drug 1 week before entering a region where malaria is common, and continue it until at least 4 weeks after leaving that region. It must be taken for the entire length of time prescribed, and other precautions to protect against mosquito bites must be undertaken while traveling.

Primaquine

Primaquine is an antimalarial agent that is very important for the radical cure of relapsing *P. vivax* or *P. ovale* malaria. It is not used for suppressive therapy or for the control of the acute clinical attacks of the disease.

How does it work?

Primaquine acts directly on the preformed nucleic acid DNA in the microorganisms. It is also gametocidal against the four human malaria species. The mechanism of antimalarial action is unknown.

How is it used?

Primaquine is indicated for the cure of relapsing *P. vivax* malaria. It eliminates symptoms and the infection as well as prevents relapse.

What are the adverse effects?

Primaquine in recommended doses is generally well tolerated. It infrequently causes nausea and vomiting, abdominal cramps, and headache. More serious, but rare, adverse effects include leukopenia, agranulocytosis, and cardiac arrhythmias.

What are the contraindications and interactions?

Primaquine is contraindicated in patients with rheumatoid arthritis and lupus erythematosus. Primaquine should be avoided in pregnancy.

What are the important points patients should know?

Instruct patients to examine their urine after each voiding and report darkening or a red tinge or a decrease in urine volume. Advise them to report chills, fever, pain in the region of the diaphragm, and cyanosis—all of which suggest a hemolytic reaction. Instruct patients to not breastfeed while taking this drug.

Pyrimethamine

Pyrimethamine is an antiparasitic compound that is administered orally. It is a folic acid antagonist that is highly selective against plasmodia and *Toxoplasma gondii.*

How does it work?

Pyrimethamine is effective against malarial parasites. Its action against *Toxoplasma gondii* is highly increased when used along with sulfonamides.

How is it used?

Pyrimethamine is used to treat toxoplasmosis and acute malaria. It is also used for the prophylaxis of malaria, along with sulfonamides, chloroquine, or quinine.

What are the adverse effects?

Pyrimethamine may cause hypersensitivity reactions, some of which may be severe, which more often occur when it is administered with a sulfonamide. Other adverse effects may include anorexia, nausea and vomiting, megaloblastic anemia, leukopenia, thrombocytopenia, pancytopenia, glossitis, hematuria, and arrhythmias.

What are the contraindications and interactions?

Pyrimethamine is contraindicated with hypersensitivity to this drug or its components. It is also contraindicated in patients with megaloblastic anemia caused by folate deficiency. This drug may interact with other antifolic agents, myelosuppressive agents, proguanil, zidovudine, methotrexate, and lorazepam.

What are the important points patients should know?

The patient must be instructed to stop taking pyrimethamine and consult the physician if skin rash, sore throat, pale skin, unusual bruising, or tongue swelling occur. These may be early symptoms of serious adverse effects. The patient must take each dose with food to lessen nausea and vomiting.

Quinine

Quinine remains the first-line therapy for severe *P. falciparum* malaria. A chemically related drug—quinidine gluconate—is an antidysrhythmic drug that is used off-label to treat severe malaria via IV administration.

How does it work?

Quinine is an agent that is destructive to *gametes*, or germ cells, and acts rapidly against all *Plasmodium* malaria except *P. falciparum*. The actual mechanism of action of quinine is unknown.

How is it used?

Quinine is the treatment of choice for severe *P. falciparum*. It is not generally used in chemoprophylaxis owing to its toxicity.

What are the adverse effects?

The adverse effects of quinine include visual and hearing disturbances, fever, headache, flushing, fainting, and cardiovascular collapse. It may also cause nausea and vomiting, diarrhea, and abdominal pain.

What are the contraindications and interactions?

Quinine should be discontinued if signs of hypersensitivity occur. It should be avoided in those with visual or auditory problems. It must be used with great caution in those with underlying cardiac abnormalities. Aluminum-containing antacids may block absorption. Quinine can raise plasma levels of warfarin and digoxin. Dosage must be reduced in renal insufficiency.

What are the important points patients should know?

Instruct patients to report feelings of faintness to their physicians and to eat a balanced diet with no excesses of fruit juices or milk. Advise patients to not self-medicate with OTC drugs without advice from their physicians and to not increase, decrease, skip, or discontinue doses without consulting their physician.

Focus on Pediatrics

Antimalarial Drugs for Children

Children who will be traveling to countries that require antimalarial vaccinations should be vaccinated 4–6 weeks before leaving to ensure full protection. Also, for antimalarial prescription drugs, infant and child dosages must usually be specially prepared; thus, adequate time also needs to be allowed for this. Guidelines must be followed exactly because *overdosage can be fatal.* One agent in particular—hydroxychloroquine—is particularly toxic to infants and children, and extra care must be taken in administration. Taking as few as 3–4 tablets (250 mg strength) of chloroquine, which is similar to hydroxychloroquine, has resulted in the death of small children.

✳ Apply Your Knowledge 19.1

The following questions focus on what you have just learned about antimalarials.

CRITICAL THINKING

1. Describe the causes of malaria and its mode of transmission.
2. List seven generic names of antimalarial drugs.
3. Give the indication of primaquine.
4. Explain the actual mechanism of action of quinine.
5. Identify people who should be vaccinated against malaria.

AMEBIC DYSENTERY

Amebic dysentery is an infection that is also known as **amebiasis**, which is caused by *Entamoeba histolytica*. It is most common in areas of the world with poor sanitation and economic conditions, including Central America, South America, Africa, and India. In the United States, most cases occur in people who travel to and from these areas of the world. Every year between 40 and 50 million people develop *amebic colitis*, an extraintestinal disease, with between 40,000 and 70,000 deaths resulting from these conditions. The *Entamoeba* species are either **trophozoites** or cysts. The trophozoites are most common in liquid stools, but die outside the body quickly. Cysts are most common in formed stools and are able to exist outside the body for a longer time.

Amebic dysentery is spread directly or indirectly between people via food or water, as well as through oral–anal contact. Although many affected individuals are asymptomatic, signs and symptoms of this disease include intermittent constipation and diarrhea, flatulence, and cramping abdominal pain. Diarrhea may range from mild to severe. There may be tenderness above the liver or ascending colon, and the stools may contain blood and mucus. There may also be a high fever and toxic systemic symptoms. The patient may become emaciated and anemic. Amebic dysentery is diagnosed by microscopic examination or enzyme immune-assay of the stool when the disease involves only intestinal infection. If it has become an extraintestinal infection, including liver abscesses, diagnosis is more difficult, involving imaging and serologic testing or therapeutic trials.

Treatment of amebic dysentery usually begins with metronidazole or tinidazole. To eradicate cysts, additional treatment involves iodoquinol or paromomycin. Table 19-2 ■ lists the medications used for amebic dysentery, including common dosages.

Table 19-2 ■ Medications Used for Amebic Dysentery

GENERIC NAME	TRADE NAME	AVERAGE ADULT DOSAGE	ROUTE OF ADMINISTRATION
Initial Treatments			
metronidazole	Flagyl	750 mg tid for 5–10 days	PO
tinidazole	Tindamax	2 g once/d with food for 3 days	PO
Follow-Up Treatments			
iodoquinol	Yodoxin	650 mg tid for 20 days	PO
paromomycin	Paromomycin Sulfate	25–35 mg/kg/d in 3 divided doses with meals for 5–10 days	PO

tid, three times a day; PO, oral.

Focus On

Metronidazole

Metronidazole is an amebicide that is used to treat liver abscess, intestinal amebiasis, trichomoniasis, anaerobic infections, vaginosis, diarrhea, colitis, and pelvic inflammatory disease and prevent postoperative infection after colorectal surgery.

How does it work?

Metronidazole is a direct-acting trichomonacide and amebicide that works at intestinal and extraintestinal sites. It apparently enters cells of microorganisms that contain the enzyme nitroreductase, forming unstable compounds that bind to DNA, inhibiting synthesis and causing cell death.

How is it used?

Metronidazole is prescribed for asymptomatic and symptomatic trichomoniasis in female and male patients. It is also used for acute intestinal amebiasis and amebic liver abscess. Metronidazole is usually indicated for preoperative prophylaxis in colorectal surgery, elective hysterectomy or vaginal repair, and emergency appendectomy.

What are the adverse effects?

The adverse effects of metronidazole include nausea and vomiting, anorexia, abdominal cramps, metallic or bitter taste, skin rashes, pruritus, flushing, fever, vertigo, headache, confusion, depression, restlessness, and insomnia. The urine sometimes turns a dark color.

What are the contraindications and interactions?

Metronidazole should not be used in patients with diseases of the central nervous system. The drug has been found to be carcinogenic in mice and rats. It has been used in pregnancy without consequence, but it is advisable to withhold it during pregnancy, if possible. Metronidazole interacts with cimetidine, disulfiram, lithium, oral anticoagulants, phenobarbital, phenytoin, and alcohol. For safety, alcohol should be completely avoided while taking metronidazole and for 3 days after stopping administration of the medication. Interaction between metronidazole and alcohol may result in tachycardia, skin warmth or redness, tingling sensations, and nausea and vomiting.

What are the important points patients should know?

Instruct patients to adhere closely to the established regimen without schedule interruptions or dose change. They must refrain from intercourse during therapy for trichomoniasis unless a condom is used to prevent reinfection. Inform patients that sexual partners should receive concurrent treatment. Asymptomatic trichomoniasis in men is a frequent source of reinfection in their female partners. Also, instruct patients to avoid alcohol while taking this drug.

(continued)

Focus On (*continued*)

Tinidazole

Tinidazole is a synthetic antiprotozoal and antibacterial agent. It is rapidly and completely absorbed via oral administration.

How does it work?

Tinidazole acts by releasing nitrates, damaging bacterial DNA in vitro. It also causes DNA changes in bacterial cells as well as breaking DNA strands. The actual mechanism of action in which tinidazole works against *Giardia* and *Entamoeba* species is not known.

How is it used?

Tinidazole is used to treat trichomoniasis in women and men, giardiasis and amebiasis in adults and children older than 3 years of age, and bacterial vaginosis in nonpregnant women.

What are the adverse effects?

Tinidazole may cause convulsions, numbness, paresthesia, vertigo, ataxia, giddiness, insomnia, drowsiness, tongue discoloration, stomatitis, diarrhea, urticaria, pruritus, rash, flushing, sweating, dry mouth, fever, burning sensations, thirst, salivation, angioedema, darkened urine, palpitations, transient neutropenia or leukopenia, and other, less common effects.

What are the contraindications and interactions?

Tinidazole is contraindicated with hypersensitivity to this drug or other nitroimidazole derivatives, women during the first trimester of pregnancy, and during lactation. Tinidazole may interact with warfarin and other oral coumarin anticoagulants, alcohol, disulfiram, lithium, phenytoin, fosphenytoin, cyclosporine, tacrolimus, and fluorouracil.

What are the important points patients should know?

Patients must be instructed not to take tinidazole if possible allergy exists, during the first 3 months of pregnancy, while breastfeeding, or if the patient has kidney disease, is on dialysis, has seizure disorders, has blood cell disorders, or is immunocompromised. Tinidazole must be taken for the entire prescribed length of time. Alcoholic beverages must not be consumed while taking tinidazole.

Iodoquinol

Iodoquinol is an anti-infective, antiamebicide, and antiprotozoal agent.

How does it work?

Iodoquinol is a direct-acting amebicide that works in the intestinal lumen. When it enters the cells of protozoa, it affects the DNA, inhibiting synthesis and causing cell death.

How is it used?

Iodoquinol is used only as a luminal amebicide and has no effect against extraintestinal amebic infections. It is commonly prescribed either concurrently or in alternating courses with another intestinal amebicide.

What are the adverse effects?

Infrequent adverse effects of iodoquinol include diarrhea—which usually stops after several days—nausea and vomiting, abdominal pain, anorexia, headache, rash, and pruritus. Iodoquinol can cause blurred vision, optic atrophy, permanent loss of vision, and thyroid hypertrophy.

What are the contraindications and interactions?

Iodoquinol is contraindicated in patients with hypersensitivity to any iodine-containing preparations or foods and those with hepatic or renal damage. Safe use during pregnancy or lactation is not established.

What are the important points patients should know?

Instruct patients to report skin rash and symptoms of a sudden decrease in their leukocyte count, such as chills, fever, weakness, and fatigue, and to complete the full course of treatment. Their stools need to be examined at 1, 3, and 6 months after the termination of treatment to ensure the infection has not returned.

Paromomycin

Paromomycin is a broad-spectrum antibiotic produced by *Streptomyces riomosus*, specifically the variant known as *paromomycinus*. It is poorly absorbed after oral administration.

How does it work?

Paromomycin works very similarly to the drug known as neomycin, which is actively transported across cell membranes to bind with receptor proteins, interfering with DNA and RNA of the target microorganisms.

How is it used?

Paromomycin is used to treat acute and chronic intestinal amebiasis. It is not effective in extraintestinal amebiasis.

What are the adverse effects?

Paromomycin may cause nausea, abdominal cramps, or diarrhea. However, these effects have only been reported when doses exceed more than 3 grams per day. The drug may also cause dizziness.

What are the contraindications and interactions?

Paromomycin is contraindicated with hypersensitivity to this drug and if the patient has intestinal obstruction. There are no significant drug interactions.

What are the important points patients should know?

Patients taking paromomycin must be instructed to use caution when driving, operating machinery, or performing other hazardous activities because this drug may cause dizziness.

GIARDIASIS

Giardiasis is an infection caused by the flagellated protozoan *Giardia lamblia*, also called *Giardia intestinalis*. *Giardia* trophozoites attach to the mucosa of the duodenum and jejunum, and then multiply using **binary fission**. Some transform into cysts that can survive in the external environment, which are spread via the fecal–oral route. Most cases of giardiasis are transmitted through contaminated water or food, sexual contact, and other direct contact.

Although many cases of giardiasis are asymptomatic, the cysts are still passed from these individuals, and symptoms appear between 1 and 2 weeks following

infection. These include watery, foul-smelling diarrhea, abdominal cramps with distention, **eructation**, flatulence, epigastric discomfort, intermittent nausea, and, occasionally, slight malaise and anorexia. The acute form of giardiasis lasts for between 1 and 3 weeks. When severe, weight loss may be significant due to malabsorption of sugars and fats. Chronic giardiasis may cause failure to thrive in children.

Treatment of giardiasis is with metronidazole, nitazoxanide, and tinidazole, which are described in Table 19-3 ■. However, it must be noted that the FDA has not officially approved metronidazole for the treatment of giardiasis.

Table 19-3 ■ Medications Used for Giardiasis

GENERIC NAME	TRADE NAME	AVERAGE ADULT DOSAGE	ROUTE OF ADMINISTRATION
metronidazole	Flagyl	250 mg tid for 5–7 days	PO
nitazoxanide	Alinia	In immunocompetent patients, 500 mg bid with food for 3 days; in AIDS patients, 1000 mg bid with food for 14 days or until diarrhea resolves	PO
tinidazole	Tindamax, Fasigyn	2 g once/d with food	PO

tid, three times a day; PO, oral; bid, twice a day.

Focus On

Nitazoxanide

Nitazoxanide is a synthetic antiprotozoal agent for oral administration. It is recommended to be administered with food.

How does it work?

Nitazoxanide is rapidly hydrolyzed to its active metabolite, tizoxanide, which is then conjugated. The drug is then able to interfere with the enzymes needed by the protozoa for energy metabolism.

How is it used?

Nitazoxanide is used to treat giardiasis in patients 1 year of age and older and for diarrhea that is caused by *Cryptosporidium parvum* in patients between 1 and 11 years of age.

What are the adverse effects?

Nitazoxanide, in its oral tablet form, most commonly causes abdominal pain, diarrhea, headache, and nausea. In its oral suspension form, the most common adverse effects include abdominal pain, diarrhea, vomiting, and headache, but these are usually mild and transient.

What are the contraindications and interactions?

Nitazoxanide is contraindicated in patients with a prior hypersensitivity to this drug or its components. It may interact with other highly plasma protein-bound drugs with narrow therapeutic indices, including warfarin.

What are the most important points patients should know?

The patient should be instructed to take nitazoxanide with food and to discuss with the physician all other prescription or OTC medications being taken, including vitamins, minerals, and herbal products.

TOXOPLASMOSIS

Toxoplasmosis is an infection caused by **Toxoplasma gondii**, and is common where cats cohabit with humans. Between 20 and 40% of healthy Americans are seropositive for this organism. Risks for developing toxoplasmosis are highest in fetuses infected *in utero* and in immunocompromised individuals. The causative parasite multiplies in the cytoplasm of nucleated cells. When the host become immune, multiplication of **tachyzoites** stops and cysts form in tissue, mostly in the muscles and brain. When an infected cat passes feces into moist soil, the cysts may remain infectious for several months. Infection develops from ingestion of cysts, via transplacental transmission, via blood transfusion, or during organ transplantation.

The most common mode of oral infection is through ingestion of cysts present in food or water that has become contaminated with cat feces. Infection also occurs by consuming raw or undercooked lamb, pork, and sometimes beef that contain cysts. In immunocompromised patients, once cysts become present in their tissues, they can reactivate at any time. In AIDS patients who are not receiving antibiotics as prophylaxis, 30–40% of patients develop toxoplasmosis. The disease can be transmitted transplacentally if the mother becomes infected during pregnancy, or if she was previously infected and her infection becomes reactivated due to immunosuppression. Transmission is also through transfusion of white blood cells or whole blood, and through organ transplantation from a donor who is seropositive. A severe complication of congenital toxoplasmosis is blindness in infants. Treatment of toxoplasmosis, when indicated, is usually with pyrimethamine/sulfadiazine, though other medications may also be used (see Table 19-4 ■).

Table 19-4 ■ Medications Used for Toxoplasmosis

GENERIC NAME	TRADE NAME	AVERAGE ADULT DOSAGE	ROUTE OF ADMINISTRATION
Most Common Treatment			
pyrimethamine*/ sulfadiazine	Daraprim/ (Generic only)	Initial: 50–75 mg pyrimethamine with 1–4 g of sulfadiazine, for 1–3 weeks prn; dosage may then be reduced by $1/2$ and continued for 4–5 weeks	PO

Table 19-4 ■ Medications Used for Toxoplasmosis

GENERIC NAME	TRADE NAME	AVERAGE ADULT DOSAGE	ROUTE OF ADMINISTRATION
Additional Treatment			
pyrimethamine*/ sulfadoxine	Daraprim/ (generic only)	Initial: 50–75 mg pyrimethamine with 1–4 g of sulfadoxine, for 1–3 weeks prn; dosage may then be reduced by $\frac{1}{2}$ and continued for 4–5 weeks	PO
For Patients Hypersensitive to Sulfonamides			
pyrimethamine*/ clindamycin	Daraprim/ Cleocin	50–75 mg pyrimethamine, with 600–800 mg tid	PO
pyrimethamine*/ atovaquone	Daraprim/ Mepron	Initial: 200 mg pyrimethamine, with 1500 mg atovaquone q12h; Maintenance: 75 mg/d pyrimethamine with atovaquone 1500 mg q12h, for 6 weeks	

*Note: All patients receiving pyrimethamine should also receive folinic acid. If bone marrow suppression occurs from pyrimethamine, this can be minimized with folinic acid. The dosage of folinic acid would be 10–25 mg, PO, once/d. Also, in pregnant women with primary infection, spiramycin (an experimental drug in the U.S.) may be used to reduce transmission during the first trimester. The dosage is 1 g PO tid or qid.

PO, oral; tid, three times a day; qid, four times a day.

Focus Point

Prevention of Toxoplasmosis

The best way to prevent transmission of toxoplasmosis is to wash the hands thoroughly after handling cat litter, soil, or raw meat. No food that could possibly be contaminated with cat feces should be consumed. Safe cooking of meats requires temperatures of 165–170°F.

CHAGAS DISEASE

Chagas disease is an infection with ***Trypanosoma cruzi***, which is transmitted by Triatominae insect bites. These insects are commonly known as conenose bugs, kissing bugs, assassin bugs, or triatomines. The bites of these insects transmit infected feces that enter either through the bite wound or penetrate the mucous membranes or conjunctivae. Eventually, the infective agents enter the bloodstream and tissue spaces and infect other body cells. The most commonly affected cells are those of the myocardium, reticuloendothelial system, muscles, and nervous system. Infection can also be transmitted via blood transfusion, ingestion of raw foods or drinks, organ transplantation, and through transplacental transmission. Animals that may act as reservoirs for this infection include cats, dogs, opossums, rats, and others. Treatment of Chagas disease is outlines in Table 19-5 ■.

Table 19-5 ■ Medications Used for Chagas Disease

GENERIC NAME	TRADE NAME	AVERAGE ADULT DOSAGE	ROUTE OF ADMINISTRATION
benznidazole	(Generic only)	2.5–3.5 mg/kg bid for 1–3 months	PO
nifurtimox	(Generic only)	2–2.5 mg/kg qid for 3–4 months	PO

Note: Both of these medications are only available through the Centers for Disease Control and Prevection.

bid, twice a day; PO, oral; qid, four times a day.

Focus On

Benznidazole

Benznidazole is only available from the Centers for Disease Control and Prevention (CDC), and is not commercially available in the United States. It is a systemic antiprotozoal.

How does it work?

Benznidazole is trypanocidal and appears to inhibit protein and RNA synthesis in the trypanosome parasite.

How is it used?

Benznidazole is used as an alternative agent in the treatment of Chagas disease, also known as *American trypanosomiasis*, which is caused by *Trypanosoma cruzi*.

What are the adverse effects?

Benznidazole may cause peripheral neuropathy, progressive purpuric dermatitis, and seizures. Less common adverse effects include blood dyscrasias such as leukopenia and thrombocytopenia, skin rash, gastrointestinal disturbances, fatigue, headache, confusion, insomnia, inability to concentrate, restlessness, amnesia, temporary memory loss, and dizziness.

What are the contraindications and interactions?

Benznidazole is contraindicated with hypersensitivity to this drug or its components, during the first trimester of pregnancy, and with medical conditions such as hematological, liver, or kidney abnormalities. It may interact with alcohol, aspirin, and coumarin-derivative anticoagulants such as warfarin.

What are the important points patients should know?

The patient should be informed about potential tumorigenicity and mutagenicity, avoidance of use during the first trimester of pregnancy, and to monitor for the more serious adverse effects.

. . . .

Nifurtimox

Nifurtimox is only available from the CDC and is not commercially available in the United States. It is a systemic antiprotozoal.

How does it work?

Nifurtimox is trypanocidal, but its mechanism of action is not fully understood. It may cause significant breakage in the parasite's DNA, or may produce toxic agents that damage the parasite's protective enzymes. It is rapidly absorbed from the gastrointestinal tract.

How is it used?

Nifurtimox is considered the primary agent in the treatment of Chagas disease, especially in the acute, early stage of the disease.

What are the adverse effects?

Nirfutimox may cause adverse effects that actually mimic the symptoms of Chagas disease. Common adverse effects include anorexia with weight loss, epigastric pain, nausea and vomiting, headache, and dizziness. Less common adverse effects include confusion, disturbances of equilibrium, nystagmus, excitation, forgetfulness, insomnia, irritability, psychoses, seizures, tremor, fever, impotence or loss of libido, leukopenia, muscle weakness, and peripheral neuropathy.

What are the contraindications and interactions?

Nifurtimox is contraindicated with alcohol or drug abuse, allergies, peripheral neuropathy, seizures, behavioral disorders, epilepsy, psychoses, and liver or kidney abnormalities. It may interact with alcohol.

What are the important points patients should know?

The patient should be informed about potential carcinogenicity or mutagenicity, hypersensitivity, and impaired fertility. The patient must have his or her weight monitored every 14 days since changes in body weight affect dosage.

✺ Apply Your Knowledge 19.2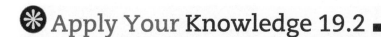

The following questions focus on what you have just learned about antiprotozoal infections and agents.

CRITICAL THINKING

1. Compare *Entamoeba histolytica* with *Giardia lamblia*.
2. Give the trade names of metronidazole and iodoquinol.
3. Identify the contraindications of metronidazole.
4. Discuss the classification of iodoquinol.
5. Explain the adverse effects of iodoquinol.
6. Describe congenital toxoplasmosis.
7. Explain Chagas disease and how it can be diagnosed.

PRACTICAL SCENARIO 1

A 51-year-old businessman traveled to an undeveloped country. After 1 week, he returned to the United States and developed a gastrointestinal infection. His symptoms included diarrhea, abdominal cramps, intermittent nausea, malaise, and anorexia. After a stool culture, his physician diagnosed him with giardiasis.

Courtesy of the author

Critical Thinking Questions

1. What is giardiasis?
2. What are the treatments for giardiasis?
3. Why is giardiasis more common in developing countries?

PRACTICAL SCENARIO 2

A medical assistant called a patient named Laila to tell her about her recent examination and laboratory test results. Laila had a vaginal infection and needed a specific medication. The medical assistant said she would call in the prescription for the medication to Laila's local pharmacy. Laila asked what type of vaginal infection she had and was told that it was caused by a type of protozoa. The medical assistant also told her the medication should be taken twice daily for a maximum of 7 days.

Andrey Kiselev/Fotolia

Critical Thinking Questions

1. What is the drug of choice for this type of protozoal infection?
2. If the physician ordered this drug of choice, what are its potential adverse effects?

Chapter Capsule

This section repeats the objectives from the beginning of the chapter and then provides a summary of the most important concepts for that objective. Use this section as a quick review and to check your knowledge.

Objective 1: Describe the causes of protozoal infections.

- Protozoal infections are actually caused by only a small number of species often restricted geographically to the tropics and subtropics.
- Two protozoal organisms—*Entamoeba histolytica* and *Giardia lamblia*—are frequently responsible for causing dysentery in humans.
- Another important protozoal infection is *Trichomonas vaginalis*, which causes a sexually transmitted disease called *trichomoniasis*.
- The most commonly reported intestinal protozoal infection in the United States is giardiasis, caused by the flagellated protozoan *G. lamblia*.

Objective 2: Describe the most common cause of malarial infections and the most serious type of infection.

- Malaria is caused by several species of the protozoan *Plasmodium*, of which *Plasmodium vivax* and *Plasmodium falciparum* are the most common.
- The most serious infections involve *P. falciparum*, which causes a higher incidence of complications and death.

Objective 3: Describe the general drug indications of antimalarial agents.

- Chloroquine: control of acute attacks of vivax malaria; suppression against all *Plasmodia spp.* except chloroquine-resistant *P. falciparum*; oral treatment of all malaria except that caused by resistant *P. falciparum*
- Primaquine: cure of relapsing vivax malaria
- Quinine: treatment of severe *P. falciparum*
- Hydroxychloroquine: suppressive prophylaxis agent; treatment of acute malarial attacks caused by all forms of susceptible malaria; used adjunctively with primaquine for the eradication of *P. vivax* and *P. malariae*

Objective 4: Describe the indications of chloroquine and its adverse effects.

- Chloroquine is used for the control of acute attacks of *P. vivax* malaria and for suppression against all plasmodia except chloroquine-resistant *P. falciparum*. Chloroquine is the drug of choice for the oral treatment of all malaria except that caused by resistant *P. falciparum*.
- The adverse effects of chloroquine include pigmentation of the skin and nail beds, pruritus, fatigue, toxic psychosis, and ototoxicity. It may also cause corneal opacities and retinopathy.

Objective 5: Explain the indications of doxycycline.

- Doxycycline should be used only to treat or prevent infections that are proven or strongly suspected to be caused by bacteria in order to reduce development of drug-resistant bacteria and maintain effectiveness of this and other antibacterial drugs.
- This drug is primarily indicated for Rickettsial infections such as Rocky Mountain spotted fever and typhus fever and for chlamydia.

Objective 6: Explain amebic dysentery.

■ Amebic dysentery is also known as *amebiasis*, which is caused by *Entamoeba histolytica*. It is most common in areas of the world with poor sanitation and economic conditions. In the United States, most cases occur in people who travel to such areas. The *Entamoeba* species are either trophozoites or cysts. Amebic dysentery is spread directly or indirectly between people via food or water, as well as through oral–anal contact. Often asymptomatic, it may also manifest as constipation, diarrhea, flatulence, and cramping abdominal pain. There may be tenderness above the liver or ascending colon and the stools may contain blood and mucus. There may also be a high fever and toxic systemic symptoms. The patient may become emaciated and anemic.

Objective 7: Explain the drugs that are most frequently used in the treatment of amebiasis and their contraindications.

■ Metronidazole—a direct-acting trichomonacide and amebicide that works at intestinal and extraintestinal sites; contraindicated in patients with central nervous system diseases and should be withheld during pregnancy

■ Iodoquinol—a direct-acting amebicide that works in the intestinal lumen; contraindicated in patients with hypersensitivity to any iodine-containing preparations or foods and those with hepatic or renal damage; safe use during pregnancy or lactation is not established

Objective 8: List three generic and trade names of medications used for giardiasis.

■ The medications used for giardiasis include metronidazole (Flagyl), nitazoxanide (Alinia), and tinidazole (Tindamax, Fasigyn).

Objective 9: Describe the mode of transmission of toxoplasmosis.

■ When an infected cat passes feces into moist soil, the cysts may remain infectious for several months. The most common mode of oral infection is through ingestion of cysts present in food or water that has become contaminated with cat feces. Infection also occurs by consuming raw or undercooked lamb, pork, and sometimes beef that contain cysts.

■ The disease can be transmitted transplacentally if the mother becomes infected during pregnancy, or if she was previously infected and her infection becomes reactivated due to immunosuppression.

■ Transmission is also through transfusion of white blood cells or whole blood and through organ transplantation from a donor who is seropositive.

Objective 10: Briefly explain Chagas disease.

■ Chagas disease is an infection with *Trypanosoma cruzi*, which is transmitted by Triatominae insect bites (conenose bugs, kissing bugs, assassin bugs, or triatomines). Their bites transmit infected feces, and the infection can also be transmitted via blood transfusion, ingestion of raw foods or drinks, and organ transplantation, as well as through transplacental transmission.

Internet Sites of Interest

- The CDC offers tips for travelers who may visit areas where malaria is a concern: **www.cdc.gov/malaria**
- Antiprotozoal Agents: **http://www.merckmanuals.com/professional/infectious-diseases/intestinal-protozoa/overview-of-intestinal-protozoan-infections**
- A fact sheet on trichomoniasis that contains reliable patient education information provided by the CDC: **www.cdc.gov/std/Trichomonas/STDFact-Trichomoniasis.htm**
- Amebiasis (amebic dysentery): **www.nlm.nih.gov/medlineplus/ency/article/000298.htm**
- The Mayo Clinic's information on giardiasis: **www.mayoclinic.org/diseases-conditions/giardia-infection/basics/definition/con-20024686**
- Learn about the symptoms of toxoplasmosis and its treatment: **www.medicinenet.com/toxoplasmosis/article.htm**
- Frequently asked questions about the seriousness of Chagas disease: **www.webmd.com/news/20120531/chagas-disease-faq**

Chapter 20

Vaccines and Immunoglobulins

Chapter Objectives

After completing this chapter, you should be able to:

1. State the names and functions of blood cells involved in immunity.
2. List the major components of the lymphatic system.
3. Discuss and contrast the various types of immunities.
4. Explain the differences between active and passive immunity.
5. State the main action of immunizing agents.
6. Contrast inactivated and attenuated vaccines.
7. List the most common adverse effects associated with vaccinations.
8. Describe the most common childhood immunizations.
9. List the most common adult immunizations.
10. Explain how immunoglobulins work to provide immunity.

Key Terms

active immunity (p. 332)
antibodies (p. 330)
antigens (p. 330)
asplenia (p. 337)
attenuated (p. 332)
booster (p. 338)
cell-mediated immunity (p. 330)
globulins (p. 339)
humoral immunity (p. 330)

immune response (p. 330)
immunity (p. 330)
immunogen (p. 332)
immunoglobulins (p. 332)
isotypes (p. 339)
lymph (p. 330)
lymphatic vessels (p. 330)
lymphocytes (p. 330)

lymphoid organs (p. 330)
macrophages (p. 330)
passive immunity (p. 332)
pathogens (p. 330)
toxin (p. 333)
toxoids (p. 333)
vaccination (p. 332)
vaccine (p. 332)

Introduction

Immunizing agents and allergenic extracts are two of the main groups of drugs that are classified as biologics by the FDA. Biologics are chemical agents that produce biological responses in the body. As a group, particularly the active immunizing agents, biologics possibly have prevented more morbidity and mortality than all other drugs combined. The *Vaccinia* vaccine may be considered the most effective drug to date because it has virtually eradicated smallpox from our world. A similar success for the poliomyelitis virus vaccines appears imminent.

The Immune System

The human immune system is a truly amazing constellation of responses to attacks from outside the body. The immune system is part of the lymphatic system, which is composed of the lymph vessels; lymph nodes; and other organs, such as the thymus gland, spleen, and tonsils. This system rids foreign substances from the blood and lymph, combats infectious diseases, maintains tissue fluid balance, and absorbs fats.

When microorganisms or foreign substances invade the body, the body responds by producing more **lymphocytes**, which are the second most numerous white blood cells. The body continues to fight the invaders by forming special proteins manufactured by the lymphocytes, called **antibodies**. The dominant cells of the lymphatic system, lymphocytes are vital to our ability to resist or overcome infection and disease. They respond to the presence of (1) invading **pathogens**, such as bacteria or viruses; (2) abnormal body cells, such as cancer cells; and (3) foreign proteins, such as the toxins released by some bacteria. Lymphocytes attempt to eliminate these threats or render them harmless by a combination of physical and chemical attack.

Lymphocytes respond to specific threats, such as a bacterial invasion of a tissue, by organizing a defense against that specific type of bacterium. Such a specific defense of the body is known as an **immune response**. **Immunity** is the ability to resist infection and disease through the activation of specific defenses.

The lymphatic system, shown in Figure 20-1 ■, includes three components:

1. A network of **lymphatic vessels** begins in peripheral tissues and ends at connections to the venous system

2. A fluid called **lymph** flows through the lymphatic vessels

3. **Lymphoid organs** are connected to the lymphatic vessels and contain large numbers of lymphocytes; examples of the organs are the lymph nodes, spleen, and thymus

The blood contains three classes of lymphocytes:

1. T cells (thymus-dependent)
2. B cells (bone marrow–derived)
3. Natural killer (NK) cells

T cells comprise approximately 80% of circulating lymphocytes. *Cytotoxic* T cells attack foreign cells or body cells infected by viruses directly. These lymphocytes are the primary cells that provide **cell-mediated immunity**.

B cells constitute 10–15% of circulating lymphocytes. B cells can differentiate into *plasma cells*, which are responsible for the production and secretion of *antibodies*. Antibodies are globular proteins that are often called *immunoglobulins (Igs)*. Antibodies react with specific chemical targets called **antigens**. Antigens are usually pathogens, parts or products of pathogens, or other foreign compounds.

NK cells make up the remaining 5–10% of circulating lymphocytes. These lymphocytes attack foreign cells, normal cells infected with viruses, and cancer cells that appear in normal tissues.

Cell-Mediated Immunity and Humoral Immunity

Cell-mediated immunity depends on the functions of the T cells, which are responsible for a delayed type of immune response. The T lymphocyte becomes sensitized by the first contact with a specific antigen. T cells and **macrophages** (immune cells derived from monocytes) work together in cell-mediated immunity to destroy the antigen. T cells attack the antigens directly rather than producing antibodies. Cell-mediated immunity may also occur without macrophages. T cells defend the body against viral, fungal, and some bacterial infections. If cell-mediated immunity is lost, as in the case of acquired immunodeficiency syndrome (AIDS), the body is unable to protect itself against many viral, bacterial, and fungal infections.

Humoral immunity is based on the antigen–antibody response. B cells, which are responsible for humoral immunity, produce circulating antibodies to act against an antigen. B cells arise from a separate population of stem cells of the bone marrow than that which produces T cells. These cells undergo multiplication and processing in lymphoid tissue elsewhere than in the thymus gland. B cells, similar to T cells, have surface receptors that enable them to recognize the appropriate antigen. But unlike T cells, B cells do not themselves interact to neutralize or destroy the antigen. On recognition of the antigen, they take up residence in secondary lymphoid tissue and proliferate to form daughter lymphocytes. These B cells then develop into plasma cells. The plasma cells produce antibodies and release them into the circulation at the lymph nodes. Some of the activated B cells do not become plasma cells. Instead, they turn into memory cells, which continue to produce small amounts of the antibody long after the infection has been overcome.

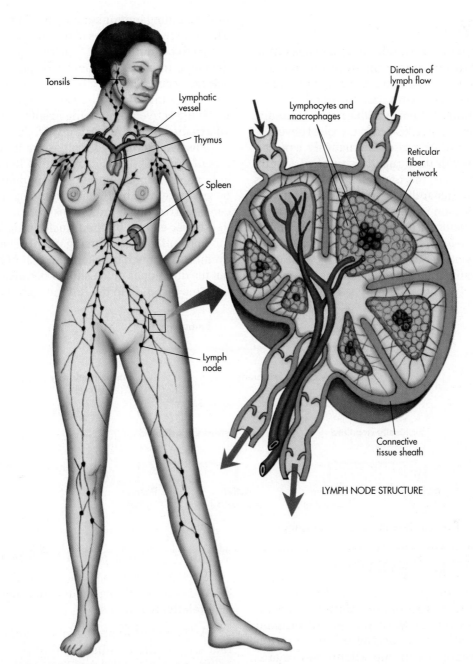

Figure 20-1 ■ The lymphatic system includes the tonsils, lymph nodes, spleen, and lymphatic vessels. Within the lymph nodes are the macrophages and lymphocytes.

✳ Apply Your **Knowledge 20.1**

The following questions focus on what you have just learned about white blood cells and immunity.

CRITICAL THINKING

1. Explain natural killer cells and their functions.
2. Describe the types of lymphocytes that are responsible for humoral immunity.
3. Discuss cell-mediated immunity.
4. Differentiate between antigens, antibodies, and macrophages.
5. Explain cytotoxic T cells.

Immunity

Immunity is the state or condition of being resistant to invading microorganisms. It is normally acquired either by contracting a disease and then developing immunity to it or by being vaccinated with proteins from the causative agent. For example, a person with a normal immune system who contracts rubella (German measles) develops a lifelong immunity to the disease. Alternatively, a person may be vaccinated with dead rubella viruses to acquire immunity. In both cases, the immune system responds to proteins in the virus and develops a *memory* for it. The next time the person is exposed to the live virus, the immune system *remembers* its past exposure and attacks and kills the virus before it can cause an infection.

Immunizing agents are broadly classified on the basis of the type of immunity they induce. Knowing the properties of the different types of immunity is fundamental to understanding immunizing agents and their applications. There are two main types of immunity: active and passive.

Active immunity is a form of acquired immunity that develops in an individual in response to an **immunogen** (antigen). This may be naturally acquired by exposure to an infectious disease or artificially acquired by receiving active immunizing agents (vaccines). The term **vaccination** is used as a synonym for active immunization.

Passive immunity involves the transfer of the effectors of immunity, which are called **immunoglobulins** or antibodies, from an immune individual to another. This occurs naturally by the active transport across the placental barrier of IgG antibodies from mother to fetus and, to a lesser extent, by the transfer of IgA antibodies in a mother's milk to her nursing infant. The onset of passive immunity is much quicker than that of active immunity, but the duration is much shorter because there is no active immune response to the immunogen (Figure 20-2 ■).

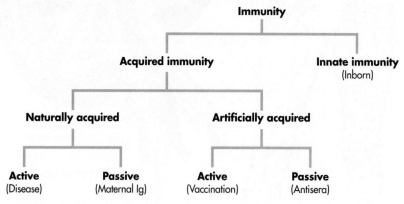

Figure 20-2 ■ Types of immunity.

Immunizing Agents

Immunizing agents are among the oldest of modern drugs and can be traced to the beginning of immunology in 1798, when Edward Jenner introduced his vaccine for smallpox. A **vaccine** is a preparation of killed microorganisms, living **attenuated** organisms that have reduced virulence, or living virulent organisms that are administered to produce or artificially increase immunity to a particular disease. They are the most successful and powerful drugs yet developed. Active immunizing agents have these advantages:

✳ Their main action is to *prevent* rather than to treat disease; most of the commonly used vaccines are highly effective.

✳ They have been proven to be remarkably *safe* in actual practice.

✳ Active immunizing agents are generally available at a relatively *low cost*.

Active immunizing agents are immunogenic drugs that are usually administered to patients before their being exposed to diseases to provide long-term, even permanent protection against the diseases. Perhaps active immunization will one day be used for a variety of conditions, ranging from cancer to drug abuse.

Passive immunizing agents date to the early part of the twentieth century after the discovery of *Igs* (antibodies). Various antitoxins derived from animals held an important place in therapy before the development of antibiotics, but these products—in contrast to the vaccines—had a number of problems with respect to efficacy and safety.

Focus on Pediatrics

Routine Immunization Reduces Disease

Immunization for diphtheria, tetanus, and pertussis (DTP) has been routinely given in the United States since the late 1940s, resulting in dramatic reductions in the incidence of all these diseases.

Focus On

Vaccines

Most vaccines consist of entire microorganisms that may be either *attenuated* (live; see Table 20-1 ■) or *inactivated* (killed; see Table 20-2 ■). One way to attenuate a virus is through laboratory manipulation, in which a bacterium is developed that lacks a **toxin** (a chemical produced by a microorganism that can be harmful), an enzyme, or some other normal constituent that causes symptoms of disease. The bacterium's virulence is thereby lessened.

Most bacterial vaccines contain killed bacteria or their components. It is important to understand that the live vaccines contain less immunogen than the killed vaccines and must actually cause an infection within the patient to induce a protective immune response.

Another type of vaccine contains **toxoids**, which are protein toxins that have been modified to reduce their hazardous properties without significantly altering their antigenic properties. The oldest and best-known active immunizing agents are diphtheria toxoid and tetanus toxoid, which protect against the bacterial exotoxins.

Whereas a *simple vaccine* is one that protects against a single disease, a *combined vaccine* is a combination product that protects against two or more diseases.

How do they work?

The principle underlying vaccination is that exposure to an antigen (a virus or bacterium) in a relatively harmless form sensitizes immune cells for possible subsequent exposure to the organism. On re-exposure, the memory of the previous challenge triggers an immune response more quickly. Because the person's own immune processes are stimulated by this agent, this is a form of active immunity. Usually, more than one dose of the vaccine is required to trigger a rapid and full immune response. The number of doses needed reflects the potency of the vaccine.

How are they used?

The indications and recommendations for the use of vaccines depend on several factors, such as safety and efficacy, as with other drugs. The FDA approves the indications for each licensed product. Vaccines are used against a range of bacterial infections, including diphtheria, tetanus, pertussis, pneumonia, tuberculosis, typhoid, cholera, meningitis, plague, and Q fever. Vaccines are also available against such viral infections as measles, mumps, and rubella (MMR); poliomyelitis; hepatitis A and B; influenza; rabies; and yellow fever (see Table 20-1 and 20-2).

What are the adverse effects?

The most common adverse effects associated with vaccinations include localized inflammation at the site of injection, a mild fever, headache, malaise, nausea, and dizziness. Convulsions resulting in permanent brain damage have been reported after administration of pertussis vaccine, but these reactions are rare. In some individuals, an allergic reaction may occur immediately after vaccination. The recipient should be observed for a short time after the vaccine is administered, and adrenaline should always be available in case anaphylaxis occurs.

What are the contraindications and interactions?

Immunizations are contraindicated in people with acute febrile illness, during pregnancy and lactation, and in those who are known to have developed anaphylactoid reactions with previous vaccines.

When several vaccines are given at the same time, the potential for drug interaction is increased. An example of this situation would be when typhoid, cholera, and plague vaccines are administered together.

What are the important points patients should know?

Instruct patients to monitor the injection site for reactions. Advise women to avoid breastfeeding until checking with their physician.

✱ Apply Your Knowledge 20.2

The following exercise focuses on what you have just learned about various types of immunities, vaccines, and toxoids.

CRITICAL THINKING

1. Differentiate between inactivated and attenuated vaccines, and name two examples of each.
2. Compare active immunity and passive immunity.
3. Explain immunity.
4. Discuss toxoids, and name two examples.
5. Name vaccines that may be administered subcutaneously.

Table 20-1 ■ Bacterial Vaccines

VACCINE	ROUTES OF ADMINISTRATION
Live Attenuated Vaccines	
Bacillus Calmette Guérin (BCG) vaccine*	Intradermal
Typhoid vaccine	PO or IM
Inactivated Vaccines	
Anthrax vaccine, adsorbed	SC or IM
Cholera vaccine	PO
Haemophilus influenzae type b (Hib)	IM
Lyme disease vaccine (removed from U.S. market due to low demand)	IM
Meningococcal polysaccharide vaccine	SC
Pertussis vaccine, adsorbed	IM
Pneumococcal conjugate vaccine (Prevnar 13)	IM
Tetanus toxoid, adsorbed	IM

*Bacillus Calmette Guerin (BCG) vaccine is not generally recommended for use in the United States because of a low risk of infection with *Mycobacterium tuberculosis* and other reasons. It should be considered only for people who meet specific criteria determined by a tuberculosis expert.

PO, oral; IM, intramuscular; SC, subcutaneous.

Table 20-2 ■ Inactivated Virus Vaccines

VACCINE	ROUTES OF ADMINISTRATION
Hepatitis A vaccine	IM
Hepatitis B vaccine	IM
Influenza virus vaccine (types A and B)	IM
Poliovirus vaccine, inactivated	SC or IM
Rabies virus vaccine	IM

Note: The measles, mumps, and rubella (MMR) vaccine contains live attenuated viruses and must be administered subcutaneously.

IM, intramuscular; SC, subcutaneous.

Standards for Childhood Immunization

The Advisory Committee on Immunization Practices (ACIP) currently recommends that children be immunized against eight infectious diseases as well as against hepatitis A in areas of high incidence (Table 20-3 ■). Childhood immunization remains one of the most important public health measures in the United States.

Haemophilus influenzae type b (Hib) was the leading cause of invasive bacterial disease (e.g., meningitis) among children until pediatric immunization was introduced in 1988. The vaccine contains inactivated bacteria (HibTiter, PedvaxHIB).

The Salk inactivated vaccine (IPV, IPOL; 1954) and the Sabin live vaccine (1961) are two types of polio immunizations that have been very effective against

Table 20-3 ■ Recommended Immunization Schedule for Persons Ages 0–6 Years—United States, 2016

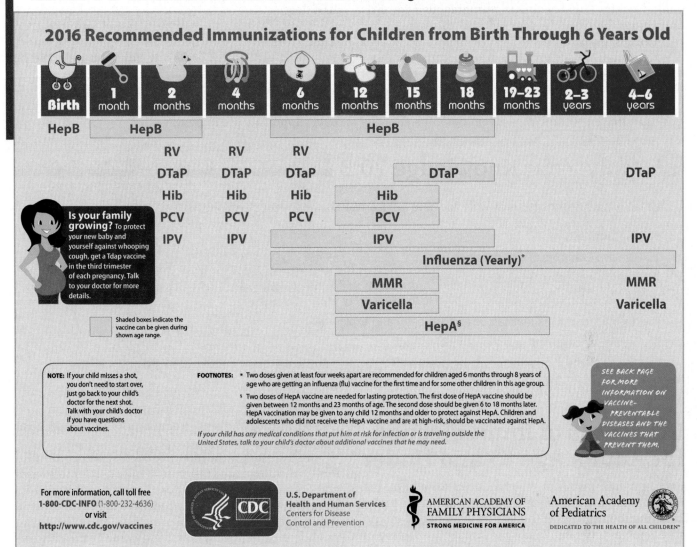

These recommendations must be read along with the footnotes, which can be found in Appendix D.

Courtesy of Centers for Disease Control and Prevention. *Recommended Immunization Schedule for Persons Aged 0 Through 6 Years—United States, 2016.* Available at www.cdc.gov/vaccines/parents/downloads/parent-ver-sch-0-6yrs.pdf.

poliomyelitis. There has been no poliomyelitis in the Americas in recent years except when vaccine associated and in a few importation cases.

Measles, mumps, and rubella (German measles) are three important viral diseases that can potentially be eradicated by mass active immunization. The combined vaccine (MMR) was licensed in 1971 and has been recommended for routine immunizations since 1977.

Hepatitis B infection is a major worldwide health problem with many facets, including acute and chronic disease, liver failure and cirrhosis, hepatic carcinoma, and chronic carriers. Neonates born to mothers who are positive for hepatitis B should be immunized immediately with the vaccine (Energix-B) and hepatitis B Ig.

Varicella (*chickenpox*) is a highly communicable disease that is generally benign but also causes herpes and sometimes may be accompanied by serious complications, such as encephalitis and bacterial super-infection. Varicella is more serious in adults, particularly in immunodeficient individuals, in whom it can cause devastating disease. The varicella vaccine (Varivax) was licensed in 1995 and appears to be very effective in protecting against chickenpox, but it is much too early to completely evaluate the impact of the immunization program on the epidemiology of varicella-zoster.

The ACIP recommends hepatitis A vaccination (Havrix, VAQTA) for children residing in communities where the incidence of hepatitis A is high and common.

In June 2006, the FDA licensed the first vaccine developed to prevent cancer and other diseases in women that are caused by certain types of the genital human papillomavirus (HPV). This vaccine (trade name Gardasil) protects against four HPV types (6, 11, 16, and

18) that are responsible for cervical cancer and 90% of genital warts. This vaccine is recommended for girls and women between the ages of 9 and 26 years.

The best time for girls to receive this vaccine is ages 10–11 years (this age group is used because, ideally, the vaccine should be administered before the onset of sexual activity). The recommendations for HPV vaccine are three intramuscular injections over a 6-month period, with the second dose given 2 months after the first dose and the third dose given 6 months after the first dose.

The HPV vaccine has been tested in more than 11,000 women in many countries throughout the world, including the United States. It has been found to be safe and without any serious side effects. The vaccine appears to be effective for at least 5 years. Efficacy studies for this vaccine in men are ongoing, but currently no data support its use in men.

✳ Apply Your **Knowledge 20.3**

The following questions focus on what you have just learned about the various childhood immunizations.

CRITICAL THINKING

1. Give five examples of viral vaccines.
2. Give five examples of bacterial vaccines.
3. Explain which vaccine should be given to toddlers every year.
4. Identify the vaccine that can be given at birth, and explain why.
5. Explain varicella, and give the name of its vaccine.
6. Discuss the best time for girls to receive the HPV vaccine, and explain how many vaccines should be received.

Standards of Immunization for Adults Age 65 and Under

Pertussis vaccine is not recommended for adults, but the other nine vaccines are commonly indicated under certain circumstances if there is no evidence of immunity, such as a reliable history of having the disease or positive serologic tests. Three circumstances in which it is particularly important that the pediatric immunizations are up to date are:

1. Individuals who travel internationally because some of these diseases remain prevalent in other parts of the world
2. Women of childbearing age who may become pregnant because the immunity (such as IgG) women transfer to the fetus depends on their immune status
3. Individuals with chronic illnesses because they may be more susceptible to a disease or its adverse effects

The only routine immunization recommended for all normal adults between the ages of 18 and 65 is a **booster** dose (a dose given to increase the effectiveness of the original medication) of adult diphtheria and tetanus toxoid every 10 years. Unfortunately, many adults in this country do not comply with this recommendation and may not even be aware of it. Sometimes, patients with traumatic injury are given a tetanus booster in the emergency room or physician's office at the time of injury.

Annual influenza immunization (Fluzone, FluShield) is recommended for those at high risk for influenza complications as well as those capable of *nosocomial* (hospital) transmission of influenza to high-risk patients (e.g., physicians, nurses, pharmacists, and others who provide inpatient, outpatient, and home health care services as well as nonprofessional caregivers).

Pneumococcal polysaccharide vaccine (Pneumovax 23, Pnu-Immune 23) should be administered to people with any major immunosuppression condition, such as human immunodeficiency virus (HIV) infection, organ transplant, and some cancers. This vaccine should also be administered to patients with pulmonary or cardiovascular diseases, chronic hepatic or renal disorders, and diabetes mellitus. Meningococcal vaccine (Menomune A/C/Y/W-135) is recommended for some travelers and some closed populations in which outbreaks may occur.

The only disease for which an *International Certificate of Vaccination* may still be required is yellow fever. Travelers to underdeveloped countries (and some developed countries) may find other vaccines recommended. Hepatitis A vaccine (Havrix, VAQTA) is most likely, but cholera, typhoid, and plague vaccines may occasionally be suggested.

Hepatitis B vaccine (Energix-B, Recombivax HB) is essential for health care workers with exposure to human blood and tissues, and a number of other immunizations are recommended for those in high-risk occupations.

Bacillus Calmette Guérin (BCG) vaccine is recommended only in extremely high-risk individuals in whom other controls are impractical. Besides for tuberculosis, BCG vaccine is also used to treat bladder cancer by direct instillation into the bladder. This is sometimes called nonspecific immunotherapy, but the precise mechanism is unknown. The vaccine does promote a local inflammatory response that may be responsible for the antitumor effects.

In 2009, H1N1 influenza A first appeared in Mexico, spreading to many countries all over the world. The World Health Organization named H1N1 (which was initially referred to as the "swine flu") a pandemic virus. A vaccine against H1N1 became available in October 2009. It is available in killed and inactivated forms—either by injection or as a nasal spray. For children younger than age 10 years, the vaccine is administered in two separate doses—given 21–28 days apart. In those age 10 years and older, it is administered as a single dose. Severe infections and even deaths have occurred in every age group contracting the disease.

In the first quarter of 2010, approximately 57 million cases of H1N1 occurred in the United States alone, causing nearly 12,000 deaths. Most of these deaths occurred in people younger than age 65 years. Pregnant women should receive this vaccine, which will also help their babies to be more resistant to developing symptoms of the flu. For the 2010–2011 flu season, the H1N1 vaccine was combined with the seasonal flu vaccine.

✱ Apply Your Knowledge 20.4

The following questions focus on what you have just learned about immunizations for adults younger than age 65.

CRITICAL THINKING

1. Explain how many boosters of adult diphtheria a person should receive between ages 18 and 65.
2. Describe which type of patients should receive the BCG vaccine.
3. Give the name of the "cancer vaccine" in women.
4. Discuss when the hepatitis B immunoglobulin is required in infants,
5. Give another name for German measles.

Standards of Immunization for Adults Age 65 and Older

Evaluation of immune status and appropriate vaccination at age 65 is important to the quality of the later years of life. Every individual should continue to receive adult diphtheria and tetanus toxoid boosters every 10 years. If this has not been done, it is important to update these vaccinations at age 65. Unfortunately, many older Americans are susceptible to these diseases. Those at highest risk of fatal pneumococcal disease, such as individuals with **asplenia** (loss of the spleen), should receive a booster dose 5 years after the initial dose of the pneumococcal polysaccharide vaccine (Pneumovax 23, Pnu-Immune 23) (Table 20-4 ■).

The herpes zoster (shingles) vaccine causes an acute, inflammatory eruption of very painful vesicles, which affect the nerves in the skin. Shingles is caused by the varicella-zoster virus (VZV), which also causes chickenpox. The virus lies dormant in the dorsal root ganglia and is usually reactivated after age 65. Stress appears to play a role in its reactivation, but the full reason is not understood. The subcutaneous Zostavax vaccine for shingles, licensed in 2006, is effective in approximately 50% of patients over age 60. Serious adverse reactions to the vaccine include chills, fever, breathing problems, sore throat, flu-like symptoms, severe or painful skin rash, and weakness. The patient's physician should be contacted if any of these serious reactions occur. This vaccine is contraindicated in hypersensitive patients, with allergies to gelatin or neomycin, with immune system disorders, with use of immunosuppressants, and in women who have any possibility of becoming pregnant. Zostavax is also used to reduce the severity and incidence of posttherapeutic neuralgia.

Focus on Geriatrics

Influenza and Pneumonia Immunization

All individuals age 65 and older should receive annual influenza immunization and a single dose of pneumococcal polysaccharide vaccine. Those who received this vaccine before age 65 should receive a booster dose if it has been 5 or more years since the first dose.

Table 20-4 ■ Recommended Adult Immunization Schedule, 2016

Recommended Adult Immunization Schedule—United States - 2016

Note: These recommendations must be read with the footnotes that follow containing number of doses, intervals between doses, and other important information.

Figure 1. Recommended immunization schedule for adults aged 19 years or older, by vaccine and age group[1]

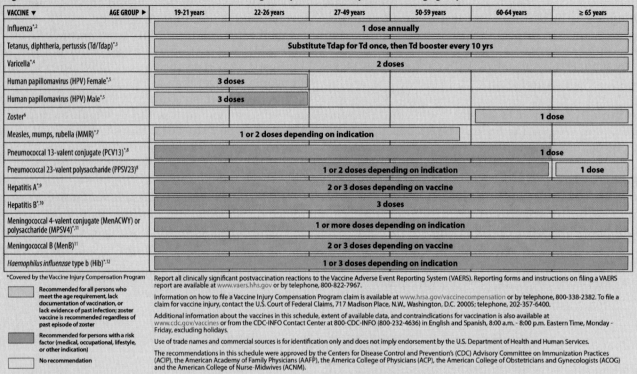

VACCINE ▼ / AGE GROUP ►	19-21 years	22-26 years	27-49 years	50-59 years	60-64 years	≥ 65 years
Influenza*,[2]	1 dose annually					
Tetanus, diphtheria, pertussis (Td/Tdap)*,[3]	Substitute Tdap for Td once, then Td booster every 10 yrs					
Varicella*,[4]	2 doses					
Human papillomavirus (HPV) Female*,[5]	3 doses	3 doses				
Human papillomavirus (HPV) Male*,[5]	3 doses					
Zoster[6]					1 dose	1 dose
Measles, mumps, rubella (MMR)*,[7]	1 or 2 doses depending on indication					
Pneumococcal 13-valent conjugate (PCV13)*,[8]						1 dose
Pneumococcal 23-valent polysaccharide (PPSV23)[8]	1 or 2 doses depending on indication					1 dose
Hepatitis A*,[9]	2 or 3 doses depending on vaccine					
Hepatitis B*,[10]	3 doses					
Meningococcal 4-valent conjugate (MenACWY) or polysaccharide (MPSV4)*,[11]	1 or more doses depending on indication					
Meningococcal B (MenB)[11]	2 or 3 doses depending on vaccine					
Haemophilus influenzae type b (Hib)*,[12]	1 or 3 doses depending on indication					

*Covered by the Vaccine Injury Compensation Program

Recommended for all persons who meet the age requirement, lack documentation of vaccination, or lack evidence of past infection; zoster vaccine is recommended regardless of past episode of zoster

Recommended for persons with a risk factor (medical, occupational, lifestyle, or other indication)

No recommendation

Report all clinically significant postvaccination reactions to the Vaccine Adverse Event Reporting System (VAERS). Reporting forms and instructions on filing a VAERS report are available at www.vaers.hhs.gov or by telephone, 800-822-7967.

Information on how to file a Vaccine Injury Compensation Program claim is available at www.hrsa.gov/vaccinecompensation or by telephone, 800-338-2382. To file a claim for vaccine injury, contact the U.S. Court of Federal Claims, 717 Madison Place, N.W., Washington, D.C. 20005; telephone, 202-357-6400.

Additional information about the vaccines in this schedule, extent of available data, and contraindications for vaccination is also available at www.cdc.gov/vaccines or from the CDC-INFO Contact Center at 800-CDC-INFO (800-232-4636) in English and Spanish, 8:00 a.m. - 8:00 p.m. Eastern Time, Monday - Friday, excluding holidays.

Use of trade names and commercial sources is for identification only and does not imply endorsement by the U.S. Department of Health and Human Services.

The recommendations in this schedule were approved by the Centers for Disease Control and Prevention's (CDC) Advisory Committee on Immunization Practices (ACIP), the American Academy of Family Physicians (AAFP), the America College of Physicians (ACP), the American College of Obstetricians and Gynecologists (ACOG), and the American College of Nurse-Midwives (ACNM).

Figure 2. Vaccines that might be indicated for adults aged 19 years or older based on medical and other indications[1]

VACCINE ▼ / INDICATION ►	Pregnancy	Immuno-compromising conditions (excluding HIV infection) [4,6,7,8,13]	HIV infection CD4+ count (cells/μL) [4,6,7,8,13] < 200	HIV infection CD4+ count ≥ 200	Men who have sex with men (MSM)	Kidney failure, end-stage renal disease, on hemodialysis	Heart disease, chronic lung disease, chronic alcoholism	Asplenia and persistent complement component deficiencies [8,11,12]	Chronic liver disease	Diabetes	Healthcare personnel
Influenza*,[2]	1 dose annually										
Tetanus, diphtheria, pertussis (Td/Tdap)*,[3]	1 dose Tdap each pregnancy	Substitute Tdap for Td once, then Td booster every 10 yrs									
Varicella*,[4]	Contraindicated	2 doses									
Human papillomavirus (HPV) Female*,[5]	3 doses through age 26 yrs	3 doses through age 26 yrs									
Human papillomavirus (HPV) Male*,[5]	3 doses through age 26 yrs	3 doses through age 21 yrs									
Zoster[6]	Contraindicated	1 dose									
Measles, mumps, rubella (MMR)*,[7]	Contraindicated	1 or 2 doses depending on indication									
Pneumococcal 13-valent conjugate (PCV13)*,[8]	1 dose										
Pneumococcal polysaccharide (PPSV23)[8]	1, 2, or 3 doses depending on indication										
Hepatitis A*,[9]	2 or 3 doses depending on vaccine										
Hepatitis B*,[10]	3 doses										
Meningococcal 4-valent conjugate (MenACWY) or polysaccharide (MPSV4)*,[11]	1 or more doses depending on indication										
Meningococcal B (MenB)[11]	2 or 3 doses depending on vaccine										
Haemophilus influenzae type b (Hib)*,[12]	3 doses post-HSCT recipients only	1 dose									

*Covered by the Vaccine Injury Compensation Program

Recommended for all persons who meet the age requirement, lack documentation of vaccination, or lack evidence of past infection; zoster vaccine is recommended regardless of past episode of zoster

Recommended for persons with a risk factor (medical, occupational, lifestyle, or other indication)

No recommendation

Contraindicated

These schedules indicate the recommended age groups and medical indications for which administration of currently licensed vaccines is commonly recommended for adults aged ≥19 years, as of February 2016. For all vaccines being recommended on the Adult Immunization Schedule: a vaccine series does not need to be restarted, regardless of the time that has elapsed between doses. Licensed combination vaccines may be used whenever any components of the combination are indicated and when the vaccine's other components are not contraindicated. For detailed recommendations on all vaccines, including those used primarily for travelers or that are issued during the year, consult the manufacturers' package inserts and the complete statements from the Advisory Committee on Immunization Practices (www.cdc.gov/vaccines/hcp/acip-recs/index.html). Use of trade names and commercial sources is for identification only and does not imply endorsement by the U.S. Department of Health and Human Services.

U.S. Department of Health and Human Services
Centers for Disease Control and Prevention

Courtesy of Centers for Disease Control and Prevention. *Recommended Adult Immunization Schedule—United States, 2016.* Available at www.cdc.gov/vaccines/schedules/downloads/adult/adult-combined-schedule.pdf.

Focus On

Immunoglobulins

Globulins are proteins that contain antibodies and are present in blood. Igs are derived from human plasma containing antibodies that have been formed by the body to specific antigens. The antibody content is primarily IgG (90–98%) and their **isotypes** (atoms of a chemical element that have the same atomic number with nearly identical chemical properties but different physical properties). There are two types of Igs: one that should be administered intramuscularly and one that should be administered intravenously.

The Ig intramuscular (IGIM) products are aqueous solutions containing 15% protein, of which more than 90% is IgG. They are standardized for antibodies to measles, diphtheria, and poliovirus to ensure reasonable uniformity of product, but they contain antibodies specific for numerous bacteria, viruses, and fungi. Ig is given by injection into a muscle.

How do they work?

The Igs are given to provide passive immunity to one or more infectious diseases. Individuals receiving Igs receive antibodies only to the diseases to which the donor blood is immune. The onset of protection is rapid but of short duration (1–3 months).

How are they used?

The main indications of IGIM are for IgG replacement therapy in disorders where there is a deficiency of IgG antibodies and for the passive prevention or modification of hepatitis A and measles in susceptible persons when given shortly after exposure. Passive immunization for measles is particularly important in children younger than 1 year of age because they are prone to measles complications and have not yet been vaccinated. IGIM is not standardized for hepatitis B, and the specific Ig should be used in this case. IGIM can be used for the prevention of varicella in immunocompromised patients if varicella-zoster Ig is not available. It has also been used to prevent fetal damage in women who are exposed to rubella during the first trimester of pregnancy. Igs (intramuscular [IM] or intravenous [IV]) are recommended to HIV-positive patients who are exposed to measles regardless of their immunization status.

What are the adverse effects?

Few adverse reactions are associated with IGIM except for local pain and tenderness at the injection site. As with all Ig products, serious anaphylactic reactions occur occasionally and are the most common selective Ig deficiency.

What are the contraindications and interactions?

IGIM must not be injected intravenously because it can cause serious anaphylactic reactions.

What are the important points patients should know?

Instruct patients to report signs and symptoms of hypersensitivity and infusion symptoms of nausea, chills, headache, or chest tightness. Advise women to avoid breastfeeding unless consulting a physician.

Focus Point

Site of Injection

The dosage and the site for the injection vary according to the amount of Ig required and the size of the person (typically, the site is in the buttocks for adults and the leg or arm for children).

❇ Apply Your **Knowledge** 20.5

The following questions focus on what you have just learned about immunoglobulins.

CRITICAL THINKING

1. Give the classifications of immunoglobulins.
2. Explain the route of administration of immunoglobulins.
3. Discuss the type of immunity that may be provided by the immunoglobulins.
4. Identify the contraindication of immunoglobulins.
5. Describe the reasons that the shingles vaccine is recommended more commonly after age 65 years.

Focus Point

Two New Vaccines

New vaccines under development include those for the Ebola virus and the Zika virus. Many companies worldwide are developing various types of vaccines against *Ebola virus disease*, which is a type of hemorrhagic fever that is often lethal. It is hoped one or more of these vaccines will reach the market within several years. The Zika virus is transmitted by the bites of infected mosquitoes and through sexual contact. It initially causes Zika fever and may be spread from a pregnant woman to her baby, resulting in microcephaly and other severe brain abnormalities. Two vaccines are under development, using recombinant and inactivated methods, but may be a decade away from reaching the market.

PRACTICAL SCENARIO 1

A young mother of an infant is seen at the pediatrician's office for the child's first visit. While you are taking a history, the mother confides that she does not want her infant to receive any vaccinations because she has heard that immunizations cause autism, diabetes, and seizures. She asks you why her infant needs to be vaccinated.

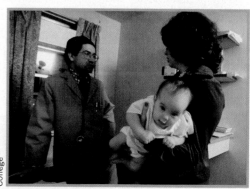

Laima Druskis/Pearson Education/PH College

Critical Thinking Questions

1. What would you tell her is the purpose of vaccinations?
2. Are there reasons why her child should not be vaccinated?
3. What questions would you suggest she ask the pediatrician to allay her concerns?

PRACTICAL SCENARIO 2

A mother brought her 2-month-old baby to the pediatrician's office to receive her first vaccines. She asked the medical assistant how many vaccines the baby should receive at this time.

Jaimie Duplass/Shutterstock

Critical Thinking Questions

1. What is the appropriate answer that the medical assistant should give?
2. Which are the vaccines that should be administered at this time?

Chapter Capsule

This section repeats the objectives from the beginning of the chapter and then provides a summary of the most important concepts for that objective. Use this section as a quick review and to check your knowledge.

Objective 1: State the names and functions of blood cells involved in immunity.

- White blood cells (lymphocytes)—manufacture antibodies to overcome infection and disease

- T cells, B cells, and natural killer cells—attack viruses, fungi, bacteria, and other foreign cells that invade the body

Objective 2: List the major components of the lymphatic system.

- Lymphatic vessels, lymph fluid, lymph nodes, thymus gland, spleen, and tonsils

Objective 3: Discuss and contrast the various types of immunities.

- Humoral immunity—B cells produce circulating antibodies to act against an antigen

- Cell-mediated immunity—T cells attack the antigens directly rather than producing antibodies

Objective 4: Explain the differences between active and passive immunity.

- Active immunity—a form of acquired immunity that develops in response to an antigen either naturally acquired by exposure to an infectious disease or artificially acquired by receiving active immunizing agents (vaccines)

- Passive immunity—the transfer of immunoglobulins (antibodies) from an immune individual to another, occurring naturally in the active transport across the placental barrier of immunoglobulin G (IgG) antibodies from mother to fetus or by the transfer of IgA antibodies in the mother's milk

Objective 5: State the main action of immunizing agents.

- Prompt the body's immune system to become resistant to a specific disease or several diseases

- Sensitize immune cells for a possible subsequent re-exposure to the organism, thus triggering an immune response

Objective 6: Contrast inactivated and attenuated vaccines.

■ Inactivated vaccines—microorganisms in the vaccine are killed, prompting immunity in the injected individual; most bacterial vaccines are inactivated

■ Attenuated (live) vaccines—these vaccines cause an infection within the patient to induce a protective immune response; they contain less immunogen than killed vaccines

Objective 7: List the most common adverse effects associated with vaccinations.

■ Localized inflammation at the site of injection, mild fever, headache, malaise, nausea, and dizziness

Objective 8: Describe the most common childhood immunizations.

■ *Haemophilus influenzae* type b (Hib) (meningitis, other bacterial diseases), Salk inactivated vaccine and the Sabin live vaccine (poliomyelitis), MMR (measles, mumps, rubella), diphtheria, tetanus, pertussis, hepatitis B, varicella-zoster (chickenpox)

Objective 9: List the most common adult immunizations.

■ Influenza vaccine annually; booster dose of adult diphtheria and tetanus toxoid every 10 years; after the initial dose of pneumococcal polysaccharide vaccine, a booster dose should be given 5 years later (adults older than age 65 need only one vaccine without a booster)

Objective 10: Explain how immunoglobulins work to provide immunity.

■ Derived from human plasma containing antibodies against specific antigens, immunoglobulins provide passive immunity

 Internet Sites of Interest

■ The Immunization Action Coalition provides numerous articles offering vaccination information for health care professionals: **www.immunize.org**

■ Safe injections are discussed on the World Health Organization's website: **www.who.int/vaccine_safety/en**

■ The National Immunization Program of the Centers for Disease Control and Prevention offers a quick reference chart, including frequently asked questions, a list of side effects, and current news related to various types of vaccines: **www.cdc.gov/vaccines/vpd-vac/vaccines-list.htm**

■ All that you need to know about getting vaccinated for travel to other countries: **wwwnc.cdc.gov/travel**

■ The Johns Hopkins Bloomberg School of Public Health provides independent assessment of studies related to vaccine safety: **www.vaccinesafety.edu**

■ State and local vaccination requirements are quite varied. For a strong collection of information: **www.cdc.gov/vaccines/imz-managers/laws/state-reqs.html**

Chapter 21

Analgesic, Antipyretic, and Anti-Inflammatory Drugs

Chapter Objectives

After completing this chapter, you should be able to:

1. List the antipyretic properties of anti-inflammatory and analgesic drugs.
2. Describe the role of prostaglandins in inflammation.
3. Outline the dangers of aspirin use.
4. List the uses and side effects of anti-inflammatory drugs.
5. Identify the different types of analgesics.
6. Describe the function of naturally occurring opioids and their receptors.
7. Explain the rationale behind the use of narcotic analgesics.
8. Describe the problems associated with the use of narcotic analgesics.
9. Explain the mechanism of action for buprenorphine and fentanyl.
10. Describe the indications of methadone.

Key Terms

acute (p. 344)
analgesic (p. 344)
antipyretics (p. 344)
aura (p. 352)
bradykinin (p. 344)

chronic (p. 344)
cyclooxygenase (p. 350)
endogenous (p. 353)
endorphins (p. 344)
enkephalins (p. 344)

migraine (p. 352)
narcotic (p. 353)
neurotransmitters (p. 344)
opiates (p. 353)
prostaglandins (p. 344)

Introduction

Analgesics are agents that relieve pain without significantly disturbing consciousness or altering the actions of the sensory nerves, which carry impulses to the brain. Therefore, many drugs that are used to relieve pain are not truly analgesics. For example, general anesthetics reduce pain but interfere with consciousness (see Chapter 25), local anesthetics reduce pain by blocking peripheral nerve fibers that carry other sensory input (see Chapter 25), antispasmodics indirectly relieve certain types of pain by relaxing smooth muscle (see Chapter 36), and steroids relieve pain associated with rheumatoid arthritis via their anti-inflammatory action (see Chapter 36). The two types of analgesics are nonopioid and opioid.

Antipyretics are drugs that reduce elevated body temperature (fever) to normal levels. Certain analgesics and antipyretics also possess anti-inflammatory properties; such agents are used in the treatment of patients with arthritis and other inflammatory conditions. The drugs considered in this chapter have demonstrated **analgesic**—or pain-relieving—action, with or without antipyretic or anti-inflammatory action.

What is Pain?

Pain is considered to be the central nervous system's (CNS's) reaction to potentially harmful stimuli characterized by physical discomfort. It has been described by the International Association for the Study of Pain as an "unpleasant sensory and emotional experience associated with actual or potential tissue damage."[1] **Acute** pain (severe pain with a sudden onset) serves as an early-warning alert to seek medical help for preventing any further damage to our bodies. Although pain can play a beneficial role as a warning system and aid in diagnosis, some pain (such as that associated with the postoperative period or cancer patients) and types of **chronic** pain (lasting a long time or marked by frequent recurrence) have very few positive effects.

Pain stimuli may result from the process of inflammation that causes tissue injury and the release of such different substances as histamine, **prostaglandins** (hormone-like substances that control blood pressure, contract smooth muscle, and modulate inflammation), serotonin, and **bradykinin** (a polypeptide that mediates inflammation, increases vasodilation, and contracts smooth muscle). Such chemical substances initiate an action potential along a sensory nerve fiber or sensitize pain receptors. These pain receptors, called *nociceptors*, are free nerve endings strategically located throughout the body. The pain enters from a pain receptor and sensory fibers, moving into the spinal cord and the brain. After being perceived, interpretation of the pain impulse occurs in the brain cortex, and appropriate autonomic and reflex responses occur to deal with the pain (Figure 21-1 ■).

The transmission of pain impulses relates to the actions of certain chemical substances called **neurotransmitters** that are concentrated in various parts of the CNS and allow communication from nerve cell to nerve cell. These neurotransmitters are known as **endorphins** and **enkephalins** and are capable of binding with opiate receptors in the CNS and thereby inhibit the transmission of pain impulses, providing an analgesic

[1] From IASP Taxonomy. Published by International Association for the Study of Pain.

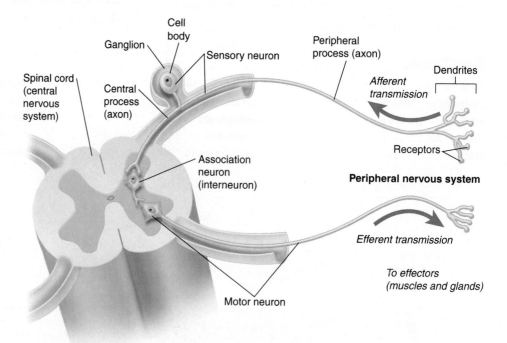

Figure 21-1 ■ Reflex responses to pain.

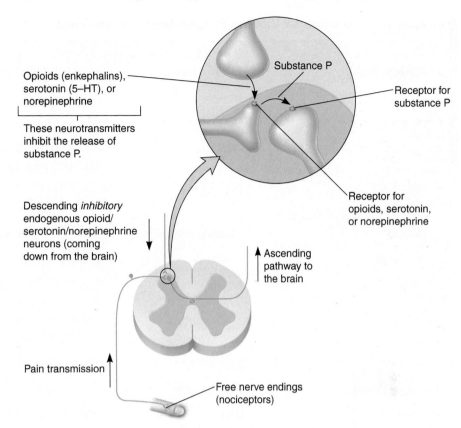

Opioids (enkephalins), serotonin (5–HT), or norepinephrine

These neurotransmitters inhibit the release of substance P.

Descending *inhibitory* endogenous opioid/ serotonin/norepinephrine neurons (coming down from the brain)

Substance P

Receptor for substance P

Receptor for opioids, serotonin, or norepinephrine

Ascending pathway to the brain

Pain transmission

Free nerve endings (nociceptors)

Figure 21-2 ■ Endogenous analgesic compounds released after pain stimuli.

effect. These analgesic compounds are released when painful stimuli affect the body (Figure 21-2 ■).

It is believed that a gating mechanism exists within the dorsal horn of the spinal cord. Small nerve fibers (pain receptors) and large nerve fibers ("normal" receptors) synapse on projection cells, which go up the spinothalamic tract to the brain and inhibitory interneurons within the dorsal horn.

The interplay among these connections determines when painful stimuli go to the brain:

1. When there is no input, the inhibitory neuron prevents the projection neuron from sending signals to the brain (the gate is closed).

2. Normal somatosensory input happens when there is more large-fiber stimulation (or only large-fiber stimulation). The inhibitory neuron and the projection neuron are stimulated, but the inhibitory neuron prevents the projection neuron from sending signals to the brain (the gate is closed).

3. Nociception (pain reception) happens when there is more small-fiber stimulation or only small-fiber stimulation. This inactivates the inhibitory neuron, and the projection neuron sends signals to the brain, informing it of pain (the gate is open).

Descending pathways from the brain close the gate by inhibiting the projector neurons and diminishing pain perception. This theory does not tell us everything about pain perception, but it does explain some things.

If you rub or shake your hand after you bang your finger, you stimulate normal somatosensory input to the projector neurons. This opens the gate and reduces the perception of pain.

Nonsteroidal Anti-Inflammatory Drugs

Nonsteroidal anti-inflammatory drugs (NSAIDs) are used to relieve some symptoms caused by arthritis, such as inflammation, swelling, stiffness, and joint pain. However, these medicines do not cure arthritis and help patients only as long as they continue to take them. Some of these drugs are also used to relieve other kinds of pain or to treat other painful conditions, such as menstrual cramps, gout attacks, bursitis, tendonitis, sprains, and muscle strains.

The salicylate group of analgesics and antipyretics is a subset of NSAIDs and are commonly used. These agents are consumed at a rate in excess of 10,000 tons annually, primarily for antiplatelet effects. Aspirin and other salicylate products should not be used in children younger than 12 years of age because of the potential for developing Reye's syndrome. Because there are so many NSAIDs available and they have similar properties, we discuss only three drugs as examples: aspirin, ibuprofen, and indomethacin. Table 21-1 ■ lists commonly used NSAIDs.

Table 21-1 ■ Commonly Used Non-Steroidal Anti-Inflammatory Drugs

GENERIC NAME	TRADE NAME	AVERAGE ADULT DOSAGE	ROUTE OF ADMINISTRATION
aspirin (acetylsalicylic acid)	Bayer	25 mg tid	PO
diclofenac	Cataflam	50 mg tid	PO
diclofenac/misoprostol	Arthrotec	100–150 mg diclofenac/ 400–600 mcg per day	PO
diflunisal	Dolobid	Initial: 1000 mg, followed by 500 mg q8h	PO
etodolac	(Generic only)	200–400 mg q6–8h	PO
fenoprofen	Nalfon	200 mg q4–6h prn	PO
flurbiprofen	Ansaid, Ocufen	Oral: 200–300 mg/d, divided into bid–qid prn; Ophthalmic: 1 drop q30min beginning 2 hours before surgery	PO, ophthalmic drops
ibuprofen	e.g., Motrin	300–800 mg tid–qid	PO
indomethacin	e.g., Tivorbex	20–40 mg bid–tid	PO
ketorolac	Generic (PO, IM, IV); Acular LS (ophthalmic)	Oral: 20 mg, followed by 10 mg q4–6h prn; IM or IV: 10 mg, followed by 10–30 mg q4–6h prn Ophthalmic: 1 drop qid prn for up to 4 days	PO, IM, IV, ophthalmic drops
nabumetone	(Generic only)	1000–2000 mg	PO
naproxen	Anaprox, Naprosyn, Naprelan	250–500 mg bid	PO
oxaprozin	Daypro	600–1200 mg/d	PO
piroxicam	Feldene	20 mg/d	PO

tid, three times a day; qid, four times a day; PO, oral; bid, twice a day; IM, intramuscular; IV, intravenous.

Focus On

Aspirin

Of all the salicylate drugs, aspirin—or acetylsalicylic acid—is the most commonly used. All commercially available salicylates have similar pharmacologic properties, so aspirin is discussed as the prototype for this group.

How does it work?

Aspirin's mechanism of action is unknown. It may produce analgesia and block pain impulses by inhibiting synthesis of prostaglandin in the CNS. It is thought to relieve fever by central action in the hypothalamic heat-regulating center. In low doses, aspirin also appears to impede clotting in the blood by blocking prostaglandin synthesis, which prevents formation of the platelet-aggregating substance, thus helping to prevent stroke and heart attack.

How is it used?

Aspirin is used as an antipyretic and analgesic in a variety of conditions. It is used for the relief of pain from simple headache, discomfort, and fever associated with the common cold and minor muscular aches and pains. When aspirin is used for lowering a fever, it is one of the most effective and safest drugs. Aspirin is also used for anti-inflammatory conditions, such as rheumatoid arthritis.

What are the adverse effects?

Although uncommon, adverse effects of aspirin taken in usual doses may include dyspepsia, nausea and vomiting, and *occult bleeding* (blood in the stool). Prolonged administration of large doses (3.6 g/day or higher) results in occult bleeding and anemia. Massive gastrointestinal (GI) hemorrhage can also occur, particularly in older adults.

What are the contraindications and interactions?

In general, salicylates are contraindicated in hypersensitive people and in patients who have GI disturbances, particularly hemorrhaging ulcers. Salicylates should also be used with caution in patients on anticoagulant therapy and avoided in patients who are taking *uricosurics* (agents that promote excretion of uric acid in the urine). Salicylates interact with a wide variety of agents, including antidiabetic drugs (causing increased hypoglycemia) and oral anticoagulants (causing increased anticoagulant effects).

What are the important points patients should know?

Aspirin can worsen any condition that involves bleeding. Advise menstruating women to avoid aspirin if menstrual bleeding is heavy, during the last 3 months of pregnancy, and while breastfeeding. Instruct patients to discontinue aspirin use 1 week before or after surgery, including oral surgery. Advise patients not to use aspirin if symptoms of meningitis exist and to avoid alcohol when taking large doses of aspirin.

Focus on Pediatrics

Aspirin and Reye's Syndrome

The use of aspirin in the treatment of fever in children who have varicella (chickenpox), a common cold, influenza virus infections, or who are younger than 12 years of age may result in the development of Reye's syndrome. The current opinion is that aspirin should not be prescribed for children who have upper respiratory viral infections. If the control of fever, aches, and pains is necessary, alternative measures should be used.

Focus on Geriatrics

Salicylates and Gastrointestinal Bleeding

Administration of salicylates to elderly patients who are vulnerable to GI bleeding may cause this bleeding to become severe. Emergency help should be requested if any of the following symptoms occurs: bloody urine, loss of hearing or vision, confusion, convulsions, diarrhea, difficulty swallowing, dizziness, severe drowsiness, severe excitement, abnormal respiration, change in skin color, hallucinations, sweating, increased thirst, nausea or vomiting, stomach pain, swelling, fever, or a "flapping" movement of the hands.

Focus On

Ibuprofen

Ibuprofen is an NSAID that possesses analgesic, anti-inflammatory, and antipyretic activities.

How does it work?

Ibuprofen, similar to other NSAIDs, has a mechanism of action that is likely related to its inhibition of prostaglandin synthesis.

How is it used?

Ibuprofen is used for rheumatoid arthritis, osteoarthritis, and arthritis. It is also indicated for patients with mild to moderate pain, dysmenorrhea, and fever.

What are the adverse effects?

Ibuprofen may cause headache, dizziness, nervousness, peripheral edema, fluid retention, and tinnitus. Common adverse effects of ibuprofen include nausea, occult blood loss, peptic ulceration, diarrhea, constipation, abdominal pain, dyspepsia, flatulence, heartburn, and decreased appetite. Severe adverse effects from ibuprofen are *azotemia* (abnormally high nitrogen-type wastes in the bloodstream), cystitis, hematuria, aplastic anemia, hypoglycemia, and hyperkalemia. In women who consume significant amounts of ibuprofen (as well as a similar agent called *naproxen*), their risk of hypertension may increase by as much as 78%.

What are the contraindications and interactions?

Ibuprofen is contraindicated in patients who are hypersensitive to the drug and in those with angioedema, nasal polyps, or bronchospastic reaction to aspirin or other NSAIDs. Pregnant women should avoid ibuprofen. Individuals with GI disorders, history of peptic ulcer, hepatic or renal disease, hypertension, and preexisting asthma should use ibuprofen cautiously. Ibuprofen may interact with antihypertensives, furosemide, and thiazide diuretics and may decrease the effectiveness of diuretics or antihypertensive drugs.

What are the important points patients should know?

Advise patients to notify their physicians if blood appears in the stool, vomitus, or urine or if there is onset of skin rash, pruritus, or jaundice. Driving a vehicle is not advised until the individual patient response to ibuprofen has been assessed. Instruct patients to not take ibuprofen with aspirin, alcohol, or NSAIDs. Breastfeeding women should not take ibuprofen.

Use of Aspirin and Ibuprofen

The FDA has issued a caution about the potential for attenuation of the antiplatelet effect of low-dose aspirin when ibuprofen is used for pain relief. This makes aspirin less effective when used for cardioprotection and stroke prevention. Patients using ibuprofen for pain relief should take this drug at least 30 minutes after taking immediate-release aspirin, or at least 8 hours before taking immediate-release aspirin. Ibuprofen and aspirin use the same receptors, meaning that they compete.

Indomethacin

Indomethacin is a nonsteroidal drug with anti-inflammatory, antipyretic, and analgesic properties. It is not a simple analgesic because of its potential serious adverse effects and should not be used for minor pain.

How does it work?

Indomethacin produces anti-inflammatory, analgesic, and antipyretic effects by inhibiting prostaglandin synthesis.

How is it used?

Indomethacin is indicated for the treatment of patients with rheumatoid arthritis, rheumatoid spondylitis, osteoarthritis, bursitis, tendonitis, gouty arthritis, and *patent ductus arteriosus* (abnormal fetal connection of the left pulmonary artery and the descending aorta) in premature neonates.

What are the adverse effects?

The most common adverse effects of indomethacin include GI ulcerations, hemorrhage, GI bleeding, increased pain in ulcerative colitis, gastritis, and nausea and vomiting. Indomethacin may also cause blurred vision, hepatic toxicity, aplastic anemia, hemolytic anemia, asthma, pruritus, urticaria, and skin rashes. Depression, mental confusion, coma, and convulsions are also reported.

What are the contraindications and interactions?

Indomethacin is contraindicated in patients who are hypersensitive to the drug and in those with a history of aspirin- or NSAID-induced asthma, rhinitis, or urticaria (hives). It must be avoided by pregnant and breastfeeding women and by neonates with untreated infection, active bleeding, and significant renal impairment. Indomethacin should be used cautiously in patients with epilepsy, parkinsonism, and hepatic or renal disease. Aminoglycosides, cyclosporine, and methotrexate may enhance the toxicity of indomethacin. Antihypertensives, furosemide, and thiazide diuretics may impair response to both drugs.

What are the important points patients should know?

Advise patients taking NSAIDs to notify their physicians promptly if they develop signs of skin rash, breathing problems, or visual disturbances. These are signs of hypersensitivity to NSAIDs.

Focus Point

Allergy to Analgesics

If the patient is allergic to one analgesic, be cautious in giving another over-the-counter (OTC) analgesic.

✳ Apply Your Knowledge 21.1

The following questions focus on what you have just learned about pain and NSAIDs.

CRITICAL THINKING

1. Explain neurotransmitters.
2. Describe the process of inflammation.
3. Define *prostaglandins*.
4. Explain endorphins and enkephalins.
5. Compare analgesics with antipyretics.
6. Define *NSAIDs*.
7. Explain Reye's syndrome.
8. Identify the mechanism of action of aspirin.
9. Discuss the indications of ibuprofen.
10. Describe the mechanism of action of indomethacin.

Focus On

Selective Cyclooxygenase-2 Inhibitors

NSAIDs play a major role in the management of inflammation and pain caused by arthritis. A new class of NSAIDs that selectively inhibits the **cyclooxygenase**-2 (COX-2) enzyme has been developed. COX is the name for a group of enzymes required to produce prostaglandins from arachidonic acid. Two subtypes of COX have been identified: COX-1 and COX-2. COX-1 is available in all cells, especially in the platelets, GI tract, and kidneys, and helps maintain homeostasis in these cells. On the other hand, COX-2 appears to be made in macrophages in response to damage to local tissues. One of the first COX-2 inhibitors—celecoxib—is said to provide therapeutic benefit with less toxicity than traditional NSAIDs. Another COX-2 selective inhibitor—meloxicam—has recently been introduced. COX-2 inhibitors and traditional NSAIDs do not appear to differ significantly in their effectiveness in alleviating pain or inflammation. They have similar GI side effects. However, short-term studies show fewer GI ulcers in patients treated with COX-2 inhibitors compared with traditional NSAIDs. On the other hand, at least one COX-2 inhibitor—rofecoxib (Vioxx)—was voluntarily removed from the market by its manufacturer because of a safety concern of increased risk of cardiovascular events (including heart attack and stroke).

How do they work?

COX-2 inhibitors affect the synthesis of prostaglandins by selectively targeting only the COX-2 enzymes. These agents have similar anti-inflammatory activity without the adverse GI effects associated with COX-1 inhibition. COX-2 inhibitors exert anti-inflammatory and analgesic effects through the inhibition of prostaglandin synthesis by blocking COX activity. The isoenzyme COX-2 is primarily associated with inflammation. Cytokines increase the expression of COX-2—mainly at inflammatory sites—producing prostaglandins that mediate inflammation, pain, and fever.

How are they used?

The FDA has labeled celecoxib for the treatment of osteoarthritis and rheumatoid arthritis in adults. It is also used for juvenile rheumatoid arthritis, ankylosing spondylitis, and the acute pain and treatment of primary dysmenorrhea. This agent is recommended in the lowest effective dosage for the shortest duration possible. Meloxicam—the newest COX-2 inhibitor—has been labeled by the FDA for the treatment of osteoarthritis (see Table 21-2 ■).

What are the adverse effects?

Similar to traditional NSAIDs, COX-2 inhibitors commonly cause abdominal pain, dyspepsia, and diarrhea. There is an increased risk of serious cardiovascular thrombotic events and even myocardial infarction and stroke, which can be fatal. This risk may increase with a longer duration of use. COX-2 inhibitors have been linked to cardiovascular problems, especially in older adults, and rofecoxib (Vioxx) was removed from the market for this reason. However, many believe that the other COX-2 inhibitors should be used cautiously in patients with a history of heart disease.

What are the contraindications and interactions?

Treatment with COX-2 inhibitors is contraindicated in patients who have hypersensitivity to these drugs, asthma, urticaria, or previous anaphylactic reactions after taking aspirin or NSAIDs. Because of the potential aggravation of hypertension and lower-extremity edema, caution should be exercised in prescribing COX-2 inhibitors to patients with congestive heart failure, fluid retention, or hypertension. COX-2 inhibitors are contraindicated in elderly patients, patients younger than 18 years, and pregnant (third-trimester) or lactating women. These agents should be avoided in patients with severe hepatic impairment or advanced renal disease. COX-2 inhibitors may diminish effectiveness of angiotensin-converting enzyme inhibitors. Fluconazole, an antifungal, can increase celecoxib concentrations. COX-2 inhibitors may increase lithium concentrations.

What are the important points patients should know?

Advise patients to tell their physicians immediately if they experience unexplained weight gain, skin rash, nausea, fatigue, lethargy, jaundice, flu-like symptoms, black tarry stool, or upper GI distress and to avoid alcohol, tobacco, and aspirin and other NSAIDs when taking meloxicam. Instruct women to avoid celecoxib during the third trimester of pregnancy. Neither celecoxib nor meloxicam should be used by women who are breastfeeding.

Table 21-2 ■ **Selective COX-2 Inhibitors**

GENERIC NAME	TRADE NAME	AVERAGE ADULT DOSAGE	ROUTE OF ADMINISTRATION
celecoxib	Celebrex	100–200 mg bid	PO
meloxicam	Mobic	7.5 mg/d	PO
bid, twice a day; PO, oral.			

✳ Apply Your Knowledge 21.2

The following questions focus on what you have just learned about selective COX-2 inhibitors and acetaminophen.

CRITICAL THINKING

1. Explain selective COX-2 inhibitors.
2. Identify the connection between COX-2 inhibitors and cardiovascular risks.
3. Differentiate between COX-1 and COX-2, and explain where these substances are especially found in the body.
4. Explain the properties and cautions of aspirin and acetaminophen.
5. Describe the adverse effects of long-term overuse of acetaminophen.

Focus Point

Differences Among Over-the-Counter Analgesics

OTC analgesics include salicylates, acetaminophen, and NSAIDs. All are antipyretics, but acetaminophen does not have an anti-inflammatory effect. Salicylates are also used to prolong clotting time by preventing platelets from binding together.

Focus On

Acetaminophen

The analgesic efficacy of acetaminophen (e.g., Tylenol) is essentially equivalent to that of NSAIDs, but acetaminophen is not anti-inflammatory. Similar to aspirin, acetaminophen has analgesic and antipyretic actions.

How does it work?

The mechanism of action of acetaminophen is unknown. As with most nonopioid analgesics, the mechanism of action is thought to be the inhibition of prostaglandin in the peripheral nervous system, making the sensory neurons less likely to receive pain signals. Acetaminophen blocks the peripheral pain impulses to a lesser degree than other NSAIDs. It lacks the anti-inflammatory action of the salicylates; hence, it is of only limited usefulness in inflammatory rheumatic disorders and is often not considered to be an NSAID agent.

How is it used?

Acetaminophen is effective in the treatment of a wide variety of arthritic and rheumatic conditions involving musculoskeletal pain as well as headache, dysmenorrhea, myalgias, and neuralgias. This agent is also useful in diseases accompanied by fever, discomfort, and pain, such as the common cold and other viral infections. Acetaminophen is particularly useful as an analgesic and antipyretic agent in patients who experience adverse reactions to aspirin.

(continued)

Focus On (continued)

. . . .

What are the adverse effects?

The adverse effects of acetaminophen are rare in therapeutic doses, and the drug is usually well tolerated by aspirin-sensitive patients. Sensitivity reactions may occur; in this case, the drug should be stopped. Over long-term use, adverse effects include skin eruptions and urticaria, hypotension, and hepatotoxicity. Daily use of acetaminophen increases the likelihood of developing hypertension. Acetaminophen is frequently combined with other drugs, such as caffeine, aspirin, and such opiates as codeine and oxycodone. An overdose can cause hepatotoxicity, coma, and internal bleeding. If overdose occurs, the antidote for acetaminophen is acetylcysteine (Acetadote).

What are the contraindications and interactions?

Acetaminophen is contraindicated in patients with a history of hypersensitivity to this drug. It must be used cautiously in children younger than 3 years of age unless directed by a physician. Repeated administration to patients with anemia, hepatic or renal impairment, or to children younger than 12 years of age who are affected by rheumatoid conditions should be avoided. Acetaminophen should be avoided in patients with alcoholism, malnutrition, or *thrombocytopenia* (a platelet deficiency often caused by anticancer drugs). Safety during pregnancy or lactation is not established.

What are the important points patients should know?

Acetaminophen may cause acute liver damage or failure in patients who consume three or more alcoholic drinks per day, but a person does not have to be a chronic drinker to experience damage. Taking acetaminophen after a weekend of drinking can prove fatal. Advise patients to avoid this combination of drugs if possible. The use of acetaminophen with barbiturates, carbamazepine, phenytoin, and rifampin may increase potential hepatotoxicity. With other drugs, such as cholestyramine, the absorption of acetaminophen is decreased. The maximum dose of acetaminophen should never exceed 4 grams per day.

Migraine

A **migraine** is the most painful type of headache, signified by pain that is pulsating or throbbing, usually in one area of the head. It may sometimes be preceded by an **aura**, which includes visual manifestations such as flashing lights, crooked lines, or blind spots. Additional perceptions may include sounds, odors, tastes, or tingling in the arms and legs. A patient with a migraine headache often becomes nauseous and may even vomit, as well as being highly sensitive to light and sound. The patient is advised to rest in a dark, quiet room. Migraines are triggered by food additives such as monosodium glutamate and nitrates. These ingredients are found in caffeinated beverages, aged cheeses, chocolate, red wine, the artificial sweetener aspartame, and also in products such as perfumes.

There are many different medications used for the treatment and future prevention of migraines. Table 21-3 ■ focuses on the selective 5-HT receptor agonists (also known as triptans), and other miscellaneous drugs. The abbreviation "5-HT" stands for 5-hydroxytriptamine, or serotonin. Other drugs that may be used for migraines include beta-adrenergic blockers, calcium channel blockers, and antiseizure drugs.

Table 21-3 ■ Drugs Used to Treat Migraines

GENERIC NAME	TRADE NAME	AVERAGE ADULT DOSAGE	ROUTE OF ADMINISTRATION
Selective 5-HT Receptor Agonists			
almotriptan	Axert	Single dose: 6.25–12.5 mg	PO
eletriptan	Relpax	Single dose: 20–40 mg	PO
frovatriptan	Frova	Single dose: 2.5 mg	PO
rizatriptan	Maxalt	Single dose: 5–10 mg	PO
sumatriptan	Imitrex	Nasal: 5–20 mg sprayed into one nostril (max: 40 mg/d)	Nasal spray
		Subcutaneous injection: 1-6 mg, may repeat (max: 12 mg/d);	SC injection

GENERIC NAME	TRADE NAME	AVERAGE ADULT DOSAGE	ROUTE OF ADMINISTRATION
sumatriptan/ naproxen	Treximet	Single dose: one tablet (85 mg sumatriptan, 500 mg naproxen)	PO
zolmitriptan	Zomig	1.25–2.5 mg/d	PO
Miscellaneous Migraine Medications			
aspirin, butalbital, caffeine, codeine	Fiorinal with Codeine	1–2 capsules q4h (max: 6 capsules/d)	PO
butorphanol nasal	Stadol	IM: 2 mg q3–4h prn IV: 1 mg q3–4h prn Nasal: one spray in one nostril of 1 mg q3–4h prn	IM, IV, nasal spray
ergotamine, caffeine	Cafergot	Initial: 2 tablets, then 1 tablet q30min (max: 6 tablets/attack)	PO

PO, oral; SC, subcutaneous; IM, intramuscular; IV, intravenous.

Opiates

The analgesic properties of opium and its derivatives have been known for centuries. **Opiates** are drugs derived from opium poppies and include morphine and codeine. *Opioid* is a general term referring to natural, synthetic, or **endogenous** (related to internal structures of function) morphine-related substances. Narcotics are drugs of certain legal status and in general are considered Schedule II drugs. They are controlled substances (see Chapter 5) and are used to treat patients with moderate to severe pain. Narcotics obtained from the raw opium plant include opium, morphine, and codeine.

Raw opium consists of the air-dried milky exudates obtained by the incision of unripe capsules of *Papaver somniferum*, which contains approximately 9.5% morphine. Opium has been known as a medicinal drug for many centuries.

Traditionally, the principal opium-exporting countries have been Iran, Turkey, India, and Yugoslavia. Drugs derived from opium, called *opiates*, owe their activity to the opioid alkaloids. Opium's chief pharmacologic effects are attributable to its morphine content and the presence of other alkaloids in amounts insufficient to significantly modify the morphine type of action. Thus, opium has many of the same uses as morphine, but morphine is nearly always preferred. Opiates have analgesic and other opioid effects.

Focus On

Morphine

Morphine can be treated chemically to produce such semisynthetic narcotics as hydromorphone, oxycodone, oxymorphone, and heroin. These are classified as Schedule II drugs, except for heroin, which is a Schedule I drug (see Chapter 5) that is an illegal **narcotic** (a medication that induces sleep or stupor and alters mood and behavior) in the United States and is not used in medicine. The properties and actions of synthetic opioids are similar to those of the natural opiates. Synthetic narcotic analgesics include meperidine (Demerol), methadone (Dolophine), remifentanil (Ultiva), and levorphanol (Levo-Dromoran).

Natural, synthetic, and semisynthetic narcotics are listed in Table 21-4 ■.

How does it work?

Morphine produces its effects by binding to the opioid receptors. Opioid receptors are located presynaptically and postsynaptically along the pain transmission pathways. High densities of receptors are found in the dorsal horn of the spinal cord and higher CNS. Opioid receptors in the brainstem are responsible for the respiratory depressant effects produced by opioid analgesics. Opioid

(continued)

Focus On (continued)

receptors in the higher CNS probably account for the effect of opioid analgesics on pain perception.

There are three major types of opioid receptors: mu, kappa, and delta. Most of the currently used opioid analgesics act primarily at mu receptors; some have varying degrees of activity at the other types of receptors.

How is it used?

Morphine is used in the management of almost all types of moderate to severe pain. Derivatives of morphine are also prescribed for cough inhibition, for treatment of GI pain, and for relieving pain associated with myocardial infarction.

What are the adverse effects?

Morphine causes nausea and vomiting, constipation, dry mouth, biliary tract spasms, dizziness, sedation, and pruritus. The major adverse effect of opioid analgesics, such as morphine, is respiratory depression. Physical and psychological dependence can occur with opioid analgesics. For this reason, health care providers often hesitate to administer the proper doses, fearing the patient will become dependent or respiratory depression will occur. When used as directed, these drugs are safe and do not cause dependent or adverse effects. Patients should always be properly medicated for pain alleviation.

What are the contraindications and interactions?

Opioid analgesics are contraindicated in patients with known hypersensitivity. They are also contraindicated in patients who have asthma, emphysema, or head injury. Opioid analgesics must be avoided in patients with increased intracranial pressure, severe liver or kidney dysfunction, acute ulcerative colitis, or convulsive disorders. Opioid analgesics must be used cautiously in patients with prostatic hypertrophy because urine retention can occur.

Opioids or opiates can interact with alcohol, causing CNS depression with subsequent respiratory depression. Meperidine undergoes a potentially fatal reaction with monoamine oxidase inhibitors (MAOIs) (antidepressants). Morphine and meperidine should not be mixed because they potentiate each other and are physically incompatible.

What are the important points patients should know?

Inform patients that the most serious adverse effect of narcotic analgesics is respiratory depression. Narcotic analgesics should not be taken if respirations are less than 12 per minute or systolic blood pressure is less than 110 mm Hg in adults. Narcotic analgesics may cause constipation, so advise patients to request symptomatic relief from their health care provider.

Table 21-4 ▪ Classifications of Opioid Analgesics

GENERIC NAME	TRADE NAME	AVERAGE ADULT DOSAGE	ROUTE OF ADMINISTRATION
Natural Opioid Analgesics			
codeine	Codeine Sulfate, also generic	15–60 mg analgesic	PO, IM, SC
morphine	Avinza	10–30 mg q4h prn or 15–30 mg sustained release of 8–12 h	PO
	Duramorph	2.5–15 mg q4h or 0.8–10 mg/h by continuous infusion	IV, epidural, intrathecal
opium tincture	Opium Tincture, Deodorized, Paregoric	Opium tincture, deodorized: 0.6 mL qid Paregoric: 5–10 mL, 1–4 times/d or as directed by physician	PO
Semisynthetic Opioid Analgesics			
hydrocodone with homatropine	Hycodan	Combination drug: 1 tablet or 1 tsp (5 mL) of syrup q4–6h prn (do not exceed 6 tablets or 6 tsp in 24 hours)	PO

GENERIC NAME	TRADE NAME	AVERAGE ADULT DOSAGE	ROUTE OF ADMINISTRATION
hydrocodone with acetaminophen	Lortab, Vicodin	Combination drug: 5–10 mg hydrocodone/ 325 mg acetaminophen q4–6h (daily dosage should not exceed 60 mg hydrocodone/ 1950 mg acetaminophen)	PO
levorphanol	Levo-Dromoran	2–3 mg q6–8h prn	PO
		1–2 mg q6–8h prn	SC, IM
		Up to 1 mg q3–6h prn	IV
oxycodone	OxyContin, Oxecta	5–15 mg q4–6h	PO
oxycodone with acetaminophen	Endocet, Percocet	Combination drug: 2.5–10 mg oxycodone/ 325 mg acetaminophen. For the 2.5 mg/ 325 mg combination, dosage is 1–2 tablets q6h prn. For the other formulations, dosage is 1 tablet q6h prn. (Total daily dose should not exceed 40 mg oxycodone/4 grams acetaminophen.)	PO
oxycodone with aspirin	Endodan, Percodan	Combination drug: 4.8 mg oxycodone/325 mg aspirin q6h prn (maximum daily dose should not exceed 12 tablets)	PO
Synthetic Opioid Agonists			
fentanyl	Duragesic, Sublimaze	Duragesic: 25 mcg/h patch q3d Sublimaze: 50–100 mcg q1–2h PRN	Transdermal IV
meperidine	Demerol	50–150 mg q3–4h prn	PO, SC, IM, IV
methadone	Dolophine, Metha- done Injection	2.5–20 mg q3–8h prn	PO, SC, IM
Synthetic Opioid Antagonists			
naloxone	Narcan	0.1–2 mg q2–3 min up to three doses if necessary	IV, IM, SC
naltrexone	ReVia	25 mg, followed by another 25 mg in 1 h if no withdrawal response (maximum: 800 mg/d)	PO
Synthetic Opioid Agonist/Antagonists			
buprenorphine	Buprenex	0.3 q6h up to 0.6 mg q4h or 25–50 mcg/h by IV infusion	IV, IM
butorphanol	Stadol	1–4 mg q3–4h prn (maximum: 4 mg/dose)	IM
		0.5–2 mg q3–4h prn	IV
	Stadol NS	1 mg (1 spray in one nostril) and, if needed, one additional dose in 60–90 minutes	Nasal spray
pentazocine with naloxone	Talwin NX	Combination drug: 50 mg pentazocine/0.5 mg naloxone. Take 1 tablet q3–4h, which may be increased to 2 tablets prn. (Total daily dosage should not exceed 12 tablets.)	PO

PO, oral; IM, intramuscular; SC, subcutaneous; IV, intravenous; qid, once a day.

Focus Point

Age Differences in Narcotic Metabolism

The metabolism of narcotics is slower in elderly patients. Therefore, opioid use may have undesirable effects, such as confusion and respiratory depression. In pediatric patients, dosing is difficult because elimination occurs at a different rate. Premature infants with chronic lung disease often have depressed hypoxic drive and require careful monitoring after the administration of opioids.

Focus On

Codeine

Although some codeine is obtained from opium directly, the quantity is not sufficient to meet the extensive use of this alkaloid as a valuable medicinal agent. Much more codeine must be used to obtain the same effects as morphine. The need for sufficient quantities of codeine is met by producing it via partial synthesis from morphine. Codeine does not produce proportionately greater analgesia as the dose is increased.

How does it work?

Similar to morphine and all other opiates, codeine binds to opioid receptors in the brain and spinal cord, thereby relieving pain.

How is it used?

Codeine is useful for inducing sleep in the presence of mild pain. Similar to morphine, this drug is used as an analgesic, sedative, hypnotic, antiperistaltic, and antitussive agent. It is commonly given in combination with aspirin, acetaminophen, or other agents. Administered alone, codeine is a Schedule II drug. In combination with aspirin-like drugs, it is classified as a Schedule III drug (see Chapter 5).

What are the adverse effects?

Codeine is less apt than morphine to cause nausea and vomiting, constipation, and *miosis* (contraction of the pupils). Tolerance, dependence, and addiction can occur. Similar to morphine, codeine produces cortical and respiratory depression, but serious degrees of either are practically unknown. Patients may also have postural hypotension.

What are the contraindications and interactions?

Codeine is contraindicated in advanced respiratory insufficiency, bronchial asthma, and patients with raised intracranial pressure. Its effects are increased by use with other drugs that have centrally suppressing effects, including alcohol, or with cimetidine (Tagamet). Antidepressive agents and neuroleptics can completely halt the analgesic effects of codeine.

What are the important points patients should know?

Instruct patients to comply with the physician-ordered drug regimen because overuse may lead to dependence and to avoid alcohol and other CNS depressants. Advise patients to report urine retention or severe constipation and to rise slowly from a lying position to prevent postural hypotension.

✳ Apply Your Knowledge 21.3

The following questions focus on what you have just learned about opioid analgesics.

CRITICAL THINKING

1. Differentiate between opioids and opiates, and give examples of each.
2. List four generic names and trade names of synthetic opioids.
3. What are three major types of opioid receptors?
4. What are three classes of opioid analgesics?
5. What are the major adverse effects of opioid analgesics?

Semisynthetic Opioid Analgesics

Semisynthetic opioid analgesics are modifications of the natural alkaloids of opium. These agents have the same advantages of morphine or codeine without their disadvantages. Examples of semisynthetic opioids include hydrocodone, oxycodone, and oxymorphone (see Table 21-4).

Focus On

Hydrocodone

Hydrocodone is a morphine derivative similar to codeine but is more addicting and has slightly greater antitussive activity and analgesic effects. This CNS depressant relieves moderate to severe pain. Hydrocodone is a Schedule III drug. Hydrocodone is combined with other drugs, such as aspirin-like analgesics, antihistamines, expectorants, and *sympathomimetics* (drugs that increase cardiac output, dilate bronchioles, and constrict blood vessels). Examples of its combinations include hydrocodone with homatropine (Hycodan) and hydrocodone with chlorpheniramine (Tussionex).

How does it work?

Hydrocodone suppresses the cough reflex by direct action on the cough center in the medulla of the brain. It also acts as a CNS depressant, which relieves moderate to severe pain.

How is it used?

Hydrocodone is used for relief of nonproductive cough and for moderate to severe pain.

What are the adverse effects?

The most common adverse effects include dry mouth, nausea and vomiting, constipation, sedation, dizziness, and drowsiness. Other adverse effects are euphoria, dysphoria, respiratory depression, pruritus, and skin rashes.

What are the contraindications and interactions?

Hydrocodone is contraindicated in patients with a history of hypersensitivity to this drug and in women who are lactating. It should be used cautiously in patients with asthma, emphysema, a history of drug abuse, and respiratory depression. This drug can be prescribed with caution in children younger than 1 year and in pregnant women. Hydrocodone with alcohol and other CNS depressant compounds may interact and cause severe CNS depression.

What are the important points patients should know?

Instruct patients taking hydrocodone to avoid hazardous activities until response to the drug is determined. Advise patients to drink plenty of liquids to ensure adequate hydration. Because the abuse potential of hydrocodone is high, advise patients to take only the dose prescribed. Patients should never breastfeed while taking this drug.

Oxycodone

Although oxycodone has less analgesic capability than morphine, it possesses comparable addiction potential and is a Schedule II drug. It frequently is used in combination with aspirin or acetaminophen. Examples include combinations of oxycodone with acetaminophen and oxycodone with aspirin.

How does it work?

The most prominent actions of oxycodone affect the CNS and organs composed of smooth muscle. Oxycodone binds with specific receptors in various sites of the CNS to alter perception of pain and emotional response to pain, but its precise mechanism of action is not clear. Oxycodone is as potent as morphine and 10–12 times more potent than codeine.

How is it used?

This agent is used for relief of moderate to severe pain, such as the type that may occur with bursitis, dislocations, simple fractures, and other injuries. Oxycodone is also indicated to relieve postoperative and postpartum pain.

What are the adverse effects?

The adverse effects of oxycodone include euphoria, dysphoria, lightheadedness, dizziness, sedation, anorexia,

(continued)

Focus On (*continued*)

nausea and vomiting, constipation, jaundice, hepatotoxicity, and respiratory depression.

What are the contraindications and interactions?

Oxycodone is contraindicated in patients with hypersensitivity to this drug and during pregnancy and lactation. It is also contraindicated in children younger than 6 years of age. It must be used cautiously in people with alcoholism, renal or hepatic disease, and viral infections. Oxycodone is also prescribed with caution in patients with chronic ulcerative colitis, gallbladder disease, head injury, acute abdominal conditions, hypothyroidism, prostatic hypertrophy, and respiratory disease.

What are the important points patients should know?

Instruct patients to take oxycodone in the form prescribed without crushing, chewing, or breaking the medication, it is formulated to be released into the blood slowly. Advise patients to avoid driving, operating heavy machinery, and performing other hazardous activities because oxycodone causes drowsiness and dizziness. Alcohol must also be avoided. This drug may increase the effects of antidepressants, antihistamines, pain relievers, anxiety medications, seizure medications, and muscle relaxants. Instruct patients to take only the dose that was prescribed; taking too much of this drug could result in serious adverse effects and even death.

Synthetic Opioid Antagonists

The term *antagonist*, as used in this section, applies to naloxone and naltrexone, which are antagonists with little or no agonist actions. These competitive opioid antagonists are effective in the management of severe respiratory depression induced by opioid drugs, of *asphyxia neonatorum* (respiratory distress in the newborn) caused by administration of these drugs to the expectant mother, and for the diagnosis or treatment of opioid addiction.

Focus On

Naloxone

Naloxone is a synthetic opioid antagonist essentially devoid of opioid-agonist properties. Hence, it does not possess morphine-like properties, such as respiratory depression, psychotomimetic effects, and pupillary constriction, which are characteristic of other opioid antagonists.

How does it work?

Available evidence suggests that naloxone antagonizes these opioid effects by competing for the same receptor sites.

How is it used?

Naloxone is prescribed for narcotic overdose and complete or partial reversal of narcotic depression, including respiratory depression induced by natural and synthetic narcotics. Naloxone is a drug of choice when the nature of a depressant drug is not known and for the diagnosis of suspected acute opioid overdose.

What are the adverse effects?

Naloxone may cause reversal of analgesia, tremors, slight drowsiness, hyperventilation, sweating, nausea and vomiting, hypertension, and tachycardia.

What are the contraindications and interactions?

Naloxone is contraindicated in patients with respiratory depression caused by nonopioid drugs. Safety during pregnancy or lactation is not established. Naloxone must be used cautiously in neonates and children. It must be avoided in patients who are suspected to be dependent on narcotics and for those with cardiac irritability.

What are the important points patients should know?

Naloxone reverses the analgesic effects of narcotic agents and may cause withdrawal symptoms or the patient may experience a return of the pain that the narcotic agents were originally prescribed to treat. Instruct patients to tell their physician about postoperative pain that emerges after naloxone is administered.

Naltrexone

Naltrexone generally has little or no agonist activity. Its opioid antagonist activity is reported to be two to nine times that of naloxone.

How does it work?

The mechanism of action of naltrexone is not clearly known, but it appears that its competitive binding at opioid receptor sites reduces euphoria.

How is it used?

Naltrexone is used as an adjunct to the maintenance of an opioid-free state in detoxified addicts who are and desire to remain narcotic-free. It is also used in the management of alcohol dependence as an adjunct to social and psychotherapeutic methods.

What are the adverse effects?

Naltrexone causes dry mouth, anorexia, nausea and vomiting, constipation, abdominal cramps, and hepatotoxicity. This agent may also cause muscle and joint pains, headache, nervousness, irritability, dizziness, and depression.

What are the contraindications and interactions?

Naltrexone is contraindicated in patients receiving opioid analgesics and in acute opioid withdrawal and opioid-dependent patients. It must be avoided in patients with acute hepatitis and liver failure. Naltrexone is also contraindicated in any individual who has a positive urine screen for opioids. Safety during pregnancy, lactation, or in children younger than age 18 years is not established.

Phenothiazines are antipsychotics that may interact with the administration of naltrexone and cause increased somnolence and lethargy. Naltrexone reverses the analgesic effects of narcotic agonists and narcotic agonist–antagonists. Examples of phenothiazines include chlorpromazine (Thorazine) and thioridazine (Mellaril).

What are the important points patients should know?

Naltrexone may put patients in danger of fatally overdosing if they are using opiates. Advise patients to check with their physician before taking OTC drugs with naltrexone because opioids are present in many OTC preparations, including cough medicines. Instruct patients to tell their physician or dentist that they are taking naltrexone before undergoing treatment and to wear medical alert jewelry to indicate naltrexone use. Warn female patients to avoid breastfeeding while using naltrexone without first consulting their physician. Patients taking methadone for treatment of opioid dependency or addiction may be able to transfer from methadone to naltrexone after gradual withdrawal and final discontinuation of methadone.

❋ Apply Your Knowledge 21.4

The following questions focus on what you have just learned about synthetic and semisynthetic opioid antagonists.

CRITICAL THINKING

1. Describe synthetic opioid antagonists, and name two examples.
2. Give three examples of semisynthetic opioids.
3. Identify the most prominent action of oxycodone.
4. Explain adverse effects of naloxone.
5. Give the trade names of naltrexone, oxycodone, and naloxone?

Synthetic Opioid Analgesics

Synthetic opioid analgesics have the properties of morphine as analgesics but have fewer undesirable effects and less addiction potential. Currently available synthetic agents have valuable analgesic and pharmacologic properties that are described in this section.

Focus On

Buprenorphine

Buprenorphine is a centrally acting synthetic and narcotic analgesic. This opiate agonist–antagonist has agonist activity approximately 30 times that of morphine and antagonist activity equal to or up to three times greater than that of naloxone.

How does it work?

Dose-related analgesia results from a high affinity of buprenorphine for mu-opioid receptors and an antagonist at the kappa-opiate receptors in the CNS.

How is it used?

Buprenorphine is used principally for patients with moderate to severe postoperative pain. It is also administered for pain associated with cancer, accidental trauma, urethral calculi, and myocardial infarction.

What are the adverse effects?

Buprenorphine may cause sedation, drowsiness, vertigo, dizziness, headache, amnesia, euphoria, and insomnia.

This agent can also cause hypotension, miosis, nausea and vomiting, diarrhea, and constipation.

What are the contraindications and interactions?

Buprenorphine is contraindicated in known hypersensitivity to this agent or to naloxone. Safety during pregnancy, lactation, and in children younger than 13 years is not established. Buprenorphine may interact with alcohol and cause CNS depression. Diazepam (Valium) may cause respiratory or cardiovascular collapse.

What are the important points patients should know?

Instruct patients to avoid driving or engaging in hazardous activities until response to this drug is known and to avoid alcohol and other CNS depressants. Advise female patients to avoid breastfeeding while using this drug without consulting their physician.

Fentanyl

Fentanyl is a potent and synthetic narcotic agonist analgesic agent with pharmacologic actions similar to those of morphine and meperidine.

How does it work?

The principal mechanism of action of fentanyl is most likely due to its conversion to morphine. However, its action is more prompt and less prolonged than that of morphine or meperidine.

How is it used?

Fentanyl is a short-acting analgesic drug used during operative and perioperative periods. This agent is prescribed as a narcotic analgesic supplement in general and as a regional anesthesia with diazepam or droperidol to produce *neuroleptanalgesia* (a form of analgesia accompanied by the general quieting of the patient and indifference to environmental stimuli without loss of consciousness). Fentanyl is also given with oxygen and a skeletal muscle relaxant to select high-risk patients, such as those undergoing open-heart surgery.

What are the adverse effects?

The adverse effects of fentanyl include sedation, euphoria, dizziness, *delirium* (excitement and mental confusion

with hallucinations), and convulsions with high doses. This agent may also cause hypotension, bradycardia, cardiac arrest, and respiratory arrest. In some patients, blurred vision and miosis are reported. Other common adverse effects of fentanyl include nausea and vomiting and constipation.

What are the contraindications and interactions?

Fentanyl is contraindicated in the management of acute or postoperative pain and in mild or intermittent pain that can be otherwise managed by less potent agents. It is also contraindicated at high doses at the initiation of opioid therapy and in patients with hypersensitivity to this agent. This agent may interact with alcohol and other CNS depressants, increasing their effects. Fentanyl may also interact with MAOIs to cause hypertensive crisis.

What are the important points patients should know?

Instruct patients to report muscle rigidity or weakness; unusual postoperative muscle movement of the extremities, eyes, or neck; and any problems breathing after taking this drug.

Meperidine

Meperidine is a synthetic opioid agonist analgesic with multiple actions qualitatively similar to those of morphine.

How does it work?

The most prominent of drug actions are on the CNS and on organs composed of smooth muscle. It acts principally to induce analgesia and sedation.

How is it used?

Meperidine is indicated for preoperative use, relief of moderate to severe pain, supportive anesthesia, and obstetric analgesia.

What are the adverse effects?

Major adverse effects include respiratory depression or arrest, circulatory depression, shock, and cardiac arrest. The most common untoward effects include dizziness, sedation, nausea and vomiting, and sweating. Other adverse effects include euphoria, headache, weakness, agitation, tremor, seizures, disorientation, and hallucinations.

What are the contraindications and interactions?

Meperidine is contraindicated in patients taking MAOIs; it has inconsistently precipitated severe and occasionally fatal reactions within 14 days. The drug should be used with caution and in reduced dosage in patients taking other opioid analgesics, general anesthetics, phenothiazines, sedatives, tricyclic antidepressants, and other CNS depressants.

What are the important points patients should know?

Advise patients to ambulate carefully and to avoid smoking. Instruct patients to avoid driving or engaging in hazardous activities until drowsiness and dizziness have passed. CNS depressants and alcohol should be avoided. Female patients should not breastfeed while using this drug.

Focus on Geriatrics

Oversedation in Elderly Patients

Sedatives and narcotics must be given with extreme caution to older adults, who may easily become oversedated.

Focus On

Methadone

Methadone is a synthetic opioid agonist with multiple analgesic actions quantitatively similar to morphine.

How does it work?

Methadone binds with opiate receptors in the CNS, altering the perception of and emotional response to pain.

How is it used?

Methadone is indicated for the relief of moderate to severe chronic pain. It is also used for the detoxification of opioid addiction and for temporary or sometimes long-term maintenance treatment of opioid addiction.

What are the adverse effects?

The adverse effects of methadone are similar to those for other opioid analgesics, especially meperidine.

What are the contraindications and interactions?

Methadone is contraindicated in patients with known hypersensitivity. The drug should be used with caution and in reduced dosage in patients taking other opioid analgesics, general anesthetics, phenothiazines and other tranquilizers, sedative–hypnotics, tricyclic antidepressants, MAOIs, and other CNS depressants. The safe use of methadone in pregnancy has not been established. It is not recommended for obstetric analgesia because its long duration may induce respiratory depression in newborns.

What are the important points patients should know?

Instruct patients to make position changes slowly, especially from a supine to an upright position, and to sit or

(continued)

Focus On (*continued*)

lie down if they feel dizzy or faint. Advise patients to avoid driving or engaging in potentially hazardous activities until the response to this drug is known. Female patients should not breastfeed while taking this drug without consulting their physician.

Pentazocine

Pentazocine is a synthetic narcotic agonist–antagonist analgesic that is classified as a controlled substance (Schedule IV drug). It is often combined with other agents. Examples include pentazocine with naloxone and pentazocine with aspirin.

How does it work?

Pentazocine has a similar mechanism of action to that of morphine but with only one-third the strength. Large doses of pentazocine may increase blood pressure and heart rate. When given in usual parenteral doses, it is as effective in relieving moderate to severe pain as the usual parenteral doses of morphine, meperidine, butorphanol, or nalbuphine.

How is it used?

Pentazocine is indicated for the control of moderate to severe pain. It is also used for preoperative analgesia or sedation and as a supplement to surgical anesthesia.

What are the adverse effects?

Pentazocine causes nausea and vomiting, diarrhea, constipation, dry mouth, and alterations of taste. This agent may also cause dizziness, lightheadedness, sedation, euphoria, headache, disturbed dreams, insomnia, syncope (fainting), and visual blurring. Hypotension, tachycardia, and respiratory depression have also been included among its adverse effects.

What are the contraindications and interactions?

Pentazocine is contraindicated in patients with a history of hypersensitivity. This agent must be avoided in patients with head injuries or increased intracranial pressure, in emotionally unstable patients, and in those with a history of drug abuse. Safety during pregnancy or lactation or in children younger than age 12 years is not established. Pentazocine must be used cautiously in patients with impaired kidney or liver function, respiratory depression, biliary surgery, and myocardial infarction with nausea and vomiting. Alcohol and other CNS depressants add to CNS depression with the use of pentazocine.

What are the important points patients should know?

Instruct patients to avoid driving and other hazardous activities until the response to this drug is known. Pentazocine should not be discontinued abruptly after extended use, and female patients should not breastfeed while taking this drug.

✳ Apply Your Knowledge 21.5

The following questions focus on what you have just learned about synthetic opioid analgesics.

CRITICAL THINKING

1. Identify the characteristics of buprenorphine.
2. Give the principal mechanism of action of fentanyl.
3. Explain the most prominent actions of meperidine.
4. Briefly discuss the effects of large doses of pentazocine on the cardiovascular system.
5. Give the trade names of meperidine, methadone, and fentanyl.

PRACTICAL SCENARIO 1

Janet is a 4-year-old girl who is found unconscious. Her grandmother calls the physician's office and speaks to the medical assistant, who instructs her to call 911 immediately, which she does. When emergency help arrives, the grandmother states that she put her granddaughter down for a nap around 1:00 P.M. in the grandmother's bedroom. At about 2:30 P.M., she checked on Janet and found her on the floor of the bedroom, unconscious and unresponsive, with an open bottle of acetaminophen beside her. The grandmother says the bottle of 60 tablets was empty, and there were seven to 10 tablets on the floor.

Pearson Education/PH College

Critical Thinking Questions

1. In counseling the grandmother about this incident, what teaching information should be provided by health care personnel?
2. What are some of the complications of an overdose of acetaminophen?

PRACTICAL SCENARIO 2

A 48-year-old man had back surgery for disc herniations. His physician prescribed oxycodone for pain relief. Two weeks after surgery, he was released on his 40th birthday. To celebrate, he drank several glasses of wine at the party. Upon going to bed, he took several doses of oxycodone for his back pain. The next morning, his wife could not wake him.

Darren Baker/Shutterstock

Critical Thinking Questions

1. What was the cause of his death?
2. Why should oxycodone never be taken with alcohol?

Chapter Capsule

This section repeats the objectives from the beginning of the chapter and then provides a summary of the most important concepts for that objective. Use this section as a quick review and to check your knowledge.

Objective 1: List the antipyretic properties of anti-inflammatory and analgesic drugs.

- Inhibition of prostaglandin synthesis in the CNS
- Central action in the hypothalamic heat-regulating center

Objective 2: Describe the role of prostaglandins in inflammation.

- Prostaglandins are hormone-like substances that modulate inflammation. They initiate an action potential along a sensory nerve fiber or sensitize pain receptors.

Objective 3: Outline the dangers of aspirin use.

- Possible massive GI hemorrhage, dyspepsia, nausea and vomiting, and occult bleeding

Objective 4: List the uses and side effects of anti-inflammatory drugs.

- Used for rheumatoid arthritis, osteoarthritis, arthritis, moderate pain, and fever
- Side effects—dizziness, nervousness, occult blood loss, peptic ulceration, GI bleeding, and others

Objective 5: Identify the different types of analgesics.

- Nonopioid analgesics
- Opioid analgesics

Objective 6: Describe the function of naturally occurring opioids and their receptors.

- Naturally occurring opioids bind to opioid receptors to block pain transmission

Objective 7: Explain the rationale behind the use of narcotic analgesics.

- Effective for almost all types of moderate and severe pain and for cough inhibition
- Mimic endogenous opioids to block pain transmission

Objective 8: Describe the problems associated with the use of narcotic analgesics.

- Can cause respiratory depression
- Can produce physical and psychological dependence

Objective 9: Explain the mechanism of action for buprenorphine and fentanyl.

- Buprenorphine causes dose-related analgesia because of a high affinity for mu-opioid receptors and an antagonist at the kappa-opiate receptors in the CNS.
- The principle mechanism of action of fentanyl is most likely due to its conversion to morphine. However, its action is more prompt and less prolonged than that of morphine or meperidine.

Objective 10: Describe the indications of methadone.

- Methadone is indicated for the relief of moderate to severe chronic pain. It is also used for the detoxification of opioid addiction and for temporary or sometimes long-term maintenance treatment of opioid addiction.

 Internet Sites of Interest

- A discussion about tolerance to opioids: **www.practicalpainmanagement.com/ treatments/pharmacological/opioids/tolerance-opioids**
- Pain management information, including treatment and education facts: **www.painedu.org/index.asp**
- The National Institutes of Health offers information on drugs and other medical conditions on its MedLine Plus website: **www.nlm.nih.gov/medlineplus**. Search for "NSAIDs."
- An explanation of antipyretics: **http://drugs.nmihi.com/fever-reducers.htm**
- The World Health Organization (WHO) has developed a widely recognized protocol for use of pain medications, called the WHO Pain Ladder. For an example: **www.who.int/cancer/palliative/painladder/en**

Chapter 22

Antineoplastic Agents

Chapter Objectives

After completing this chapter, you should be able to:

1. List the seven warning signs of cancer.
2. Summarize the basic cell cycle and its importance in the use of antineoplastic agents.
3. List commonly used antineoplastic agents in each class.
4. Describe the indications of mercaptopurine and vinblastine.
5. Explain the mechanism of action of each class of antineoplastic agents.
6. Discuss how steroids, estrogens, progestins, antiestrogens, and antiandrogens work in the treatment of cancer.
7. Explain how biologic response modifiers are created and how they work.
8. Identify how monoclonal antibodies function in the treatment of cancer.
9. Identify the common side effects of chemotherapy treatment.
10. Describe immunotherapy to treat cancers.

Key Terms

adenocarcinoma (p. 366)
adjuvant (p. 369)
alkylating agents (p. 372)
alopecia (p. 372)
angiogenesis (p. 366)
antimetabolites (p. 373)
antitumor antibiotics (p. 376)
benign (p. 366)

carcinogenic (p. 367)
hybridomas (p. 377)
hyperplasia (p. 366)
malignant (p. 366)
metastasis (p. 366)
mitosis (p. 367)
monoclonal antibodies (p. 377)
nucleotides (p. 367)

oncogenes (p. 367)
palliative (p. 369)
partial response (p. 369)
plant alkaloids (p. 374)
sarcomas (p. 366)
stable disease (p. 369)
teratogenic (p. 372)
tumor suppressor genes (p. 367)

Introduction

Approximately 14.5 million individuals in the United States have some form of cancer. The American Cancer Society estimated that more than 1.6 million new cancer cases would be diagnosed in 2015. Advances in chemotherapy and radiation therapy, along with better understanding of treatment principles, allow patients to receive the majority of their treatment in clinics or at home. Cancer is the second-most common cause of death in the United States after cardiovascular disease, with more than 589,000 fatalities annually. The most common cancers are breast, prostate, lung, and colorectal. The leading cause of cancer death is lung cancer. Cancer is a group of more than 100 different diseases, characterized by uncontrolled cellular division and **hyperplasia**, local tissue invasion, and **metastasis**. Leukemia is a very common cancer in children, particularly in African Americans. Tumors can be benign or malignant.

Neoplasms

Tumors arise from any of the four basic tissue types: epithelial, connective (blood, bone, and cartilage), muscle, and nerve. **Benign** tumors are generally slow growing and resemble normal cells. They are localized and not harmful. **Malignant** tumors often proliferate more rapidly and have an atypical appearance. This atypical appearance is because cancer cells, unlike normal cells, do not continue to mature. Instead, their rapid multiplication causes them to become more and more atypical— a process often called *differentiation*. They invade and destroy surrounding tissues, and they induce the formation of new blood vessels that act as the tumor's own blood supply to help spread malignant cells to other tissues. This process is known as **angiogenesis**.

Benign tumors are named by adding the suffix *-oma* to the name of the cell type. For example, *adenomas* are benign growths of glandular origin. On the other hand, *carcinomas* are malignant growths arising from epithelial cells. An **adenocarcinoma** is a malignant tumor arising from glandular origin. Malignant growths of muscle or connective tissue are called **sarcomas**. Another term used frequently in the description of malignancy is *carcinoma in situ*. In this instance, the cancer is limited to the epithelial cells where it began. Because cancers are most curable with surgery or radiation before they have metastasized, early detection and treatment is very important. In addition, small tumors are more responsive to chemotherapy than are large tumors. Early diagnosis is difficult for many cancers because they do not produce clinical signs or symptoms until they have become large or have metastasized.

Tumors are constantly shedding neoplastic cells into the systemic circulation or surrounding lymphatic nodules. Cells of benign tumors resemble the cells from which they developed. These masses seldom metastasize, and after they are removed, they rarely recur. In contrast, malignant tumors invade and destroy the surrounding tissues. Malignant tumors tend to metastasize, so recurrences are common after the removal or destruction of the primary tumor.

What Causes Cancer?

Cancer is actually a complex group of diseases. There are many possible causes of cancer. A variety of carcinogens may cause cancer. Carcinogens are present in tobacco, radiation exposure, sun and ultraviolet exposure, various chemical substances, and viruses. Cigarette smoking remains the major individual cause of cancer death in the United States. The use of tobacco causes nearly one out of every five deaths. Since smoking is a chosen habit, it is the most preventable cause of death from cancer. Smoking is linked to cancers of not only the lungs, but also the oral cavity, nose, sinuses, pharynx, larynx, esophagus, stomach, pancreas, kidney, bladder, cervix, ovary, colorectum, and also acute myeloid leukemia. Secondhand smoke is also significant in causing cancer.

Exposure to many different types of radiation is also a potential cause of cancer. Radiation includes x-rays, gamma rays, radon, and others. X-rays and gamma rays come from natural sources, such as radon gas, radioactive elements in the earth itself, and cosmic rays from outer space. These rays can also be man-made, as when they are used in nuclear power plants, medical imaging tests, airport security scanners, and even in cancer treatment itself. Radon is a colorless and odorless radioactive gas that develops when radioactive elements in the environment are broken down. Ultraviolet radiation is primarily emitted from the sun, though it is also found in man-made sources, including tanning beds and welding torches. The majority of ultraviolet radiation from the sun occurs between the hours of 10:00 A.M. and 3:00 P.M.

Various chemicals are also carcinogenic, such as benzene, pesticides, chlorine, and toluene. Chemicals that are added to foods may also be carcinogens. The foods that are most likely to contain these chemicals include genetically modified foods, processed meats, microwave popcorn, soda, foods containing artificial sweeteners, refined flour and sugar, and hydrogenated oils.

Genetics plays an important role in the development of cancer because certain types of cancer occur in families. Gene changes that begin in a single cell over the course of an individual's lifetime cause most of these cancers. Abnormal genes may be passed within a family from one generation to another. Though cancer may or may not develop, the passage of these abnormal genes between family members is called *inherited cancer*.

Viruses may also cause cancer. The human papillomavirus (HPV) is linked to cervical, penile, anal, vaginal, and valvular cancers. The HPV vaccine is approved for use in females between the ages of 9 and 25. The HPV vaccine is also approved for boys and young men. The Epstein-Barr virus, which causes mononucleosis, may remain in the B-lymphocytes, and may later cause nasopharyngeal cancer or lymphoma. It may also be linked to Hodgkin's lymphoma and stomach cancer. Hepatitis B and C may also cause primary liver cancer. Various cancers, such as Kaposi sarcoma, cervical cancer, and non-Hodgkin lymphoma, may be caused by the human immunodeficiency virus (HIV).

ONCOGENES

Recent explorations into the causes of cancer have centered on the role of genes that cause cancer. There are two major classes of genes involved in carcinogenesis: oncogenes and tumor suppressor. **Oncogenes** develop from normal genes, termed *protooncogenes*, which are present in all cells. Protooncogenes are essential regulators of normal cellular functions, including the cell cycle. Genetic alteration of the protooncogenes may activate the oncogenes. These genetic alterations may be caused by such **carcinogenic** (cancer-causing) agents as radiation, chemicals, or viruses. **Tumor suppressor genes** are another category of genes involved in carcinogenesis. The normal function of these genes is to regulate and inhibit inappropriate cellular growth and proliferation. Gene loss or mutation can result in the loss of control over normal cell growth.

THE CELL CYCLE AND MOLECULAR BIOLOGY

The ability of chemotherapy to kill cancer cells depends on its ability to stop cell division. Usually, cancer drugs work by damaging the ribonucleic acid (RNA) or deoxyribonucleic acid (DNA) that tells the cell how to copy itself for division. If the cancer cells are unable to divide, they die. The faster cancer cells divide, the more likely it is that chemotherapy will kill the cells, causing the tumor to shrink. Both cancer cells and normal cells reproduce themselves in a series of steps known as the *cell cycle*. There are usually four steps after the resting (G_0) stage:

✳ G_0: The resting or dormant stage when cells have not started to divide. Cells spend much of their lives in this phase. Depending on their type, different cells can last just a few hours or a few years. When cells receive a signal to reproduce, they move into the G_1 phase (Figure 22-1 ■).

✳ G_1: The first gap phase. The cell starts making proteins to prepare for division. This phase lasts about 18–30 hours.

✳ S: DNA synthesis occurs. The chromosomes containing the genetic code are copied so both of the new cells formed have the right amount of DNA. This phase lasts about 18–20 hours.

✳ G_2: The second gap phase. This occurs just before the cell starts splitting into two cells. It lasts from 2 to 10 hours.

✳ M: **Mitosis** (when one cell splits into two new cells) occurs. This lasts only 30–60 minutes.

Most human cells exist in the G_0 phase, and most cancer cells in this stage are not sensitive to the effects of chemotherapy. Not all cancer cells proliferate faster than normal cells. Many anticancer drugs target rapidly proliferating cells, and these agents may act at selective or multiple sites of the cell cycle. Agents with major activity in a particular phase of the cell cycle are known as *cell cycle phase–specific agents*. Many antineoplastic agents interfere with the cellular synthesis of DNA, RNA, and proteins. The genetic information is encoded in DNA by the precise sequencing of basic structural subunits of DNA, known as **nucleotides**. The goal of chemotherapy is to selectively destroy tumor cells, which can be achieved by targeting specific growth characteristics of most tumors. Agents used in cancer chemotherapy are commonly categorized by their mechanism of action or by their origin.

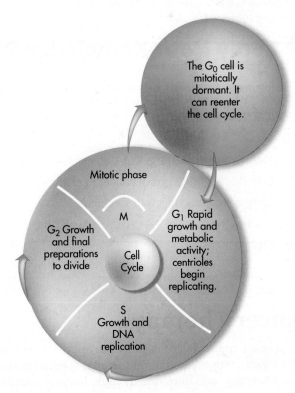

Figure 22-1 ■ The four steps of the cell cycle.

Focus Point

The Seven Warning Signs of Cancer

1. Change in bowel or bladder habits
2. A sore that does not heal
3. Unusual bleeding or discharge
4. Thickening or lump in breast or elsewhere
5. Indigestion or difficulty swallowing
6. Obvious change in a wart or mole
7. Nagging cough or hoarseness

Focus on Pediatrics

Warning Signs of Cancer in Children

1. Unexplained or persistent lump
2. Unexplained or persistent limping
3. Unexplained normocytic anemia
4. Unexplained thrombocytopenic bruising
5. Unexplained weight loss
6. Abdominal mass
7. Unexplained persistent headache or vomiting on awakening

✳ Apply Your Knowledge 22.1

The following questions focus on what you have just learned about various cancer cells and molecular biology.

CRITICAL THINKING

1. Explain oncogenes.
2. Identify and explain the four steps of the cell cycle.
3. Give the warning signs of cancer in children.
4. Compare carcinomas with sarcomas.
5. Discuss the stage of the cell cycle in which DNA synthesis occurs.
6. Explain mitosis.

Cancer Therapy

Five primary methods are used in the approach to cancer treatment: surgery, radiation therapy, chemotherapy, immunotherapy, and hormone therapy. Surgery remains the treatment of choice for many solid tumors. Radiation was first used for cancer treatment in the late 1800s. Although very effective for treating many types of cancer, surgery and radiation are local treatments. Systemic diseases, such as leukemia, cannot be treated this way. Chemotherapy and hormone therapy access the systemic circulation. Immunotherapy uses the stimulation of the host's immune system to fight against the cancer. The response to chemotherapy may be described as cure, complete response, **partial response**, **stable disease**, or progression of disease. A *cure* implies that the patient is entirely free of disease and has the same life expectancy as a cancer-free individual. *Complete response* means total disappearance of all cancer and no evidence of new disease for at least 1 month after treatment. A *partial response* is defined as a 50% or greater decrease in the tumor size or other objective disease markers and no evidence of any new disease for at least 1 month. A patient whose tumor size neither grows nor shrinks significantly has *stable disease*.

ANTINEOPLASTIC AGENTS

Depending on the type of cancer and the drug used, antineoplastic (chemotherapy) agents may be administered orally (PO), intramuscularly (IM), subcutaneously (SC), or intravenously (IV). IV administration is the most common method. Oral chemotherapy is becoming more popular than ever because of its ease of use. Chemotherapy uses chemical agents to interact with cancer cells to stop or control the growth of the cancer. For example, during World War II, soldiers exposed to nitrogen mustard experienced low white blood cell (WBC) counts. Today, nitrogen mustard is used to treat patients with lymphoid leukemia and lymphomas. However, because chemotherapeutic drugs cannot distinguish between normal cells and cancer cells, both types of cells are affected by chemotherapy. But the killing effect of chemotherapeutic agents has selectivity for cancer cells over normal host cells and thus normal host cells are able to repair themselves and continue to grow.

Chemotherapy, as used for the treatment of cancer, may be termed a *primary*, *palliative*, *adjuvant*, or *neoadjuvant* agent. For some cancers, chemotherapy alone can destroy all the cancer cells and cure the cancer, which is *primary* treatment. As an **adjuvant** treatment (one that aids or contributes), chemotherapy is given before or after other methods of treatment, such as surgery and radiation, to reduce the risk of recurrence or to prolong survival. **Palliative** treatment, which eases a disease's effects but does not cure it, may be used if a cure is not possible to minimize the discomfort caused by cancer or to slow the progression of the disease and prolong the patient's life. Chemotherapy may also be given in the *neoadjuvant* or preoperative setting. The goal in this setting is to make other treatments more effective by reducing tissue damage, decreasing tumor size, or destroying micrometastases. The most common antineoplastic agents are listed in Table 22-1 ■.

Table 22-1 ■ Common Agents Used in the Treatment of Cancer

GENERIC NAME	TRADE NAME	AVERAGE ADULT DOSAGE	ROUTE OF ADMINISTRATION
Alkylating Agents			
chlorambucil (nitrogen mustard)	Leukeran	0.1–0.2 mg/kg/d	PO
cyclophosphamide	Cytoxan	1–5 mg/kg/d	PO
		10–15 mg/kg q7–10d or 3–5 mg/kg twice weekly	IV
ifosfamide	Ifex	1.2 g/m^2/d for 5 d	IV
mechlorethamine (nitrogen mustard)	Mustargen	0.4 mg/kg in 1–4 divided doses	IV or intracavitary
melphalan	Alkeran	2–10 mg/d (0–15 mg/kg/d) for 7 d	PO
Ethyleneimines			
altretamine	Hexalen	260 mg/m^2/d for 14 or 21 d in a 28-d cycle	PO
thiotepa (injection)	Thiotepa	0.3–0.4 mg/kg	IV
		0.6–0.8 mg/kg	Intravesicular, directly into the bladder

(continued)

Table 22-1 ■ **Common Agents Used in the Treatment of Cancer** (*continued*)

GENERIC NAME	TRADE NAME	AVERAGE ADULT DOSAGE	ROUTE OF ADMINISTRATION
Alkyl Sulfonate			
busulfan	Busulfex	4–8 mg/d	PO
		0.8 mg/kg q6h for 4 d	IV
Miscellaneous			
carboplatin	Paraplatin	On day 1 every 4 wk	IV infusion
cisplatin (injection)	Platinol-AQ	20–100 mg/m^2/d (schedule depends on type of cancer; up to 360 mg/m^2)	IV
procarbazine	Matulane	2–4 mg/kg/d for 1 wk and then 4–6 mg/kg/d until WBCs are less than 4,000/mm^3	PO
Antimetabolites			
capecitabine	Xeloda	2,500 mg/m^2/d in two divided doses for 2 wk	PO
fluorouracil	Adrucil	6–2 mg/kg/d	IV
mercaptopurine	Purinethol	1.5–2.5 mg/kg/d	PO
methotrexate	Rheumatrex, Trexall	10–30 mg/kg/d for 4–8 d with 7–10-d rest interval	PO
		10–30 mg	IM
		20–500 mg/m^2	IV
Mitotic Inhibitors (Plant Alkaloids)			
etoposide	VePesid, Etopophos	35–100 mg/m^2/d	PO, IV
teniposide	Vumon	165 mg/m^2 in combination twice weekly for 4.5 wk	IV
vinblastine sulfate (injection)	Vinblastine Sulfate	3.7–11.1 mg/m^2	IV
vincristine	Vincasar PFS	1.4 mg/m^2	IV
vinorelbine	Navelbine	15–30 mg/m^2	IV
Antitumor Antibiotics			
bleomycin	Blenoxane	0.25–0.50 units/kg/d	IM, IV, SC
daunorubicin	Cerubidine	30–60 mg/m^2/d	IV
doxorubicin	Adriamycin PFS	20–75 mg/m^2	IV

GENERIC NAME	TRADE NAME	AVERAGE ADULT DOSAGE	ROUTE OF ADMINISTRATION
epirubicin	Ellence	100–120 mg/m^2 infused over 3–5 min on day 1 of a 3–4 wk cycle or 50–60 mg/m^2 on day 1 and day 8 of a 3–4 wk cycle	IV
idarubicin	Idamycin	12 mg/m^2/d for 3 d	IV
mitomycin	Mutamycin	10–20 mg/m^2	IV
plicamycin	Mithracin	20–30 mcg/kg day for 8–10 d	IV
valrubicin	Valstar	800 mg in 75 mL of solution once a week for 6 wk	Instilled into the urinary bladder
Hormone Therapy			
Corticosteroids			
dexamethasone	Decadron	0.25–4 mg bid to qid	PO
prednisone	Deltasone	5–60 mg/d in single or divided doses	PO
Estrogens			
estramustine	Emcyt	10–16 mg/kg/d in 3–4 divided doses for up to 3 y	PO
tamoxifen	Nolvadex	10–20 mg 1–2 times/d	PO
Progestins			
megestrol	Megace	40–320 mg/d in divided doses	PO
Gonadotropins			
goserelin	Zoladex	3.6 mg once every 4 wk or 10.8 mg depot every 3 mo	SC implants
leuprolide	Lupron	1 mg/d	SC
	Eligard	7.5 mg monthly as depot injection	IM
Antiandrogens			
bicalutamide	Casodex	50 mg/d	PO
flutamide	Eulexin	250 mg three times/d at 8-h intervals	PO
nilutamide	Nilandron	300 mg/d for 3 d	PO

PO, oral; bid: twice a day; IV: intravenous; IM, intramuscular; SC, subcutaneous; qid: four times a day.

IMMUNOTHERAPY

Immunotherapy may be used to treat cancer and involves several methods. These include stimulating the immune system to be more efficient or to be smarter to attack cancer cells or the use of man-made immune system proteins to boost the immune system against cancer. Immunotherapy is also called *biologic therapy* or *biotherapy*. Duke University Medical Center has developed a technique in which the poliovirus is genetically modified with a portion of a rhinovirus, which causes the common cold. The poliovirus receptor is found on most tumor cells. Therefore, when this viral combination is injected at the site of a tumor, in this case glioblastoma multiforme in the brain, it finds and destroys tumor cells while boosting the immune system to fight the cancer. Continuing studies will include this type of treatment against other cancers, such as prostate, melanoma, pancreas, lung, breast, and metastasized brain cancers that originated from other tumors.

There are three primary types of immunotherapy: monoclonal antibodies, cancer vaccines, and nonspecific immunotherapies. Monoclonal antibodies are man-made versions of immune system proteins that are designed to attack specific parts of cancer cells. They may work individually, along with other chemotherapy agents, or by binding to multiple proteins at one time. Cancer vaccines are designed to cause immune responses against certain cancers. They are not yet a major type of treatment for cancer, but research is very encouraging. Types of cancer vaccines include tumor cell, antigen, dendritic cell, and vector-based vaccines. Nonspecific immunotherapies provide an overall boost to the immune system, which may help it to attack cancer cells more effectively. These therapies include cytokines such as interleukins, interferons, and granulocyte-macrophage colony-stimulating factor; drugs that target certain immune system molecules, and immune boosting agents.

Focus Point

Bone Marrow Depression

Depression of bone marrow is usually the most serious limiting toxicity of cancer chemotherapy.

Focus On

Alkylating Agents

Alkylating agents cause replacement of hydrogen by an alkyl group, specifically one that inhibits cell division and growth. There are five major types of alkylating agents:

1. Nitrogen mustards
2. Ethyleneimines
3. Alkyl sulfonates
4. Nitrosoureas
5. Temozolomide

Acquired resistance to alkylating agents is a common event, but resistance of a cancer to one alkylating agent does not always imply cross-resistance to others.

How do they work?

Alkylating agents act directly on DNA, causing cross-linking of DNA strands, abnormal base pairing, or DNA strand breaks, thus preventing the cells from dividing. They are cell cycle phase–nonspecific but are most active in the resting phase.

How are they used?

Alkylating agents are generally of greatest value in treating slow-growing cancers. They are not as effective on rapidly growing cells.

What are the adverse effects?

This class has a dose-limiting toxicity to bone marrow and intestinal mucosa. Alkylating agents cause oral mucosa ulceration and intestinal denudations. All alkylating agents can cause instances of pulmonary fibrosis and venoocclusive disease in the liver; renal failure; or central neurotoxicity with seizures, coma, and, at times, death. Most alkylating agents cause **alopecia** (hair loss). Central nervous system toxicity is indicated by nausea and vomiting. Ifosfamide is the most neurotoxic of this class, producing altered mental status, coma, generalized seizures, and paralysis. All alkylating agents have toxic effects on the reproductive system.

What are the contraindications and interactions?

Alkylating agents are contraindicated during pregnancy, especially during the first trimester, because they are **teratogenic** (able to cause birth defects in fetuses). Alkylating agents may interact with antidepressants; other anticancer medications; warfarin (Coumadin); and such prescription and nonprescription medications as certain vaccines, aspirin, and vitamins.

What are the most important points patients should know?

Teach patients about the manifestation of bone marrow depression. Advise patients to avoid contact with people who have colds or other infections during susceptible times (e.g., after a course of therapy). Warn patients that hair loss may occur from the head, eyelashes, nose, and pubic area, but reassure them that their hair will grow back after the course of therapy is complete.

Focus Point

Tyramine and Procarbazine

Procarbazine (Matulane) is available as a 50-mg capsule. It can cause an acute disulfiram-like reaction (flushing, headache, acute vomiting, and chest or abdominal pain) with alcohol. Avoid tyramine-containing foods (e.g., aged cheese, chocolate, pickles, aged meat, wine), which can cause a life-threatening elevation in blood pressure.

Focus On

Antimetabolites

Antimetabolites prevent cancer cell growth by affecting DNA production. They are only effective against cells that are actively participating in cell metabolism. The classes of antimetabolites include:

1. Purine antagonists: mercaptopurine
2. Adenosine antagonists: fludarabine
3. Pyrimidine antagonists: fluorouracil
4. Folic acid antagonists: methotrexate

How do they work?

Antimetabolites replace natural substances as building blocks in DNA molecules, altering the function of enzymes required for cell metabolism and protein synthesis. They are cell cycle phase–specific and are most effective during the S-phase of cell division.

How are they used?

Mercaptopurine is useful in the maintenance therapy of children with acute and chronic myelocytic leukemia. Fludarabine is used in the treatment of chronic lymphocytic leukemia and non-Hodgkin's lymphoma. Capecitabine is used for metastatic breast and colorectal cancers. It is a *prodrug* (a modified, pharmacologically inactive form of a pharmacologic agent) of fluorouracil and undergoes hydrolysis in the liver to form the active drug. Fluorouracil is prescribed for the treatment of *keratoses* (overgrowths of horny skin tissue) and *basal cell carcinomas* (skin cancer). Methotrexate is used for acute lymphoblastic leukemia, meningeal leukemia, and head and neck cancers (and for such noncancerous disorders as rheumatoid arthritis and psoriasis).

What are the adverse effects?

The adverse effects of mercaptopurine include anorexia, nausea and vomiting, hepatotoxicity, bone marrow depression, and hyperuricemia. Fludarabine may cause headache, hearing loss, sleep disorders, and depression. It may also cause bone marrow toxicity, pneumonia, *dyspnea* (difficulty breathing), *epistaxis* (nosebleed), and edema. Fluorouracil causes marked myelosuppression. It can also result in gastrointestinal (GI) disturbances, alopecia, dermatitis, and nail changes.

Methotrexate commonly causes skin rashes, hyperpigmentation, photosensitivity, hyperuricemia, inflammation of the tongue, and alopecia. Serious adverse effects include severe leukopenia, bone marrow aplasia, and thrombocytopenia.

What are the contraindications and interactions?

Mercaptopurine is contraindicated in patients with a history of resistance to this agent. It must be avoided in the first trimester of pregnancy, in women who are lactating, and in patients who have acute infectious diseases. Fluorouracil, mercaptopurine, and methotrexate are contraindicated in patients with severe bone marrow depression and renal dysfunction. Mercaptopurine may interact with allopurinol; warfarin; and certain drugs used to treat ulcerative colitis, such as mesalamine, olsalazine, and sulfasalazine. Patients should be instructed not to start or stop any prescription or nonprescription medications while taking this drug and to tell their health care providers about all medications they are currently taking before taking mercaptopurine.

What are the most important points patients should know?

Advise patients that antimetabolites may cause bone marrow suppression and damage to the GI lining, such as stomatitis (a group of diseases affecting the mucous membranes of the mouth) and ulceration.

Focus on Natural Products

Green Tea as an Antioxidant

Green tea has a reputation as a healthful drink, with studies suggesting it may reduce the incidence of a variety of cancers, including cancers of the colon, pancreas, and stomach. Green tea contains high levels of polyphenols, which exhibit antioxidant and chemopreventive properties. However, green tea is not a proven cure for cancer. As often happens with natural supplements that are supported primarily by observational trials, results of these studies are inconsistent. Also, green tea should not be given to infants or young children.

Focus On

Mitotic Inhibitors (Plant Alkaloids)

Plant alkaloids are typically physiologically active organic bases containing nitrogen (and usually oxygen) that occur in seed plants. They are called *mitotic inhibitors* because they prevent *meiosis* (cell division). The primary plant alkaloids are vincristine and vinblastine; examples are listed in Table 22-1.

How do they work?

Mitotic inhibitors act throughout the cell cycle, and some of these agents are more effective during the S- and M-phases of the cell cycle. They inhibit DNA and RNA synthesis.

How are they used?

Mitotic inhibitors are used to treat cancer of the breast, bladder, ovaries, and lungs as well as leukemias, lymphomas, and testicular cancer.

What are the adverse effects?

These agents may cause nausea and vomiting, diarrhea, alopecia, dizziness, weakness, headache, depression, and stomatitis. The adverse effects of mitotic inhibitors may also cause anemia and hyperpigmentation of the nails, tongue, or oral mucosa.

What are the contraindications and interactions?

Mitotic inhibitors are contraindicated in severe cardiac disease, hypocalcemia, bleeding disorders, myelosuppression, and pregnancy. Some of these drugs, such as plicamycin, must be used cautiously in patients with hepatic or renal impairment. Mitomycin may cause acute shortness of breath and severe bronchospasm if it is used with mitotic inhibitors. These agents may decrease phenytoin levels. Erythromycin and itraconazole may increase vinblastine toxicity.

What are the important points patients should know?

Be sure patients are aware that mitotic inhibitors may produce serious toxicity with bone marrow depression and GI damage. Advise them that if they have diarrhea to avoid foods that are likely to cause GI irritation, such as coffee, spicy foods, fruits, and raw vegetables.

Focus on Geriatrics

Toxicity of Antineoplastic Drugs in Elderly Patients

Older adults—many of whom may have such chronic diseases as cardiovascular disease or kidney impairment—are at higher risk for adverse effects when they are being treated with antineoplastic drugs. As a result, lower dosages of antineoplastics should be administered to these patients. Creatinine clearance is used to monitor renal function in elderly patients.

Focus On

Hormone Therapy

Hormonal agents are frequently prescribed in antineoplastic therapy. These agents may selectively suppress the growth of certain tissues of the body without causing a cytotoxic action. The sex hormones, such as estrogens, progestins, and androgens, are generally used to change the hormonal environment of tissues dependent on these agents for their growth. For example, the administration of antiandrogens or estrogens is beneficial in the treatment of prostatic cancer. On the other hand, these hormones can be useful in treating breast or endometrial cancers.

How do they work?

Hormonal agents are a class of heterogeneous compounds that have various effects on cells. These agents block either hormone production or hormone action. Their action on malignant cells is highly selective. Steroids inhibit the migration of WBCs and inhibit the production of products of the arachidonic acid cascade. Estrogen works by promoting the release of calcitonin and by enhancing the availability of vitamin D_3 to increase bone formation in postmenopausal patients with breast cancer.

Progestins inhibit secretion of pituitary gonadotropins by positive feedback. Antiestrogens bind to estrogen receptors, which prevents estrogen from binding to these receptors. Antiandrogens act by blocking the synthesis of endogenous testosterone.

How are they used?

Hormones and their antagonists have various uses in the treatment of malignant tumors. Steroids are especially useful in treating acute lymphocytic leukemia. They are also used in conjunction with radiation therapy to reduce radiation edema. Sex hormones are used in carcinomas of the reproductive tract; for example, estrogen may be given to patients with testicular cancer or to patients with certain carcinomas of the breast.

What are the adverse effects?

GI disturbances are common adverse effects associated with these drugs. Impaired fertility may result from treatment with sex hormone antagonists. In women, menstrual irregularities may develop depending on premenopausal or menopausal stages of life.

What are the contraindications and interactions?

Most hormones are contraindicated during pregnancy because they are harmful to fetuses. These drugs should be used during pregnancy only in circumstances in which the benefits of treatment far outweigh the risk of harm to the fetus. Interactions with hormone therapies occur with tamoxifen, alcohol, St. John's wort, zinc, magnesium, vitamin B, and thyroid supplements.

What are the important points patients should know?

Warn patients that hormonal agents are contraindicated during pregnancy and that menstrual irregularities are common. If appropriate, advise female patients to use strict contraception and to avoid pregnancy for 3–4 months after completing the course. Some sources advise that men and women should avoid conceiving a child for about 2 years after treatment.

Focus Point

Possibility of Infertility

It is important to instruct patients that infertility, which may occur with antineoplastic agents, may not be reversible.

Focus On

Antitumor Antibiotics

Antitumor antibiotics are made from natural products produced by species of the soil fungus *Streptomyces*. They are very effective in the treatment of certain tumors. The classifications of these agents are listed in Table 22-1.

How do they work?

The majority of antitumor antibiotics inhibit DNA and RNA synthesis, causing cell death.

How are they used?

Antitumor antibiotics are used only to treat cancer and are not used to treat infections. The effects of each of the antitumor antibiotics are:

✳ Doxorubicin is used in the treatment of breast, ovarian, and bone cancers. It is also used in the therapy for acute lymphoblastic and myeloblastic leukemias. Doxorubicin is generally used in combination with surgery, radiation, and immunotherapy.

✳ Daunorubicin is the first-line treatment for advanced HIV-associated Kaposi's sarcoma. It is also used for testicular cancer, Wilms' tumor, and choriocarcinoma.

✳ Idarubicin can be used for treating acute monocytic leukemia and solid tumors.

✳ Plicamycin is used to treat hypercalcemia associated with advanced neoplasms and testicular cancer.

✳ Bleomycin is used in *squamous cell carcinomas* (skin cancer) of the head, neck, penis, and cervix. It is also used for the treatment of lymphomas and testicular carcinoma.

✳ Mitomycin is used in combination with other chemotherapeutic agents in palliative and adjunctive treatment of breast, stomach, and pancreatic cancers.

What are the adverse effects?

Bone marrow suppression is a major adverse effect of antitumor antibiotics. Stomatitis, GI upset, and alopecia can occur during treatment but cease when treatment is discontinued. Bleomycin is less toxic to bone marrow but tends to cause hyperpigmentation, redness, and sometimes ulceration of the skin. Pulmonary fibrosis can occur during therapy. Mitomycin may induce serious renal impairment.

What are the contraindications and interactions?

Antitumor antibiotics are contraindicated in patients with known hypersensitivity to these agents. Some antitumor antibiotics have toxic effects on the heart, kidneys, and liver. Therefore, they are contraindicated in patients with diseases of these organs. Plasma digoxin levels may decrease when administered with bleomycin. When bleomycin is used with cisplatin, there is an increased risk of bleomycin toxicity. Mitomycin and plicamycin may have an additive bone marrow depressant effect when used with other antineoplastic agents. There is an increased risk of bleeding when plicamycin is administered with aspirin, heparin, warfarin, or NSAIDs.

What are the important points patients should know?

Advise patients that bone marrow suppression is a major adverse effect of these drugs. Because cardiac toxicity is observed with antitumor antibiotics, instruct patients to report to their physician if they experience cardiac problems.

✳ Apply Your Knowledge 22.2

The following questions focus on what you have just learned about various cancer therapies.

CRITICAL THINKING

1. Identify the five primary methods used to treat cancer.
2. Point out the most common method of administration of chemotherapy agents for the treatment of cancer.
3. Give the trade names of nitrogen mustard, melphalan, busulfan, and bleomycin.
4. Identify the most serious toxicity of cancer chemotherapy.
5. Point out the five major types of alkylating agents.
6. Give four examples of antimetabolites.
7. Explain why green tea may reduce the incidence of colon, pancreas, and stomach cancers.
8. Discuss the mechanisms of action of antitumor antibiotics.

BIOLOGIC RESPONSE MODIFIERS

Biologic response modifiers include agents that affect the patient's biologic response to a neoplasm in a beneficial way. Included in this class are agents that act indirectly to mediate antitumor effects or directly on the tumor cells. Recombinant DNA technology has greatly facilitated the identification and production of a number of human proteins, with potent effects on the function and growth of normal and neoplastic cells. Interferons, interleukin-2, tumor necrosis factor, and monoclonal antibodies are types of human proteins.

An example of how the biologic response modifiers are produced is that of **monoclonal antibodies**. These are produced by fusing a single immune cell to tumor cells that are grown in cultures, known as **hybridomas**. Large quantities of these identical antibody cells are produced (rather like clones)—all with the same specific antigen as their target. The advantage of monoclonal antibodies is they can be used to target and then purify the *specific* protein that induced their formation. Interferons are another type of biologic response modifiers that are discussed in detail in this chapter.

Focus On

Interferons

Interferons are a group of blood proteins that have antiviral effects. The genes that produce some of the interferons have been isolated, and those interferons are now commercially produced by means of genetic engineering. Interferons are naturally produced in response to viral infections or other biological inducers, such as some tumors.

There are three types of interferons:

✳ Alfa 2a and 2b (called alfa when referring to drugs)—produced by WBCs

✳ Beta—produced by connective tissue cells

✳ Gamma—produced by T-lymphocytes

Only interferon alfa-2b (Intron A) is effectively used for some cancers. Thus, only alfa-2b is discussed here.

How does it work?

Interferon alfa-2b is a natural product induced virally in peripheral WBCs. Interferon alfa-2b is obtained by the recombinant DNA technology of *Escherichia coli*, bearing an interferon alfa-2b gene from human leukocytes.

How is it used?

Interferon alfa-2b is a chemotherapy agent that has been used for years to treat kidney cancers, lymphoma, and melanoma. It is given IV or IM, with the method and schedule of administration determined by the actual cancer type and the extent of its growth. It is usually administered daily for a specific period of days.

What are the adverse effects?

Patients receiving high IV doses of this agent are closely monitored in a hospital for adverse effects, which may include nausea and vomiting; weight gain; fluid retention; and damage to the liver, lungs, nerves, or kidneys.

What are the contraindications and interactions?

Contraindications include hypersensitivity to interferon alfa-2b or to any components of this product. Safe use during pregnancy, lactation, or in children younger than 18 years has not been established.

Interferon alfa-2b should be used cautiously in severe, preexisting cardiac, renal, or hepatic disease; pulmonary disease; diabetes mellitus; and in those prone to ketoacidosis. This agent may increase theophylline levels, and zidovudine may increase hematologic toxicity.

What are the important points patients should know?

Teach patients techniques for reconstituting and administrating these drugs. Warn them not to change brands of interferon without first consulting their physicians. Advise patients about adverse effects and when to notify their physicians about those that cause significant discomfort. Advise women not to breastfeed while taking these drugs without consulting their physician.

Focus Point

Interferon Administration Changes

All changes in interferon administration must be directed by a physician. Patients should never change the times or doses specified for taking interferons.

✳ Apply Your **Knowledge 22.3**

The following questions focus on what you have just learned about biologic response modifiers.

CRITICAL THINKING

1. Explain interferons.
2. Describe interleukin-2.
3. Discuss tumor necrosis factor.
4. Explain monoclonal antibodies.
5. Identify the advantage of monoclonal antibodies.

PRACTICAL SCENARIO 1

A 68-year-old man has undergone adjuvant chemotherapy for completely resected colon cancer that involved several pericolonic lymph nodes at the time of his surgical resection. After a few days of experiencing diarrhea, he calls his physician and tells him that he has experienced approximately five to six loose, watery stools per day over the past few days. He is mildly lightheaded when walking around.

Mark Harmel/The Image Bank/Getty Images

Critical Thinking Questions

1. What is the most likely cause of this patient's ongoing diarrhea?
2. What are the consequences of ongoing diarrhea, and why do you think the physician might instruct this patient to report to the clinic or emergency room immediately?
3. What advice on diet might you offer this patient after he has been seen by his physician?

PRACTICAL SCENARIO 2

A 38-year-old woman complained of pain in the left iliac region of her pelvis, which worsened over several months. She went to her physician and after a laparoscopy and biopsy, it was discovered she had ovarian cancer.

Critical Thinking Questions

1. If the cancer has not metastasized, what would be the common treatments after surgical removal of the ovary?
2. If the cancer has metastasized to other sites, what would be the most appropriate treatments?

Jami Rae/Shutterstock

Chapter Capsule

This section repeats the objectives from the beginning of the chapter and then provides a summary of the most important concepts for the objective. Use this section as a quick review and to check your knowledge.

Objective 1: List the seven warning signs of cancer.

- Changes in bowel or bladder habits
- A sore that does not heal
- Unusual bleeding or discharge
- Thickening or lump in breast or elsewhere
- Indigestion or difficulty swallowing
- Obvious change in a wart or mole
- Nagging cough or hoarseness

Objective 2: Summarize the basic cell cycle and its importance in the use of antineoplastic agents.

- The basic cell cycle—G_0 (resting or dormant stage), G_1 (the first gap phase), S (DNA synthesis occurs), G_2 (the second gap phase), and M (mitosis occurs)
- Some antineoplastic agents target cancer cells in various stages of the cell cycle, which, in part, determines how and when they are used

Objective 3: List commonly used antineoplastic agents in each class.

- Alkylating agents: nitrogen mustards, ethyleneimines, alkyl sulfonates, nitrosoureas, and triazenes
- Antimetabolites: purine antagonists, adenosine antagonists, pyrimidine antagonists, and folic acid antagonists
- Mitotic inhibitors (plant alkaloids): vincristine and vinblastine
- Hormone therapy: estrogens, progestins, and androgens
- Antitumor antibiotics: doxorubicin, daunorubicin, idarubicin, plicamycin, bleomycin, and mitomycin
- Biologic response modifiers: interferons, interleukin-2, tumor necrosis factor, and monoclonal antibodies

Objective 4: Describe the indications of mercaptopurine and vinblastine.

- Mercaptopurine is useful in the maintenance therapy of children with acute and chronic myelocytic leukemia.
- Vinblastine, a mitotic inhibitor, is used to treat cancer of the breast, bladder, ovaries, and lungs as well as leukemias, lymphomas, and testicular cancer.

Objective 5: Explain the mechanism of action of each class of antineoplastic agents.

- Alkylating agents: cell cycle phase–nonspecific; most active in resting phase; act directly on DNA, causing cross-linking of DNA strands, abnormal base pairing, or DNA strand breaks, thus preventing the cell from dividing
- Antimetabolites: cell cycle phase–specific; most effective during S-phase; replace natural substances as building blocks in DNA molecules, altering the function of enzymes required for cell metabolism and protein synthesis

- Mitotic inhibitors: act throughout cell cycle; some are most effective during S- and M-phases; inhibit DNA and RNA synthesis
- Hormonal agents: highly selective; either block hormone production or block hormone action
- Antitumor antibiotics: most inhibit DNA and RNA synthesis, causing cell death
- Biologic response modifiers: affect biologic responses to a neoplasm in beneficial ways, sometimes acting indirectly to mediate antitumor effects or directly on the tumor cells

Objective 6: Discuss how steroids, estrogen, progestins, antiestrogens, and antiandrogens work in the treatment of cancer.

- Steroids: inhibit migration of WBCs and inhibit production of products of the arachidonic acid cascade
- Estrogens: promote the release of calcitonin and enhance the availability of vitamin D_3 to increase bone formation in postmenopausal patients with breast cancer
- Progestins: inhibit secretion of pituitary gonadotropins by positive feedback
- Antiestrogens: bind to estrogen receptors, preventing estrogen from binding to these receptors
- Antiandrogens: block the synthesis of endogenous testosterone

Objective 7: Explain how biologic response modifiers are created and how they work.

- Human proteins modified by recombinant DNA technology to produce agents with potent effects on the function and growth of normal and neoplastic cells
- Examples: interferon, interleukin-2, tumor necrosis factor, and monoclonal antibodies

Objective 8: Identify how monoclonal antibodies function in the treatment of cancer.

- Monoclonal antibodies can be used to specifically track down and purify the specific protein that induced their formation

Objective 9: Identify the common side effects of chemotherapy treatment.

- Alkylating agents: oral mucosal ulceration and intestinal denudations, pulmonary fibrosis and venoocclusive disease in the liver, renal failure, or central neurotoxicity with seizures, coma, and, at times, death; most of these agents cause hair loss; some cause nausea and vomiting; ifosfamide is the most neurotoxic of this class, producing altered mental status, coma, generalized seizures, and paralysis. All these agents have toxic effects on the reproductive system.
- Antimetabolites: nausea and vomiting, hepatotoxicity, bone marrow depression, headache, hearing loss, sleep disorders, depression, myelosuppression, GI disturbances, hair loss, dermatitis, nail changes, skin rashes, hyperpigmentation, photosensitivity, hyperuricemia, and inflammation of the tongue. Methotrexate may cause serious adverse effects, including severe leukopenia, bone marrow aplasia, and thrombocytopenia.
- Mitotic inhibitors (plant alkaloids): nausea and vomiting; diarrhea; hair loss; dizziness; weakness; headache; depression; stomatitis; anemia; and hyperpigmentation of the nails, tongue, and oral mucosa
- Hormone therapy: GI disturbances, possible impaired fertility, menstrual irregularities
- Antitumor antibiotics—bone marrow suppression, stomatitis, GI upset, hair loss, hyperpigmentation, skin ulceration, pulmonary fibrosis, serious renal impairment

■ Biologic response modifiers: nausea and vomiting; weight gain; fluid retention; and damage to the liver, lungs, nerves, or kidneys

Objective 10: Describe immunotherapy to treat cancers.

■ Immunotherapy involves several methods. These include stimulating the immune system to be more efficient or to be smarter to attack cancer cells, or the use of man-made immune system proteins to boost the immune system against cancer. Immunotherapy is also called *biologic therapy* or *biotherapy*. There are three primary types of immunotherapy, which include monoclonal antibodies, cancer vaccines, and nonspecific immunotherapies.

 Internet Sites of Interest

■ Health care workers who are exposed to antineoplastic agents when working with patients are at risk for toxicity. See the Centers for Disease Control and Prevention (CDC) publication about occupational hazards: **www.cdc.gov/niosh/docs/2004-102**

■ Information on the cell cycle: **www.pnas.org/content/94/7/2776.full**

■ The Mayo Clinic discusses hormone therapy for treatment of reproductive cancers: **www.mayoclinic.com**. Search for "hormone therapy for reproductive cancer."

■ The American Cancer Society has a wealth of information for patients and health care providers: **www.cancer.org**

■ Good information about oncogenes: **www.news-medical.net/health/ What-are-Oncogenes.aspx/**

■ The National Cancer Institute's treatment guidelines: **www.cancer.gov/ about-cancer/treatment**

Checkpoint Review 3

Select the best answer for the following questions.

MULTIPLE CHOICE

1. Vitamin requirements are measured by which of the following units?

   a. Milligrams
   b. Centigrams
   c. Micrograms
   d. a and c

2. Vitamin B_1 is also called:

   a. Riboflavin
   b. Cobalamin
   c. Thiamine
   d. Retinol

3. Which of the following is the newest COX-2 inhibitor for the treatment of osteoarthritis?

   a. Celecoxib (Celebrex)
   b. Meloxicam (Mobic)
   c. Oxycodone/acetaminophen (Percocet)
   d. Fentanyl (Duragesic)

4. Which of the following vaccines is used for the prevention of viral infections?

   a. Q fever
   b. Pertussis
   c. Yellow fever
   d. Plague

5. Which of the following minerals acts in bone formation, impulse conduction, myocardial contractions, and the blood-clotting process?

   a. Sodium
   b. Phosphorus
   c. Iodine
   d. Calcium

6. Which of the following is the trade name of naloxone, when it is not part of a combination agent?

   a. Demerol
   b. Talwin Nx
   c. Narcan
   d. Stadol

7. Zinc is a very important trace element for which of the following conditions?

   a. During hemoglobin synthesis and energy production
   b. During periods of rapid tissue growth
   c. Significant weight gain
   d. Kidney failure

8. Which of the following vitamins is an antioxidant?

   a. Tocopherol (vitamin E)
   b. Cholecalciferol (vitamin D)
   c. Phylloquinone (vitamin K)
   d. Cobalamin (vitamin B_{12})

9. Patients should be instructed to drink several full glasses of water when taking which of the following antimicrobial drugs?

   a. Penicillins
   b. Sulfonamides
   c. Fluoroquinolones
   d. Aminoglycosides

10. Acetaminophen should be avoided in which of the following patients?

    a. Those taking antacids
    b. Those drinking milk
    c. Those drinking alcohol
    d. Those taking antibiotics

11. The sulfonamides block the biosynthetic pathway of which of the following?

    a. Folic acid
    b. Bacterial proteins
    c. Bacterial nucleic acid
    d. Bacterial lipids

12. The presence of food in the GI tract reduces the absorption of many anti-infective agents including which of the following?

    a. Penicillin V
    b. Doxycycline
    c. Minocycline
    d. All of the above

13. Which of the following foods contains very high amounts of tyramine, which may interact with MAOIs and cause hypertensive crises?

    a. Bananas
    b. Cottage cheese
    c. Red meat
    d. Red apples

14. Ethanol impairs absorption of which of the following vitamins?

    a. Thiamine (vitamin B_1)
    b. Cobalamin (vitamin B_{12})
    c. Ascorbic acid (vitamin C)
    d. Tocopherol (vitamin E)

15. *Black "hairy" tongue* (temporary overgrowth of harmless bacteria or yeast in the mouth) is a side effect of oral administration of which of the following antibacterials?

    a. Tetracycline
    b. Erythromycin
    c. Penicillin
    d. Streptomycin

16. Opioid receptors in the brainstem are responsible for the respiratory depressant effects produced by which of the following?

    a. Nonopioid analgesics
    b. Nonopioid antagonists
    c. Opioid antagonists
    d. Opioid analgesics

17. Fluoride's main function in human nutrition is to prevent:

    a. Retarded physical growth
    b. Formation of kidney stones
    c. Dental caries
    d. Wilson's disease

18. Which of the following is the major adverse effect of aminoglycosides?

    a. Hepatotoxicity
    b. Nephrotoxicity
    c. Neurotoxicity
    d. GI toxicity

19. Most of the currently used opioid analgesics act primarily at which of the following receptors?

    a. Mu
    b. Delta
    c. Kappa
    d. Gamma

20. Which of the following is the major adverse effect of meperidine?

    a. Hypertensive crisis
    b. Agitation
    c. Hallucinations
    d. Respiratory depression

21. Essential fatty acids are required for the formation of:

    a. Prostaglandins
    b. Insulin
    c. Vitamin K
    d. Enzymes

22. Aspirin appears to impede clotting by blocking which of the following?

    a. Opioid receptors
    b. Calcium channels
    c. Prostaglandin formation
    d. All of the above

23. Which of the following antibiotics may impair bone growth and discolor the teeth in children?

    a. Macrolides
    b. Aminoglycosides
    c. Sulfonamides
    d. Tetracyclines

24. Cytoxan is the trade name of:

    a. Estramustine
    b. Cyclophosphamide
    c. Fludarabine
    d. Idarubicin

25. Patients should notify their physicians if blood appears in their stools, vomitus, or urine if they are taking:

    a. Indomethacin
    b. Antacids
    c. Acetaminophen
    d. Benzodiazepines

26. All the following infections may be transmitted by mosquitoes except:

    a. West Nile virus
    b. Malaria
    c. Rabies
    d. Encephalitis

27. Which of the following antibiotics is in the class of macrolides?

    a. Erythromycin
    b. Ciprofloxacin
    c. Doxycycline
    d. Rifampin

28. Which of the following is the most common adverse effect of vaccinations?

    a. Convulsions
    b. Liver impairment
    c. Malaise
    d. Allergic reaction

29. A booster dose of adult diphtheria and tetanus toxoid is recommended every:

    a. 2 years
    b. 5 years
    c. 10 years
    d. Not required

30. Ganciclovir is used for the prophylaxis and systemic treatment of which of the following infections?

    a. Respiratory syncytial virus
    b. Hepatitis C virus
    c. Advanced HIV
    d. Cytomegalovirus

31. Which of the following was the leading cause of invasive bacterial disease (meningitis) among children until pediatric immunization was introduced in 1988?

    a. Measles
    b. Polio
    c. *Haemophilus influenzae* type b
    d. Varicella

32. Which of the following are trade names for doxycycline?

    a. Minocin and Solodyn
    b. Vibramycin and Quinidine
    c. Monodox and Oracea
    d. Sumycin and Actisite

33. Which of the following vaccines may be given at birth?

    a. Varicella (chickenpox)
    b. Rubella (German measles)
    c. Hepatitis B
    d. Influenza

34. Which of the following agents may cause a reddish-orange discoloration of body fluids, including tears, urine, and saliva?

    a. Isoniazid
    b. Chloramphenicol
    c. Spectinomycin
    d. Rifampin

35. Amantadine is used to prevent or treat symptoms of:

    a. Mumps
    b. Influenza A
    c. Hepatitis A
    d. Hepatitis C

36. Which of the following vaccines is recommended every year for those at a high risk for complications?

    a. Influenza
    b. Meningococcal
    c. Typhoid
    d. Cholera

37. Meningococcal polysaccharide vaccine must be administered via which of the following routes?

    a. Subcutaneously
    b. Intramuscularly
    c. Intravenously
    d. Inhalation

38. The second most common cause of death in the United States is:

    a. Cardiovascular disease
    b. Car accidents
    c. Cancer
    d. Infectious diseases

39. The ability of chemotherapy to kill cancer cells depends on which of the following factors?

    a. Its ability to destroy specific tissues
    b. Its ability to stop cell division
    c. Its ability to cause necrosis of tissues
    d. All of the above

40. Which of the following vaccines is recommended only in extremely high-risk individuals in whom other controls are impractical?

    a. Q fever
    b. Rabies
    c. Tuberculosis
    d. Typhoid

41. DNA synthesis occurs in which of the following phases of the cell cycle?

    a. G_0
    b. G_1
    c. S
    d. M

42. Chemotherapy agents may be administered by which of the following routes?

    a. Intramuscularly
    b. Orally
    c. Subcutaneously
    d. All of the above

43. Which of the following vaccines is recommended between 12 and 15 months of age?

    a. Hepatitis B
    b. *Haemophilus influenzae* b
    c. Diphtheria, tetanus, pertussis
    d. Measles, mumps, rubella

44. Which of the following is an antimetabolite?

    a. Nitrogen mustards
    b. Ethyleneimines
    c. Adriamycin
    d. Fluorouracil

45. Which of the following antitumor antibiotics is the first-line treatment for advanced HIV-associated Kaposi's sarcoma?

    a. Doxorubicin (Adriamycin PFS)
    b. Daunorubicin (Cerubidine)
    c. Idarubicin (Idamycin)
    d. Plicamycin (Mithracin)

46. Interferons are a group of blood proteins that have which of the following effects?

    a. Antiviral
    b. Antiprotozoal
    c. Antibiotic
    d. None of the above

47. Acyclovir is used to treat all the following except:

    a. Chickenpox
    b. Hepatitis B
    c. Herpes zoster (shingles)
    d. Herpes simplex encephalitis

48. Which of the following is the major adverse effect of didanosine (antiviral drug)?

    a. Hepatitis and heart failure
    b. Peripheral neuropathies and pancreatitis
    c. Nephritis and pulmonary edema
    d. Ototoxicity and glaucoma

For questions 49–53, match the lettered drug to the numbered description.

DESCRIPTION

49. _____ Used for the relief of nonproductive cough and for moderate to severe pain

50. _____ Related to its inhibition of prostaglandin

51. _____ Used for the treatment of osteoarthritis and rheumatoid arthritis in adults

52. _____ Has caused liver damage in patients who consume three or more alcoholic drinks per day

53. _____ Used for narcotic overdose

TERM

    a. celecoxib
    b. naloxone
    c. acetaminophen
    d. ibuprofen
    e. hydrocodone

For questions 54–58, match the lettered term to the numbered description.

DESCRIPTION

54. _____ Another name for fungal

55. _____ Another name for a common opportunistic infection (candidiasis)

56. _____ Caused by *Plasmodium vivax*

57. _____ Responsible for causing dysentery

58. _____ Caused by the flagellated protozoan lamblia

TERM

    a. *Entamoeba histolytica*
    b. Giardiasis
    c. Moniliasis

    d. Malaria
    e. Mycosis

Select terms from your reading to fill in the blanks.

DESCRIPTION

59. _____ is prescribed for asymptomatic and symptomatic trichomoniasis in females and males.

60. Iodoquinol is an anti-infective, antiamebicide, and _____ agent.

61. Substances produced by microorganisms that, in low concentrations, are able to inhibit or kill other microorganisms are called _____.

62. The most common sources of natural antibiotics are molds and _____.

63. Systemic antibacterial agents that are able to kill microbes are called _____.

64. Today, sulfamethoxazole is the most commonly used sulfonamide and is usually combined with trimethoprim and abbreviated _____.

65. The cephalosporins are a group of antibiotics closely related to the _____.

66. First-generation cephalosporins have their highest activity against _____ bacteria.

67. The serious adverse effects of aminoglycosides include ototoxicity and _____.

68. Macronutrients are needed by the body in relatively _____ and constitute the bulk of the diet.

69. The daily requirement for carbohydrates is _____% to _____% of one's total caloric intake.

70. Deficiency of thiamine (vitamin B_1) leads to a disease called _____.

71. Pyridoxine (vitamin B_6) is prescribed to treat _____ during pregnancy.

72. _____ is the ability to resist infection and disease through the activation of specific defenses.

73. Active immunity is a form of acquired immunity that develops in an individual in response to an _____.

74. Immunoglobulin is produced by _____.

75. The treatment of patients with diphtheria requires a specific _____.

UNIT 4

The Effects of Drugs on Specific Systems

> **"** The nervous and endocrine systems involve high-level integration in the brain and have the ability to influence processes in distant regions of the body and to extensively use negative feedback. **"**

Chapter 23

Drugs Used to Treat Central Nervous System Conditions

Chapter Objectives

After completing this chapter, you should be able to:

1. Describe the four major parts of the brain.

2. Name three benzodiazepine hypnotic drugs, and explain the mechanism by which they produce hypnotic effects.

3. List three different types of epilepsy and two drugs used specifically to treat each type of epilepsy.

4. Explain the onset of Alzheimer's disease, identifying common signs and symptoms.

5. Describe the mechanisms of action of drugs that increase dopamine or decrease acetylcholine levels in the basal ganglia.

6. Describe five adverse effects associated with antianxiety drugs.

7. Describe the common adverse effects and the specific neurologic conditions caused by antipsychotic drugs.

8. Explain the use of lithium in mania and the adverse effects associated with its use.

9. Describe the main adverse effects of antipsychotic drugs.

10. Identify three of the most common types of drugs used to treat patients with depression.

Key Terms

absence seizures (p. 392)
akathisia (p. 408)
antipsychotics (p. 398)
anxiety (p. 391)
ataxia (p. 392)
basal ganglia (p. 390)
bradykinesia (p. 408)
central nervous system (CNS) (p. 389)

cerebrum (p. 390)
convulsion (p. 395)
efflux (p. 399)
epilepsy (p. 394)
neuroleptic (p. 405)
neurons (p. 389)
neurotransmitters (p. 389)
parkinsonism (p. 403)

peripheral nervous system (PNS) (p. 389)
porphyria (p. 394)
seizures (p. 392)
substantia nigra((p. 403)
synapses (p. 391)
tardive dyskinesia (p. 408)
tonic–clonic (p. 395)

Introduction

Thinking, remembering, feeling, moving, and being aware of the world require activity from the nervous system. The human brain has about 100 billion **neurons**, which help to coordinate all other body functions to maintain homeostasis and to enable the body to respond to changing conditions. The neurons release chemical substances called **neurotransmitters** that allow communication from one nerve cell to another. The most common neurotransmitters are acetylcholine, norepinephrine, dopamine, serotonin, gamma-aminobutyric acid (GABA), and glutamate. Some mental disorders or conditions are associated with abnormal changes in the activity or amount of a specific neurotransmitter.

The Nervous System

The organs of the nervous system can be divided into two groups. One group, consisting of the brain and spinal cord, forms the **central nervous system (CNS)**. The other group, composed of the nerves (peripheral nerves) that connect the central nervous system to other body parts, is called the **peripheral nervous system (PNS)**. Together, these systems provide three general functions: sensory, integrative, and motor (see Figure 23-1 ■).

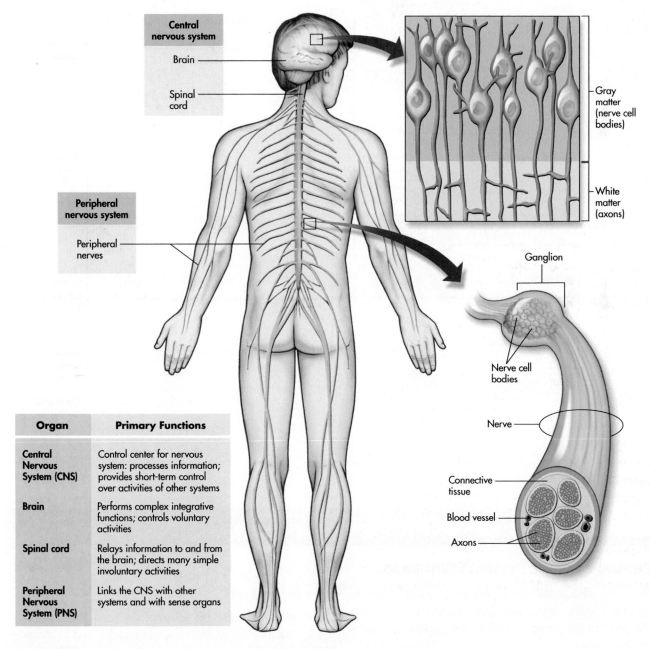

Organ	Primary Functions
Central Nervous System (CNS)	Control center for nervous system: processes information; provides short-term control over activities of other systems
Brain	Performs complex integrative functions; controls voluntary activities
Spinal cord	Relays information to and from the brain; directs many simple involuntary activities
Peripheral Nervous System (PNS)	Links the CNS with other systems and with sense organs

Figure 23-1 ■ The central nervous system includes the brain and spinal cord. The peripheral nervous system includes the nerves throughout the body that exit from the spinal cord.

The brain can be divided into four major portions: the cerebrum, diencephalon, brainstem, and cerebellum. The **cerebrum**, the largest part of the brain, includes nerve centers associated with sensory and motor functions and provides higher mental functions, including memory and reasoning. The cerebrum is composed of an outer cerebral cortex and inner cerebral medulla. In the medulla, there is a group of cell bodies—gray matter—known as the **basal ganglia**, which is involved in the regulation of motor activity. Degeneration of certain neurons within the basal ganglia is responsible for Parkinson's disease. The *diencephalon*

also processes sensory information. Nerve pathways in the brainstem connect various parts of the nervous system and regulate certain visceral activities. The cerebellum includes centers that coordinate voluntary muscular movements.

The spinal cord is a slender nerve column that passes downward from the brain into the vertebral canal, continuing on to the peripheral organs and skeletal muscle, carrying motor impulses. Nerve axons travel from the peripheral parts of the body, such as the skin, muscles, and visceral organs, to the brain, carrying sensory information (see Figure 23-2 ■).

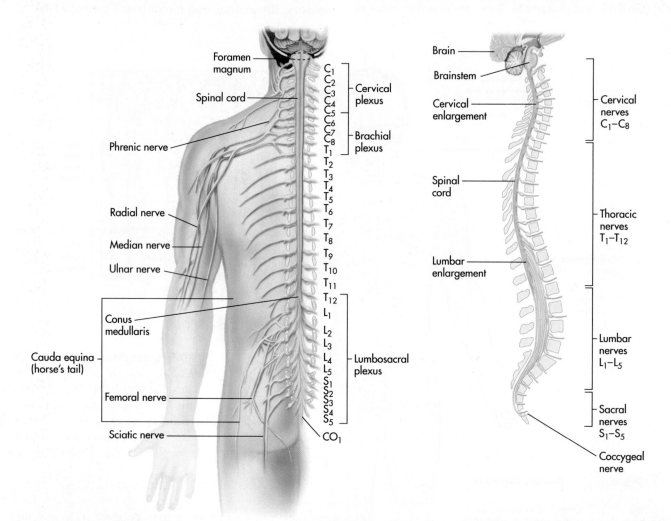

Figure 23-2 ■ The spinal cord.

Focus On

Central Nervous System Stimulants

The CNS stimulants are a diverse group of pharmacologic agents. Many are used therapeutically and are prescription drugs, such as the psychostimulant amphetamines.

How do they work?

The exact mechanism of action of CNS stimulants is not clear, but they stimulate the cerebral cortex and increase the activity of norepinephrine, dopamine, and other catecholamines at CNS **synapses**, which are the point of contact between nerve cells with each other or other types of cells. This increased activity can lead to many effects, including euphoria, reduced appetite, insomnia, and wakefulness.

How are they used?

The indirect-acting sympathomimetics (e.g., methylphenidate and the amphetamines) are more potent CNS stimulants than caffeine but have limited therapeutic use. They are used in the treatment of attention-deficit/hyperactivity disorder (ADHD), narcolepsy, and obesity. However, because these CNS stimulants convey a sense of self-confidence, well-being, and euphoria, they are highly addictive. Some of these agents are widely abused, such as amphetamines and especially methamphetamine.

What are the adverse effects?

The most common adverse effects include headache, palpitations, cardiac dysrhythmias, hypertension, nervousness, and nausea.

What are the contraindications and interactions?

CNS stimulants are contraindicated in persons who are hypersensitive to sympathomimetic amines; have a history of drug abuse; are severely agitated; have hyperthyroidism, diabetes mellitus, moderate to severe hypertension, advanced arteriosclerosis, angina pectoris, or other cardiovascular disorders; or have glaucoma. Safety during pregnancy and lactation is not established. These agents should be used cautiously in those with mild hypertension. Acetazolamide and sodium bicarbonate decrease amphetamine elimination, whereas ammonium chloride and ascorbic acid increase amphetamine elimination.

What are the important points patients should know?

Advise patients that when taking CNS stimulants for a prolonged period, withdrawal symptoms could occur. A gradual decrease is essential to prevent withdrawal effects.

Focus on Pediatrics

The Need for Counseling in Attention-Deficit/Hyperactivity Disorder

Families of children with ADHD should be encouraged to seek counseling for support and reassurance. Drug treatment alone is an insufficient form of therapy.

Anxiety

Anxiety is a very common disorder defined as a persistent and irrational fear of specific objects, activities, or situations. In many cases, anxiety is self-limiting, and recourse to medications is not necessary. Occasionally, however, anxiety is so stressful and mentally painful that drug therapy is required. Anxiety and stress are part of everyday life, and it is important that education programs include life skills that help people develop coping mechanisms. Furthermore, anxiety may be accompanied by mild reactive or even endogenous depression. When exposed to chronic stress, some people develop excessive anxiety. In others, the response may simply be inappropriate to the stressor. Anxiety may cause the affected person to become unable to live a normal life. According to the Anxiety Disorders Association of America, anxiety disorders are the most common psychiatric illnesses in the United States, affecting 40 million people, with a higher incidence in women than in men.

Anxiety is an uncomfortable state that has both psychological and physical components. The psychological component is characterized by emotions such as fear, apprehension, dread, and uneasiness. The physical components include tachycardia, palpitations, trembling, dry mouth, sweating, weakness, fatigue, and shortness of breath. Untreated, anxiety disorders often lead to severe disorders such as depression and alcoholism. Fortunately, anxiety disorders respond well to treatment such as behavior therapy, psychotherapy, or drug therapy.

In general, treatments for the various anxiety disorders include increased physical activities, relaxation exercises, and anxiolytic drugs. Selective serotonin reuptake inhibitors (SSRIs) are used first, often with amitriptyline/nortriptyline. Benzodiazepines are often prescribed, including lorazepam, clonazepam, and alprazolam. These are used on an "as-needed" basis for only a short time due to dependence potential.

Insomnia

Sleep and its importance for normal living is a process that is still little understood. Sleep disturbances are extremely common and, if continuous, they have the potential to seriously disrupt normal day-to-day living.

Many people with sleep disorders want to turn to drugs to solve their problem.

Insomnia is the inability to fall asleep or stay asleep. Difficulty in falling asleep or disturbed sleep patterns both result in insufficient sleep. Sleep disorders are common and may be short in duration or of long standing. They may have little or no apparent relationship to other immediate disorders. Sleep disorders can be secondary to emotional problems, pain, physical disorders, and the use or withdrawal of drugs. Excess alcohol consumed in the evening can shorten sleep and lead to withdrawal effects in the early morning.

SEDATIVES AND HYPNOTICS

A sedative diminishes the activity of the CNS. This effect on the CNS can, in many circumstances, relieve anxiety, which is why sedatives are often referred to as *anxiolytics*. *Hypnotic* is the term used to describe a substance that induces sleep. Many of the drugs in these categories are addictive if taken regularly for even short periods. In some cases, addiction has been known to occur in about 10 days. Thus, the use of these drugs is controversial. If prescribed, they should be taken for only limited periods, for no more than 7 days under normal circumstances.

The use of hypnotics in the treatment of short-term insomnia is often beneficial in cases in which the insomnia can be predicted. There are at least two stages of sleep: the first is *rapid eye movement (REM)*, which is the dreaming stage, and the second is *non-REM* stage. It seems that many hypnotics upset the REM stage of sleep.

The difference between most hypnotics and anxiolytics is the dosage, not the drug. Therefore, the drugs are dealt with according to their chemical classification and not their therapeutic classification, except when there is no overlap.

Focus Point

Sleep with Hypnotics

It is important to remember that no currently available hypnotics induce what could be termed "natural sleep."

Focus On

Benzodiazepines

Benzodiazepines may be used as sedatives or hypnotics. However, it is wise to attempt treatment options with less addictive potential before using a benzodiazepine for this purpose. Table 23-1 ■ shows some of the most commonly prescribed benzodiazepines.

How do they work?

The mechanism of action of benzodiazepines on the CNS appears to be closely related to their ability to increase the action of the neurotransmitter GABA.

How are they used?

Indications for the use of benzodiazepines include generalized anxiety disorders, panic disorders, insomnia, myoclonic and **absence seizures**, status epilepticus, and muscle relaxation. In **seizures**, injectable forms of diazepam and lorazepam are commonly used initially to stop the repetitive seizure activity and then long-acting drugs, such as phenytoin, are given to prevent the recurrence of seizures.

What are the adverse effects?

The adverse effects of benzodiazepines include drowsiness, **ataxia**, impaired judgment, rebound insomnia, and the development of tolerance. Overdosage may result in CNS and respiratory depression as well as hypotension and coma. Gradual withdrawal of these drugs is recommended. Sudden withdrawal of benzodiazepines may cause such serious problems as seizures, severe anxiety, sensory disturbances, schizophrenia, and suicidal thoughts.

What are the contraindications and interactions?

If taken during pregnancy, benzodiazepines are likely to cause fetal abnormalities, and flurazepam is entirely contraindicated during pregnancy. Benzodiazepines are also contraindicated in individuals with severe liver and kidney disorders and in children who are hyperactive.

Benzodiazepines increase CNS depression with alcohol and omeprazole. They also increase pharmacologic effects if combined with cimetidine, disulfiram, or hormonal contraceptives. The effects of benzodiazepines decrease with theophylline and ranitidine.

What are the important points patients should know?

Instruct patients about methods, such as relaxation, they can use to decrease anxiety. Advise patients not to stop the medication abruptly after prolonged use because withdrawal symptoms may occur. Warn patients not to drink alcohol or take other CNS depressants while taking hypnotics or anxiolytics.

Instruct patients about methods to assist with sleep, such as avoiding coffee, heavy meals, and excessive stimuli close to bedtime. Caution them against driving or operating machinery because dizziness or drowsiness might occur.

Table 23-1 ■ Commonly Used Benzodiazepines

GENERIC NAME	TRADE NAME	AVERAGE ADULT DOSAGE	ROUTE OF ADMINISTRATION
alprazolam	Xanax	0.25–0.5 mg tid up to 4 mg/d in divided doses	PO
chlordiazepoxide	Librium	5–25 mg tid–qid	PO
		25–100 mg; then 25–50 mg tid–qid prn	IM, IV
clorazepate	Tranxene	7.5–60 mg in divided doses tid	PO
diazepam	Valium	2–10 mg bid–qid	PO
		2–20 mg; may be repeated in 1–4 h prn	IM, IV
		0.2 mg/kg only once q5d	Rectal
eszopiclone	Lunesta	1–3 mg at bedtime	PO
estazolam	ProSom	1–2 mg at bedtime	PO
flurazepam	Dalmane	30 mg at bedtime; 15 mg may suffice	PO
lorazepam	Ativan	1–10 mg/d in divided doses, with largest dose at bedtime	PO
		0.05–4 mg/kg	IM
		0.004 mg/kg but no greater than 2 mg/kg total	IV
midazolam	Midazolam Injection	0.07–0.08 mg/kg 30–60 min before procedure	IM
		1–1.5 mg; may repeat in 2 min prn	IV
oxazepam	Serax	10–30 mg tid–qid	PO
quazepam	Doral	7.5–15 mg until desired response is seen	PO
ramelteon	Rozerem	8 mg at bedtime	PO
temazepam	Restoril	15–30 mg at bedtime	PO
triazolam	Halcion	0.125–0.5 mg at bedtime	PO
zaleplon	Sonata	5–10 mg at bedtime	PO
zolpidem	Ambien, Ambien CR	5–12.5 mg at bedtime	PO

tid, three times a day; PO, oral; qid, four times a day; IM, intramuscular; IV, intravenous; bid, twice a day.

Focus Point

Oral Contraceptives and Benzodiazepines

Women who are taking benzodiazepines should not use oral contraceptives because the drug combination may cause increased sedative effects, and high levels of the benzodiazepine may accumulate in the blood plasma.

Focus on Geriatrics

Diazepam

Elderly patients usually require lower dosages of diazepam to decrease ataxia and avoid oversedation. Apnea and cardiac arrest may occur when diazepam is given to elderly patients, people with severe illness, and individuals with limited pulmonary reserve.

Focus On

Barbiturates

Barbiturates are classified as CNS agents, anticonvulsants, and sedative–hypnotic drugs.

How do they work?

The sedative and hypnotic effects of barbiturates, such as phenobarbital, appear to be primarily attributable to interference with impulse transmission of the cerebral cortex by the inhibition of the *reticular activating system*, which is a part of the brain that appears to control sleep and wakefulness. CNS depression may range from mild sedation to coma depending on the dosage, route of administration, degree of nervous system excitability, and drug tolerance. Initially, barbiturates suppress REM sleep, but with chronic therapy, REM sleep returns to normal. In seizure disorders, phenobarbital limits the spread of seizure activity by increasing the threshold for motor cortex stimuli. Barbiturates are habit forming.

How are they used?

Barbiturates are primarily used to treat insomnia, although they are also used for partial **epilepsy** and tonic–clonic seizures.

What are the adverse effects?

The most common adverse effect associated with barbiturates is sedation, which can range from mild sleepiness or drowsiness to somnolence. The barbiturate phenobarbital may also cause nausea and vomiting, constipation or diarrhea, bradycardia, skin rash, fever, and headache. The toxic effects of barbiturates include respiratory depression, circulatory shock, and renal or hepatic damage.

What are the contraindications and interactions?

Barbiturates are contraindicated in anyone with a familial history of **porphyria**, a genetic disorder caused by deficiency of enzymes of the heme biosynthetic pathway, and in cases of severe respiratory or kidney disease. They should be avoided in patients with a history of previous addiction to sedative–hypnotics or uncontrolled pain and in women who are pregnant or lactating. Alcohol may interact with barbiturates because of these agents' similar CNS depressant qualities. The barbiturate phenobarbital may decrease absorption and increase metabolism of oral anticoagulants and may also increase metabolism of corticosteroids and oral contraceptives.

What are the important points patients should know?

Instruct patients about methods, such as relaxation, they can use to decrease anxiety. Advise patients not to stop the medication abruptly after prolonged use because withdrawal symptoms may occur. Warn patients not to drink alcohol or take other CNS depressants while taking hypnotics or anxiolytics.

Instruct patients about methods to assist with sleep, such as avoiding coffee, heavy meals, and excessive stimuli close to bedtime. Caution them against driving and operating machinery because dizziness or drowsiness might occur.

Attention-Deficit Disorder and Attention-Deficit/Hyperactivity Disorder

Attention-deficit disorder (ADD) and attention-deficit/hyperactivity disorder (ADHD) may begin in childhood and continue into adulthood. The two disorders are signified by inattentiveness and impulsive actions, often causing problems at work, in relationships, in school, and at home. The patient with either of these disorders finds it difficult to pay attention, even when they try to concentrate. They find it hard to get organized, control their behavior, remember details, or listen to instructions. Both ADD and ADHD may run in families and are more common in males than in females. Many patients grow out of the hyperactive symptoms of ADHD, but continue to be easily distracted as adults, often having mood imbalances and the tendency to become angry quickly. Drugs used to treat ADD and ADHD are listed in Table 23-2 ■.

Table 23-2 ■ Drugs Used for ADD/ADHD

GENERIC NAME	TRADE NAME	AVERAGE ADULT DOSAGE	ROUTE OF ADMINISTRATION
amphetamine/dextroamphetamine	Adderall	5–40 mg in 1–3 divided doses	PO
atomoxetine	Strattera	80 mg/d in A.M.	PO
dexmethylphenidate	Focalin	2.5–10 mg bid	PO
dextroamphetamine	Dexedrine	5–40 mg/d in A.M.	PO
lisdexamfetamine	Vyvanse	30 mg/d in A.M.	PO
methylphenidate	Ritalin	5–15 mg bid–tid	PO

PO, oral; bid, twice a day; tid, three times a day.

✳ Apply Your Knowledge 23.1

The following questions focus on what you have just learned about the nervous system, CNS stimulants, and sedatives and hypnotics.

CRITICAL THINKING

1. Identify the four major portions of the brain.
2. Explain the disorder that will result from degeneration of the basal ganglia.
3. Point out the two major functions of the brain.
4. Describe the mechanism of action of CNS stimulants.
5. Discuss the differences between sedatives and hypnotics.
6. Identify the significant adverse effects of overdosage of benzodiazepines.
7. Give the trade names of oxazepam, diazepam, and alprazolam.
8. Describe the contraindications of barbiturates.
9. Discuss the treatments for ADD and ADHD.

Epilepsy

The terms **convulsion** and *seizure* are often used interchangeably and basically have the same meaning. A seizure is a periodic attack of disturbed cerebral function. A seizure may also be defined as an abnormal disturbance in the electrical activity in one or more areas of the brain. Seizures may be classified as generalized **tonic–clonic** (contraction–relaxation) seizures (previously termed *grand mal*); generalized absence seizures (previously called *petit mal*); generalized myoclonic seizures; and partial seizures. Status epilepticus is an emergency condition that may result in brain injury or death if not treated immediately.

Epilepsy is a permanent, recurrent seizure disorder. Examples of the known causes of epilepsy include brain injury at birth, head injuries, and inborn errors of metabolism. In some patients, the cause of epilepsy is never determined.

ANTISEIZURE DRUGS (ANTICONVULSANTS)

The categorizations of antiseizure drugs that follow are based on chemical structure and mechanism of action.

Chemical groupings include the hydantoins, succinimides, benzodiazepines, and barbiturates.

In addition, several miscellaneous drugs are used as anticonvulsants, such as carbamazepine, valproic acid or valproate, primidone, gabapentin, and lamotrigine. All can depress abnormal neural discharges in the CNS, resulting in an inhibition of seizure activity. Drugs that control generalized tonic–clonic seizures are not effective for absence seizures. If both conditions are present, then combined drug therapy is required. Table 23-3 ■ lists the most commonly used antiseizure medications.

Table 23-3 ■ Most Commonly Prescribed Antiseizure Drugs

GENERIC NAME	TRADE NAME	AVERAGE ADULT DOSAGE	ROUTE OF ADMINISTRATION
Hydantoins			
fosphenytoin	Cerebyx	Individualized	IM, IV
phenytoin	Dilantin	50–200 mg bid–tid	PO
Succinimides			
ethosuximide	Zarontin	500 mg/d	PO
methsuximide	Celontin	300–1,200 mg/d	PO
Benzodiazepines			
diazepam	Valium	5–10 mg; repeat if needed at 10- to 15-min intervals to 30 mg and then repeat if needed q2–4h	IM, IV
lorazepam	Ativan	4 mg injected slowly at 2 mg/min; may repeat once after 10 min	IV
Barbiturates			
mephobarbital	Mebaral	400–600 mg/d in divided doses	PO
		Anticonvulsant: 100–300 mg/d	PO
phenobarbital	Luminal	Anticonvulsant: 200–600 mg up to 20 mg/kg	IM, IV
		Status epilepticus: 15–18 mg/kg in single or divided doses (maximum, 20 mg/kg)	IV
Miscellaneous Antiseizure Drugs			
carbamazepine	Tegretol	100–400 mg tid	PO
divalproex	Depakote	125–250 mg tid–qid	PO
gabapentin	Neurontin	100–800 mg tid–qid	PO
lamotrigine	Lamictal	500 mg bid (maintenance)	PO
		Starting dosage depends on patient weight and other variables	
levetiracetam	Keppra	500 mg bid	PO
pregabalin	Lyrica	100 mg tid based on creatinine clearance	PO

GENERIC NAME	TRADE NAME	AVERAGE ADULT DOSAGE	ROUTE OF ADMINISTRATION
primidone	Mysoline	250 mg–2 g in divided doses	PO
topiramate	Topamax	200–400 mg/day in two divided doses	PO
valproate	Depacon	10–15 mg/kg/d, increased by 5–10 mg/kg/week prn (max: 60 mg/kg/d)	IV
valproic acid	Depakene	100–200 mg bid–tid	PO
zonisamide	Zonegran	100–400 mg/d	PO

IM, intramuscular; IV, intravenous; bid, twice a day; tid, three times a day; PO, oral; bid, twice a day.

Focus on Natural Products

Drug Interactions with Kava

The dried, crushed roots and rhizome of the kava plant, an Australasian shrubby pepper found in abundance on the islands of the South Pacific, are often used as an antiepileptic and dietary supplement to reduce stress and anxiety. Kava is available in many different oral forms, such as teas, cold drink powders, and paste. It should not be used in patients who have Parkinson's disease, and concurrent use with carbidopa and levodopa is contraindicated. Antipsychotics taken with kava may result in neuroleptic movement disorders. Barbiturates, benzodiazepines, and CNS depressants in general may cause increased sedation when taken with kava.

Focus On

Phenytoin

The most commonly used and recognizable drug in this group is phenytoin, which was first synthesized in 1908. It is the sole clinical representative of the hydantoins in use as an antiseizure drug.

How does it work?

Phenytoin is a hydantoin derivative chemically related to phenobarbital. The precise mechanism of anticonvulsant action is not known, but use of this drug is accompanied by reduced voltage, frequency, and spread of electrical discharges within the motor cortex.

How is it used?

Phenytoin is approved by the U.S. Food and Drug Administration (FDA) for partial seizures with complex symptomatology and tonic–clonic, psychomotor, and nonepileptic seizures, such as those caused by head trauma. It is also used to prevent or treat seizures occurring during or after neurosurgery. Phenytoin is prescribed as an antiarrhythmic agent, especially in the treatment of digitalis-induced arrhythmias.

What are the adverse effects?

Phenytoin may cause blurred vision, dizziness, drowsiness, fatigue, thrombocytopenia, and aplastic anemias. Patients should be advised to use caution when driving or operating machinery and performing tasks that require mental alertness. Serum levels above the optimal range may produce confusion, delirium, or psychosis. Dose adjustments may be necessary in patients with renal disease. Chronic use may cause gingival hyperplasia.

What are the contraindications and interactions?

Phenytoin is contraindicated in patients who are hypersensitive to the drug. It must be avoided in patients with seizures caused by hypoglycemia, sinus bradycardia, and complete or incomplete heart block and in pregnant and lactating patients.

(*continued*)

Focus On (*continued*)

There are numerous drug–drug interactions with phenytoin, including antacids, antidiabetic agents, **antipsychotics**, anxiolytics, barbiturates, calcium channel blockers, cardiac glycosides, corticosteroids, estrogens, neuromuscular-blocking agents, opiate agonists, oral contraceptives, progestins, salicylates, sulfonamides, thyroid hormones, tricyclic antidepressants (TCAs), vinca alkaloids, and vitamin D analogues. Phenytoin should be used cautiously in patients with impaired liver or kidney function, alcoholism, blood disorders, and hypotension.

What are the important points patients should know?

Advise patients taking phenytoin that their urine might become discolored to a pink or red-brown color. This discoloration is harmless. For patients with diabetes who are taking phenytoin, advise them that their blood glucose level should be checked more closely because phenytoin can inhibit insulin release. Also, advise patients about the importance of oral hygiene and regular dental checkups to prevent gingivitis and gingival hyperplasia.

Focus on Geriatrics

Phenytoin

Phenytoin should be used cautiously and at lower doses in elderly patients to avoid toxicity.

Focus On

Valproic Acid

Valproic acid is used to treat patients with simple and complex absence seizures. It has been used for other generalized seizures, including primary generalized tonic–clonic, atypical absence, myoclonic, and atonic seizures.

How does it work?

The mechanism of action of valproic acid is unknown. It may be related to the increased bioavailability of the inhibitor neurotransmitter GABA to brain neurons.

How is it used?

Valproic acid is used alone or with other anticonvulsants in the management of absence and mixed seizures and mania and in migraine headache prophylaxis. It is the drug of choice for symptomatic and idiopathic generalized seizures, juvenile myoclonic epilepsy, and childhood absence seizures.

What are the adverse effects?

Adverse effects of valproic acid include nausea and vomiting, hypersalivation, abdominal cramps, liver failure, and cases of life-threatening pancreatitis. Sedation and drowsiness are the most frequently reported adverse effects. There are considerable hematologic effects, and because valproic acid inhibits the secondary phase of platelet aggregation, it may prolong bleeding time.

What are the contraindications and interactions?

Safe use of valproic acid during pregnancy has not been established. Patients taking valproic acid may develop clotting abnormalities. Additive CNS depression may occur when valproic acid is administered with other CNS depressants. Valproic acid may potentiate the effects of monoamine oxidase inhibitors (MAOIs) and other antidepressant drugs. This drug may alter some laboratory tests, such as thyroid function and urinary ketones. Alcohol and other CNS depressants potentiate its depressant effects. Haloperidol, loxapine, phenothiazines, and TCAs can increase CNS depression or lower seizure thresholds. Aspirin and warfarin (Coumadin) increase the risk of spontaneous bleeding and decrease clotting. Cimetidine (Tagamet) may increase valproic acid levels and toxicity.

What are the important points patients should know?

Valproic acid may irritate the mouth, throat, and stomach, so if patients are taking the capsule form, instruct them to swallow the capsules whole and not chew, crush, or break them. The syrup form of valproic acid may be added to foods or liquids for a better taste. It is advisable to take valproic acid with meals or snacks to reduce stomach upset.

Ethosuximide

Succinimides are anticonvulsant agents. Only one member of this group still used in clinical practice, ethosuximide, is the drug of choice for control of uncomplicated absence seizures. It is generally considered to be the safest of the succinimide drugs. The FDA approved ethosuximide in 1960 as a succinimide-derived anticonvulsant.

How does it work?

Ethosuximide acts to stabilize neuronal excitability, thereby raising the threshold of uncontrolled cerebral discharges, especially within the motor cortex. It does this by delaying the entry of calcium into neuron cells by blocking calcium channels. It suppresses the electroencephalogram pattern associated with lapses of consciousness in absence seizures. Its actual mechanism of action is not understood, but it may act to inhibit neuronal systems.

How is it used?

Ethosuximide is used to manage absence seizures in adults and children older than 6 years of age, myoclonic seizures, and akinetic epilepsy. This agent may be administered with other anticonvulsants when other forms of epilepsy coexist with absence seizures. It is the drug of choice for absence seizures during pregnancy because it is much less teratogenic than other drugs in this category.

What are the adverse effects?

Common adverse effects of ethosuximide include drowsiness, hiccups, ataxia, dizziness, headache, euphoria, restlessness, anxiety, blurred vision, and aggressiveness. *Pancytopenia* (an abnormal reduction in red and white blood cells and platelets), nausea and vomiting, anorexia, abdominal pain, weight loss, diarrhea, and gingival hyperplasia are also seen. Vaginal bleeding, *agranulocytosis* (depression of granulocyte-producing bone marrow), aplastic anemia, *alopecia* (hair loss), and muscle weakness have been associated with ethosuximide therapy. Abnormal liver and kidney function test results are sometimes seen.

What are the contraindications and interactions?

Contraindications include hypersensitivity to succinimides and severe liver or kidney disease. Safety during pregnancy, lactation, and in children younger than 3 years has not been established. Ethosuximide decreases the serum levels of primidone. Carbamazepine decreases ethosuximide levels, and isoniazid significantly increases ethosuximide levels.

What are the important points patients should know?

Advise patients about the possibility of blood disorders, and instruct them to report any signs of a sore throat, fever, or bruising of unknown cause to their physician. Warn them against driving or working with heavy machinery because of the adverse effects of succinimides.

Carbamazepine

Carbamazepine is an oral anticonvulsant drug similar to TCAs. It is used to treat partial seizures—simple and complex—and for tonic–clonic seizures. It is the drug of choice in symptomatic partial seizures. This drug is preferred over phenobarbital because it has fewer adverse effects on behavior and alertness. Carbamazepine is also the drug of choice for the treatment of neuralgias, particularly trigeminal neuralgia (intense pain in the lips, eyes, nose, scalp, forehead, and upper or lower jaw).

How does it work?

Carbamazepine promotes sodium **efflux** (the process of flowing out) across the nerve membranes. As a consequence, carbamazepine reduces neuronal excitability, especially repeated firing of the same neuron. Unlike phenytoin, carbamazepine leaves the motor cortex relatively unaffected.

How is it used?

FDA-approved uses are for partial seizures, tonic–clonic seizures, and trigeminal neuralgia. However, this drug is often used to treat many other disorders, such as depression and bipolar disorder.

What are the adverse effects?

Severe cardiovascular disturbances, blood disorders, altered urination, and liver or kidney dysfunctions are adverse effects of carbamazepine in addition to those generally associated with antiseizure drugs. Elderly patients may be more susceptible to confusion or agitation. Carbamazepine commonly causes blurred vision, dizziness, drowsiness, and fatigue.

(continued)

Focus On (continued)

What are the contraindications and interactions?

Absolute contraindications for use of carbamazepine are hypersensitivity and cardiac or liver impairment. It should be used with extreme caution in pregnant women because it crosses the placenta and has been implicated in a number of fetal abnormalities.

Drug interactions occur with antineoplastic agents, antiretroviral protease inhibitors, barbiturates, calcium channel blockers, corticosteroids, MAOIs, neuromuscular blockers, opiate agonists, oral contraceptives, progestins, estrogens, halogenated anesthetics, thyroid hormones, and TCAs.

What are the important points patients should know?

Inform patients about the possibility of blood disorders. Advise them to report any signs of a sore throat, mucosal ulceration, *petechiae* (minute hemorrhagic spots in the skin), or bruising of unknown cause.

✳ Apply Your Knowledge 23.2

The following questions focus on what you have just learned about antiseizure medications.

CRITICAL THINKING

1. Identify the classifications of seizures.
2. Explain the causes of epilepsy.
3. Identify the most commonly prescribed antiseizure drugs.
4. Give the trade names of ethosuximide, phenytoin, valproic acid, and carbamazepine.
5. Describe the indications of phenytoin.
6. Identify the indications of valproic acid.
7. Point out the drug of choice for the control of uncomplicated absence seizures.
8. Explain the indications of carbamazepine.

Alzheimer's Disease

Alzheimer's disease is one of the primary causes of severe cognitive dysfunction in adults over 65 years of age, and is also known as *senile dementia*. In those over age 85, it has greatly increased incidence. Alzheimer's disease is the most common type of *dementia*, which is a term that describes a variety of diseases and conditions in which neurons of the brain die or stop functioning normally. One of every three older adults in the United States dies with this disease, or another type of dementia. Approximately 5.2 million Americans are affected. Of these, 5 million people are age 65 or older, and the remainder have younger-onset Alzheimer's. Incidence of this disease will increase dramatically by the year 2050, to approximately 21 million people in the United States.

The brain of a patient with Alzheimer's disease progressively atrophies and develops senile plaques. The disease is not fully understood, but appears to progress because of beta amyloid deposits in these neuritic plaques as well as arterial walls. Due to an abnormality on chromosome 21, the disease may be genetically linked in certain families. However, there are usually additional factors, including losses of neurotransmitter stimulation by choline acetyltransferase, changes in brain biochemistry, viral infections, autoimmune reactions, toxic chemicals, blood vessel defects, chemical deficiencies, and lack of certain neurochemicals. Sometimes, head trauma has also been linked to Alzheimer's disease (Figure 23-3 ■).

Figure 23-3 ■ An elderly woman with Alzheimer's disease.

Alzheimer's disease is signified by progressive short-term memory failure, impaired ability to think and concentrate, inability to reason normally or to learn new information, and confusion or disorientation. There may be changes in personality, speech disturbances, restlessness, and inability to perform normal tasks of daily living. Progression of the disease may result in inability to talk to other people, sit without supportive products, or walk without assistance. Disease progression occurs over 5–10 years, and the patient needs increased care. Once advanced, the disease causes the patient to be emotionally detached, and often, hostile to others. Disturbances of sleep are also common. The patient becomes bedridden, and death is often due to infections or complications.

Alzheimer's disease is not curable, and accurate diagnosis is only made after the patient's death by examining the brain. Positive diagnosis is based on loss of neurons, presence of senile plaques, and visualization of microscopic amyloid deposits. There is supportive treatment available. Cholinesterase inhibitors may alleviate cognitive symptoms. Medications include donepezil, galantamine, and rivastigmine.

Symptoms of Alzheimer's disease may be caused by chronic activation of N-methyl-D-aspartate (NDMA) receptors by glutamate, which is an excitatory amino acid. Memantine is a drug classified as an NMDA inhibitor, which may be helpful. Other medications include tacrine, haloperidol, alprazolam, lorazepam, buspirone, and SSRIs such as paroxetine. When the patient is aggressive and has delusional symptoms, risperidone or olanzapine may be used. Additional treatments include the prescription dietary supplement known as Axona, vitamin B_{12} supplements, and a combination vitamin product called Cerefolin. Table 23-4 ■ lists medications used for Alzheimer's disease.

Table 23-4 ■ Medications Used for Alzheimer's Disease

GENERIC NAME	TRADE NAME	AVERAGE ADULT DOSAGE	ROUTE OF ADMINISTRATION
Approved for all stages of disease			
donepezil	Aricept	5–23 mg once/d, h.s., with water	PO
Approved for mild to moderate disease			
galantamine	Razadyne	16–32 mg/day bid	PO
rivastigmine	Exelon	6–12 mg per day in divided doses in A.M. and P.M., with food	PO
tacrine	Cognex	Initial: 40 mg/d (10 mg qid) for 4 weeks, which may be increased to 80 mg/d (20 mg qid)	PO
Approved for moderate to severe disease			
memantine	Namenda	Initial: 5 mg (2.5 mL) once/d, increased in 5 mg increments every week, to 20 mg (5 mL) bid	PO
memantine/donepezil	Namzaric	28 mg memantine/10 mg donepezil, taken once/d in P.M.	PO
Not FDA-approved for Alzheimer's but still in use to delay disease onset			
vitamin E	Alpha Tocopherol	2,000 International Units/d	PO

PO, oral; bid, twice a day; qid, four times a day; h.s., take before bedtime.

Focus On

Donepezil

Donepezil is a reversible inhibitor of the enzyme acetylcholinesterase, and it is available for oral administration in film-coated tablets.

How does it work?

Donepezil is believed to enhance cholinergic function by increasing the concentration of acetylcholine through reversible inhibition of its hydrolysis by acetylcholinesterase.

How is it used?

Donepezil is indicated for the treatment of dementia of the Alzheimer's type, and it is effective for mild, moderate, and severe disease.

What are the adverse effects?

Donepezil may cause nausea and vomiting, diarrhea, insomnia, muscle cramps, fatigue, and anorexia.

What are the contraindications and interactions?

Donepezil is contraindicated in patients with known hypersensitivity to this drug or to piperidine derivatives. It may interact with ketoconazole, quinidine, phenytoin, carbamazepine, dexamethasone, rifampin, phenobarbital, anticholinergics, cholinomimetics, and other cholinesterase inhibitors.

What are the important points patients should know?

The patient must be instructed to report heart rhythm disorders such as *sick sinus syndrome*, enlarged prostate, urination problems, asthma, obstructive pulmonary disease, seizure disorders, and any upcoming scheduled surgeries. The patient must be told that this drug can impair thinking and reactions, and to use care driving or performing activities that require alertness.

Galantamine

Galantamine is a reversible, competitive acetylcholinesterase inhibitor that is available in extended-release capsules, and standard-release tablets and an oral solution.

How does it work?

Galantamine is believed to enhance cholinergic function by increasing the concentration of acetylcholine through reversible inhibition of its hydrolysis by cholinesterase.

How is it used?

Galantamine is indicated for the treatment of mild to moderate dementia of the Alzheimer's type.

What are the adverse effects?

Galantamine may cause serious skin reactions or even death in patients with mild cognitive impairment. The most common adverse reactions include nausea, vomiting, diarrhea, dizziness, headache, decreased appetite, and weight loss.

What are the contraindications and interactions?

Galantamine is contraindicated in patients with known hypersensitivity to this drug or its constituents. This drug may interact with anticholinergic medications, cholinomimetics, and other cholinesterase inhibitors.

What are the important points patients should know?

The patient must be instructed to tell the physician about urination problems, heart disease, heart rhythm disorders, stomach ulcers or bleeding, seizure disorders, liver or kidney disease, or asthma. The drug must be stopped if there is chest pain, slow heart rate, blood in the stool, coughing up blood, decreased urination, weakness, confusion, extreme thirst, or hot, dry skin. All other medications being used must be reviewed. Galantamine may need to be stopped during any surgical procedures, and the patient must be careful performing activities that require alertness while taking this drug.

Memantine

Memantine is an orally active NMDA receptor antagonist available as an oral solution.

How does it work?

Memantine is believed to bind to NMDA receptor-operated cation channels.

How is it used?

Memantine is used to treat moderate to severe dementia of the Alzheimer's type.

What are the adverse effects?

Memantine may cause dizziness, headache, confusion, and constipation. Less commonly, it may cause fatigue, pain, hypertension, vomiting, somnolence, hallucinations, coughing, or dyspnea.

What are the contraindications and interactions?

Memantine is contraindicated in patients with known hypersensitivity to this drug or its constituents. It may interact with carbonic anhydrase inhibitors, sodium bicarbonate, and other NMDA antagonists such as amantadine, ketamine, or dextromethorphan.

What are the important points patients should know?

The patient must tell his or her physician about any drug allergies, seizure disorders, cataracts, liver or kidney disease, or bladder or kidney infections. The patient should avoid activities requiring alertness while taking this drug.

Parkinson's Disease

Parkinson's disease was first described by English physician James Parkinson in 1817. It is a disease that principally occurs in older adults, but it can also develop in middle-aged people. Parkinson's disease is a nervous system disorder characterized by movement abnormalities, such as tremors of the extremities and head, and great difficulty in the coordination of fine muscle movement. The other salient feature is *hypokinesia*, an inability or slowness in initiating movements. Other signs and symptoms include a shuffling gait and skeletal muscle rigidity. Often, the affected person breaks into a run to stop from falling.

The incidence of Parkinson's disease is about 1% in people older than 60 years, so it is not an uncommon disease. Its cause is unknown, but a considerable amount is known about the CNS defect that leads to the illness.

This defect is in the basal ganglia portion of the midbrain known as the **substantia nigra**, which is a large cell mass involved in metabolic disturbances associated with Parkinson's disease. This part of the brain is important in the initiation and control of muscular movement. Skeletal muscle movements are initiated in the motor cortex of the brain and pass through the basal ganglia and thalamus to the spinal cord along the corticospinal tract.

In the pathways of the substantia nigra, there is a balance between dopamine and acetylcholine in normal individuals. In patients with Parkinson's disease, a lack of dopaminergic activity leads to an imbalance between these neurotransmitters (Figure 23-4 ■).

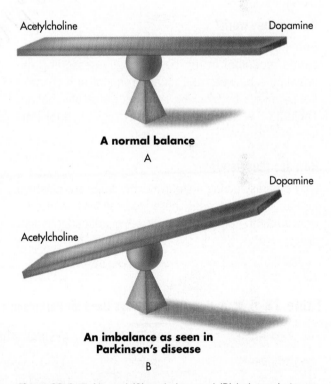

A normal balance
A

An imbalance as seen in Parkinson's disease
B

Figure 23-4 ■ Normal (**A**) and abnormal (**B**) balance between dopamine and acetylcholine.

Parkinsonism is a term that refers to the symptoms produced by certain drugs, poisons, and traumatic lesions in the basal ganglia. When the cause is known, the disease is termed *secondary parkinsonism*, as opposed to *primary parkinsonism*. Secondary parkinsonism is sometimes only temporary if the symptoms are caused by drugs. Secondary parkinsonism is not the same as Parkinson's disease.

There is no cure for Parkinson's disease. Drugs have been developed that can help patients manage many of the symptoms, but they do not stop the progression of the disease. However, patients with Parkinson's disease frequently experience dramatic swings in mobility and mood (known as being "on" or "off"), which may depend on the severity of the disease or the timing of the medication doses.

Because surgical treatment is still experimental, the usual way to treat people with this condition is to try to rebalance dopamine and acetylcholine by using drugs. Two methods are used to correct the condition: decreasing the muscarinic activity by using antimuscarinic drugs, or increasing the dopaminergic activity by increasing dopamine levels, blocking its breakdown, or mimicking its action.

Focus On

Anticholinergic Drugs (Muscarinic Antagonists)

The most commonly used agents in this class are benztropine and trihexyphenidyl. Amantadine is sometimes useful for tremor or for making levodopa work better, but exactly how it works is not clear. It may also dramatically reduce *dyskinesia* (difficulty in making voluntary movements) in some patients.

How do they work?

Anticholinergic agents work by inhibiting the muscarine receptors in the basal ganglia, lessening the imbalance between the extrapyramidal and pyramidal pathways by blocking the effect of acetylcholine. Table 23-5 ■ lists anticholinergic drugs used for Parkinson's disease.

How are they used?

Only centrally acting anticholinergic drugs are effective for Parkinson's disease. These medications can also be prescribed in combination with other antiparkinsonian drugs.

What are the adverse effects?

CNS adverse effects include anxiety, which is experienced by 30–50% of all patients, and, more seriously, agitation or confusion. The anticholinergic effects include dry mouth and decreased sweating and heat release. Other serious adverse reactions include urticaria, urine retention, paresthesias, and sinus tachycardia.

What are the contraindications and interactions?

The safe use of anticholinergic agents in pregnant patients has not been established. They should not be given with other antimuscarinics because additive effects may occur.

What are the important points patients should know?

Instruct patients to avoid alcohol consumption because this combination may intensify the CNS depressant effects. Advise patients that constipation can occur and urge them to consume a high-fiber diet. Because drowsiness is a common effect of these drugs, advise patients to avoid driving a car or operating heavy machinery.

Table 23-5 ■ Anticholinergic Drugs Used for Parkinson's Disease

GENERIC NAME	TRADE NAME	AVERAGE ADULT DOSAGE	ROUTE OF ADMINISTRATION
benztropine	Cogentin	0.5–1 mg/d; gradually increase as needed up to 6 mg/d	PO
biperiden	Akineton	2 mg 1–4 times/d	PO
diphenhydramine	Benadryl	25–50 mg tid–qid	PO
procyclidine	Kemadrin	2.5–5 mg tid	PO
trihexyphenidyl	Artane	1 mg on day 1; 2 mg on day 2; then increase by 2 mg every 3–5 d, up to 6–10 mg/d	PO

PO, oral; tid, three times a day; qid, four times a day.

Focus On

Dopaminergic Drugs

Levodopa was the first drug approved specifically for Parkinson's disease, in 1970. It is still the most commonly administered therapy. In most patients, it significantly improves mobility and allows them to function relatively normally. A number of chemicals, such as carbidopa—a drug that prevents peripheral metabolism of levodopa—are able to prolong the effects of levodopa and help reduce its side effects. The combination drug carbidopa–levodopa is marketed in the United States as Sinemet®. Dopaminergic agents used for Parkinson's disease are listed in Table 23-6 ■.

How do they work?

Dopaminergic agents, such as levodopa, are metabolic precursors of dopamine, a catecholamine neurotransmitter. Unlike dopamine, levodopa readily crosses the blood–brain barrier. Its precise mechanism of action is unknown.

How are they used?

The dopaminergic agent levodopa is used in idiopathic Parkinson's disease, postencephalitic and arteriosclerotic parkinsonism, and parkinsonism symptoms associated with manganese and carbon monoxide poisoning.

What are the adverse effects?

The debilitating side effects of dopaminergic agents include dyskinesia, hallucinations, and mental confusion. A major long-term complication is loss of efficacy after about 5 years of therapy. Abrupt discontinuation should be avoided because some patients experience a complex called *neuroleptic malignant syndrome (NMS)*, especially if they are also taking **neuroleptic** agents, which are psychotropic drugs used to treat psychosis. Manifestations of NMS include tachycardia, muscular rigidity, fever, mental status changes, diaphoresis, tachypnea, and increases in serum creatinine levels.

What are the contraindications and interactions?

Dopaminergic agents should be administered with extreme caution to patients who have cardiac disease. Other drugs work differently. The so-called *dopamine agonists*, such as bromocriptine, ropinirole, pergolide, and pramipexole, work directly on the target cells of the substantia nigra in a way that imitates dopamine. Dopamine agonists are often used in combination with levodopa.

Unfortunately, all drugs used to treat Parkinson's disease may have side effects. Although some people never experience such side effects, others are very sensitive to the medications and may be unable to tolerate them. Most commonly, the side effects of antiparkinsonian drugs are mental confusion, hallucinations, and dyskinesia. Because effective treatment of Parkinson's disease is often a matter of balancing beneficial effects of drugs against their side effects, many people prefer to see experienced specialists.

What are the important points patients should know?

Instruct patients to take dopaminergic agents with food to avoid gastrointestinal irritation. Levodopa may discolor urine and perspiration. Advise patients to avoid foods rich in vitamin B_6, such as beans and cereals, and alcohol. Bromocriptine can cause postural hypotension, so advise patients to rise slowly from a lying position. Also, instruct patients to regularly visit their dentists to prevent dental problems caused by the inhibition of salivation. Dopaminergic agents should never be stopped abruptly because of a possible rebound of parkinsonism.

Table 23-6 ■ Dopaminergic Drugs Used for Parkinson's Disease

GENERIC NAME	TRADE NAME	AVERAGE ADULT DOSAGE	ROUTE OF ADMINISTRATION
amantadine	Symmetrel	100 mg bid	PO
bromocriptine	Parlodel	1.25– 2.5 mg/d up to 100 mg/d in divided doses	PO
carbidopa–levodopa	Sinemet	1 tablet containing 10 mg carbidopa/100 mg levodopa or 25 mg carbidopa/100 mg levodopa tid; increased by 1 tablet every day or every other day, up to 6 tablets/d	PO

(continued)

Table 23-6 ■ Dopaminergic Drugs Used for Parkinson's Disease (*continued*)

GENERIC NAME	TRADE NAME	AVERAGE ADULT DOSAGE	ROUTE OF ADMINISTRATION
levodopa	Dopar	500 mg–1 g/d	PO
pergolide	Permax	Start with 0.5 mg/d for 2 d; then increase by 0.1 or 0.15 mg/d q3d for 12 d; and then increase by 0.25 mg every third day until reaching the desired effect	PO
pramipexole	Mirapex	Start with 0.125 mg tid for 1 wk; double this dose for the next week; continue to increase by 0.25 mg/dose tid q1wk to the desired dose of 1.5 mg tid	PO
ropinirole	Requip	Start with 0.25 mg tid; increase q1wk by 0.25 mg/dose to the target dose of 1 mg tid	PO
tolcapone	Tasmar	100 mg tid (maximum: 600 mg/d)	PO

bid, twice a day; PO, oral; tid, three times a day.

✳ Apply Your Knowledge 23.3

The following questions focus on what you have just learned about Parkinson's disease and antiparkinsonian drugs.

CRITICAL THINKING

1. Describe the factors that may cause Alzheimer's disease.
2. Explain the prognosis of Alzheimer's disease.
3. Identify the major signs and symptoms of Parkinson's disease.
4. Discuss the role of the substantia nigra in Parkinson's disease.
5. Describe how dopamine and acetylcholine influence Parkinson's disease.
6. Explain the difference between Parkinson's disease and parkinsonism.
7. Identify the mechanism of action of levodopa.
8. Discuss the result of abrupt discontinuation of dopaminergic agents.
9. Describe the mechanism of action of anticholinergic drugs.
10. Give the trade names of benztropine, procyclidine, levodopa, amantadine, and bromocriptine.

Schizophrenia and Psychotic Disorders

Schizophrenia is one of the most common psychotic disorders. Almost 1.6% of the population, or about 2 million people in the United States, across all cultural groups, are affected by this disorder during their lifetimes. It occurs more commonly in urban populations and in lower socioeconomic groups. The cause of schizophrenia is unknown.

Manifestations of schizophrenia include either positive or negative symptoms. Positive symptoms tend to be exaggerations of normal functioning. For example, a distortion of perceptions may manifest as hallucinations, which involve hearing or seeing things that are not real, and as distortions of thought processes that may manifest as delusions. Negative symptoms include terseness in speech, social withdrawal, *anhedonia* (the inability to experience pleasure), and apathy. Symptoms usually manifest during the early years of adulthood. The illness is chronic, and fewer than 20% of patients recover fully from a single episode of psychosis.

Today, psychotic disorders are referred to as *schizophrenia spectrum* and *other psychotic disorders*. The other mental disorders in this group include:

✳ *Brief psychotic disorder:* a short-term illness with psychotic symptoms that often develop suddenly, but last for less than 1 month

✳ *Delusional disorder:* previously called *paranoid disorder*, it features the presence of delusions, which are unshakable beliefs in something that is untrue

✳ *Schizophreniform disorder:* resembles schizophrenia and includes delusions, hallucinations, disorganized speech, pacing, walking in circles, writing constantly, lack of energy, poor hygiene, loss of interest or ability to experience pleasure, and withdrawal from other people

✳ *Schizoaffective disorder:* severe changes in mood with some schizophrenia-like symptoms such as hallucinations, delusions, and disorganized thinking

✳ *Schizotypal personality disorder:* actually a group of conditions thought of as eccentric personality disorders, including oddness, peculiar actions, and unusual thinking patterns and behaviors

✳ *Catatonia:* generally involves immobility, unresponsiveness, rigid and stiff body positions, and unwillingness to move

✳ *Psychosis caused by a medical condition:* includes brain diseases, dementia, human immunodeficiency virus, epilepsy, stroke, or personality disorders

✳ *Substance- or medication-induced psychotic disorder:* includes alcoholism or drug use or withdrawal syndrome

✳ *Postpartum psychosis:* a rare condition affecting women who have recently given birth

Mood Disorders

Also, mood disorders can become so severe that psychotic symptoms develop. Examples of mood disorders include:

✳ *Bipolar disorder:* characterized by periods of extreme excitation or mania and deep depression, which for some reason may change back and forth over several months. There may be mostly manic episodes or mostly depressive episodes.

✳ *Major depressive disorder:* characterized by one or more major depressive episodes. Also called unipolar disorder, it is a chemical deficit within the brain, and a precise diagnosis is based on biologic factors or personal characteristics. The causes of depression include genetic and psychosocial stressors.

PSYCHOACTIVE DRUGS

The past three decades of research in the neurosciences have dramatically increased our understanding of the neurobehavioral aspects of mental illness. The 1990s were referred to as the "decade of the brain," and the more recent discovery of the human genome was accomplished in 2000. Historically, the advent of the first psychotropic medications in the 1950s significantly changed the treatment of people with mental illness. Recent advances in psychoactive drugs have resulted in increased use as the primary treatments for a variety of different conditions. The amount spent on psychoactive drugs has grown much more rapidly than the amount spent on other types of drugs.

More than 1,500 compounds, classified as *psychoactive* or *psychotropic* drugs, have been described. Approximately 20% of all prescriptions written in the United States are for medications intended to alter mental processes and behavior. Those agents used in the treatment of people with psychotic illnesses and depressant disorders are the focus of this chapter. One of the major uses of antipsychotic drugs is the treatment of people with schizophrenia.

Focus On

Antipsychotic Drugs

The terms *antipsychotic* and *neuroleptic* are used interchangeably to denote a group of drugs that have been used mainly for treating schizophrenia but are also effective in some other psychoses and agitated states. A new type of antipsychotic medication became available with the introduction of clozapine in 1990. After its success, other medications with similar clinical profiles were developed. These atypical antipsychotic agents are effective against the positive and the negative symptoms of schizophrenia. Although the atypical agents are more expensive than the typical drugs,

recent evaluations of the total costs of treatment show that atypical drugs are economically superior. This is because the increased efficacy and higher rate of compliance result in fewer hospital admissions and other emergency interventions.

Typical antipsychotics are available in several different groups. Structurally, they can be divided into phenothiazines, thioxanthenes, butyrophenones, dihydroindolone derivatives, and dibenzodiazepines. Common typical and atypical antipsychotic drugs are listed in Table 23-7 ■.

(continued)

Focus On (continued)

How do they work?

The mechanism of action of the antipsychotic agents is complex, and many details remain to be established. However, the evaluation of properties shared by effective antipsychotic agents provides clues to their mechanism of action. All the typical antipsychotic agents block postsynaptic dopaminergic receptors and act as competitive antagonists of dopamine centrally and peripherally.

How are they used?

Antipsychotic drugs are effective mainly against the positive symptoms of schizophrenia. In addition to their use in treating schizophrenia, several of these drugs are also effective antiemetic and antinausea agents.

What are the adverse effects?

The main adverse effects of antipsychotic drugs include sedation, dry mouth, sexual dysfunction, **akathisia** (difficulty in initiating muscle movement), **bradykinesia** (extremely slow movement), rigidity, and sometimes **tardive dyskinesia** (slowed ability to make voluntary movements).

What are the contraindications and interactions?

Many of the contraindications to the use of these drugs are similar. They are contraindicated in comatose patients who have received large amounts of CNS depressant drugs, such as alcohol and barbiturates.

What are the important points patients should know?

Advise family members of psychiatric outpatients about the adverse effects of drug therapy and any adverse reactions that may occur because they will be responsible for administering antipsychotic drugs to the patient. They should suggest that the patient use hard candy or ice chips for a dry mouth. Advise the patient not to drive a car or operate machinery until a maintenance dose has been established. Instruct patients who are taking phenothiazines, such as chlorpromazine, that their urine may turn pink or red-brown and that this discoloration is not harmful.

Table 23-7 ■ Common Typical and Atypical Antipsychotic Drugs

GENERIC NAME	TRADE NAME	AVERAGE ADULT DOSAGE	ROUTE OF ADMINISTRATION
Typical			
chlorpromazine	Thorazine	25–100 mg tid–qid up to 1,000 mg/d	PO
		25–50 mg up to 600 mg q4–6h; switch to oral dosage as soon as possible	IM
fluphenazine	Prolixin	0.5–10 mg/d in divided doses q6–8h; usual daily dose is less than 3 mg	PO
		2.5–10 mg/d (range: 2.5–10 mg) q6–8h	IM
haloperidol	Haldol	Initial dosage range: 0.5–5 mg bid–tid	PO
		2–5 mg (up to 10–30 mg) q60min or q4–8h prn; switch to oral dose as soon as possible	IM
lithium	Eskalith	600 mg tid or 900 mg slow-release form bid to produce effective serum levels of 1–1.5 mEq/L	PO
loxapine	Loxitane	Initially, 10 mg bid, rapidly increased to 60–100 mg/d in 2–4 divided doses	IM
		12.5–50 mg q4–6h; when controlled, change to oral dose	IM

GENERIC NAME	TRADE NAME	AVERAGE ADULT DOSAGE	ROUTE OF ADMINISTRATION
molindone	Moban	50–75 mg/d in 3–4 divided doses; may be increased to 100 mg/d in 3–4 d	PO
perphenazine	Perphenazine Tablets	4–16 mg bid–qid; reduce as soon as possible; avoid dosages greater than 64 mg/d	PO
		Initially 5–10 mg q6h, not exceeding 30 mg/d	IM
		Dilute to 0.5 mg per mL; give no more than 1 mg per injection at no less than 1- to 2-min intervals; do not exceed 5-mg total dose	IV
prochlorperazine	Compazine	Initially 5–10 mg tid–qid; gradually increase q2–3h up to 50–150 mg/d	PO
		10–20 mg q2–4h; switch to oral therapy as soon as possible	IM
		2.5–10 mg q6–8h (maximum: 40 mg/d)	IV
		25 mg bid up to 40 mg/d	Rectal
thioridazine	Mellaril	50–100 mg tid; may increase up to 800 mg/d	PO
trifluoperazine	Stelazine	1–2 mg bid; may increase up to 20 mg/d in hospitalized patients	PO
		1–2 mg q4–6h (maximum, 10 mg/d)	IM
Atypical			
aripiprazole	Abilify	10–15 mg/d	PO
clozapine	Clozaril	25 mg/d in 1–2 doses; gradually increase by 25–50 mg/d, up to 300–450 mg/d, by end of week 2	PO
olanzapine	Zyprexa	5–10 mg/d; increase by 5 mg/d at 1-wk intervals	PO
quetiapine	Seroquel	25 mg bid; increase by 25–50 mg bid, up to 800 mg/d	PO
risperidone	Risperdal	2 mg/d (maximum dosage: 4–8 mg/d)	PO
ziprasidone	Geodon	40 mg/d	IM, PO

tid, three times a day; qid, four times a day; PO, oral; IM, intramuscular; bid, twice a day.

Focus On

Lithium Carbonate

Lithium carbonate can control symptoms in the manic and depressive phases of psychotic disorders and is also used to treat bipolar disorder.

How does it work?

Lithium's exact mechanism of action is unclear. Therefore, therapeutic levels of lithium must be considered individually. Therapeutic effects usually take 1–2 weeks to be observed.

How is it used?

Lithium is used in the control and the prophylaxis of acute mania and the acute manic phase of mixed bipolar disorder.

(continued)

Focus On (continued)

What are the adverse effects?

Common adverse effects of lithium include nausea and tremors, which subside with continued treatment. Overdose may cause vomiting, diarrhea, dizziness, headache, drowsiness, tinnitus, loss of equilibrium, disorientation, and short-term memory loss. Toxic levels may cause kidney and heart damage. Therefore, serum concentration levels should be monitored on a regular basis.

What are the contraindications and interactions?

Lithium should be avoided in pregnant women or patients with thyroid disorders. Carbamazepine, haloperidol, and phenothiazines increase the risk of neurotoxicity when they are used with lithium.

What are the important points patients should know?

Advise patients to drink plenty of fluids—at least 2–3 liters per day during the stabilization period and at least 1 to $1\frac{1}{2}$ liters per day during ongoing therapy. Alert them that urine output will be increased and diluted and that they may have persistent thirst. Dose reduction may be indicated. Instruct patients to contact their physicians if diarrhea or fever develops. Warn patients to avoid hot environments and excessive use of caffeinated beverages. Warn patients against driving and engaging in other potentially hazardous activities until the response to the drug is known.

Focus Point

Lithium, Contraception, and Pregnancy

Women who are taking lithium should use effective contraceptive measures. If therapy must be continued during pregnancy, serum lithium levels should be closely monitored to prevent toxicity.

✳ Apply Your Knowledge 23.4

The following questions focus on what you have just learned about psychoactive drugs.

CRITICAL THINKING

1. Identify the manifestations of schizophrenia.
2. Describe the effects of atypical antipsychotic agents.
3. Compare atypical and typical antipsychotic agents.
4. Explain the indications of lithium.
5. Identify the contraindications of lithium.
6. Give the trade names of haloperidol, lithium, olanzapine, and clozapine.

Depression

Major depression is one of the most common psychiatric disorders in the United States. About 5–6% of the population is depressed. Depression may be "reactive" (in response to a stimulus such as the loss of a loved one) or "endogenous" (a chemical disorder in the brain).

The majority of antidepressant medications are used chiefly in the management of endogenous depression. Symptoms of depression include feelings of doom, a lack of self-worth, an inability to sense pleasure, loss of energy, an inability to concentrate, changes in sleep habits, and thoughts of suicide.

ANTIDEPRESSANTS

Antidepressants are classified into several groups on the basis of their chemical structures and antidepressant action in the brain. The most commonly used drugs are listed in Table 23-8 ■ and include TCAs, MAOIs, and SSRIs.

Another class that is used less commonly is the selective serotonin–norepinephrine reuptake inhibitors (SSNRIs), also known as the serotonin–norepinephrine reuptake inhibitors (SNRIs). These include venlafaxine, duloxetine, and several other, less commonly used medications.

Table 23-8 ■ **Classifications of Antidepressants**

GENERIC NAME	TRADE NAME	AVERAGE ADULT DOSAGE	ROUTE OF ADMINISTRATION
Tricyclic Antidepressants			
amitriptyline	Elavil	Up to 300 mg/d in divided doses	PO
amoxapine	Amoxapine Tablets	Start at 50 mg bid–tid; may increase on day 3 to 100 mg tid	PO
clomipramine	Anafranil	50–150 mg/d in single or divided doses	PO
desipramine	Norpramin	100–300 mg/d	PO
doxepin	Sinequan	25–30 mg/d in divided doses	PO
imipramine	Tofranil	75–300 mg/d in divided doses	PO
nortriptyline	Pamelor	25 mg tid–qid	PO
protriptyline	Vivactil	15–40 mg/d in 3–4 divided doses (maximum: 60 mg/d)	PO
trimipramine	Surmontil	100–300 mg/d in divided doses	PO
Monoamine Oxidase Inhibitors			
phenelzine	Nardil	15 mg tid rapidly increased to at least 60 mg/d; may need up to 90 mg/d	PO
selegiline	Eldepryl	10 mg/d in divided doses at breakfast and lunch	PO
tranylcypromine	Parnate	30–60 mg/d in divided doses at 3-wk interval	PO
Selective Serotonin Reuptake Inhibitors			
citalopram	Celexa	20–40 mg/d	PO
escitalopram	Lexapro	10 mg/d; may increase to 20 mg after 1 wk	PO
fluoxetine	Prozac, Sarafem	20 mg/d in the morning; may increase by 40–80 mg/d in divided doses; weekly dose: 1 capsule/wk	PO
fluvoxamine	Luvox	50–300 mg/d in divided doses	PO
paroxetine	Paxil	20–50 mg/d	PO
sertraline	Zoloft	50–200 mg/d	PO

PO, oral; bid, twice a day; tid, three times a day; qid, four times a day.

Focus On

Tricyclic Antidepressants

Historically, drugs from this group have been the first choice in the treatment of depression and include imipramine, amitriptyline, doxepin, and related drugs.

How do they work?

TCAs increase the effect of norepinephrine and serotonin in the CNS by blocking their reuptake by the neurons.

How are they used?

TCAs are used for endogenous depression and occasionally for reactive depression.

What are the adverse effects?

Adverse effects derive from the fact that TCAs have secondary actions, including antimuscarinic, antihistamine, and antiadrenergic activity. The first action accounts for dry mouth, blurred vision, constipation, urine retention, and tachycardia. Mental confusion and sedation arise from a central antihistamine action, and postural hypotension can occur as a result of an antiadrenergic effect. When used together with antihypertensive agents, orthostatic hypotension may increase. Norepinephrine and other sympathomimetics may increase cardiac toxicity when they are used with TCAs.

What are the contraindications and interactions?

TCAs are contraindicated in patients who are hypersensitive to these drugs. They must be avoided in patients during the acute recovery period after a heart attack and in patients with severe renal or hepatic impairment. MAOIs may precipitate hyperpyrexic crisis, tachycardia, or seizures as a result of drug interaction with TCAs.

What are the important points patients should know?

Warn patients against stopping TCAs abruptly. Advise patients to take these drugs at bedtime to promote a normal sleep pattern. Instruct patients to report having severe postural hypotension to their physicians and explain that the drug's effectiveness begins after about 2 weeks of use. Antidepressant treatment needs to continue even after recovery because of the potential for a relapse.

Focus on Geriatrics

Effect of Tricyclic Antidepressants on the Prostate Gland

Elderly men with enlarged prostate glands are at higher risk for urine retention when taking TCAs.

Focus Point

Tricyclic Antidepressants and Other Medications

Patients taking TCAs should not take any medications, including over-the-counter (OTC) medications, without notifying their physicians.

Focus on Natural Products

Drug Interactions with St. John's Wort

St. John's wort is a flower grown throughout the world and is used to treat patients with mild to moderate depression and anxiety. It is administered orally for this purpose. St. John's wort should not be used during pregnancy and lactation. Interactions with St. John's wort occur with TCAs, MAOIs, SSRIs, alcohol, and foods that are high in tyramine or catecholamines. The major problem in using St. John's wort for depression and anxiety is that this herbal supplement may take 4–6 weeks to become effective. It may also cause increased photosensitivity.

Focus On

Selective Serotonin Reuptake Inhibitors

SSRIs are relatively newer antidepressants that have had a tremendous impact on prescribing patterns. They are now considered the first-line drugs in the treatment of patients with major depression.

How do they work?

SSRIs primarily block the effect of serotonin reuptake. Clinical studies have found that, generally, SSRIs have comparable efficacy to TCAs. However, TCAs have been found to be more effective in the treatment of patients with severe depression.

How are they used?

SSRIs are commonly used for depression, geriatric depression, obsessive–compulsive disorder, bulimia nervosa, and premenstrual dysphoric disorder.

What are the adverse effects?

In general, the adverse effects of SSRIs are relatively mild, of shorter duration than those of TCAs, and diminish as treatment continues. Cardiac toxicity and the risk of death after overdose are less likely than with

TCAs. Common adverse effects include headache, nausea and vomiting, tremor, insomnia, dizziness, and diarrhea.

What are the contraindications and interactions?

SSRIs must be avoided in patients who are hypersensitive to them. SSRIs should not be used concurrently with MAOIs or thioridazine. These drugs should not be used during pregnancy or in children younger than 7 years. SSRIs should be used with caution in patients with hepatic or renal impairment, renal failure, lactation, cardiac disease, or diabetes mellitus.

What are the important points patients should know?

Advise patients to report withdrawal symptoms, including abdominal pain, diarrhea, nausea, headache, sweating, and insomnia. Tell patients to take great care when driving and operating machinery while on antidepressant therapy, especially during the initial stages of treatment. Instruct patients to take SSRIs in the morning to minimize the incidence of insomnia and to avoid alcohol because of the additive CNS depressant effects.

Focus on Geriatrics

Taking SSRIs

All SSRIs should be administered with food. Patients—particularly older adults and nutritionally compromised patients—should be weighed weekly to monitor weight loss.

Focus On

Monoamine Oxidase Inhibitors

The therapeutic response rate with all antidepressants is similar, and the selection of the proper agent depends on the side effects the patient experiences from the drugs. MAOIs are second- or third-line antidepressants because of the numerous interactions with prescription and OTC medications as well as with certain foods and beverages.

How do they work?

MAOIs are thought to act by preventing the natural breakdown of neurotransmitters, but their precise mode of action is not known. It is also thought that MAOIs are able to inhibit

hepatic microsomal drug-metabolizing enzymes; thus, they may intensify and prolong the effects of many drugs.

How are they used?

Until the availability of SSRIs, MAOIs were the most effective antidepressants available. These agents are used to manage endogenous depression, the depressive phase of manic-depressive (bipolar) psychosis, and severe exogenous (reactive) depression that is not responsive to more commonly used therapies.

(*continued*)

Focus On (continued)

What are the adverse effects?

Common adverse reactions of MAOIs are less serious than those observed during TCA therapy but consist of antimuscarinic and antiadrenergic effects. Orthostatic hypotension is a common adverse effect of MAOIs. Nausea, constipation, dry mouth, diarrhea, dizziness, vertigo, and headache are also seen. A serious hypertensive crisis may occur if a patient taking MAOIs eats a food containing tyramine, an amino acid present in some foods.

What are the contraindications and interactions?

MAOIs are contraindicated in those with epilepsy, liver disease, and serious cardiovascular disease. These drugs are also contraindicated in patients with known hypersensitivity to them.

What are the most important points patients should know?

Instruct patients to avoid foods that contain tyramine and provide a list of these foods, which includes cheese, sour cream, yogurt, chicken liver, beef, coffee, tea, caffeinated sodas, chocolate, pickled herring, soy sauce, yeast extracts, and fruits and vegetables such as dried beans, fava beans, figs, raisins, avocados, bananas, and raspberries. Inform patients that the drug's effectiveness occurs after about 2 weeks of therapy.

Focus Point

Diet and Monoamine Oxidase Inhibitors

Patients taking MAOIs must avoid foods containing tyramine to avoid severe hypertension, heart attack, adverse reactions, and death.

✳ Apply Your Knowledge 23.5

The following questions focus on what you have just learned about TCAs, SSRIs, and MAOIs.

CRITICAL THINKING

1. Describe endogenous depression.
2. Identify the classifications of antidepressants.
3. Explain which class of antidepressants contains relatively newer drugs.
4. Describe the class of antidepressants that was most effective before the availability of selective serotonin reuptake inhibitors.
5. Identify the trade names of clomipramine, doxepin, phenelzine, citalopram, and paroxetine.

PRACTICAL SCENARIO 1

The father of an 18-year-old teenager calls the physician's office, stating that his son, who has been diagnosed with schizophrenia, has become increasingly withdrawn and does not seem interested in doing anything at all. He says his son is taking the antipsychotic clozapine, and he believes his son's condition should be better. His father states he is worried because his son also seems to have strange movements—he seems to move very slowly.

Michal Heron/Pearson Education/PH College

Critical Thinking Questions

1. As the medical assistant who takes the phone call, what might you say to alleviate some of the father's anxiety as you take down the details to relay to the physician?
2. What questions would you ask the father about his son's personality, mood, and physical changes?
3. What teaching points might you offer the father during the phone call?

PRACTICAL SCENARIO 2

A 45-year-old woman has had major depression. Recently, she attempted suicide. Her family history includes a sister who also had depression and committed suicide 3 years earlier.

Studio Grand Ouest/Fotolia

Critical Thinking Questions

1. In your opinion, what would be the best of the popular medications for this patient to treat her depression?
2. If she takes an MAOI, what precautions should she take concerning foods to avoid drug–food interactions?

Chapter Capsule

This section repeats the objectives from the beginning of the chapter and then provides a summary of the most important concepts for that objective. Use this section as a quick review and to check your knowledge.

Objective 1: Describe the four major parts of the brain.

- Cerebrum—the largest part, which includes nerve centers associated with sensory and motor functions and provides higher mental functions, including memory and reasoning; composed of an outer cerebral cortex and inner cerebral medulla
- Diencephalon—also processes sensory information
- Brainstem—contains nerve pathways that connect various parts of the nervous system and regulate certain visceral activities
- Cerebellum—includes centers that coordinate voluntary muscular movements

Objective 2: Name three benzodiazepine hypnotic drugs, and explain the mechanism by which they produce hypnotic effects.

- Diazepam—appears to act at the limbic and subcortical levels of the CNS
- Lorazepam—effects are mediated by GABA; it acts on the thalamic, hypothalamic, and limbic levels of the CNS
- Phenytoin—precise mechanism is not known, but it appears to reduce the voltage, frequency, and spread of electrical discharges within the motor cortex

Objective 3: List three different types of epilepsy and name two drugs used specifically to treat each type of epilepsy.

- The three different types of epilepsy include:
  - Generalized tonic–clonic seizures
  - Generalized absence seizures
  - Partial seizures
- Drugs used specifically to treat each type of epilepsy include:
  - Phenytoin, carbamazepine—generalized tonic–clonic seizures
  - Valproic acid, ethosuximide—generalized absence seizures
  - Phenytoin, carbamazepine—partial seizures

Objective 4: Explain the onset of Alzheimer's disease, identifying common signs and symptoms.

- The onset of Alzheimer's disease occurs because of progressive brain atrophy and the development of senile plaques. Though not fully understood, it appears to progress because of beta amyloid deposits in these neuritic plaques as well as arterial walls. Due to an abnormality on chromosome 21, the disease may be genetically linked in certain families. Other factors include loss of neurotransmitter stimulation by choline acetyltransferase, changes in brain biochemistry, viral infections, autoimmune reactions, toxic chemicals, blood vessel defects, chemical deficiencies, lack of certain neurochemicals, and, sometimes, head trauma.
- Common signs and symptoms include progressive short-term memory failure, impaired ability to think and concentrate, inability to reason normally or to learn new information, and confusion or disorientation. There may be changes in personality, speech disturbances, restlessness, and inability to perform normal tasks of daily living. Progression may result in inability to talk to other people, sit without supportive products, or to walk without assistance. Once advanced, the patient becomes emotionally detached and, often, hostile to others. Disturbances of sleep are also common.

Objective 5: Describe the mechanisms of action of drugs that increase dopamine or decrease acetylcholine levels in the basal ganglia.

- Anticholinergic agents—work by inhibiting the muscarine receptors in the basal ganglia, lessening the imbalance between the extrapyramidal and pyramidal pathways by blocking the effect of acetylcholine
- Dopaminergic drugs such as levodopa—the exact mechanism of action is unknown

Objective 6: Describe five adverse effects associated with antianxiety drugs.

- Drowsiness
- Nausea
- Bradycardia

- Skin rash
- Fever

Note: *There are more adverse effects, but these five are the most common.*

Objective 7: Describe the common adverse effects and the specific neurologic conditions caused by antipsychotic drugs.

- Common adverse effects—nausea and vomiting, diarrhea, dizziness, headache, drowsiness, tinnitus, disorientation, and short-term memory loss
- Neurological conditions—tremors, loss of equilibrium, and neurotoxicity, when combined with carbamazepine, haloperidol, and phenothiazines

Objective 8: Explain the use of lithium in mania and the adverse effects associated with its use.

- Lithium—controls symptoms in the manic and depressive phases of psychotic disorders; used for the control and prophylaxis of acute mania and the acute manic phase of mixed bipolar disorder
- Adverse effects—nausea and vomiting, tremors (which subside with continued treatment), diarrhea, dizziness, headache, drowsiness, tinnitus, loss of equilibrium, and short-term memory loss; at toxic levels, kidney and heart damage

Objective 9: Describe the main adverse effects of antipsychotic drugs.

- Sedation, dry mouth, sexual dysfunction, akathisia, bradykinesia, and rigidity; sometimes, tardive dyskinesia

Objective 10: Identify three of the most common types of drugs used to treat patients with depression.

- The most common types of drugs used to treat depression include the tricyclic antidepressants, monoamine oxidase inhibitors, and selective serotonin reuptake inhibitors.

 Internet Sites of Interest

- Find a concise description of sedative–hypnotic agents on the *Psychology Today* website: **www.psychologytoday.com**. Search for "sedatives."

- The National Institute of Neurological Disorders and Stroke contains a comprehensive site for information on epilepsy, including support organizations and fact sheets for patients and caregivers: **www.ninds.nih.gov/disorders/epilepsy**

- For an overview of anticonvulsant medications: **www.drugs.com/drug-class/anticonvulsants.html**

- In-depth information on a variety of topics related to schizophrenia, including symptoms and diagnosis, drug therapy, support groups, and frequently asked questions: **http://schizophrenia.com**

- Information about bipolar disorder and medications used to treat it: **www.pendulum.org**

- The National Institute of Mental Health discusses the latest treatments for schizophrenia, depression, and other psychiatric disorders: **www.nimh.nih.gov/health/topics/schizophrenia/index.shtml**

Chapter 24

Drugs Used to Treat Autonomic Nervous System Conditions

Chapter Objectives

After completing this chapter, you should be able to:

1. List the two divisions of the nervous system and their subdivisions.
2. Explain the basic functional unit cell of the nervous system.
3. Define the terms *cholinergic* and *adrenergic*.
4. Describe the fight-or-flight response.
5. List the two main adrenergic receptors and what they respond to.
6. Explain the actions of adrenergic agonists.
7. Explain the actions of receptor agonists.
8. Define *adrenergic antagonists*.
9. List the two types of cholinergic receptors.
10. Discuss parasympathomimetics (also called *cholinergic agonists*).

Key Terms

adrenergic (p. 420)
alpha-adrenergic receptors (p. 422)
anticholinergics (p. 434)
beta-adrenergic receptors (p. 422)
catecholamines (p. 422)

cholinergic (p. 419)
cholinergic blockers (p. 434)
fight-or-flight response (p. 422)
muscarinic receptors (p. 432)
nicotinic receptors (p. 432)

parasympathetic nervous system (p. 419)
parasympatholytics (p. 434)
sympathetic nervous system (p. 419)
sympathomimetics (p. 426)

Introduction

The two major systems controlling bodily functions are the nervous system and the endocrine system. These systems involve high-level integration in the brain and have the ability to influence processes in distant regions of the body as well as to extensively use negative feedback. Both use chemicals to transmit information. In the endocrine system, these chemicals (hormones) are released into the blood circulation and travel to interact with receptors in target tissue. In the nervous system, these chemicals (transmitters) are released from nerve terminals in the synaptic cleft (axons) and interact with receptors on neurons or effectors.

These two systems work closely with each other to control all the body's functions. They are the most complicated and difficult parts of the anatomy and physiology of the body. For this reason, neuropharmacology is a challenging subject for allied health care students.

Anatomy of the Autonomic Nervous System

The nervous system is divided into two main parts: the central nervous system (CNS), which comprises the brain and spinal cord, and the peripheral nervous system (PNS), that part of the nervous system that is outside the brain and spinal cord (Figure 24-1 ■). The autonomic nervous system (ANS) is a division of the PNS, which can itself be divided into two sections: motor and sensory neurons. In turn, motor neurons can be divided into two divisions that generally possess opposing functions: the **sympathetic nervous system** (which accelerates heart rate, constricts blood vessels, and raises blood pressure) and the **parasympathetic nervous system** (which slows the heart rate, increases intestinal and glandular activity, and relaxes muscles). This division is an anatomical division rather than a strict neurotransmitter division. Each division uses two efferent neurons to carry neural signals to effector tissues with the specific receptors.

The neuron is the basic functional unit cell of the nervous system. Therefore, these cells must communicate with each other and the other tissues of the body. The communication sites of neurons are called synapses, which are actually junctions that nerve impulses pass across. The nerve starting the original impulse is known as the *presynaptic nerve*. The nerve that originates after the synapse is called *postsynaptic nerve*.

The space between each synapse (called the *synaptic cleft*) is bridged by chemicals called *neurotransmitters*. The two primary neurotransmitters in the ANS are acetylcholine (ACh) and norepinephrine (NE), although many different types of neurotransmitters exist throughout the nervous system. Many drugs act as neurotransmitters. Drugs can also be used to block or enhance the activity of these neurotransmitters (Figure 24-2 ■).

Sympathetic Nervous System

A *ganglion* is an aggregation of nerve cell fibers. Sympathetic preganglionic fibers exit the CNS through the thoracic and lumbar spinal nerves. Sympathetic preganglionic fibers terminate in ganglia located in the two paravertebral chains that lie on either side of the spinal cord. Thus, sympathetic preganglionic fibers are short and can activate diffuse numbers of postganglionic neurons. ACh is the neurotransmitter released by the preganglionic sympathetic neuron. Postganglionic sympathetic neurons project long fibers to innervate the sympathetic target tissue. The major neurotransmitter released by the postganglionic neuron is NE. However, in sweat glands, the postganglionic neuron releases ACh. Dopamine serves as the postganglionic neurotransmitter in renal smooth muscle. The adrenal medulla also receives sympathetic preganglionic fibers that release ACh and bind to nicotinic receptors. This results in the release of epinephrine and NE into the blood circulation, where they act as hormones at adrenergic receptors throughout the body (Figure 24-3 ■).

Parasympathetic Nervous System

Parasympathetic preganglionic fibers exit the CNS through the cranial nerves and the sacral spinal roots and then travel to innervated tissues. Most preganglionic parasympathetic fibers terminate on ganglion cells. Innervation (neural or electrical arousal) of the target tissue is far less divergent than in the sympathetic nervous system. Just as in the sympathetic division, parasympathetic preganglionic neurons release ACh at the ganglia. The parasympathetic postganglionic neurons also release ACh, which binds to the target tissue.

Neurotransmitters of the Autonomic Nervous System

Neurons in the ANS can be classified into two groups based on the neurotransmitter they release. Neurons that release ACh are termed **cholinergic**. Cholinergic neurons include:

✳ Preganglionic neurons in the sympathetic and parasympathetic nervous systems

✳ Parasympathetic postganglionic neurons

✳ Somatic transmission at the neuromuscular junction

✳ Sympathetic postganglionic fibers that innervate sweat glands

Figure 24-1 ■ Divisions of the nervous system.

Accordingly, receptors to which ACh binds are also termed *cholinergic*. There are more specific designations for cholinergic receptor–based selectivity for agonist/ antagonist binding and anatomical location. Neurons that release NE, epinephrine, or dopamine are termed **adrenergic**. Similarly, receptors to which these adrenergic agonists bind are also termed *adrenergic*. Besides acting as direct agonists or antagonists at cholinergic and adrenergic receptors, drugs can affect the synthesis, storage, release, and termination of neurotransmitters in the ANS.

Figure 24-2 ■ In the autonomic pathway (**A**), nerve impulses (**B**); shown as arrows) travel along a presynaptic neuron to reach the junction between two neurons called the *synapses*. Chemicals called neurotransmitters (shown as triangles) must cross the synapses to carry the nerve impulse to the postsynaptic neuron. When the neurotransmitters cross the synapses, they reach a receptor (**C**). Many drugs act as neurotransmitters or they act by blocking the neurotransmitters from reaching a receptor or enhancing the activity of neurotransmitters so that more of them reach the receptor.

Figure 24-3 ■ Receptors in the autonomic nervous system.
(**A**) Sympathetic pathways (acetylcholine [ACh] and norepinephrine [NE]).
(**B**) Parasympathetic pathway (ACh).

❋ Apply Your **Knowledge 24.1** ▬▬▬▬▬

The following questions focus on what you have just learned about the anatomy of the ANS.

CRITICAL THINKING

1. Describe the two major systems in the human body that control and coordinate the other systems.
2. Identify the divisions of the nervous system.
3. Explain the two primary neurotransmitters in the autonomic nervous system.
4. Give the definitions of adrenergic and cholinergic neurons.
5. Describe the neurotransmitters that are released from the parasympathetic and sympathetic postganglionic neurons.

FUNCTIONS OF THE AUTONOMIC NERVOUS SYSTEM

The parasympathetic nervous system is required for life; it maintains such essential body functions as digestion and excretion. Its actions generally oppose those of the sympathetic system. At times of "rest-and-digest," the parasympathetic nervous system dominates the sympathetic nervous system. Rather than discharging as a complete system, the parasympathetic nervous system operates in discrete units based on the specific needs of the body. Discharging as a complete system would produce massive, undesirable symptoms (such as in organophosphate poisoning).

The sympathetic nervous system adjusts body functions in response to such stressors as trauma, fear, hypoglycemia, cold, or exercise. The **fight-or-flight response**, the reaction in the body when faced by a sudden threat or source of stress, has been used to describe activation of the sympathetic nervous system during emergencies (Figure 24-4 ■).

Remember that because of the sympathetic nervous system's anatomic wiring and release of epinephrine from the adrenal medulla, all the sympathetic effector organs and tissues are activated. Heart rate, cardiac output, and blood pressure are increased; blood flow is diverted from the skin and internal organs to skeletal muscle; energy stores are mobilized; and pupils and bronchioles dilate. Autonomic regulation of target organs and tissues is listed in Table 24-1 ■.

ADRENERGIC RECEPTORS

The effects of stimulation of the sympathetic nervous system are mediated by the release of NE from postganglionic nerve terminals and epinephrine from the adrenal medulla. NE and epinephrine are two types of endogenous **catecholamines** (chemical compounds containing nitrogen that are derived from the amino acid *tyrosine*) that bind to adrenergic receptors and produce sympathetic effects.

The two main adrenergic receptors are alpha and beta. Whereas alpha-adrenergic receptors are divided into α_1 and α_2, beta-adrenergic receptors are divided into β_1 and β_2. **Alpha-adrenergic receptors** (parts of cells that respond to adrenaline) are found in vascular smooth muscle and, when stimulated by NE or epinephrine, cause vasoconstriction.

Beta-adrenergic receptors (receptors that respond to NE or epinephrine) are found on smooth and cardiac muscle membranes. In the heart, the predominant beta-adrenergic receptors are β_1 receptors, which, when stimulated by NE and epinephrine, increase the heart rate and force of contraction. In smooth muscle, the predominant beta-adrenergic receptors are β_2 receptors. When stimulated by epinephrine, β_2 receptors produce vasodilation, particularly in the coronary arteries and skeletal muscle blood vessels. β_2 receptors can produce the relaxation of bronchiolar smooth muscle. NE does not affect β_2 receptors (Table 24-2 ■).

CHOLINERGIC RECEPTORS

The parasympathetic nervous system, also known as the *cholinergic nervous system*, releases the neurotransmitter ACh. Receptors that respond to cholinergic stimulation are called *cholinergic receptors*. These receptors are subdivided into *muscarinic* and *nicotinic* receptors (see Table 24-2). Drugs that bind to cholinergic receptors are referred to as *cholinergic drugs* and exhibit effects similar to those of ACh. Agents that bind to cholinergic receptors and prevent ACh from acting on its receptors (antagonism) are called *cholinergic-blocking drugs* (see Figure 24-3).

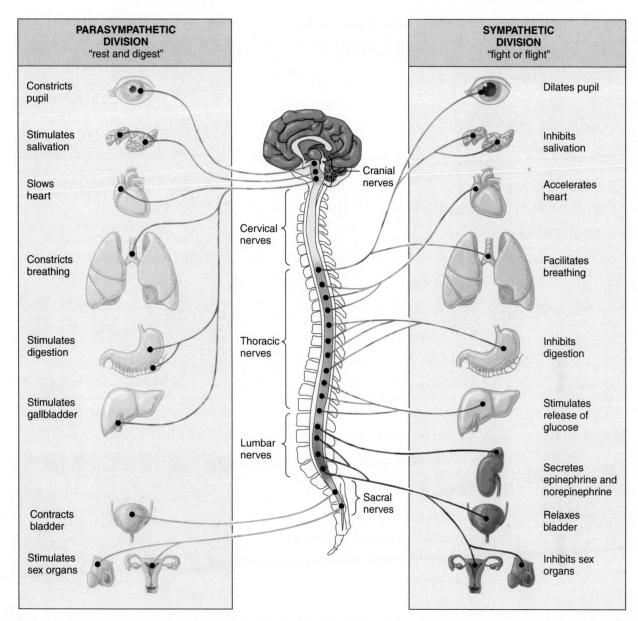

Figure 24-4 ■ "Rest-and-digest" effects of the parasympathetic nervous system; "fight-or-flight" effects of the sympathetic nervous system.

Table 24-1 ■ Autonomic Regulation of Target Organs and Tissues

ORGANS OR TISSUES	PARASYMPATHETIC	SYMPATHETIC
Eyes		
Pupillary response	Causes constriction (miosis)	Causes dilation (mydriasis)
Heart		
	Decreases heart rate	Increases heart rate
	No effect	Increases arrhythmias
Blood Vessels		
Skin	No effect	Causes vasoconstriction
Skeletal muscle vessels	No effect	Relax; cause vasodilation

(*continued*)

Table 24-1 ■ Autonomic Regulation of Target Organs and Tissues (*continued*)

ORGANS OR TISSUES	PARASYMPATHETIC	SYMPATHETIC
Bronchial Smooth Muscle		
	Causes bronchoconstriction	Causes bronchodilation
Gastrointestinal Tract		
Smooth muscle walls	Contract; increase motility and tone	Relax; decrease motility and tone
Smooth muscle sphincter	Relaxes	Contracts
Secretion	Increases	No effect
Genitourinary Smooth Muscle		
Bladder wall	Contracts; increases pressure	Relaxes; decreases pressure
Sphincter	Relaxes	Contracts
Uterus (pregnant)	No effect	Relaxes and contracts
Penis	Causes erection	Causes ejaculation
Skin		
Sweat glands	No effect	Increases

Table 24-2 ■ Sympathetic and Parasympathetic Receptors and Effects

PARASYMPATHETIC NERVOUS SYSTEM	
Receptors	**Effects**
Alpha$_1$ receptors	Closure of urinary bladder sphincter
	Contraction of arrector pili muscles
	Increased peripheral resistance / increased blood pressure
	Male sexual emission
	Pupil dilation
	Thickened salivary secretions
	Vasoconstriction
Alpha$_2$ receptors	Moderation of insulin release from pancreas
	Negative feedback control of norepinephrine release from presynaptic neurons
Beta$_1$ receptors	Increased conduction through atrioventricular node
	Increased heart rate
	Increased myocardial contraction
	Lipolysis in peripheral tissues
Beta$_2$ receptors	Bronchial dilation
	Decreased gastrointestinal muscle tone and activity, decreased secretions
	Increased breakdown of muscle and liver glycogen
	Relaxation of urinary bladder detrusor muscle
	Relaxation of uterine smooth muscle
	Release of glucagon from pancreas
	Vasodilation

PARASYMPATHETIC NERVOUS SYSTEM	
Receptors	**Effects**
Muscarinic receptors	Accommodation of lenses
	Decreased heart rate
	Increased gastrointestinal motility and secretions
	Increased urinary bladder contraction
	Male erection
	Pupil constriction
	Sweating
Nicotinic receptors	Autonomic ganglia stimulation
	Muscle contractions
	Release of norepinephrine from adrenal medulla

✳ Apply Your Knowledge 24.2

The following questions focus on what you have just learned about the functions of the ANS.

CRITICAL THINKING

1. What is the definition of the *fight-or-flight response*?
2. What are endogenous catecholamines?
3. What are the two main adrenergic receptors and their subdivisions?
4. What is the "rest-and-digest" response?
5. What is the effect of the sympathetic nervous system on the eyes, heart, and bronchial smooth muscle?
6. What is the effect of the parasympathetic nervous system on the bladder wall, penis, bronchial smooth muscle, and uterus (in pregnant women)?
7. What are cholinergic receptors?
8. What is another name of the parasympathetic nervous system?

Focus on Geriatrics

Effects of Stress in Older Adults

Older adults experience many losses and changes in their lives. These changes may be incremental and, over time, become stressful and possibly overwhelming. Stress can have physical, emotional, intellectual, social, and spiritual consequences. Usually, the effects are mixed because stress affects every person uniquely.

DRUG EFFECTS ON THE AUTONOMIC NERVOUS SYSTEM

Autonomic drugs are categorized based on which receptors can be stimulated or blocked.

1. **Sympathomimetics** (or adrenergic agonists) produce symptoms of the fight-or-flight response and stimulate the sympathetic nervous system.

2. *Parasympathomimetics* (or cholinergic agonists) produce symptoms of the rest-and-digest response and stimulate the parasympathetic nervous system.

3. *Adrenergic blockers* produce actions opposite to sympathomimetics and inhibit the sympathetic nervous system.

4. *Anticholinergics* (or cholinergic blockers) produce actions opposite to parasympathomimetics and inhibit the parasympathetic nervous system.

Focus on Natural Products

Essential Fatty Acids

Essential fatty acids, which cannot be manufactured by the body, are most commonly found in polyunsaturated vegetable oils. Both omega-3 and omega-6 fatty acids are converted in the body into *prostaglandins*, powerful hormone-like substances that affect almost every biologic function, including the regulation of smooth muscle and autonomic reflexes. Omega-6 fatty acids are present in food sources, and it is important to balance their intake with omega-3 fatty acids, which are found in fish and flaxseed oil. Adding 1 tablespoon of flaxseed oil to your daily diet is beneficial.

ADRENERGIC AGONISTS OR SYMPATHOMIMETIC DRUGS

The adrenergic agonists are categorized as catecholamines and noncatecholamines. The catecholamines include NE, which is released at the nerve terminals; epinephrine, from the adrenal medulla; and dopamine, from sites in the brain, kidneys, and gastrointestinal (GI) tract. These types of drugs can be made synthetically to produce the same effects as those of the naturally secreted neurotransmitters. The noncatecholamines have somewhat similar actions to the catecholamines but are more selective of receptor sites, are not quite as fast acting, and have a longer duration. The medications of the adrenergic agonist class mimic the sympathetic nervous system and are also called *sympathomimetics* or *adrenergic agonists*. Classifications of sympathomimetic drugs are listed in Table 24-3 ■.

As previously discussed, there are two principal types of adrenoreceptors: alpha (α) and beta (β). These receptors have been further subdivided into the main subtypes of α_1, α_2, β_1, and β_2. The activation of alpha and beta receptors through the administration of adrenergic agonists produces effects consistent with sympathetic (fight-or-flight) stimulation.

Table 24-3 ■ Classifications of Sympathomimetic Drugs

GENERIC NAME	TRADE NAME	PRIMARY USE
Catecholamines		
dopamine hydrochloride	Dopamine (α_1 and β_1)	Shock
epinephrine	Adrenalin, Primatene Mist (α and β)	Asthma, cardiac arrest
isoproterenol	Isuprel (β_1 and β_2)	Asthma, dysrhythmias, heart failure
norepinephrine bitartrate	Levophed (α and β)	Shock
Alpha₁ Agonists		
midodrine	ProAmatine	Orthostatic hypotension
oxymetazoline	Afrin	Nasal congestion
phenylephrine	Neo-Synephrine Nasal	Nasal congestion

GENERIC NAME	TRADE NAME	PRIMARY USE
Alpha$_2$ Agonists		
apraclonidine	Iopidine Eye	Operative eye pressure, glaucoma
clonidine	Catapres (in the CNS)	Hypertension
guanfacine	Tenex	Hypertension
methyldopa	(Generic only) (in the CNS)	Hypertension
Beta$_1$ Agonists		
dobutamine	Dobutamine	Cardiac stimulant
Beta$_2$ Agonists		
albuterol	Ventolin HFA, Ventolin Solution, Ventolin Syrup	Asthma
metaproterenol	Alupent	Asthma
salmeterol xinafoate	Serevent Diskus	Decongestant
terbutaline sulfate	Terbutaline Sulfate	Asthma
Miscellaneous Adrenergic Agonists		
amphetamine*	(Generic only)	Narcolepsy, ADD, obesity
ephedrine	Ephedrine Sulfate Injection	Allergies, asthma, narcolepsy
methylphenidate*	Ritalin	ADHD, obesity
pemoline	Cylert	ADHD
pseudoephedrine	Sudafed (α and β)	Rhinitis, coryza, sinusitis

* Discussed in Chapter 23 as central nervous system (CNS) stimulants. These agents are primarily used for their CNS effects and are not used for the same indications as pseudoephedrine and other similar agents. Ephedrine has strictly controlled uses within the United States.

ADD, attention-deficit disorder; ADHD, attention-deficit/hyperactivity disorder.

Focus On

Alpha$_1$-Receptor Agonists

Alpha$_1$ receptors are located on blood vessels and influence blood pressure and blood flow into the tissues (called *tissue perfusion*). Resistance to blood flow is determined by the diameter of the vessels. Alpha$_1$ receptors are also found on the muscles of the iris; on smooth muscle of the GI tract and male and female reproductive tracts; and in liver cells, sweat glands, and sphincters of the urinary bladder.

How do they work?

The stimulation of receptors causes vasoconstriction of blood vessels, dilation of the pupils (mydriasis), decreased GI motility, contraction of the external sphincter of the bladder, decreased bile secretion, and stimulation of sweat glands.

How are they used?

Alpha$_1$-receptor agonists are used to treat hypotension, nasal congestion, and subconjunctival hemorrhage (red eye).

What are the adverse effects?

The common adverse effects of α_1-receptor agonists are hypertension, blurred vision, constipation, urine retention, gooseflesh, and sweating.

What are the contraindications and interactions?

Alpha$_1$-receptor agonists are contraindicated for severe coronary or cardiovascular disease; glaucoma; hypovolemia (within 2 weeks of taking monoamine oxidase inhibitors [MAOIs]); acute kidney disease; urine retention;

(continued)

Focus On (continued)

pheochromocytoma (adrenal tumor); thyrotoxicosis (hyperthyroidism or Graves' disease); sensitivity to adrenergic substances; supine hypertension (i.e., when lying down); ventricular tachycardia; and for pregnant, lactating, and very young patients. Drug interactions occur with digoxin, doxazosin, ephedrine, guanethidine, halothane, methyldopa, oxytocin, phentolamine, phenothiazines, phenylpropanolamine, prazosin, pseudoephedrine, reserpine, alpha blockers, beta blockers, atropine, MAOIs, terazosin, tricyclic antidepressants (TCAs), vasopressin, and ergot alkaloids.

What are the important points patients should know?

Instruct patients taking receptor agonists to inform their health care provider if they have high blood pressure, thyroid disease, an enlarged prostate, glaucoma, or are breastfeeding. Also, instruct patients to inform their doctors of other prescriptions they are taking, such as antihypertensive medicines, thyroid medications, other decongestants, and TCAs. Caution them against taking more than the prescribed dosage or of combining these medications with over-the-counter (OTC) drugs without consulting their health care provider.

Alpha$_2$-Receptor Agonists

Alpha$_2$ receptors are believed to be located on the presynaptic neurons, and they seem to function as controllers of neurotransmitter release by the presynaptic neurons. They are often used in reducing blood pressure.

How do they work?

These agonists stimulate Alpha$_2$ adrenergic receptors in the CNS to inhibit sympathetic vasomotor centers. They reduce plasma concentrations of NE, decrease systolic blood pressure and heart rate, and inhibit renin release from the kidneys.

How are they used?

These agonists are used to treat hypertension—either alone or with diuretic or other hypertensive agents. They are also used epidurally as adjunct therapy for severe pain.

What are the adverse effects?

Adverse effects of these agonists include hypotension, peripheral edema, dry mouth or eyes, constipation, drowsiness, dizziness, rash, pruritus, impotence, nausea

and vomiting, hepatitis, hallucinations, depression, and recurrent herpes simplex.

What are the contraindications and interactions?

These agonists are contraindicated in pediatric, pregnant, and lactating patients; hypertension that is associated with toxemia of pregnancy; polyarteritis nodosa (swollen or damaged arteries); scleroderma (skin hardening); hepatitis; cirrhosis; pheochromocytoma; and blood dyscrasias. Interactions include alcohol and other CNS depressants, amphetamines, TCAs, ephedrine, haloperidol, levodopa, lithium, MAOIs, methotrimeprazine, opiate analgesics, phenothiazines, phenoxybenzamine, digoxin, calcium channel blockers, or beta blockers.

What are the important points patients should know?

Instruct patients with hypertension that excessive sodium leads to fluid retention and to avoid foods that are high in sodium, including canned, frozen, or dehydrated soup; processed cheese; salted biscuits; potato chips; and pretzels.

Beta$_1$-Receptor Agonists

Beta$_1$ receptors are located on the myocardium, adipocytes (fat cells), sphincters and smooth muscle of the GI tract, and renal arterioles.

How do they work?

Beta$_1$-receptor agonists increase the rate and force of contraction of the heart, increase lipolysis in adipose tissue, decrease digestion and GI motility, and increase glomerular filtration.

How are they used?

Beta$_1$-receptor agonists are used to treat circulatory shock, hypotension, and cardiac arrest. Two important drugs represent this group: dobutamine (Dobutamine), a selective β_1-receptor agonist, and isoproterenol (Isuprel), a nonselective β_1-receptor agonist.

What are the adverse effects?

The common adverse effects of receptor agonists include hypertension, tachycardia, and constipation.

What are the contraindications and interactions?

Beta$_1$-receptor agonists are contraindicated in patients with a history of hypersensitivity to other sympathomimetic amines (nitrogen compounds); in those with ventricular tachycardia; in pediatric, pregnant, or lactating patients; or after an acute myocardial infarction (MI). Interactions can occur with general anesthetics (especially cyclopropane and halothane), such beta-adrenergic blocking agents as metoprolol and propranolol, MAOIs, and TCAs.

What are the important points patients should know?

Alert patients that sputum and saliva may turn pink after the inhalation of isoproterenol. Warn patients not to breastfeed when taking these agents. Patients should not increase, decrease, or omit doses or change intervals between doses. Advise patients to immediately report anginal pain to their health care provider.

Beta$_2$-Receptor Agonists

These adrenoreceptors are distributed on the smooth muscle of the bronchioles; in skeletal muscle; in blood vessels supplying the brain, heart, kidneys, and skeletal muscle; in the uterus; and in liver cells.

How do they work?

Stimulation of β_2 receptors results in bronchodilation; increased skeletal muscle excitability; vasodilation of blood vessels to the brain, heart, kidneys, and skeletal muscle; and relaxation of the uterus in pregnancy.

How are they used?

Beta$_2$-receptor agonists are used in patients with chronic obstructive airway disease, circulatory shock, premature labor, and peripheral vascular disease.

What are the adverse effects?

The common adverse effects of β_2-receptor agonists include muscle tremor (in the hands), increased muscle tension, and feelings of warmth. These agents also cause hyperglycemia (increased blood glucose).

What are the contraindications and interactions?

β_2-receptor agonists are contraindicated in pediatric, pregnant, or lactating patients; in those who are sensitive to other sympathomimetic agents; and in patients with cardiac arrhythmias associated with tachycardia or digitalis intoxication, hyperthyroidism, preeclampsia (hypertension during pregnancy), eclampsia (coma and convulsions related to pregnancy), intrauterine infection, hypertension, diabetes mellitus, hypovolemia (decrease in volume of circulating blood), thyrotoxicosis, asthma that is treated with beta-mimetics, hypersensitivity, coronary artery disease (within 14 days of MAOI therapy), and angle-closure glaucoma. Interactions can occur with beta-adrenergic blockers, corticosteroids, epinephrine, other sympathomimetic bronchodilators, MAOIs, and TCAs.

What are the important points patients should know?

Instruct patients about using the inhaler correctly and have them demonstrate the technique for you. Warn patients not to change the dose or frequency of doses. Patients should know that these drugs may cause dizziness (albuterol) or tremor (metaproterenol), so advise them to change positions slowly. They should not take other OTC drugs or breastfeed without first consulting their health care provider. Advise patients to report if the drug fails to reduce symptoms.

Focus on Pediatrics

Stress and Childhood Asthma

Stress caused by such major events as the birth of a sibling, the death of a family member, or moving to a new home can quadruple a child's risks of an asthma attack within 2 days of the events. The asthma attack often reoccurs about 6 weeks later. The ANS of a child—together with hormones and brain chemicals—can trigger immediate and delayed stress-related effects. Other events that may relate to asthma attacks are departures of family members, illnesses, hospital visits, separations, and changes in family relationships.

ADRENERGIC ANTAGONISTS OR SYMPATHOLYTICS

Similar to sympathomimetic agents, sympatholytics can act either directly or indirectly. Direct-acting sympatholytics are antagonists that have an affinity for a receptor but block the normal response. Adrenergic antagonists can show specificity for one receptor or subtype. Indirect-acting agents block adrenergic nerve transmission—usually by inhibiting the release of neurotransmitters or depleting the stores of transmitters. Table 24-4 ■ lists common adrenergic antagonists.

Table 24-4 ■ Adrenergic Antagonists

GENERIC NAME	TRADE NAME	AVERAGE ADULT DOSAGE	ROUTE OF ADMINISTRATION	PRIMARY USE
Alpha-Receptor Antagonists				
doxazosin	Cardura	Start 1 mg at bedtime and titrate up to max of 16 mg/d in 1–2 divided doses	PO	Hypertension
phenoxybenzamine	Dibenzyline	5–10 mg bid; may increase by 10 mg/d at 4-d intervals to desired response	PO	Pheochromocytoma
phentolamine	Phentolamine Myslate	2–5 mg as needed	IV, IM	Hypertensive episode during surgery
prazosin	Minipress	Start 1 mg at bedtime and then 1 mg bid or tid; may increase to 20 mg/d in divided doses	PO	Hypertension
terazosin	Hytrin	Start 1 mg at bedtime and then 1–5 mg/d (maximum: 20 mg/d)	PO	Hypertension, urinary obstruction
Beta-Receptor Antagonists (Nonselective)				
labetalol	Trandate	100 mg bid (maximum: 2,400 mg/d)	PO	Hypertension
		20 mg slowly (maximum: 300 mg total dose)	IV	Hypertension
nadolol	Corgard	40 mg/d (maximum: 320 mg/d in 1–2 divided doses)	PO	Hypertension, angina
pindolol	Visken	5 mg bid (maximum: 60 mg/d in 2–3 divided doses)	PO	Hypertension
		15–40 mg/d in 3–4 divided doses	PO	Angina pectoris
propranolol	Inderal	10–40 mg bid (maximum: 480 mg/d)	PO	Hypertension, angina, acute MI, and dysrhythmias
timolol	Blocadren	10–45 mg in bid–tid/d (maximum: 60 mg/d in 2 divided doses)	PO	Hypertension, angina
Beta-Receptor Antagonists (Selective)				
acebutolol	Sectral	200–800 mg/d in 1–2 divided doses (maximum: 1,200 mg/d)	PO	Hypertension, dysrhythmias

GENERIC NAME	TRADE NAME	AVERAGE ADULT DOSAGE	ROUTE OF ADMINISTRATION	PRIMARY USE
atenolol	Tenormin	25–50 mg/d (maximum: 100 mg/d)	PO	Hypertension, angina pectoris
		5 mg q5min in 2 doses	IV	MI
esmolol	Brevibloc	25–50 mg/d (maximum: 100 mg/d)	IV	Supraventricular tachydysrhythmias
metoprolol	Lopressor	50–100 mg/d in 1–2 divided doses (maximum: 450 mg/d)	IV	Hypertension
		100 mg/d in 2 divided doses (maximum: 400 mg/d)	PO	Angina pectoris
		5 mg q2min for 3 doses and then PO therapy	PO	MI
		50 mg q6h for 48 h and then 100 mg bid	PO	MI

PO, oral; bid, bid twice a day; IV: intravenous; IM: intramuscular; tid: three times a day; MI: myocardial infarction.

Focus On

Alpha-Receptor Antagonists

Alpha-receptor antagonists can work in a reversible or an irreversible manner. Some are nonselective and antagonize α_1 and α_2 receptors. Others are highly selective for α_1 receptors. All antagonize the effects of endogenous catecholamines.

How do they work?

These antagonists selectively inhibit the actions of alpha adrenoreceptors, producing vasodilation in arterioles and veins, with the result that peripheral vascular resistance and blood pressure are reduced.

How are they used?

Applications for alpha-receptor antagonists include control of hypertension and treatment of patients with peripheral vascular disease, adrenal medulla tumor (pheochromocytoma), and urinary retention.

What are the adverse effects?

The common adverse effects of alpha-receptor antagonists include nasal congestion and stuffiness, postural hypotension (which occurs on sitting or standing), inhibition of ejaculation, and lack of energy.

What are the contraindications and interactions?

A contraindication for the use of alpha-receptor antagonists is known hypersensitivity to any of these drugs. Interactions can occur with diuretics, ephedrine, epinephrine, NE, other hypotensive agents, nonsteroidal anti-inflammatory drugs, and phenylephrine.

What are the important points patients should know?

Because these drugs may cause dizziness, advise patients to change positions slowly. Patients should avoid driving for at least 12 hours after taking the first dose to determine side effects. Patients should not breastfeed while taking these drugs or take OTC drugs for coughs, colds, or allergies without discussing it with their health care providers.

(continued)

Focus On (*continued*)

Beta-Receptor Antagonists

Beta$_2$ antagonists work against the effects of catecholamines at beta adrenoreceptors. Beta-blocking drugs reduce receptor occupancy by beta agonists. Most of these agents are pure antagonists and occupy beta receptors, causing no activation of the receptors.

How do they work?

Beta blockade by these antagonists results in vasodilation, decreased peripheral resistance, and orthostatic hypotension. These agents work primarily on cardiac muscle, competitively blocking β-adrenergic receptors within the heart.

How are they used?

These agents are used in the management of hypertension—sometimes with a thiazide diuretic—for patients who have failed to respond to diet, exercise, and weight reduction. They are also used to treat cardiac arrhythmias, MI, tachyarrhythmias, *hypertrophic subaortic stenosis* (thickening of the ventricular septum or wall), angina pectoris, pheochromocytoma, and hereditary essential tremor.

What are the adverse effects?

Common adverse effects of beta-receptor antagonists are dizziness, lethargy, insomnia, and diarrhea.

What are the contraindications and interactions?

Beta-blockers are contraindicated in patients with known hypersensitivity, heart block, severe heart failure, cardiogenic shock, and other severe circulatory disorders. These agents should be avoided in patients with a history of asthma or chronic obstructive airway disease unless no alternative is available. Interactions can occur with phenothiazines, beta-adrenergic agonists, atropine, TCAs, diuretics and other hypotensive agents, tubocurarine, cimetidine, and antacids.

What are the important points patients should know?

Teach patients to take their heart rate and blood pressure and to report a decrease in either. Because these drugs may cause dizziness, advise patients to change positions slowly. Patients should avoid driving for at least 12 hours after taking the first dose to determine side effects. Patients should not breastfeed while taking these drugs or take OTC drugs for coughs, colds, or allergies without discussing it with their health care provider. Warn patients not to discontinue these drugs suddenly. Advise patients to check with their health care provider before taking OTC medications.

Parasympathomimetics or Cholinergic Agonists

Cholinergic agonists (also called *parasympathomimetics* or *cholinomimetics*) stimulate the parasympathetic nervous system because they mimic the parasympathetic neurotransmitter ACh. This neurotransmitter is located at the ganglions and the parasympathetic terminal nerve endings. It stimulates the receptors in tissues, organs, and glands. There are two types of cholinergic receptors: (1) **muscarinic receptors** (which innervate smooth muscle and slow the heart rate) and (2) **nicotinic receptors** (which affect the skeletal muscles). Many cholinergic drugs are nonselective and can therefore affect the muscarinic and the nicotinic receptors. However, selective cholinergic drugs for the muscarinic receptors do not affect the nicotinic receptors.

How do they work?

The rapid destruction of systemically administered ACh by cholinesterases makes the *endogenous* (self-produced) neurotransmitter of limited clinical value. Clinically useful cholinomimetic drugs are either cholinergic agonists that are resistant to the hydrolytic (water-eliminating) action of cholinesterases or agents that inhibit cholinesterases. Based on their mechanisms of action, cholinomimetic drugs may be classified as direct-acting agents (agonists) or indirect-acting agents (anticholinesterases).

How are they used?

Pilocarpine (Isopto-Carpine) is a direct-acting cholinergic drug that is used most commonly in ophthalmology to reduce elevated intraocular pressure in patients with glaucoma and induce miosis. Specific muscarinic agonist drugs that are nonspecific may be used in the treatment of constipation that is caused by a lack of muscle tone (called *atonic*), congenital megacolon, and postoperative and postpartum *intestinal ileus* (obstructed bowel). Bethanechol (Bethanechol Chloride) has been used to increase the tone of the lower esophageal sphincter in the treatment of patients with reflux esophagitis. In the genitourinary tract, muscarinic agonists are useful in the treatment of those with postoperative and postpartum nonobstructive urine retention and neurogenic urinary bladder with retention. The primary use of the drug in the cardiovascular field is in the diagnosis of atrial tachycardia. In pulmonary practice, the hypersensitivity of patients with asthma to bronchiolar constriction induced by cholinomimetics makes methacholine useful in the diagnosis of asthma. Muscarinic agonists are also known to increase secretion of the salivary and lacrimal glands. They are used to treat symptoms of dry mouth caused by radiotherapy for cancer of the head and neck. The most common cholinomimetic drugs are summarized in Table 24-5 ■.

What are the adverse effects?

Adverse effects produced by the cholinomimetics can be predicted based on the pharmacodynamic activity of the drugs. Thus, undesirable effects may include flushing, sweating, abdominal cramps, difficulty in visual accommodation, headache, and convulsions at high doses. Specific

GI adverse effects include nausea and vomiting, diarrhea, and abdominal pain. Other adverse effects are bronchospasm, excessive salivation, and urinary frequency.

What are the contraindications and interactions?

Muscarinic drugs are contraindicated in the presence of atrioventricular arrhythmias, coronary insufficiency, hyperthyroidism, asthma, and peptic ulcer. Interactions can occur with ambenonium, neostigmine, and other cholinesterase inhibitors; mecamylamine; procainamide; quinidine; atropine; epinephrine; beta-adrenergic agonists; and parasympathomimetic drugs.

What are the important points patients should know?

Advise patients to inform their health care provider of any other drugs they are taking. Because these drugs may cause dizziness, caution patients to change positions slowly. Warn patients not to breastfeed without a health care provider's approval. Explain to patients that they may experience increased sweating and urinary frequency.

Table 24-5 ■ Cholinergic Agents

GENERIC NAME	TRADE NAME	AVERAGE ADULT DOSAGE	ROUTE OF ADMINISTRATION	PRIMARY USE
Direct-Acting Cholinergic Agonists				
bethanechol	Bethanechol Chloride	Individualized, but ranges from 10 to 50 mg tid or qid	PO	Acute postoperative and postpartum nonobstructive urinary retention, neurogenic atony of urinary bladder with retention
carbachol	Miostat	1–2 drops q4–8h; 0.5 mL injected	Intraocular solution	Glaucoma
cevimeline	Evoxac	30 mg tid	PO	Dry mouth from Sjögren's syndrome
pilocarpine	Isopto-Carpine	1 drop in eye or eyes up to qid	Ophthalmic solution	Glaucoma, prevention of postoperative elevated intraocular pressure, induction of miosis
Indirect-Acting Cholinergic Agonists				
ambenonium	Mytelase	5–75 mg qid	PO	Myasthenia gravis
edrophonium	(Generic only)	2 mg injected over 15–30 sec; if no reaction, inject 8 mg after 45 sec	IV	Diagnosis of myasthenia gravis

(continued)

Table 24-5 ■ Cholinergic Agents *(continued)*

GENERIC NAME	TRADE NAME	AVERAGE ADULT DOSAGE	ROUTE OF ADMINISTRATION	PRIMARY USE
neostigmine	Prostigmin	15–375 mg/d in 3–6 divided doses	PO	Myasthenia gravis, urine retention
pyridostigmine	Mestinon	60 mg–1.5 g/d 180–540 mg 1–2 times/d by sustained release	PO	Myasthenia gravis
tacrine	Cognex	10–40 mg/d (maximum: 160 mg/d)	PO	Alzheimer's disease

tid, three times a day; qid: four times a day; PO, oral.

CHOLINERGIC BLOCKERS

Drugs that inhibit the actions of ACh by occupying the ACh receptors are called *cholinergic antagonists* or **cholinergic blockers** (also called **anticholinergics** or **parasympatholytics**). The major body tissues and organs affected by the cholinergic-blocking agents include the heart, respiratory tract, urinary bladder, eyes, GI tract, and sweat glands.

Focus On

Atropine

Atropine (Atropine, AtroPen) is a classic anticholinergic or muscarinic antagonist drug. Atropine was first derived from the belladonna plant. Scopolamine was the second belladonna alkaloid produced. Atropine and scopolamine act on the muscarinic receptor, but they have little effect on the nicotinic receptor.

How does it work?

Atropine acts by selectively blocking all muscarinic responses to Ach—whether excitatory or inhibitory. Selective depression of the CNS relieves the rigidity and tremor of Parkinson's syndrome.

How is it used?

Atropine is used adjunctively to treat the symptoms of GI disorders; to treat ophthalmic disorders, various cardiac conditions, bronchial conditions, chronic obstructive airway disease, and upper respiratory infections; and to counteract mushroom poisoning. It is also used in preoperative situations.

What are the adverse effects?

The common adverse effects of atropine and atropine-like drugs include dry mouth, decreased perspiration, blurred vision, tachycardia, constipation, and urine retention. Other adverse effects are nausea, headache, dry skin, abdominal distension, hypotension or hypertension, impotence, photophobia, and coma.

What are the contraindications and interactions?

Atropine is contraindicated for patients with hypersensitivity to belladonna alkaloids; with angle-closure glaucoma, *parotitis* (inflammation of the saliva glands), obstructive uropathy, *intestinal atony* (muscular weakness), paralytic ileus, GI obstructions, severe ulcerative colitis, toxic megacolon, tachycardia, acute hemorrhage, and *myasthenia gravis* (muscle weakness brought on by movement); and in pregnant or lactating patients. Interactions include amantadine, antihistamines, TCAs, quinidine, disopyramide, procainamide, levodopa, methotrimeprazine, and phenothiazines.

What are the important points patients should know?

Encourage patients receiving atropine to use frequent mouth rinses, chew gum, or suck on sugarless sour hard candy to relieve dry mouth. Meticulous dental hygiene should be encouraged. Caution patients to avoid driving. Warn patients not to breastfeed while taking this drug. Tell patients to report a fast heartbeat or palpitations.

Focus Point

Ecstasy and the Autonomic Nervous System

MDMA (3,4-methylenedioxymethamphetamine) is an illegal drug known as Ecstasy. Other names for MDMA are "Adam," "XTC," "Doves," and just "E." Originally patented as an appetite suppressant, data now show that MDMA may be toxic to the brain. This drug is a serious problem in the United States because of its trendiness among teenagers, who may be unaware of its harmful effects. Studies have shown a 20–60% reduction in healthy serotonin cells in the brains of MDMA users, damaging their ability to remember and to learn. Tests on the brains of monkeys showed brain damage that remained visible 7 years after the monkeys were given MDMA.

✳ Apply Your Knowledge 24.3

The following questions focus on what you have just learned about drug effects on the ANS.

CRITICAL THINKING

1. Describe the mechanism of action of α_1-receptor agonists.
2. Explain the indications of β_1-receptor agonists.
3. Discuss the contraindications of β_2-receptor agonists.
4. Identify the mechanism of action of beta-receptor antagonists.
5. Give the trade names of propranolol, prazosin, atenolol, and metaproterenol.
6. Describe the mechanism of action of cholinergic blockers.
7. Identify the two types of cholinergic receptors and their effect on the body.
8. Give the trade names of pilocarpine, nadolol, and metoprolol.

PRACTICAL SCENARIO 1

The emergency medical services (EMS) team has brought a 54-year-old female patient to the emergency department where you are working. The EMS personnel state that the patient was found wandering in a nearby park by a jogger, who called 911 from her cell phone after the woman screamed obscenities at her and then fell, seriously scraping her arm and face. The woman is bleeding, disoriented, combative, and accusing the EMS team of stealing her purse. Her hands are shaking severely, and she is shouting at the doctors and nurses that she needs a bottle. The woman's clothing is dirty, and you can smell stale body odor and urine.

Laima Druskis/Pearson Education/PH College

Critical Thinking Questions

1. Based on your first impressions of this patient's actions and appearance, what do you suspect she is suffering from?
2. What short- and long-term health risks would you suspect this patient faces?
3. Why do you think the patient's hands are shaking, and what do you think causes her confusion and combativeness?
4. What assessments do you think are needed for this patient?

PRACTICAL SCENARIO 2

A 62-year-old woman with a history of glaucoma went to her family physician with symptoms of the common cold. Her physician prescribed medication for her nasal congestion. After 2 days of use, she noticed that her vision was blurred and she had a severe headache. She was taken to the emergency room of a local hospital.

Critical Thinking Questions

1. What is the relationship between nasal decongestants and the woman's history of glaucoma?

2. List the other contraindications of α_1-receptor agonists.

dundanim/Shutterstock

Chapter Capsule

This section repeats the objectives from the beginning of the chapter and then provides a summary of the most important concepts for that objective. Use this section as a quick review and to check your knowledge.

Objective 1: List the two divisions of the nervous system and their subdivisions.

- Central nervous system (CNS): brain and spinal cord
- Peripheral nervous system (PNS)
  - ❏ Autonomic nervous system (ANS)
    - Motor neurons
      - ◆ Sympathetic nervous system
      - ◆ Parasympathetic nervous system
    - Sensory neurons

Objective 2: Explain the basic functional unit cell of the nervous system.

- Neurons: carry nervous system signals throughout body

Objective 3: Define the terms *cholinergic* and *adrenergic*.

- Cholinergic: liberated or activated by the neurotransmitter acetylcholine
- Adrenergic: liberated or activated by norepinephrine, epinephrine, or dopamine

Objective 4: Describe the fight-or-flight response.

- The body's reaction to a sudden threat or source of stress, such as trauma, fear, hypoglycemia, cold, or exercise
- Activates the sympathetic nervous system during emergencies

Objective 5: List the two main adrenergic receptors and what they respond to.

- Alpha receptor: responds to adrenaline
- Beta receptor: responds to norepinephrine and epinephrine

Objective 6: Explain the actions of adrenergic agonists.

- Mimic the sympathetic nervous system
- Produce fight-or-flight symptoms

Objective 7: Explain the actions of receptor agonists.

- Alpha-receptor agonists: influence blood pressure and tissue perfusion
- Beta-receptor agonists: work against catecholamines, reducing receptor occupancy by beta agonists

Objective 8: Define *adrenergic antagonists*.

- Block adrenergic nerve transmission (usually by inhibiting the release of neurotransmitters or depleting the stores of transmitters)

Objective 9: List the two types of cholinergic receptors.

- Muscarinic receptors: innervate smooth muscle and slow the heart rate
- Nicotinic receptors: affect skeletal muscle

Objective 10: Discuss parasympathomimetics (also called *cholinergic agonists*).

- Parasympathomimetics stimulate the parasympathetic nervous system because they mimic the parasympathetic neurotransmitter acetylcholine, which is located at the ganglions and parasympathetic terminal nerve endings.
- There are two types of cholinergic receptors: muscarinic and nicotinic. Many parasympathomimetics are nonselective, but those that are selective affect only one of these types of receptors.
- They are characterized based on their mechanisms of action as either direct-acting agents (agonists) or indirect-acting agents (anticholinesterases).
- The most common direct-acting cholinergic agonists are bethanechol, carbachol, cevimeline, and pilocarpine.
- The most common indirect-acting cholinergic agonists are ambenonium, edrophonium, neostigmine, pyridostigmine, and tacrine.

Internet Sites of Interest

- For recent research and graphics that illustrate the concepts of neurotransmitters, the autonomic nervous system, and more: **http://faculty.washington.edu/ chudler/ehceduc.html**
- Autonomic nervous system disorders are discussed at: **www.nlm.nih.gov/ medlineplus/autonomicnervoussystemdisorders.html**
- An explanation of how the ANS controls heart rate can be found at: **http://circres. ahajournals.org/content/19/2/400.short**
- The body's control of blood pressure is explained at: **http://ehealthmd.com/ content/how-body-controls-blood-pressure#axzz3eZScrKQb**
- Understanding stress and its relation to the ANS: **www.dgward.com/physo101/ web_pages/section_8/lab_stress.htm**

Chapter 25

Anesthetic Agents

Chapter Objectives

After completing this chapter, you should be able to:

1. Outline the stages of anesthesia.
2. Define the importance of premedications before anesthesia.
3. Explain the action of anesthetics within the central nervous system.
4. List the effects of general anesthetics.
5. Describe the common local anesthetics and their uses.
6. Compare ester and amide local anesthetics
7. List the problems associated with the use of local anesthetics.
8. Explain the indications for spinal anesthesia.
9. Discuss various techniques for local anesthetics.
10. Compare epidural anesthesia with field block anesthesia.

Key Terms

analgesia (p. 439)
anesthesia (p. 439)
anesthetics (p. 439)
cryoanesthesia (p. 449)

epidural anesthesia (p. 450)
lipophilic (p. 443)
preanesthetics (p. 440)
regional anesthesia (p. 439)

spinal anesthesia (p. 450)
subarachnoid (p. 450)
volatile liquids (p. 442)

Introduction

It was not until the 1840s that surgical anesthesia became possible with the introduction of three agents in quick succession: chloroform, ether, and nitrous oxide. These three agents, when inhaled quickly, led to unconsciousness, and surgical anesthesia was produced. Today, patients having surgery receive medication before, during, and after surgery to achieve specific therapeutic outcomes. Usually, all other medication orders are withheld when a patient goes to surgery.

Anesthesia

General **anesthetics** are normally used to produce loss of consciousness before and during surgery. However, for certain minor procedures, an anesthetic may be given in small amounts to relieve anxiety or pain without causing unconsciousness. These are called *local anesthetics*. They numb small areas of tissue where a minor procedure is to be done and are commonly used in dentistry and for minor surgery. **Regional anesthesia** affects a larger, but still limited, part of the body and is often used in obstetrics, during labor and delivery. It does not make the person unconscious. Spinal and epidural anesthesia are examples of regional anesthesia.

The ideal anesthetic agent should possess the following characteristics:

✳ Rapid and pleasant induction and withdrawal from **anesthesia**—loss of sensation, consciousness, or both

✳ Skeletal muscle relaxation

✳ **Analgesia**—pain relief while still conscious

✳ High potency

✳ A wide therapeutic index

✳ Nonflammability

✳ Chemical inertness with regard to anesthetic delivery devices

However, in practice, it is common to use a variety of drugs because no single agent meets all these criteria.

Stages of Anesthesia

Before patients reach surgical anesthesia, they go through four stages: analgesia, excitement or delirium, surgical anesthesia, and medullary paralysis.

STAGE 1: **Analgesia.** Pain is the first sense to be abolished, and consciousness is still retained. This type of anesthesia is often used in childbirth and in trauma, as a mixture of nitrous oxide and oxygen. The patient inhales the gas until pain recedes but does not inhale enough to reach the unconscious state, thus maintaining some control over the situation. The sense of hearing is often enhanced in this stage.

STAGE 2: **Excitement.** This stage may not be a pleasant time of anesthesia. More or less unconscious, the patient may experience shaking and become violent. A sense of extreme fear may be felt, which can produce a phobic response to any suggestion of anesthetics in the future. It is important that the passage from stage 1 to stage 3 be attained as quickly as possible. Sudden death can occur during stage 2, possibly because of vagal nerve inhibition, since the vagus nerve extends from the cranium to the abdomen.

STAGE 3: **Surgical anesthesia.** This stage is characterized by progressive muscular relaxation. Muscle relaxation is important during many surgical procedures because reflex movements can occur when a scalpel slices through the tissues. This muscular relaxation ends in respiratory paralysis, and unless the patient is on a respirator, death may ensue fairly quickly. These reflexes are abolished with high delivery rates of gaseous anesthetics, but the dividing line between the desired state and respiratory paralysis is narrow. Early anesthetists used various reflexes of the body, such as corneal reflexes and pupillary size, to help them determine when to reduce the amount of anesthetic given to maintain surgical anesthesia but not so much as to return to stage 2. To prevent the danger of respiratory depression, the use of a respirator during surgical procedures is usually obligatory. An endotracheal tube is passed into the trachea, which is connected to the respirator. Unfortunately, the laryngeal reflex, also called the gag reflex, is one of the last reflexes to disappear before stage 4 is reached.

STAGE 4: **Medullary paralysis.** This stage begins with respiratory failure and can lead to circulatory collapse. Through careful monitoring, this stage is avoided. If it is reached, it is called an *anesthetic accident*. In the induction of anesthesia with intravenous (IV) anesthetic agents, stages 1–3 merge so quickly into one another that they are not apparent.

Focus on Geriatrics

Respiratory Apnea

During the recovery period, the patient must be observed for underventilation by monitoring for respiratory apnea. It is very important to watch elderly patients and those with pre-existing respiratory insufficiency.

Preoperative Medications as Adjuncts to Surgery

Surgical patients are usually given preoperative medications—called **preanesthetics**—45–70 minutes before the scheduled surgery. Any delay in administration should be reported promptly to the surgical department.

A combination of preoperative drugs may be ordered to achieve the desired outcomes with minimal side effects. Such outcomes include sedation, reduced anxiety, amnesia to minimize unpleasant surgical memories, increased comfort during preoperative procedures, reduced gastric acidity and volume, increased gastric emptying, decreased nausea and vomiting, and reduced incidence of aspiration by drying oral and respiratory secretions. Table 25-1 ■ lists commonly prescribed preoperative medications.

Table 25-1 ■ Preoperative Medications as Adjuncts to Surgery

GENERIC NAME	TRADE NAME	AVERAGE ADULT DOSAGE	ROUTE OF ADMINISTRATION
Benzodiazepines			
diazepam	Valium	2–10 mg bid–qid or 15–30 mg/d sustained release	PO
		2–10 mg; repeat if needed in 3–4 h	IM, IV
lorazepam	Ativan	2–4 mg at least 2 h before surgery	IM
		0.044–2 mg/kg 15–20 min before surgery	IV
midazolam	Midazolam Injection	Premedicated: 0.15–0.25 mg/kg over 20–30 sec; allow 2 min for effect	IV
		Nonpremedicated: 0.3–0.35 mg/kg over 20–30 sec; allow 2 min for effect	IV
Opioid Analgesics			
meperidine	Demerol	50–150 mg 30–90 min before surgery	IM, SC
morphine	DepoDur	10–15 mg as single dose 30 min before surgery (maximum: 20 mg)	Epidural
Antacids			
sodium citrate/ citric acid	Bicitra	15–30 mL	PO
H₂-Receptor Antagonists			
cimetidine	Tagamet	300 mg	IM, IV, or PO
famotidine	Pepcid	20 mg	IV
ranitidine	Zantac	50 mg	IM, IV, or PO

GENERIC NAME	TRADE NAME	AVERAGE ADULT DOSAGE	ROUTE OF ADMINISTRATION
Gastric Acid Pump Inhibitors (see Chapter 34 for a complete list)			
lansoprazole	Prevacid	15–60 mg	PO
omeprazole	Prilosec	20–40 mg	PO
Antiemetics			
droperidol	Inapsine	2.5–10 mg 30–60 min before surgery	IM, IV
metoclopramide	Reglan	10 mg administered over 1–2 min	IM, IV
Anticholinergics			
atropine	Atropine	0.4–0.6 mg	IM, IV, SC
glycopyrrolate	Robinul	0.1–0.3 mg	IM, IV

bid, twice a day; qid, four times a day; PO, oral; IM, intramuscular; IV, intravenous; SC, subcutaneous.

✳ Apply Your Knowledge 25.1

The following questions focus on what you have just learned about the types of anesthesia and the use of preoperative medications as adjuncts to surgery.

CRITICAL THINKING

1. Explain the differences between general anesthetics and regional anesthesia.
2. Identify the characteristics of anesthetic agents.
3. Describe many stages of anesthesia exist, and which stage is dangerous.
4. Discuss why preanesthetics are used before surgery.
5. Explain why a combination of preoperative drugs may be ordered.

General Anesthetics

General anesthesia affects the entire body and makes the patient unconscious by depressing the central nervous system (CNS). The unconscious patient is completely unaware of what is going on and does not feel pain from the surgery or procedure. Skeletal muscles relax and reflexes also diminish.

The advantages of general anesthesia include rapid excretion of the anesthetic agent and prompt reversal of its effects when desired. In addition, general anesthesia can be used with all age groups and in any type of surgical procedure.

An ideal anesthetic drug would induce anesthesia smoothly and rapidly while allowing for prompt recovery after its administration is discontinued. The drug would also possess a wide margin of safety and be devoid of adverse effects. No single anesthetic agent is capable of achieving all these desirable effects without some disadvantages when used alone. For this reason, modern anesthesiology practice commonly uses combinations of IV and inhaled drugs, taking advantage of each drug's individual favorable properties while attempting to minimize any potential for adverse reactions.

Focus Point

Choosing Appropriate Anesthesia

The choice of anesthetic drug depends on many factors, including the patient's general physical condition; the area, organ, or body system being operated on; and the anticipated length of the surgical procedure.

(continued)

Focus Point (*continued*)

The anesthetic technique varies depending on the proposed type of diagnostic, therapeutic, or surgical intervention. For minor procedures, conscious sedation is achieved by using oral or parenteral sedatives in conjunction with local anesthetics. These techniques provide profound analgesia but retain the patient's ability to maintain his or her own airway and to respond to verbal commands. For more extensive surgical procedures, anesthesia frequently includes the use of preoperative benzodiazepines, the induction of anesthesia with IV thiopental or propofol, and the maintenance of anesthesia with a combination of inhaled and IV anesthetic drugs.

Focus on Geriatrics

Adverse Drug Reactions

Older adults are more likely to experience adverse drug reactions than younger adults because, in general, they take more prescription medications. These adverse reactions may be drug–drug interactions; drug–disease interactions, in which a drug may adversely affect a patient with a certain condition; or drug–food interactions.

TYPES OF GENERAL ANESTHETICS

General anesthetics are usually given by inhalation or by IV injection.

Drugs given to induce or maintain general anesthesia are given either as gases or vapors (inhalation anesthetics) or injections (IV anesthetics). Most commonly, these two forms are combined, although it is possible to deliver anesthesia solely by inhalation or injection.

Inhalation anesthetic agents are either **volatile liquids**, which are easily vaporized, or gases. They are usually delivered by using an anesthesia machine. These machines allow mixtures of anesthetic agents with oxygen. Anesthetics and ambient air are delivered to the patient, who is monitored along with the machine's parameters. Liquid anesthetics are vaporized in the machine.

Many compounds have been used for inhalation anesthesia, but only a few are still in widespread use. Today, desflurane (Suprane) and sevoflurane (Ultane) are the most widely used volatile anesthetics. They are often combined with nitrous oxide. Older, less popular volatile anesthetics include isoflurane (Forane), halothane (Fluothane), and enflurane (Ethrane). The major inhalation anesthetics are listed in Table 25-2 ■.

Intravenous anesthetics are discussed in the following Focus On box.

Table 25-2 ■ General Anesthetics Used by Inhalation

GENERIC NAME	TRADE NAME	PHYSICAL STATE AT ROOM TEMPERATURE
desflurane	Suprane	Volatile liquid
enflurane	Ethrane	Volatile liquid
halothane	Fluothane	Volatile liquid
isoflurane	Forane	Volatile liquid
nitrous oxide (laughing gas)	(Generic only)	Gas
sevoflurane	Ultane	Volatile liquid

Focus Point

The Dangers of Malignant Hyperthermia

Malignant hyperthermia is a life-threatening, acute pharmacogenetic disorder that develops during or after anesthesia. This is a disorder that presents itself in some patients undergoing anesthesia and, in some cases, in the postoperative care unit. Hyperthermia is characterized by a rapid increase in body temperature, unexplained tachycardia, unstable blood pressure, muscle rigidity, and cyanosis. The body temperature may increase to above 115°F (46°C).

Focus On

Intravenous Anesthetics

Injectable anesthetics are used for the induction and maintenance of a state of unconsciousness. Anesthetists prefer to use IV injections because they are faster, less painful, and more reliable than intramuscular or subcutaneous injections. Among the most widely used drugs (Table 25-3 ■) are propofol (Diprivan); etomidate (Amidate); such barbiturates as methohexital (Brevital Sodium) and thiopental (Pentothal); such benzodiazepines as midazolam (Midazolam Injection) and diazepam (Valium); and ketamine (Ketalar).

How do they work?

The mechanism of action of most of the IV agents is principally confined to the CNS. A common property of all general anesthetics is that they are all very **lipophilic** (able to dissolve much more easily in lipids than in water). This property is essential because the drug must cross the blood–brain barrier to be effective. Cell membranes are, by nature, lipophilic and hydrophilic depending on the site in the membrane. When the lipophilic anesthetic enters the lipid membrane, the whole membrane is slightly distorted and closes the sodium channels, causing a marginal blockage, which prevents neural conduction (Figure 25-1 ■).

How are they used?

Volatile anesthetics are rarely used as the sole agents for the induction and maintenance of anesthesia. Most commonly, IV and volatile anesthetics are combined in regimens of so-called balanced anesthesia. Of the inhaled anesthetics, nitrous oxide, desflurane, sevoflurane, and isoflurane are the most commonly used in the United States. Use of the more soluble volatile anesthetics has declined during the past decade because more surgical procedures are being performed on an outpatient or short-stay basis. Desflurane and sevoflurane allow a more rapid recovery and produce fewer postoperative adverse effects than halothane or isoflurane. Although halothane is still used in pediatric anesthesia, sevoflurane is rapidly replacing halothane in this setting.

In the past two decades, there has been an increased use of IV drugs in anesthesia—as adjuncts to inhaled anesthetics and in techniques that do not include inhaled anesthetics. IV drugs such as thiopental, etomidate, ketamine, and propofol have faster onsets of anesthetic action than the fastest of the inhaled gaseous agents such as desflurane and sevoflurane. Therefore, IV agents are commonly used for induction of anesthesia.

What are the adverse effects?

Because intravenous and inhaled anesthetics affect the CNS, patients may feel drowsy, weak, or tired for as long as a few days after having general anesthesia. Fuzzy thinking, blurred vision, and coordination problems are also possible. For these reasons, anyone who has had general anesthesia should not drive, operate machinery, or perform other activities that could endanger themselves or others for at least 24 hours or longer if necessary.

(continued)

Focus On (continued)

· ·

After general anesthesia, patients may also complain of headache, shivering, muscle pain, mental or mood changes, nausea and vomiting, sore throat, and nightmares.

What are the contraindications and interactions?

IV anesthetics are contraindicated in patients who have received monoamine oxidase inhibitors (MAOIs) within 14 days. Those who are intolerant to benzodiazepines or have hypersensitivity, myasthenia gravis, acute narrow-angle glaucoma, increased intracranial pressure, impaired cerebral circulation, acute alcohol intoxication, intra-arterial injection, a history of paradoxic excitation, status asthmaticus, and acute intermittent or other hepatic porphyrias should not receive general anesthetics. They are contraindicated in shock and coma and during obstetric procedures, labor and delivery, and lactation. They must be used carefully during pregnancy and in children younger than age 12 years. Interactions occur with alcohol and other CNS depressants, MAOIs, anticonvulsants, cimetidine, levodopa, phenytoin, and phenothiazines and in patients who smoke. The general anesthetic propofol interacts with alfentanil; midazolam and thiopental interact with the herbal supplements kava-kava and valerian.

What are the important points patients should know?

Because these drugs can interact with medications administered in the perioperative period, ask the patient about the use of over-the-counter medications, including herbal supplements. Instruct the patient in deep breathing and coughing, which reopens the lung alveoli and helps to clear secretions from the lower respiratory tract. Encourage the patient to perform these maneuvers as soon as possible after emergence from deep sedation or general anesthesia.

Table 25-3 ■ General Anesthetics Commonly Given by Injection

GENERIC NAME	TRADE NAME	AVERAGE ADULT DOSAGE	ROUTE OF ADMINISTRATION
etomidate	Amidate	0.3 mg/kg over 30–60 sec	IV
fentanyl	Sublimaze	Up to 150 mcg/kg prn	IV
ketamine	Ketalar	100 mg	IM
methohexital	Brevital Sodium	5–12 mL of 1% solution at a rate of 1 mL q5min and then 2–4 mL q4–7min prn	IV
midazolam	Midazolam Injection	Premedicated: 0.15–0.25 mg/kg over 20–30 sec; allow 2 min for effect	IM, IV
		Nonpremedicated: 0.3–0.35 mg/kg over 20–30 sec; allow 2 min for effect	IV
propofol	Diprivan	2–2.5 mg/kg q10sec until induction onset	IV
thiopental	Pentothal	Test dose: 25–75 mg and then 50–75 mg at 20–40 sec intervals; additional 50 mg may be given if needed	IV

IV, intravenous; IM, intramuscular.

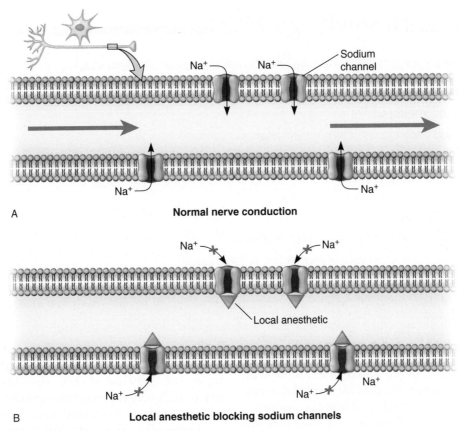

A   **Normal nerve conduction**

B   **Local anesthetic blocking sodium channels**

Figure 25-1 ■ Mechanism of action of anesthetics: normal nerve conduction (**A**) and anesthetic blocking sodium channels (**B**).

Focus on Natural Products

Stopping Herbal Medications Before Surgery

The recent increased use of natural products has been an issue raised by the American Society of Anesthesiologists concerning anesthesia. It is recommended that patients stop taking herbal medications at least 2 to 3 weeks before surgery to decrease the risk of adverse effects resulting from an enhancement or prolongation of anesthetic effects.

Focus Point

Diabetes and Surgery

The stress of surgery in patients with diabetes may increase their blood glucose levels, rather than decrease them. Insulin injections and hypoglycemic medications should be coordinated with the patient, surgeon, and anesthesiologist.

✳ Apply Your Knowledge 25.2

The following questions focus on what you have just learned about general anesthetics.

CRITICAL THINKING

1. Explain balanced anesthesia.
2. Give generic and trade names of inhaled anesthetics.
3. Point out the trade names of propofol, ketamine, and fentanyl.
4. Describe how long a patient should stop taking herbal medications before surgery to decrease the risk of adverse effects.
5. Explain volatile liquids.
6. Discuss the factors that affect the anesthetic technique.
7. Identify the most widely used volatile anesthetics in current use.
8. Describe the advantages of intravenously injected anesthetics.

TYPES OF LOCAL ANESTHETICS

Local anesthesia is used to provide regional or topical anesthesia to relieve pain and to provide localized nerve block for surgical procedures without loss of consciousness. Generally, local anesthesia is safer than general anesthesia and allows for more rapid recovery. Local anesthetics are divided into two groups: esters and amides.

Ester-type local anesthetics have been in use longer than amides. Esters, except for tetracaine, tend to have a rapid onset and short duration of activity. Esters are associated with a higher incidence of allergic reactions because of one of their metabolites: para-amino benzoic acid, or PABA, which is structurally similar to methylparaben. Ester-type agents include benzocaine, cocaine, procaine, propoxycaine, chloroprocaine, and tetracaine. Because of these possible hypersensitivity reactions, many manufacturers have reformulated some of their products to eliminate methylparaben.

Generally, they are used topically. Procaine 2% is still marketed for use with epinephrine but is rarely used. Tetracaine is most efficacious as a topical anesthetic but is also 10 times more toxic than procaine. However, amides are often recommended over esters. They are safer and can also be used for topical applications.

Amide-type agents are discussed in the Focus On box below.

Focus On

Amide-Type Agents

The most commonly recognized drug in the class of amides is lidocaine, which was synthesized in 1943. The amides have several advantages over the esters. Amide local anesthetics do not undergo metabolism to PABA as esters do; therefore, hypersensitivity to amide local anesthetics is rare. Also, they can undergo repeated high-temperature sterilization without losing potency. Most of the local anesthetics in common use today belong to the amide class. Along with lidocaine, these include bupivacaine, mepivacaine, etidocaine, prilocaine, and the most recent, ropivacaine.

Lidocaine is supplied in many formulations, including an ointment, a water-soluble jelly, and a 4% solution for topical use; a 5% solution with dextrose for spinal administration; and 0.5%, 1%, 1.5%, and 2% solutions for injection. It is also widely available in a 1% multidose vial and prepared with epinephrine. The most common local anesthetics are summarized in Table 25-4 ■.

How do they work?

Local anesthetics appear to work by inhibiting the movement of sodium through channels in the membrane of a neuron, which in turn inhibits the transmission of nerve impulses. The action of the local anesthetics is dose dependent. The more of the drug that is present, the more the inhibition—until a complete block is produced.

Local anesthetics can also affect sodium channels in other parts of the body, such as the conduction system of the heart. This can lead to an abnormal heartbeat; thus, systemic distribution of local anesthetics is best kept to a minimum.

How are they used?

Local anesthesia is useful in a wide variety of clinical situations. It increases patient comfort and facilitates patient cooperation during procedures. As a diagnostic aid, it helps localize or identify the source of pain. Local anesthesia is warranted for any clinical procedure with a potential for pain, such as incision and drainage of abscesses, laceration repair, biopsy, wart treatment, vasectomy, neonatal circumcision, and dental procedures. Local anesthesia is also used during labor and delivery and for diagnostic procedures, such as gastrointestinal endoscopy. Occasionally, local anesthetics are used to relieve pain associated with pathologic conditions.

What are the adverse effects?

True allergic reactions to local anesthetics are rare and usually involve the ester agents. Allergic reactions are seldom caused by amide anesthetics. There is no cross-reactivity between amide and ester agents.

It is important to keep track of the total anesthetic dose given because toxic effects are dose related. Adverse effects are related to the CNS and, to a lesser degree, the cardiovascular system. Symptoms of toxicity include lightheadedness, dizziness, *nystagmus* (rhythmic oscillation of the eyeballs), restlessness, disorientation, and psychosis. Slurred speech and tremors often precede seizures. Hypotension, bradycardia, and cardiac arrest may occur.

What are the contraindications and interactions?

Local anesthetics are contraindicated in older adults and debilitated patients and should be used cautiously in children younger than 14 years of age. They should not be used during pregnancy, labor, or lactation. They are contraindicated in patients who are hypersensitive to these agents and who have sepsis, acidosis, heart or spinal block, severe hemorrhage, hypotension and shock, hypertension, cerebrospinal deformities or diseases, blood dyscrasias, supraventricular dysrhythmias, untreated sinus bradycardia, or bowel pathology. They should not be used concurrently with long-term ophthalmic preparations, bupivacaine or chloroprocaine, obstetric paracervical anesthesia, spinal anesthesia, or topical or IV regional anesthesia. Avoid use on infected application or injection sites, on a perforated eardrum or ear discharge, and on large areas. They are contraindicated in patients with a history of malignant hyperthermia and during severe trauma. These drugs interact with the sulfonamides, epinephrine, MAOIs, antihypertensive agents, isoproterenol, ergonovine, tricyclic antidepressants, phenothiazines, other local anesthetics, barbiturates, cimetidine, beta-blockers, quinidine, phenytoin, and procainamide.

What are the important points patients should know?

Instruct patients who have received local anesthetics to report such symptoms as lightheadedness, dizziness, disorientation, or slurred speech and to avoid driving and operating heavy machinery.

Table 25-4 ■ Local Anesthetics

GENERIC NAME	TRADE NAME	AVERAGE ADULT DOSAGE	ROUTE OF ADMINISTRATION
Esters			
benzocaine	Americaine	Lowest effective dose	Topical
cocaine hydrochloride (solution)	Cocaine	1–10% solution (use greater than 4% solution with caution) (maximum: single dose of 1 mg/kg)	Topical
procaine	Novocain	0.25–0.5% solution	SC
tetracaine	Pontocaine	1–2 drops of 0.5% solution diluted with equal volume of 10% dextrose	Topical

(continued)

Table 25-4 ■ Local Anesthetics (*continued*)

GENERIC NAME	TRADE NAME	AVERAGE ADULT DOSAGE	ROUTE OF ADMINISTRATION
Amides			
bupivacaine	Marcaine, Sensorcaine	0.25–0.75% solution	IM local infiltration, sympathetic block, lumbar epidural, caudal block, peripheral nerve block, retrobulbar block
etidocaine	Duranest	0.5–1.5% solution (maximum: 300 mg; 400 mg if given with epinephrine)	Percutaneous infiltration, peripheral nerve block (caudal), central neural block
lidocaine	Xylocaine	0.5–5% solution; solution with glucose (spinal); solution with dextrose (saddle block); jelly, ointment, cream, or solution (topical)	Infiltration, nerve block, epidural, caudal, spinal, saddle block, topical
mepivacaine	Carbocaine	1–2% solution	Infiltration, nerve block, caudal and lumbar epidurals
ropivacaine	Naropin	5–250 mg (0.5–1% solution)	Epidural, nerve block

SC, subcutaneous; IM, intramuscular.

✳ Apply Your **Knowledge** 25.3 ▬▬▬▬

The following questions focus on what you have just learned about local anesthesia.

CRITICAL THINKING

1. Identify the main groups of local anesthetics.
2. Describe the most common uses of local anesthetics today.
3. Explain why it is important to keep track of the total amount of anesthetics being administered.
4. Identify the type of local anesthetic that has been used for the longest time.
5. Give the trade names of procaine, tetracaine, bupivacaine, lidocaine, and ropivacaine.

SPECIFIC APPLICATIONS

Several local anesthetics can be used with different techniques or specific applications. They include topical anesthesia, local infiltration anesthesia, field block and nerve block anesthesia, spinal anesthesia, and epidural anesthesia. Techniques for applying local anesthesia are illustrated in Figure 25-2 ■.

Topical Anesthesia

Topical anesthesia involves the placement of a nerve conduction–blocking agent onto a tissue layer (skin or mucous membrane). This method is used to provide anesthesia on mucous membranes of the urethra, vagina, rectum, and skin. The tissue affected is limited to the area in contact with the topical anesthetic. Topical

Figure 25-2 ■ Techniques for applying local anesthesia: topical (**A**), nerve block (**B**), infiltration (**C**), spinal (**D**), and epidural (**E**).

anesthesia is usually administered by the physician and is achieved with either the use of **cryoanesthesia** or a pharmacologic agent.

Cryoanesthesia involves the reduction of nerve conduction by localized cooling. This may be accomplished with ice or by the use of a cryoanesthesia machine to produce the cooling action. Reduced skin temperature may also be a result of a pharmaceutical agent sprayed onto the skin, such as ethyl chloride. Lidocaine and cocaine are examples of topical anesthetic agents. Although the amount of agent applied is limited, the patient must be monitored for toxic reactions.

Local Infiltration Anesthesia

Local infiltration anesthesia, which works by blocking nerves, is produced by the injection of a local anesthetic solution directly into an area that is painful or about to be operated on. Local infiltration is probably the most common route used to administer local anesthetics and is the simplest form of regional anesthesia. Local infiltration is used primarily for minor surgical procedures, such as the removal of superficial skin lesions; suturing of a wound; or slightly more invasive surgeries, such as the insertion of chest tubes. In this technique, a local anesthetic agent is injected into superficial tissues to produce a small area of

Focus Point

Contact with Topical Anesthetics

Patients should be advised that when using topical anesthetics for skin conditions, they must not touch their eyes. Also, topical medications should never be applied to areas where there is an open lesion or cut.

analgesia and anesthesia. When a local anesthetic is to be administered by infiltration, epinephrine may be added to it to decrease its dosage and prolong its duration of action. However, epinephrine should not be used to anesthetize fingers, toes, and other tissues with end arteries. Lidocaine is a popular choice for infiltration anesthesia, but bupivacaine is used for longer procedures.

Field Block and Nerve Block Anesthesia

Field block anesthesia affects a single nerve, a deep plexus, or a network of nerves. Field block and nerve block anesthesia are forms of regional anesthesia. For example, a radial nerve block may be used to anesthetize the structures innervated by the radial nerve, including portions of the forearm and hand. Intraorbital block is often used for ocular surgery. A local anesthetic is administered in a series of injections to form a wall of anesthesia encircling the operative field.

Spinal Anesthesia

During **spinal anesthesia**, an anesthetic agent is injected into the **subarachnoid** space, which is located beneath the arachnoid membrane, or between the arachnoid and pia mater. The subarachnoid space is filled with cerebrospinal fluid (CSF) through a spinal needle. Spinal anesthesia can be used for many procedures but is most often used for gynecologic, obstetric, orthopedic, and genitourinary surgery. Spinal anesthesia may cause marked vasodilation (hypotension), headaches, and respiratory depression. Lidocaine, tetracaine, and bupivacaine are often used for spinal anesthesia.

Epidural Anesthesia

Epidural anesthesia involves the injection of a local anesthetic into the epidural space, lumbar or caudal, via a catheter that allows repeated infusions. After injection, the anesthetic agent is very slowly absorbed into the CSF. This is popular for labor and delivery. High concentrations of local anesthetic can get into the blood circulation and may increase the risk of systemic toxicity. Therefore, they can cause cardiac depression and neurotoxicity in the mother and neonate. Highly lipid-soluble locals, such as lidocaine, tend to get into the blood more than the less lipid-soluble agents, such as bupivacaine.

Focus Point

Alleviating Headache After Spinal Block

Patients should be advised to lay flat for approximately 12 hours after a spinal block or epidural to prevent the leakage of CSF, which may increase the risk of a postanesthetic headache.

✳ Apply Your Knowledge 25.4

The following questions focus on what you have just learned about specific applications of anesthesia.

CRITICAL THINKING

1. Explain cryoanesthesia.
2. Describe field block anesthesia.
3. Discuss spinal anesthesia.
4. Explain local infiltration anesthesia.
5. Describe epidural anesthesia.

PRACTICAL SCENARIO 1

A nurse reports she was reprimanded for being late in giving a preanesthetic medication. She administered the drug 10 minutes before the patient was taken to surgery. The patient was placed under general anesthesia for the surgical procedure. Several hours after the surgery, the patient experienced complications and reported that no one told him ahead of time what to expect in the recovery room.

Michal Heron/Pearson Education/PH College

Critical Thinking Questions

1. Why is it important to administer the preanesthetic medication at the proper time before surgery?
2. When the nurse realized she was delayed in giving the preanesthetic, what should she have done?
3. In what way did the nurse neglect her responsibilities toward the patient?

PRACTICAL SCENARIO 2

A 31-year-old pregnant woman went into labor at the local hospital. After 12 hours, her physician ordered epidural anesthesia. A high concentration of this anesthetic caused cardiac depression in the mother and neonate.

michaeljung/Shutterstock

Critical Thinking Questions

1. Besides cardiac depression, what other toxicity may manifest?
2. Explain the procedure used for epidural anesthesia.

Chapter Capsule

This section repeats the objectives from the beginning of the chapter and then provides a summary of the most important concepts for that objective. Use this section as a quick review and to check your knowledge.

Objective 1: Outline the stages of anesthesia.

- **Stage 1**—Analgesia: pain is abolished; consciousness is retained; sense of hearing is often enhanced
- **Stage 2**—Excitement: may be unpleasant; patient may experience shaking and become violent or feel extreme fear; passage from stage 1 to stage 3 must be attained as quickly as possible because sudden death can occur during stage 2, possibly caused by vagal nerve inhibition
- **Stage 3**—Surgical anesthesia: characterized by progressive muscular relaxation, which must be controlled to avoid respiratory paralysis; various body reflexes, corneal reflexes, and pupillary size are helpful indicators; patients are usually put on a respirator during this stage
- **Stage 4**—Medullary paralysis: begins with respiratory failure; can lead to circulatory collapse; through careful monitoring, this stage is avoided

Objective 2: Define the importance of premedications before anesthesia.

- Also known as *preoperative medications* or preanesthetics, premedications help to:
  - Achieve sedation
  - Reduce anxiety
  - Induce amnesia to minimize unpleasant surgical memories
  - Increase comfort during preoperative procedures
  - Reduce gastric acidity and volume
  - Increase gastric emptying
  - Decrease nausea and vomiting
  - Reduce incidence of aspiration by drying oral and respiratory secretions

Objective 3: Explain the action of anesthetics within the central nervous system.

- Depress the CNS to cause unconsciousness
- Create unawareness of surroundings and block pain from surgery or procedure
- Relax patients' skeletal muscles and diminish reflexes

Objective 4: List the effects of general anesthetics.

- Loss of consciousness before and during surgery
- Relief of anxiety or pain without causing unconsciousness

Objective 5: Describe the common local anesthetics and their uses.

- Ester-type agents—generally used topically
- Amide-type agents—most commonly used; used to increase patient comfort, to facilitate patient cooperation, as diagnostic aids, and for the following specific procedures:
  - Incision and drainage of abscesses
  - Laceration repair
  - Biopsy
  - Wart treatment
  - Vasectomy
  - Neonatal circumcision
  - Dental procedures
  - Labor and delivery
  - Diagnostic procedures, such as gastrointestinal endoscopy
  - Pain relief associated with pathologic conditions

Objective 6: Compare ester and amide local anesthetics.

- Ester-type agents: attributable to allergic reactions caused by para-amino benzoic acid (PABA), these agents are generally not preferred; amide-type agents are often recommended instead
- Amide-type agents: safer than ester-type agents with less allergic reaction potential; they are available in many forms, including ointments, jellies, and solutions for injection

Objective 7: List the problems associated with the use of local anesthetics.

- Allergic reactions involving the ester-type agents, caused by the ingredient PABA, are common
- Toxic effects are possible and dose related
- Lightheadedness, dizziness, nystagmus, restlessness, disorientation, and psychosis may be experienced
- Slurred speech and tremors often precede seizures
- Hypotension, bradycardia, and cardiac arrest may occur

Objective 8: Explain the indications for spinal anesthesia.

- Gynecologic, obstetric, orthopedic, and genitourinary surgery

Objective 9: Discuss various techniques for local anesthetics.

- Local anesthesia is used to provide regional or topical anesthesia to relieve pain and provide localized nerve block without a loss of consciousness. They are commonly used topically or by injection. The amide-type local anesthetics are safer than the ester-type local anesthetics.
- Local anesthesia increases patient comfort and facilitates patient cooperation, helps to localize or identify sources of pain, and is used in all the following procedures:
  - Incision and drainage of abscesses, laceration repair, biopsy, wart treatment, vasectomy, neonatal circumcision, dental procedures, during labor and delivery, for gastrointestinal procedures such as endoscopy, and sometimes to relieve pain associated with pathologic conditions

Objective 10: Compare epidural anesthesia with field block anesthesia.

- Epidural anesthesia: involves injection of the local anesthetic into the epidural space via a catheter that allows repeated infusions. It is often used in labor and delivery. Care must be taken to avoid systemic toxicity.
- Field block anesthesia: affects a single nerve, a deep plexus, or a network of nerves. It is a form of regional anesthesia, wherein a local anesthetic is administered in a series of injections to form a wall of anesthesia encircling the operative field.

Internet Sites of Interest

- The journal of the Anesthesia & Analgesia organization can be searched at: **http://journals.lww.com/anesthesia-analgesia/pages/default.aspx**
- Excellent patient information can be found at the website of the American Society of Anesthesiologists: **http://asahq.org**
- *Scientific American* online offers an article titled "How Does Anesthesia Work?" Search at: **www.scientificamerican.com**
- The difference between local and general anesthesia is discussed at: **www.differencebetween.net/science/health/drugs-health/difference-between-local-and-general-anesthesia**
- The stages of anesthesia are explained at: **www.ahc.umn.edu/rar/anesthesia.html**

Chapter 26

Drugs Used to Treat Skin Conditions

Chapter Objectives

After completing this chapter, you should be able to:

1. Describe the top two layers of the skin.
2. Compare the causes and symptoms of eczema and psoriasis.
3. Identify the mainstay of treatment for acute or chronic inflammatory disorders of the skin.
4. Describe the mechanism of action of topical corticosteroids.
5. Identify the drugs used to treat psoriasis.
6. List the drugs used to treat acne.
7. Explain the action and uses of keratolytics.
8. Describe the treatments for scabies and pediculosis.

Key Terms

candidiasis (p. 462)
dermatitis (p. 455)
eczema (p. 455)
emollients (p. 458)
erythema (p. 455)

keratinization (p. 459)
keratinocytes (p. 458)
keratolytic (p. 458)
pediculicides (p. 463)

pruritus (p. 458)
psoriasis (p. 457)
scabicides (p. 463)
scabies (p. 463)

Introduction

The integumentary system is the largest of all organs in the human body. It consists of the skin, hair, nails, sweat glands, and oil glands. The skin forms a barrier between ourselves and our environment and, as such, is fundamental to the functioning of all other organs. The skin is vital in maintaining homeostasis. In addition to providing a protective covering, the skin helps regulate body temperature, retards water loss from deeper tissues, houses sensory receptors, synthesizes various biochemicals, and excretes small quantities of wastes.

The Skin

The skin consists of two distinct layers (Figure 26-1 ■). The outer layer is called the *epidermis*. The inner layer, or *dermis*, is thicker than the epidermis. Beneath the dermis are masses of loose connective and adipose tissues that bind the skin to the underlying organs. These tissues form the subcutaneous layer, which lies beneath the skin but is not a true layer of skin.

Figure 26-1 ■ The two layers of the skin.

EPIDERMIS

The epidermis has either four or five sublayers. The outermost sublayer is the *stratum corneum* (horny layer). The deepest layer of epidermal cells, called the *stratum basale* or *stratum germinativum*, is close to the dermis and is nourished by dermal blood vessels. As the cells of this layer divide and grow, the older epidermal cells are pushed away from the dermis toward the skin surface. The farther the cells move, the poorer their nutrient supply becomes and, in time, they die. Specialized cells in the epidermis called *melanocytes* produce melanin, a dark pigment that provides skin color. Melanin absorbs ultraviolet (UV) radiation in sunlight, preventing mutations in the DNA of skin cells and other damaging effects. Melanocytes lie in the deepest portion of the epidermis.

DERMIS

The dermis binds the epidermis to underlying tissues. It is largely composed of dense, irregular connective tissue that gets its name from its irregular arrangement of thick protein fibers.

Dermal blood vessels supply nutrients to all skin cells. These vessels also help regulate body temperature. Nerve cell processes are scattered throughout the dermis. The dermis also contains hair follicles, oil glands, and sweat glands. Embedded in the skin are structures called *appendages*, such as the nails, hair follicles, and sweat and sebaceous glands—all of which are subject to disease.

SUBCUTANEOUS LAYER

The subcutaneous layer or *hypodermis*, which lies beneath the dermal layer of the skin, consists of loose connective and adipose tissues. The adipose tissue of the subcutaneous layer insulates, helping to conserve body heat and impede the entrance of heat from the outside. The subcutaneous layer also contains the major blood vessels that supply the skin and underlying adipose tissue.

Disorders of the Skin

Disruptions in skin integrity may be precipitated by trauma, abnormal cellular function, infection and inflammation, and systemic diseases. Many of these diseases are caused by infections, and most of the drugs used to treat such infections are discussed in Chapters 16, 17, and 18. Other common diseases of the skin are caused by inflammatory conditions resulting from allergies.

ECZEMA AND MISCELLANEOUS INFLAMMATORY DISORDERS

The most common inflammatory disorder of the skin is **eczema**, a response of the skin caused by endogenous and exogenous agents; it is often considered synonymous with **dermatitis**, which is inflammation of the skin. Endogenous eczemas include dermatitis and seborrheic dermatitis. Exogenous eczemas include irritant dermatitis and allergic contact dermatitis. Eczematous dermatitis is characterized by **erythema**, which is skin redness caused by capillary dilation, as well as vesicles, scales, and itching.

The mainstay of treatment of acute or chronic inflammatory disorders is topical or oral corticosteroids. Systemic corticosteroids were discussed in other chapters. Only topical corticosteroids are discussed here (Table 26-1 ■).

Table 26-1 ■ **Selected Topical Corticosteroids**

GENERIC NAME	TRADE NAME	AVERAGE ADULT DOSAGE	ROUTE OF ADMINISTRATION
alclometasone	Aclovate	Apply 0.05% cream or ointment sparingly bid–tid.	Topical
amcinonide	Amcinonide Lotion, Amcinonide Cream	Apply thin film bid–tid.	Topical
betamethasone dipropionate	Diprolene	Apply thin film bid–tid.	Topical
betamethasone valerate	Luxiq (foam)	Apply sparingly bid to scalp.	Topical
desoximetasone	Topicort	Apply thin layer bid.	Topical
dexamethasone	Baycadron	Apply thin layer tid–qid.	Topical
diflorasone	Florone	Apply thin layer of cream 2–4 times/d.	Topical
fluocinolone	Flurosyn	Apply thin layer bid–qid.	Topical
fluocinonide	Vanos	Apply thin layer bid–qid.	Topical
flurandrenolide	Cordran	Apply thin layer bid–tid; apply tape 1–2 times/d q12h.	Topical
hydrocortisone	Cortaid	Apply a small amount to affected area 1–4 times/d.	Topical
triamcinolone	Cinolar	Apply sparingly bid–tid.	Topical

bid, twice a day; tid, three times a day; qid, four times a day.

Focus on Pediatrics

Eczema Common in Pediatric Patients

Eczema, also called *atopic dermatitis*, is common in pediatric patients. Eczema in some infants is believed to be traceable to sensitivity to milk, orange juice, or certain foods.

Focus On

Topical Corticosteroids

The corticosteroids are potent anti-inflammatory agents. Topical administration goes directly to the site of inflammation. These drug preparations are available as lotions, creams, and aerosols in various concentrations.

How do they work?

Topical corticosteroids prevent the accumulation of inflammatory cells at sites of infection and inhibit phagocytosis.

When applied to inflamed skin, they reduce itching, redness, and swelling.

How are they used?

Topical corticosteroids are used for the treatment of such skin disorders as eczema, dermatitis, psoriasis, insect bite reactions, and first- or second-degree burns. Topical corticosteroids are the primary agents used to treat dermatitis.

Potency depends on the type of drug formulation and on whether it is packaged as a cream, lotion, solution, or gel.

What are the adverse effects?

Common localized adverse effects may include dryness, redness, itching, irritation, or burning of the skin. Topical corticosteroids may also produce secondary infections.

What are the contraindications and interactions?

Topical corticosteroids are contraindicated in bacterial skin infections. They must not be used in patients with known hypersensitivity. Topical corticosteroids should be used cautiously in pregnant or lactating women. Drug interactions are not significant when administered as directed.

What are the important points patients should know?

Advise patients to follow the directions of their physician regarding covering the treated area or leaving it exposed to air. The effectiveness of certain drugs depends on keeping the area covered or leaving it open. Instruct patients to not apply medications to areas other than those specified by their physician, and to use the drug as directed; for example, "apply a thin layer" or "apply liberally." Topical corticosteroids must be kept away from the eyes, unless use in or around the eyes has been recommended.

✸ Apply Your Knowledge 26.1

The following questions focus on what you have just learned about the skin.

CRITICAL THINKING

1. Describe the major functions of the skin.
2. Identify the outermost and deepest layers of the epidermis.
3. Explain the mainstay of treatment of acute or chronic inflammatory disorders of the skin.
4. Give another name for eczema.
5. Point out the trade names of amcinonide, fluocinonide, and flurandrenolide.

PSORIASIS

Psoriasis is a chronic, relapsing inflammatory skin disorder that occurs at any age; onset usually occurs by 20 years of age. The cause of psoriasis is unknown, but it has a hereditary component. The disorder is marked by a greatly increased rate of cellular proliferation, which leads to thickening of the dermis and epidermis. It is characterized by rounded plaques, covered by silvery-white scaly patches. The skin lesions of psoriasis are variably pruritic. External factors may exacerbate psoriasis, including infections, stress, and such medications as lithium, beta-blockers, and antimalarials.

The most common areas for psoriasis to occur are the elbows, knees, gluteal cleft, and scalp. Involvement tends to be symmetric. There is no cure for this disease yet, but remissions can often be produced by the available therapies, which include the use of ultraviolet light either alone or in combination with drugs and topical and systemic treatments.

Focus Point

Preventing Recurrence of Psoriasis

Keeping the skin moist and lubricated, avoiding cold and dry climates, avoiding stress and anxiety, limiting alcohol intake, and not scratching the skin help to prevent the recurrence of psoriasis.

Focus On

Topical Antipsoriatics

Treatment is related to reducing epidermal cell turnover and changes in the immune response. Mild lesions are usually treated with skin-softening agents called **emollients**, **keratolytic** agents that separate or loosen the horny layer of the epidermis, and topical corticosteroids. Systemic medications are used for moderate to severe lesions, which may respond to methotrexate, vitamin A, and vitamin D analogues. Sometimes, for the treatment of psoriasis, various techniques are used with or without other antipsoriasis medications (Table 26-2 ■). Various forms of tar treatments, such as coal tar, and a substance called anthralin are available. Phototherapy, which uses UV light, is indicated in cases of severe psoriasis.

How do they work?

The mechanism of action of acitretin, ammoniated mercury, and anthralin are unknown. Calcipotriene is a synthetic vitamin D_3 that controls psoriasis by inhibiting the proliferation of **keratinocytes**, which are the epidermal cells that produce keratin, and by decreasing the number of epithelial cells. Methoxsalen is a psoralen derivative with strong photosensitizing effects. Methoxsalen, which causes photodamage, inhibits rapid and uncontrolled epidermal psoriasis.

How are they used?

Antipsoriatic agents are used for the treatment of moderate to severe forms of psoriasis in adults.

What are the adverse effects?

The major adverse effects associated with acitretin are alopecia, skin peeling, dry skin, **pruritus**, rash, skin atrophy, and abnormal skin odor. The adverse effects of calcipotriene include facial dermatitis, burning, stinging, erythema, and itching. Methoxsalen may cause severe edema, erythema, burning, peeling, and thinning of the skin.

What are the contraindications and interactions?

Topical antipsoriatics are contraindicated in hypersensitivity to these agents. Patients with hypercalcemia or vitamin D toxicity should not use calcipotriene. The antipsoriatics are also contraindicated in pregnancy or lactating women.

What are the important points patients should know?

Instruct patients to avoid additional exposure to UV light for at least 8 hours after oral drug ingestion and UVA exposure. Warn patients against mixing calcipotriene with any other topical medicines. Advise patients to discontinue the drug and immediately report visual problems.

Table 26-2 ■ Antipsoriatic Drugs

GENERIC NAME	TRADE NAME	AVERAGE ADULT DOSAGE	ROUTE OF ADMINISTRATION
acitretin	Soriatane	10–50 mg/d with main meal	PO
anthralin	Psoriatec	Dosing is individualized. In general, both the cream and ointment formulations are applied to affected areas once per day, then washed off within 10–30 minutes.	Topical
azelaic acid	Azelex	Apply twice daily.	Topical
calcipotriene	Dovonex	Apply twice daily.	Topical
methoxsalen	Oxsoralen, Uvadex	Give 1.5–2 h before exposure to UV light 2–3 times/wk (ranging from 10–70 mg based on the weight of the patient).	PO

PO, oral; UV, ultraviolet.

ACNE

Acne vulgaris is an inflammatory disorder of the sebaceous glands that commonly occurs during puberty. The incidence of acne tends to decline with age and is unusual in adults, although it can persist for many years. Sebaceous glands secrete sebum, the natural oil of the skin.

Testosterone is partially responsible for the secretion of sebum, and it may be that acne is caused by an increased responsiveness of the sebaceous glands to varying levels of this hormone during puberty. When too much sebum is produced, the duct of the gland may become blocked, and bacteria can become trapped beneath the sebum plug. The bacteria then grow in the duct, leading to a small abscess.

Focus on Natural Products

Use Caution in Treating Acne with Zinc

A variety of natural products are used to treat acne. The most common of these are zinc, niacinamide gel, and tea tree oil. It is important to note that zinc can be toxic at high dosages, primarily because it causes copper deficiency.

Focus On

Antiacne Agents

Major drugs for acne-related disorders are listed in Table 26-3 ■. Benzoyl peroxide is a powerful oxidizing agent, which at least partially relieves some cases of acne by having bacterial action, and is the main OTC drug used for this purpose. Azelaic acid is a naturally occurring dicarboxylic acid. Such topical antibiotics as clindamycin and erythromycin are also prescribed.

How do they work?

The antimicrobial action of these agents may be attributable to the inhibition of microbial cellular protein synthesis. A normalization of **keratinization**, which is keratin formation or development of a horny layer, is caused by some of these agents, such as azelaic acid and benzoyl peroxide. This normalization of keratinization may also contribute to their clinical effectiveness.

How are they used?

These agents are used for mild to moderate inflammatory acne vulgaris. Topical applications of clindamycin are used in the treatment of acne vulgaris, and vaginal applications are used in the treatment of bacterial vaginosis in nonpregnant women.

What are the adverse effects?

Topical antiacne drugs may cause pruritus, burning, erythema, and stinging. Benzoyl peroxide can produce allergic dermatitis, excessive drying, peeling, erythema, and stinging. Topical clindamycin and erythromycin also produce dryness, burning, and excessive oil in the skin. In rare cases, clindamycin may cause bloody diarrhea and abdominal pain.

What are the contraindications and interactions?

These agents are avoided in patients with known hypersensitivity. Topical antiacne drugs are contraindicated during pregnancy and lactation.

What are the important points patients should know?

Instruct patients that proper application of these creams and gels is essential. Warn them to avoid contact with the eyes or mucous membranes and to wash out the eyes with large amounts of water if contact with the medication occurs. Advise patients to avoid breastfeeding while using these agents or to consult their physician.

Table 26-3 ■ Major Drugs Used to Treat Acne

GENERIC NAME	TRADE NAME	AVERAGE ADULT DOSAGE	ROUTE OF ADMINISTRATION
adapalene	Differin	Apply once daily, in the evening, to affected areas.	Topical
azelaic acid	Azelex	Apply twice daily.	Topical
benzoyl peroxide	BenzaClin, Benzamycin	Apply 1–2 times/d.	Topical
clindamycin	Cleocin	Apply to affected areas bid.	Topical
doxycycline	Doryx, Vibramycin	100 mg q12h on day 1 and then 100 mg/d	PO
erythromycin	Eryc	250 mg q6h taken 1h before meals	PO

(continued)

Table 26-3 ■ Major Drugs Used to Treat Acne (*continued*)

GENERIC NAME	TRADE NAME	AVERAGE ADULT DOSAGE	ROUTE OF ADMINISTRATION
tetracycline	(Generic only)	Oral: 500–1,000 mg/d in four divided doses	PO
	(Generic only)	Topical: Apply to cleansed areas bid.	Topical
tretinoin	Retin-A	Apply once daily at bedtime.	Topical

bid, twice a day; PO, oral.

KERATOSES

Keratoses are characterized by a thickening of the keratin layer of the skin. Keratoses are benign lesions that are usually associated with aging or skin damage. *Seborrheic keratoses* result from the proliferation of epidermis, leading to an oval elevation that may be smooth or rough and is often dark in color. *Actinic keratoses* occur on skin (especially fair skin) exposed to UV radiation. The lesion appears as a pigmented, scaly patch. Actinic keratoses may develop into skin cancer.

Focus On

Keratolytic Agents

Keratolytic agents promote shedding of the horny layer of the epidermis and softening of scales. The most commonly used keratolytic agents are salicylic acid, resorcinol, and sulfur. Selected keratolytic medications are summarized in Table 26-4 ■.

How do they work?

Keratolytics act by breaking down the protein structure of the keratin layer, thereby permitting easier removal of compacted cellular material.

How are they used?

Keratolytic agents are used in the treatment of corns, calluses, and plantar warts. Some of these medications, such as sulfur and ammonium lactate, are used in the treatment of patients with acne, eczema, psoriasis, and seborrheic dermatitis.

What are the adverse effects?

The adverse effects of keratolytic agents include burning, local irritation, rash, dry skin, and scaling.

What are the contraindications and interactions?

Keratolytic drugs must be avoided in patients with known hypersensitivity. They are contraindicated on moles, warts with hair growing from them, genital or facial warts, birthmarks, or infected skin. Salicylic acid may cause salicylate toxicity with prolonged use (see Chapter 21). These agents must be used cautiously during pregnancy and lactation.

What are the important points patients should know?

Instruct patients that keratolytic agents are for external use only. Tell them to avoid contact with the eye, face, mucous membranes, and normal skin around warts. Advise the patient to soak the area with warm water for 5 minutes before application to enhance the effect of the medication.

Table 26-4 ■ Selected Keratolytic Agents

GENERIC NAME	TRADE NAME	AVERAGE ADULT DOSAGE	ROUTE OF ADMINISTRATION
diclofenac	Solaraze	Apply to affected area bid for 60–90 d.	Topical
masoprocol (cream)	Actinex	Apply to lesions bid for 14–28 d.	Topical
salicylic acid	Fostex, Mediplast	Apply enough medicine to cover affected area and rub in gently or apply a patch as directed.	Topical
salicylic acid with podophyllum (also known as *podophyllum resin*)	Podocon-25, Podofin	Apply enough medicine to cover the affected area and rub in gently or apply a patch as directed.	Topical

bid, twice a day.

Focus Point

Corns and Calluses

Corns and calluses are extremely common, localized hyperplastic areas of the stratum corneum layer of the epidermis.

✳ Apply Your Knowledge 26.2

The following questions focus on what you have just learned about psoriasis, acne, and keratoses as well as the medications used to treat these conditions.

CRITICAL THINKING

1. Compare acne with psoriasis.
2. Describe actinic keratosis and its complication.
3. Give the descriptions of corns and calluses.
4. Identify the trade names of clindamycin, azelaic acid, tretinoin, and adapalene.
5. Point out the trade names of masoprocol, diclofenac, and salicylic acid with podophyllum.

Bacterial Skin Infections

Cutaneous infections are common forms of skin disease. Most bacterial infections of the skin are caused by local invasion by pathogens. Staphylococci and beta-hemolytic streptococci are the common causative microorganisms. Examples of skin and hair bacterial infections include impetigo, cellulites, and folliculitis. These infections generally remain localized, although serious complications can occur. Impetigo is a common superficial bacterial infection of skin caused by either *Streptococcus spp.* or *Staphylococcus aureus.* The primary lesion is a superficial pustule that ruptures and forms a characteristic yellow-brown crust. Lesions caused by staphylococci may be tense, clear bullae, and this less common form of the disease is called *bulbous impetigo.* Treatment of impetigo involves gentle debridement of adherent crusts, which is facilitated by the use of soaks and topical antibiotics in conjunction with appropriate oral antibiotics. Topical antibiotic drugs are listed in Table 26-5 ■. Systemic antibiotics are discussed in Chapter 16.

Table 26-5 ■ Topical Antibiotic Drugs

GENERIC NAME	TRADE NAME	AVERAGE ADULT DOSAGE	ROUTE OF ADMINISTRATION
azelaic acid	Azelex	Apply a thin film to clean and dry area bid.	Topical
bacitracin	Baciguent	Apply thin layer of ointment bid–tid as solution of 250–1,000 units/mL in wet dressing.	Topical
benzoyl peroxide	Benzac	Apply 1–2 times/d.	Topical
clindamycin (topical)	Cleocin T	Apply to affected areas bid.	Topical
gentamicin	Garamycin	1–2 drops of solution in eye q4h up to 2 drops q1h or small amount of ointment bid–tid	Topical
metronidazole	MetroGel, MetroLotion	Apply thin film to affected area bid.	Topical

(continued)

Table 26-5 ■ **Topical Antibiotic Drugs** (*continued*)

GENERIC NAME	TRADE NAME	AVERAGE ADULT DOSAGE	ROUTE OF ADMINISTRATION
mupirocin	Bactroban	Apply to affected area tid; if no response in 3–5 d, reevaluate, usually continue for 1–2 wk.	Topical
neomycin	Myciguent	Apply 1–3 times/d	Topical
sulfacetamide	Sebizon	Apply thin film to affected area 1–3 times/d.	Topical
bid, twice a day; tid, three times a day.			

Fungal Infections

Dermatophytes are fungi that infect skin, hair, and nails. An example is *tinea pedis*, which affects the feet, the most common and often chronic. It is characterized by variable erythema and edema, scaling, pruritus, and occasionally vesiculation. Involvement may be widespread or localized, but almost invariably, the web space between the fourth and fifth toes is affected. Infection of the nails, called *tinea unguium*, occurs in many patients with tinea pedis and is characterized by opacified, thickened nails and subungual debris.

The groin is the next most commonly involved area, a condition called *tinea cruris*, with men affected much more often than women. Dermatophyte infection of the scalp, called *tinea capitis*, produces an inflammatory or relatively noninflammatory condition that may present with either well-defined or irregular, diffuse areas of mild scaling and hair loss.

Candidiasis is also a fungal infection caused by a related group of yeasts—mostly *Candida albicans*. This organism is a normal flora of the gastrointestinal tract, but it may overgrow, usually because of broad-spectrum antibiotic therapy, causing disease at a number of skin sites. Other predisposing factors include diabetes mellitus, oral contraceptive use, and cellular immune deficiency. Candidiasis is a very common infection in HIV-infected individuals. In the oral cavity, the tongue or buccal mucosa is usually involved, and this type of infection is also known as *thrush*. *Candida* infection may involve vulvovaginal candidiasis, which is very common in women of reproductive age.

ANTIFUNGAL AGENTS

Topical and systemic therapies may be used to treat dermatophyte infections. Treatment depends on the site involved and the type of infection (Table 26-6 ■). Systemic therapies for fungal disorders were discussed in Chapter 18.

Table 26-6 ■ **Topical Antifungal Drugs**

GENERIC NAME	TRADE NAME	AVERAGE ADULT DOSAGE	ROUTE OF ADMINISTRATION
amphotericin B	Fungizone	100 mg swish and swallow qid	PO
ciclopirox (skin)	Loprox	Massage cream into affected area and surrounding skin bid (morning and evening).	Topical (cream, gel, or lotion)
ciclopirox (nail)	Penlac Nail	Paint affected nails under the surface and on the nail bed once daily at bedtime, at least 8 h before washing. After 7 d, remove lacquer with alcohol and remove or trim away unattached nail. Continue for 48 wk.	Nail lacquer
ciclopirox (scalp)	Ciclopirox Shampoo	Wet hair and apply approx. 1 tsp to the scalp (up to 10 mL for long hair); leave on for 3 min and then rinse. Repeat twice/wk for 4 wk, with a minimum of 3 d between applications.	Topical on scalp
econazole	Spectazole	Apply sufficient amount of 1% cream to affected areas 1–2 times/d (morning and evening).	Topical

GENERIC NAME	TRADE NAME	AVERAGE ADULT DOSAGE	ROUTE OF ADMINISTRATION
miconazole (skin)	Monistat-Derm	Apply cream sparingly to affected areas bid and once daily for tinea versicolor for 2 wk (improvement is expected in 2–3 d; tinea pedis is treated for 1 mo to prevent recurrence).	Topical
miconazole (vaginal)	Monistat Vaginal Cream	Insert suppository or vaginal cream at bedtime for 7 d (100 mg) or 3 d (200 mg).	Intravaginal
naftifine	Naftin	Apply cream once daily or apply gel bid; may use up to 4 wk	Topical
nystatin	Mycostatin	Apply 100,000 units/g cream, ointment, and powder or 1–2 tablets daily for 2 wk.	Intravaginal
oxiconazole	Oxistat	Apply to affected area once daily in the evening.	Topical
terbinafine	Lamisil	Apply 1–2 times/d to affected and immediately surrounding areas until clinical signs and symptoms are significantly improved (1–7 wk).	Topical
tolnaftate	Aftate, Tinactin	Apply 0.5–1 cm ($\frac{1}{4}$–$\frac{1}{2}$ in.) of cream or 3 drops of solution bid in morning and evening; powder may be used prophylactically in normally moist areas.	Topical

qid, four times a day; PO, oral; bid, twice a day.

Scabies and Pediculosis

Scabies is a group of dermatologic conditions caused by mites that burrow into the skin, causing intense itching. Scabies may be found anywhere on the trunk or extremities. Pediculosis is a lice infestation. Lice primarily affect hairy areas of the body, including the top of the head, eyebrows, eyelids, underarms, chest, and pubic area. Lice can infest just the head or the entire body. Another species—pubic lice—is commonly referred to as *crabs*. Lice feed on human blood and lay their eggs, called *nits*, on hair shafts. When a louse has its blood meal, irritation may be produced, which can eventually lead to a severe inflammatory reaction. The condition is highly contagious and requires treatment with specially formulated insecticides.

Focus On

Antilice Drugs

Scabicides are pharmacologic drugs that kill mites; **pediculicides** kill lice. However, either treatment may be effective for both types of parasites. The choice of drug depends on where the infestation has occurred. Table 26-7 ■ summarizes the most commonly used agents.

How do they work?

The mechanism of action of antilice drugs is related to their direct absorption by parasites and ova, which are also called *nits*. They stimulate the nervous system of the parasites, resulting in seizures and death.

How are they used?

These agents are used topically in the treatment of *Pediculus humanus* infestations.

What are the adverse effects?

The adverse effects include irritation with repeated use, causing pruritus, burning, stinging, numbness, erythema, edema, and rash.

What are the contraindications and interactions?

Lindane is contraindicated in premature neonates and patients with known seizure disorders. It should not be

(continued)

Focus On (continued)

applied to the eyes, face, mucous membranes, or open cuts. The use of pyrethrins with dyes is contraindicated. These drugs should be avoided in acute inflammation of the scalp and in pregnant or lactating women. They should be used cautiously in children younger than 2 years. There are no clinically significant interactions established with these topical agents.

What are the most important points patients should know?

Instruct patients and their families that these agents are highly toxic drugs if used in excess or if they are swallowed or inhaled. Warn patients to keep these agents out of the reach of children. Advise patients to use a fine-toothed comb that is infused with medication to remove dead lice and remaining nits or nit shells when hair is dry. Regular shampooing should be resumed after treatment; residual deposit of drug on the hair is not reduced. Warn patients not to share combs, brushes, or other grooming equipment with other people. Instruct female patients to avoid breastfeeding while using these drugs without consulting their physician.

Table 26-7 ■ Drugs Used to Treat Lice

GENERIC NAME	TRADE NAME	AVERAGE ADULT DOSAGE	ROUTE OF ADMINISTRATION
crotamiton	Eurax	Apply directly from the neck to the toes; apply a second layer 24 h later. Bathe 48 h after the last application to remove the drug.	Topical
lindane	(Generic only)	Apply to all body areas except the face; leave lotion on 8–12 h and then rinse off; leave shampoo on 5 min and then rinse thoroughly. *Do not* repeat in less than 1 wk.	Lotion, shampoo
permethrin	Acticin, Nix	Apply sufficient volume to clean, wet hair to saturate the hair and scalp; leave on 10 min and then rinse hair thoroughly.	Cream, lotion
pyrethrum	(Generic only)	Apply to affected areas and leave on 10 min and then rinse thoroughly. Reapply only as directed.	Topical

✵ Apply Your Knowledge 26.3

The following questions focus on what you have just learned about skin infections, scabies, and pediculosis.

CRITICAL THINKING

1. Identify the most common bacterial infections of the skin.
2. Describe impetigo.
3. Explain the predisposing factors for candidiasis.
4. Discuss pediculosis.
5. Describe scabicides.
6. Give the trade names of amphotericin B, haloprogin, oxiconazole, and nystatin.

PRACTICAL SCENARIO 1

A 45-year-old woman who has spent more than 20 summers at the beaches of Florida and goes to the tanning salon three times a week notices that a small spot has appeared on her arm. It is a different color than the surrounding skin and has a bumpy surface. She assumes that it is a skin infection or bite and applies an OTC antibiotic ointment for several weeks. Finally, she calls her physician's office and speaks to you, wondering if she should schedule an office visit for such a small matter.

Jpc-Prod/Shutterstock

Critical Thinking Questions

1. What questions might you ask the patient about the skin spot?
2. What should you tell the patient to do about scheduling an office visit?
3. After the patient has been seen by the physician and treated, what patient education can you provide to her?

PRACTICAL SCENARIO 2

A 7-month-old infant developed sensitivity to milk and orange juice. She began to develop a skin disorder on her face.

Courtesy of the author

Critical Thinking Questions

1. What is the most common skin condition caused by food allergies in infants?
2. What would be the most common type of skin medication prescribed for this condition?

Chapter Capsule

This section repeats the objectives from the beginning of the chapter and then provides a summary of the most important concepts for that objective. Use this section as a quick review and to check your knowledge.

Objective 1: Describe the top two layers of the skin.

- Epidermis—outer layer with four or five sublayers; contains specialized cells called *melanocytes*, which produce melanin, a dark pigment that provides skin color
- Dermis—inner layer; thicker than the epidermis. Beneath the dermis are masses of loose connective and adipose tissues that bind the skin to the underlying organs.

Objective 2: Compare the causes and symptoms of eczema and psoriasis.

- Eczema
  - Causes: endogenous and exogenous agents
  - Symptoms: erythema, vesicles, scales, itching

- Psoriasis
  - ❏ Causes: unknown, but with a hereditary component; external factors that may exacerbate psoriasis include infections, stress, and medications such as lithium, beta-blockers, and antimalarials
  - ❏ Symptoms: thickening of the dermis and epidermis, characterized by rounded plaques covered by silvery-white scaly patches that itch

Objective 3: Identify the mainstay of treatment for acute or chronic inflammatory disorders of the skin.

- Topical or oral corticosteroids are the mainstay of treatment for acute or chronic inflammatory skin disorders

Objective 4: Describe the mechanism of action of topical corticosteroids.

- Topical corticosteroids prevent accumulation of inflammatory cells at sites of infection and inhibit phagocytosis; when applied to inflamed skin, they reduce itching, redness, and swelling

Objective 5: Identify the drugs used to treat psoriasis.

- Emollients
- Keratolytic agents
- Topical corticosteroids
- Systemic medications
- Tar treatments
- Anthralin
- UV light (phototherapy)

Objective 6: List the drugs used to treat acne.

- Benzoyl peroxide
- Azelaic acid
- Clindamycin
- Erythromycin

Objective 7: Explain the action and uses of keratolytics.

- Keratolytics—promote shedding of the horny layer of the epidermis and soften scales
- Used in the treatment of corns, calluses, and plantar warts; some, such as sulfur and ammonium lactate, are used in the treatment of acne, eczema, psoriasis, and seborrheic dermatitis

Objective 8: Describe the treatments for scabies and pediculosis.

- Scabicides—pharmacologic drugs that kill mites
- Pediculicides—kill lice
- Both treatments may be effective for both types of parasites; the choice of drug depends on where the infestation has occurred

Internet Sites of Interest

- Dermatology A to Z, sun safety, and consumer information can be found at the American Academy of Dermatology's website: **www.aad.org**

- A detailed discussion of eczema, its triggers, and its treatments: **www.webmd.com/allergies/guide/eczema**

- The About.com website includes an article written by a physician on the use of corticosteroids in skin disorders, such as acne: **http://dermatology.about.com/cs/ medications/a/steroidswork.htm**

- MedlinePlus offers a discussion of scabies, including photos, treatments, and an interactive tutorial: **www.nlm.nih.gov/medlineplus/scabies.html**

- The National Psoriasis Foundation offers detailed information: **www.psoriasis.org**

Chapter 27

Drugs Used to Treat Cardiovascular Conditions

Chapter Objectives

After completing this chapter, you should be able to:

1. Name the three layers of the heart and the four heart valves.
2. Identify the electrical conduction system of the heart.
3. Define three types of *angina pectoris*.
4. Name the mainstays of angina therapy.
5. Describe the action of vasodilation.
6. Explain myocardial infarction.
7. Identify the classifications of antidysrhythmic drugs and explain their actions.
8. Define *calcium channel blockers*.
9. Describe the newest and oldest drugs that are used for congestive heart failure.
10. Explain the most common side effects of digitalis.

Key Terms

angina pectoris(p. 470)
ascites (p. 484)
atrioventricular (AV) node (p. 470)
atrium (p. 470)
automaticity (p. 479)
bradycardia (p. 476)
bundle of His (p. 470)
congestive heart failure (CHF) (p. 469)
dysrhythmia (p. 476)
electrocardiogram (ECG or EKG) (p. 470)
endocardium (p. 470)
epicardium (p. 470)

fibrillation (p. 478)
flutter (p. 478)
gingival hyperplasia (p. 479)
hypertension (p. 469)
hypotension (p. 473)
insomnia (p. 474)
ischemia (p. 471)
myocardial infarction (MI) (p. 469)
myocardium (p. 469)
nystagmus (p. 479)
Purkinje fibers (p. 470)

refractory (p. 481)
sinoatrial (SA) node (p. 470)
somnolence (SAHM-no-lents) (p. 479)
sympathetic (p. 474)
syndrome (p. 475)
tachycardia (p. 473)
tachypnea (p. 484)
vasodilation (p. 475)
vasospasms (p. 473)
ventricles (p. 470)
vertigo (p. 479)

Introduction

The circulatory system is often referred to as the *cardiovascular system* and is composed of the heart and blood vessels, collectively known as *vasculature*. Cardiovascular disease (CVD) is the most common cause of death in the United States and can result from *coronary artery disease (CAD)*, which is blockage of the arteries that supply the heart muscle itself. This can lead to a **myocardial infarction (MI)**, or heart attack. An MI occurs when part of the heart is deprived of its blood supply to such an extent that the cells of the myocardium die. Another term for CAD is *coronary heart disease (CHD)*; the terms may be used interchangeably. Other related cardiovascular conditions that can lead to or result from CAD or MI include dysrhythmias, also

called *arrhythmias*, **congestive heart failure (CHF)**, hyperlipidemia, and **hypertension**, which is blood pressure that is elevated above the normal limits. A stroke, also known as a *cerebrovascular accident (CVA)* or a *brain attack*, may be thought of as similar to an MI, except the vasculature affected is in the brain and the resulting damage occurs to brain cells.

To understand the drug therapies used to treat CVD, the health care professional must have a solid understanding of the anatomy, physiology, and electrical properties of the heart as well as the vasculature. The medications in current use can produce their effects on the **myocardium**, which is the middle layer and most important structure of the heart. It contains the heart muscles that regulate cardiac output, the conduction system, and the coronary and other blood vessels (Figure 27-1 ■).

Figure 27-1 ■ Anatomy of the heart.

Focus on Geriatrics

Lifestyle and Cardiovascular Disease

Cardiovascular disease is most prevalent in older, sedentary individuals who are overweight or obese. With the aging of the baby boom generation, many of whom grew up on a diet of fast food rich in salt and fats, the prevalence of heart disease in the United States is increasing significantly.

Angina pectoris is a common form of ischemic heart disease and often precedes and accompanies MI. It has been described as chest pain and a squeezing pressure that can radiate to the jaw and arm. Related components of CVD and their manifestations, including CHF, hypertension, hyperlipidemia, and stroke, are discussed in Chapters 28 and 29.

Cardiac drugs to be discussed in this chapter are broadly classified according to their effects on certain parts of the cardiovascular system. These drugs can affect:

1. The rate of the heart
2. The rhythm of the heartbeat
3. The amount of blood output
4. The strength of contraction

The Cardiovascular System

The cardiovascular system begins its activity when the fetus is barely 4 weeks old and is the last system to cease activity at the end of life. This body system is so vital that it helps define the presence of life.

The heart, arteries, veins, and lymphatic system form the cardiovascular network that serves as the body's transport system. This system brings life-supporting oxygen and nutrients to cells, removes metabolic waste products, and carries hormones from one part of the body to another.

The cardiovascular, or circulatory, system is divided into two branches: pulmonary circulation and systemic circulation. In pulmonary circulation, blood picks up oxygen and liberates the waste product, carbon dioxide. In systemic circulation, which includes coronary circulation, blood carries oxygen and nutrients to all active cells and transports waste products to the kidneys, liver, and skin for excretion.

Circulation requires normal heart function to propel blood through the system by continuous rhythmic contractions of the heart. Blood circulates through three types of vessels: arteries, veins, and capillaries.

The heart is a muscular pump located within the mediastinum of the thorax. It consists of three layers:

1. The **endocardium**, which is the thin membrane lining the inside of the cardiac muscle
2. The cardiac muscle, which is called the *myocardium*
3. The **epicardium**, which is a thin membrane lining the outside of the myocardium

The heart is composed of four compartments that maintain the body's blood circulation. The two smaller upper chambers are the receiving chambers, called the left **atrium** and the right atrium; together, they are known as *atria*. The two lower chambers are called the left and right **ventricles**. These are the chambers that pump blood out of the heart. The upper and lower chambers are divided by a septum.

The four valves of the heart—tricuspid, pulmonary, mitral, and aortic—are located at the entrance and exit of each ventricle. Blood pumps through the four chambers of the heart with the help of the valves, which open and close via flaps, to allow blood to flow in only one direction.

The electrical conduction system contains all the wiring to initiate and maintain the rhythmic contraction of the heart (Figure 27-2 ■). The system consists of:

✳ **Sinoatrial (SA) node.** Located just beneath the epicardium in the right atrium near the opening of the superior vena cava, this small, elongated mass of specialized cardiac muscle tissue initiates one impulse after another. Because it generates the heart's rhythmic contractions, it is known as the *pacemaker*.

✳ **Atrioventricular (AV) node.** Located in the inferior portion of the septum, which separates the atria, and just beneath the endocardium, the AV node provides the only normal conduction pathway between the atrial and ventricular syncytia, and its fibers delay impulse transmission. This delay allows more time for the atria to completely contract so they empty all their blood into the ventricles before ventricular contraction occurs.

✳ **Bundle of His.** Located between the AV node and the Purkinje fibers and also known as the *AV bundle*, the bundle of His consists of a large group of fibers that enter the upper part of the intraventricular septum and are divided into right and left bundle branches lying just beneath the endocardium.

✳ Right and left bundle branches. Located in the heart's lower chambers (ventricles), the bundle branches divide at the bundle of His and form the right and left bundle branches. An electrical impulse travels down the right and left bundle branches at the same speed and causes the left and right ventricles to contract at the same time.

✳ **Purkinje fibers.** Located about halfway down the septum, the Purkinje fibers spread from the interventricular septum into the papillary muscles toward the apex of the heart. Along this pathway, the Purkinje fibers give off many small branches, which become continuous with cardiac muscle fibers.

An **electrocardiogram (ECG or EKG)** is a tracing of the heart's electrical activity. It measures electrical activity across the myocardium. Each electrical impulse takes less than one-quarter of a second to occur. An ECG provides a visual means of examining the electrical impulses of the heart, which are labeled in a series of letters known as P, QRS, and T. An ECG graphs the atrial depolarization, ventricular depolarization, and ventricular repolarization of each electrical impulse of the heart.

Sinoatrial node
(pacemaker)

Atrioventricular
node

Atrioventricular
bundle (bundle of His)

Bundle branches

Purkinje fibers

Purkinje
fibers

Figure 27-2 ■ Electrical conduction
system of the heart.

✳ Apply Your Knowledge 27.1

The following questions focus on what you have just learned about the anatomy and physiology of the cardiovascular system.

CRITICAL THINKING

1. What are the major functions of the cardiovascular system?
2. What are the names of the heart wall layers?
3. What is the structure of the electrical conduction system?
4. What are the locations and names of the four valves in the heart?
5. What is the difference between pulmonary and systemic circulation?

Coronary Heart Disease

When the delivery of oxygen to the myocardium is inadequate to meet the heart's oxygen consumption needs, myocardial **ischemia** occurs, which is insufficient blood flow to the myocardium. One of the major causes of ischemia is CAD, including *atherosclerosis* (blockage of an artery) and *arteriosclerosis* (hardening of an artery).

Angina pectoris is an episodic, reversible oxygen insufficiency. Oxygen demand is directly related to the strength of contraction, heart rate, and resistance to blood flow. Angina pectoris may result from the obstruction or narrowing of coronary arteries by fatty deposits or clots, arterial spasm, pulmonary hypertension, and *cardiac hypertrophy* (enlargement of the heart).

Antianginal drugs are used primarily for the treatment of angina pectoris. There are several types of angina:

✳ *Classical (stable) angina* is the most common form and often occurs during exertion, emotional stress, or indigestion caused by excessive eating or a meal rich in fats and proteins. It usually causes chest discomfort, which is relieved by rest, nitroglycerin, or both. The pain typically radiates to the jaw, neck, shoulder, and left arm. Stable angina is characteristically caused by a fixed obstruction in a coronary artery.

✳ *Variant* or *vasospastic angina* is the result of a coronary artery spasm that reduces blood flow. It usually occurs at rest rather than with exertion or emotional stress.

✳ *Unstable angina* is caused by significant CAD. It occurs at rest for the first time and decreases in response to rest or nitroglycerin. Unstable angina is often a warning of an MI.

THERAPEUTIC AGENTS FOR CORONARY HEART DISEASE

Antianginal drugs are used primarily to dilate coronary blood vessels. The mainstays of treatment include the following three classes of drugs:

✳ Organic nitrates
✳ Beta-adrenergic blockers (also called beta-blockers)
✳ Calcium channel blockers

Although nitrates and calcium channel blockers dilate coronary arteries, this dilation makes a minimal contribution to their antianginal effects except in vasospastic angina.

Organic Nitrates

The oldest and most frequently prescribed drugs for the different types of angina are organic nitrates, administered to stop an acute angina attack. Inhaled amyl nitrate, translingual spray (administered onto or under the tongue), or sublingual nitrates have a rapid onset of action and are effective for short periods. Various dosage forms of organic nitrates, also called *organonitrates*, are listed in Table 27-1 ■.

Table 27-1 ■ Organic Nitrates and Other Anginal Medications

GENERIC NAME	TRADE NAME	AVERAGE ADULT DOSAGE	ROUTES OF ADMINISTRATION
Nitrates			
nitroglycerin	Nitrolingual	0.4–0.8 mg prn	Translingual spray
	Nitrostat	0.15–0.6 mg prn	Sublingual
	Nitro-Dur	0.2–0.4 mg/hr; with patch 12–14 h on and 10–12 h off	Transdermal patch
	Rectiv	375 mg q12h for up to 3 weeks	Rectal ointment
	Nitro-Bid	5 mcg/min continuous infusion, increase by 5 mcg/min q3–5min prn (maximum: 20 mcg/min)	IV
isosorbide dinitrate	Isordil, Dilatrate-SR	2.5–40 mg tid	Sublingual
isosorbide mononitrate	Imdur, ISMO	20 mg bid	PO
Beta-Adrenergic Blockers			
atenolol	Tenormin	50–200 mg/d	PO
metoprolol	Lopressor	100–400 mg bid	PO, IV
	Toprol XL	100 mg/d	PO
nadolol	Corgard	Initial: 40 mg/d; increase in 40–80 mg increments at 3–7 day intervals	PO
propranolol	Inderal	10–90 mg bid or qid	PO

GENERIC NAME	TRADE NAME	AVERAGE ADULT DOSAGE	ROUTES OF ADMINISTRATION
Calcium Channel Blockers (see Table 27-3 for other calcium channel blockers used as antidysrhythmics.)			
diltiazem	Dilacor XR	120–480 mg/d	PO
nicardipine	Cardene SR	30–60 mg bid	PO
	Cardene IV	20–40 mg q8h	IV
nifedipine	Procardia	10–20 mg tid	PO
verapamil	Calan, Covera-HS, Isoptin SR, Verelan	80 mg q6–8h; may increase up to 320–480 mg/d in divided doses (Covera-HS must be given once daily at bedtime)	PO

IV, intravenous; tid, three times a day; PO, oral; bid, twice a day; qid, four times a day.

Focus On

Nitroglycerin

The classic organic nitrate nitroglycerin was once the drug of choice for the treatment of patients with angina pectoris. Nitroglycerin is effective, inexpensive, and fast acting.

How does it work?

Nitroglycerin directly affects the vascular smooth muscle to dilate blood vessels. It decreases cardiac oxygen demand in stable angina, but in variant angina, it relaxes the spasms and increases oxygen supply.

How is it used?

Nitroglycerin preparations are administered by using a variety of routes, producing similar responses but differing in the time of onset and duration. Some of these preparations are rapidly effective within 1–5 minutes, and last about 60 minutes. For others, the effect is slower in onset but lasts several hours. Only a few medications have a rapid onset and long duration of action. They can be used to relieve acute anginal pain or prophylactically to prevent angina attack with extended-release forms.

Sublingual nitroglycerin is effective rapidly, lasts about 1 hour, and is an ideal preparation for acute anginal pain. By this route of administration, it avoids hepatic first-pass metabolism. If one dose is not sufficient, one or two additional doses should be taken at 5-minute intervals. The medication bottle should not be opened unless it is needed because its shelf-life is longer in a dark and tightly closed container.

Transdermal nitroglycerin can release its reservoir slowly for absorption through the skin. These patches should be applied once a day to a hairless site of skin. The patch sites should be rotated daily to prevent local irritation. The patch should not be worn for more than 10–12 hours per day; this so-called "off" period is necessary to prevent the development of a tolerance to the drug and allows for continued therapeutic efficacy.

Nitroglycerin is also available as a topical ointment that must be measured on a paper provided with the prescription to ensure proper dosage. See Chapter 7 for the application of percutaneous medications. Discontinuation of nitroglycerin should take place over time because discontinuation of long-acting nitroglycerin preparations can cause **vasospasms** and angina.

What are the adverse effects?

The most common adverse effects include headache, **hypotension**, which is an abnormal condition in which the blood pressure is not adequate for full oxygenation of the tissues, and **tachycardia**, which is an abnormally fast heartbeat. The dizziness and lightheadedness of hypotension are better tolerated with time.

What are the contraindications and interactions?

Nitroglycerin's contraindications include obstructive hypertrophic cardiomyopathy, pronounced *hypovolemia* (decrease in the volume of circulating blood), inferior MI with right ventricular involvement, increased intracranial

(continued)

Focus On (continued)

pressure, and *cardiac tamponade* (blockage in the heart). It should not be stopped abruptly after long therapy because there is a rebound risk of more frequent angina pectoris. Nitroglycerin reinforces the hypotensive effect of antihypertensive agents. If combined with alcohol, a sudden decrease in blood pressure can occur. Nitroglycerin increases the bioavailability of dihydroergotamine. In smokers, nicotine antagonizes the coronary dilating effect of nitroglycerin. Nitroglycerin is also contraindicated in pregnancy and lactation.

What are the important points patients should know?

Advise patients that nitroglycerin should not be carried close to the body because heat from the body can deactivate it. Tell patients to store the medication in a cool, dark place and keep it in the original container. Advise patients to avoid alcoholic beverages when taking nitroglycerin and to take one tablet sublingually every 5 minutes, not exceeding three tablets. Tell patients that if chest pain continues, they should seek emergency medical attention. Advise patients to discard unused tablets after 6 months.

Focus Point

Nitroglycerin

Nitroglycerin may cause severe low blood pressure, which is marked by dizziness or lightheadedness, especially if an individual is in an upright position or has just gotten up from sitting or lying down. The heart rate can slow, and chest pain can increase. People taking diuretic medications and those who have low systolic blood pressure of less than 90 mm Hg should use nitroglycerin with caution.

Isosorbide dinitrate and isosorbide mononitrate are other forms of organic nitrates that provide longer durations of action than nitroglycerin. These agents are effective in the treatment of all types of angina pectoris and are available in sublingual and chewable tablet forms. The most common complaint by users is headache. Both agents should be given cautiously to patients with glaucoma (see Chapter 37). The advantage of isosorbide mononitrate over isosorbide dinitrate is that there is no first-pass metabolism.

Beta-Adrenergic Blockers

Beta-adrenergic blockers are known as *beta-blockers* or *β-blockers*. Examples include propranolol and atenolol. These agents reduce the heart's oxygen demand by decreasing the heart rate. In the heart, **sympathetic** stimulation causes increased rate and force as well as increased oxygen use. The term *sympathetic* relates to the sympathetic part of the autonomic nervous system, or the *fight-or-flight* response. Beta-blockers prevent the development of myocardial ischemia and pain. Propranolol is often used for the treatment of angina, and it may be used in combination with nitrates for controlling angina. Beta-blockers should be used with caution or avoided in patients with asthma because of the potential for bronchospasm, and they may mask hypoglycemia in patients with diabetes mellitus. Beta-blockers may produce **insomnia**, bizarre dreams, and depression. See Table 27-1 for dosages and routes of transmission. Beta-blockers are discussed in more depth later in this chapter.

Focus on Natural Products

Food and Drug Interactions

Many natural substances, including food, interact with pharmaceuticals; for example, warfarin sodium interacts with such foods as beef liver, broccoli, Brussels sprouts, cabbage, spinach, and other leafy green vegetables. These foods contain large amounts of vitamin K, which decreases the effect of the drug.

Calcium Channel Blockers

Calcium channel blockers such as verapamil interfere with the movement of calcium ions through cell membranes. These drugs can affect the heart itself or the peripheral vasculature. They are used to treat the pain of angina pectoris and to lower blood pressure. Contraction of the vascular smooth muscle depends on calcium movement from extracellular to intracellular sites.

The prevention of calcium action inhibits this contraction. Therefore, it decreases vascular tone and causes **vasodilation**, which is the dilation of blood vessels. Vasodilation relaxes the smooth muscle of the peripheral arterioles. Calcium channel blockers are prescribed for vasospastic angina. They are used for the treatment of angina, dysrhythmia, and hypertension (see Tables 27-1 and 27-3 for dosages and routes of delivery). Calcium channel blockers are discussed in detail in a later section of this chapter.

✳ Apply Your Knowledge 27.2

The following questions focus on what you have just learned about CHD and related therapeutic agents.

CRITICAL THINKING

1. What are the most common types of angina?
2. What are three classes of antianginal drugs?
3. What is the mechanism of action of nitroglycerin?
4. What is the advantage of isosorbide mononitrate over isosorbide dinitrate?
5. What types of organic nitrates are used in the prophylaxis of angina pectoris?
6. What are the most common adverse effects of nitroglycerin?
7. What are some of the trade names of nitroglycerin?
8. Which type of angina occurs at rest for the first time?

Myocardial Infarction

An *acute myocardial infarction (AMI)* occurs when a part of the myocardium experiences a severe and prolonged restriction of oxygenated coronary blood. Nearly 40% of all patients experiencing AMI die before reaching acute care health centers. An AMI can occur when an area of the heart muscle dies through lack of sufficient oxygen. AMI is the leading cause of death in industrialized nations, possibly because of a diet high in cholesterol and fat and a sedentary lifestyle. The insufficient oxygen supply to the myocardium is the result of: (1) a decreased flow of oxygen-rich blood to the heart muscle, and (2) an increased demand for oxygen by the myocardium that exceeds what the circulation can supply. The main causes of AMI are CAD, clot formation in the coronary artery or spasm of these arteries, stress, heavy exertion, and an abrupt increase in blood pressure.

Focus on Pediatrics

Acute Myocardial Infarction in Children

AMI is rare in childhood. Adults usually develop CAD from the lifelong buildup of *atheroma*, which is a yellow-tinted swelling of the arteries that is characteristic of atherosclerosis, and *plaque*, which causes coronary artery spasm and thrombosis. Pediatric patients with AMI usually have either an acute inflammatory condition of the coronary arteries or an anomalous origin of the left coronary artery.

THERAPEUTIC AGENTS FOR MYOCARDIAL INFARCTION

The goal of treatment of patients with AMI is to limit damage to the myocardium, thereby preserving enough myocardial function to sustain life. In addition to intravenous (IV) fluids, pharmacotherapeutics are used as the first line of treatment for AMI. Treatment is designed to relieve distress, reverse ischemia, limit the size of *infarct* (the amount of tissue death related to lack of arterial or venous blood), reduce cardiac work, and prevent and treat complications. AMI is an acute medical emergency, and outcome is significantly influenced by rapid diagnosis and treatment. Fifty percent of deaths from AMI occur within 3–4 hours of onset of the clinical **syndrome** (a collection of signs and symptoms that together signify a specific disease). The outcome can be influenced by early treatment.

Nitroglycerin is administered to decrease the heart's workload and increase blood supply to the heart muscle. Aspirin and thrombolytic drugs are most effective if given within the first few minutes and hours after the onset of MI. The greatest risk of thrombolytic therapy is hemorrhage (bleeding), specifically inside the brain. Anticoagulants are discussed in Chapter 30.

Morphine sulfate—2–4 mg IV; repeated as needed—is a critical adjunct to nitroglycerin. Morphine is highly effective for the pain of MI. Potential side effects of morphine are the depression of respiration and reduction of myocardial contractility. Hypotension and **bradycardia**, an abnormally slow heartbeat, secondary to morphine, can usually be overcome by prompt elevation of the lower extremities. Such beta-blockers as metoprolol and atenolol reduce the heart's oxygen demand by decreasing the heart rate. Such calcium channel blockers as nifedipine and diltiazem decrease myocardial oxygen demand and increase oxygen supply. Oxygen is also reasonably administered via 40% mask or nasal prongs at 4–6 L/min for the first few hours.

✳ Apply Your Knowledge 27.3

The following questions focus on what you have just learned about MI and its therapeutic agents.

CRITICAL THINKING

1. What are causes of insufficient oxygen supply to the myocardium?
2. Why is acute MI rare in childhood?
3. What is the goal of treatment in acute MI?
4. What are the mainstays of treatment in acute MI?
5. What is the definition of bradycardia?
6. What are the adverse effects of morphine to relieve pain in MI?

Dysrhythmias

The rate of heartbeat and rhythm of the heart are controlled by the SA node, sometimes termed the *pacemaker*, in the right atrium. This node generates tiny electrical impulses to the adjacent muscle of the atrium, causing the atria to contract and pump blood into the ventricles. The impulses sent out by the SA node are received by the AV node, travel down the bundle of His, and are transported to the ventricular muscles by a network of nerves. The SA node and the AV node receive autonomic innervations that control the rate of the heart to a certain extent.

Any deviation from the normal orderly sequence of impulses is a disturbance of the rhythm and is called a **dysrhythmia** or an *arrhythmia*. Sometimes, an area of muscle in one of the atria becomes more excitable than the SA node and fires more rapid impulses. The rest of the heart then responds to this new pacemaker, and the resulting dysrhythmia is known as *atrial tachycardia*. Dysrhythmias may be benign, as in atrial tachycardia, or malignant, as in ventricular tachycardia. Benign abnormalities generally have a low risk of sudden death. Malignant abnormalities have a moderate risk of sudden death. Malignant arrhythmias indicate an immediate risk for heart disease. Table 27-2 ■ summarizes different arrhythmias and beats per minute.

ANTIDYSRHYTHMIC AGENTS

Dysrhythmias can occur from heart disease or from chronic drug therapy. Dysrhythmias can also be caused by the drugs used to regulate them because they create

Table 27-2 ■ Various Dysrhythmias

ARRHYTHMIA	BEATS PER MINUTE
Bradycardia	Less than 60
Tachycardia	150–250
Atrial flutter	200–350
Atrial fibrillation	More than 350
Ventricular fibrillation	Variable
Premature atrial contraction	Variable
Premature ventricular contraction	Variable

an alteration of the heart's electrical impulse. When severe dysrhythmia occurs, especially in ventricular disorders, the patient can be experiencing a medical emergency requiring hospital care.

Antidysrhythmic drug therapy is the mainstay of management for most important dysrhythmias. There is no universally effective drug. All these agents have important safety limitations and can aggravate or promote arrhythmias. Drug selection is difficult and often involves trial and error (Table 27-3 ■).

Antidysrhythmic drug actions based on cellular electrophysiologic effects have been classified into four groups. This classification is recognized internationally and provides a general logic for grouping drugs. Classifications of antidysrhythmic drugs are seen in Table 27-3.

Table 27-3 ■ Antidysrhythmic Medications

GENERIC NAME	TRADE NAME	AVERAGE ADULT DOSAGE	ROUTES OF ADMINISTRATION
Class Ia			
quinidine sulfate	Quinidine Sulfate	Initial: 300 mg q8–12h; followed by individualized dosage adjustments	PO
disopyramide	Norpace	400–800 mg/d in divided doses	PO
Class Ib			
lidocaine	Xylocaine	1–1.5 mg/kg; may repeat 0.5–1.5 mg/kg q5–10min, to total of 3 mg/kg	IV
	(Generic only for IM administration)	4.3 mg/kg	IM
phenytoin	Dilantin	100 mg q5min	PO
Class Ic			
flecainide	Tambocor	Initially, 100 mg q12h; increase in 50-mg increments twice daily q4d until effective	PO
propafenone	Rythmol	450 mg/d; increase dosage slowly if needed, up to 900 mg/d	PO
Class II			
esmolol	Brevibloc	50–500 mcg/min	IV
propranolol	Inderal	10–30 mg 3–4 times/d before meals and at bedtime	PO
metoprolol	Lopressor	100 mg/d in two divided doses	PO
		5 mg q2min for three doses followed by PO	IV
acebutolol	Sectral	Initially, 200 mg bid; dose is increased gradually until the optimal response is obtained.	PO
Class III			
amiodarone	Cordarone	400–1,600 mg/d	PO
	Cordarone IV	150 mg over 10 min, followed by 360 mg over the next 6 h	IV loading dose
dronedarone	Multaq	400 mg bid	PO

(*continued*)

Table 27-3 ■ **Antidysrhythmic Medications** (*continued*)

GENERIC NAME	TRADE NAME	AVERAGE ADULT DOSAGE	ROUTES OF ADMINISTRATION
sotalol	Betapace	80–320 mg/d	PO
dofetilide	Tikosyn	125–250 mcg bid	PO
ibutilide	Corvert	Weight <60 kg, 0.01 mg/kg (0.1 mL/kg) injection; weight >60 kg, 1 mg (10 mL)	IV
bretylium	Bretylium	5–10 mg/kg by rapid infusion	IM, IV
Class IV			
verapamil	Calan	240–480 mg/d divided into 3–4 doses	PO
	(Generic only for IV administration)	Initially, 5–10 mg as IV bolus over 2 min	IV
diltiazem	Cardizem, Tiazac	60–120 mg sustained-release bid	PO
	Cardizem IV	0.25 mg/kg IV bolus over 2 min	IV

PO, oral; IM, intramuscular; IV, intravenous.

Class I—Drugs That Bind to Sodium Channels

Class I drugs are sodium channel blockers, including older antidysrhythmic drugs such as quinidine. These drugs reduce the maximal rate of contraction of the myocardium and slow conduction. Class I drugs are subclassified into three classes:

Class Ia—drugs with intermediate onset and offset
Class Ib—drugs with short effects
Class Ic—drugs with prolonged effects

Focus On

Quinidine (Class Ia)

Quinidine is approved for atrial **fibrillation**, which is very rapid, irregular contractions or twitching of the individual muscle fibers of the atria or ventricles, and **flutter**, which is rapid, regular atrial contractions that often produce "sawtooth" waves in an ECG or rapid ventricular tachycardia that appears as a regular, undulating pattern in an ECG, without QRS and T waves, as would normally be found. Quinidine is related to quinine and has been used in cardiac conditions since the 1920s.

How does it work?

Quinidine depresses the myocardium and the conduction system, decreasing the contractile force of the heart and slowing the heart rate.

How is it used?

If an initial test dose of quinidine sulfate is tolerated, the maintenance dosage is usually 200–400 mg orally every 4–6 hours. A salt form of quinidine gluconate is also available in IM and IV forms. Sustained-release forms are also available for the sulfate and gluconate salts.

What are the adverse effects?

Adverse reactions include diarrhea, flatulence, and abdominal pain. Fever, reduced platelets and megakaryocyte fragments (important in the clotting of blood), and liver function abnormalities can occur. Quinidine syncope, which is sudden ventricular fibrillation in patients taking quinidine, is potentially dangerous and can be life-threatening.

What are the contraindications and interactions?

Quinidine is contraindicated in pregnancy, lactation, bacterial endocarditis, and myasthenia gravis. Quinidine has the potential to double digoxin levels in the blood. Potentially fatal interactions can occur when quinidine is given with digoxin. Quinidine also interacts with amiodarone and verapamil.

What are the important points patients should know?

Tell patients to immediately report any chest pain or change in heart rhythm to their health care provider.

Advise patients to take quinidine with food to avoid gastric upset, although this may delay absorption of the drug. A diet high in citrus fruits, vegetables, and milk may delay excretion of the drug, so advise patients not to increase their intake of these foods beyond their normal diet. Advise patients to report diarrhea to their health care provider.

DISOPYRAMIDE (CLASS Ia)

Disopyramide decreases cardiac excitability and is a cardiac depressant. Oral dosing is usually 100–150 mg every 6 hours. Adverse effects are dry mouth, constipation, visual disturbances, and urine retention.

LIDOCAINE (CLASS Ib)

Lidocaine can suppress the ventricular arrhythmias that complicate MI and reduce the incidence of primary ventricular fibrillation when given prophylactically in early AMI. Its mechanism of action appears to be the blocking of activated and inactivated sodium channels, with a great effect on depolarized or ischemic tissues. Adverse effects are neurologic, such as tremor and convulsions, rather than cardiac. Drowsiness, delirium, and *paresthesias* (abnormal burning, pricking, tickling, or tingling) may occur with too-rapid administration. Lidocaine has noted drug interactions with cimetidine (Tagamet).

PHENYTOIN (CLASS Ib)

Phenytoin was used extensively for dysrhythmia management, particularly for suppressing the ventricular dysrhythmias of digitalis toxicity, until the advent of newer drugs and the decline of digoxin toxicity. Now phenytoin is most commonly used for epilepsy. The common adverse effects are **gingival hyperplasia** (an increase in the number of cells in the gums of the mouth, causing them to have a swollen appearance), blurred vision, **vertigo** (sensation of revolving, either of the patients themselves or of their environment), and **nystagmus** (constant, involuntary movement of the eyes). Phenytoin has noted drug interactions with cimetidine, disulfiram, dopamine, and fluconazole.

FLECAINIDE (CLASS Ic)

Flecainide is an antidysrhythmic agent with electrophysiologic properties similar to those of other class Ic antidysrhythmic drugs. It is used for the treatment of patients with life-threatening ventricular dysrhythmias. Adverse effects include dizziness, headache, fatigue, chest pain, and blurred vision. Flecainide may also produce nausea, constipation, and a change in taste perception.

PROPAFENONE (CLASS Ic)

Propafenone is another class Ic antidysrhythmic drug with a direct stabilizing action on myocardial membranes. It is used for the treatment and management of patients with ventricular dysrhythmias. Adverse effects include blurred vision, dizziness, fatigue, **somnolence**, vertigo, and headache. It may also cause hypotension, nausea and vomiting, abdominal discomfort, constipation, dry mouth, and taste alterations.

Class II—Beta-Adrenergic Blockers

Beta-blockers may be the least toxic and most powerful drugs available, but their antidysrhythmic effects are often overlooked. Relatively few dysrhythmias are caused primarily by sympathetic overactivity; most are regulated by *autonomic tone*, which is the firmness of muscles as controlled by the autonomic nervous system.

Overactivity of the sympathetic nerves releases norepinephrine and epinephrine. These agents increase heart rate, heart excitability, conduction velocity, and **automaticity** (the heart impulse's automatic, spontaneous initiation, particularly of the ventricles). In general, beta-blockers are well tolerated, but they may depress left-ventricular function, particularly in antiarrhythmic doses. They are contraindicated in people with asthma. Gastrointestinal disturbances, insomnia, and nightmares may occur. Beta-adrenergic blockers are discussed in Chapter 28.

Focus On

Propranolol (Class II)

Propranolol is the most common beta-blocker used as an antidysrhythmic. Before 1978, it was the only beta-blocker approved to treat dysrhythmias. Since then, several other beta-blockers have been approved to treat dysrhythmias, but propranolol is still the mainstay of treatment.

How does it work?

Propranolol affects both types of beta receptors; because of this, it is considered a nonselective beta-blocker. It reduces or slows the heart rate and lowers blood pressure. In addition to its beta-blocking effect, it also causes a quinidine-like depression of the myocardium.

How is it used?

Propranolol is often combined with other cardiovascular drugs, such as digoxin and quinidine, to treat patients with CVD. It is most effective for tachycardia, but it is also approved to treat a broad range of other disorders, such as hypertension and angina, and for the prevention of MI.

What are the adverse effects?

Hypotension and bradycardia are the most common side effects. Patients with other cardiac disorders, such as heart failure, must be carefully monitored because propranolol can slow the heart rate. Such side effects as diminished sex drive and impotence can also occur.

What are the contraindications and interactions?

Propranolol is contraindicated in bronchial asthma or bronchospasm, severe chronic obstructive airway disease, allergic rhinitis during pollen season, and pregnancy. Propranolol interacts with clonidine, cimetidine, epinephrine, and insulin.

What are the important points patients should know?

Propranolol should not be abruptly discontinued because it may cause MI or severe dysrhythmias. Tell the patient to take his or her pulse on a regular basis; if the pulse is less than 60 beats per minute, the patient's health care provider should be notified immediately. Because of propranolol's potential to cause hypotension, advise the patient to slowly rise from a lying or sitting position.

Class III—Drugs That Interfere with Potassium Outflow

Class III antidysrhythmic agents—potassium channel blockers—interfere with potassium channels to alter the repolarization phase of the heart's contraction. This prolongs the potential contraction duration of the Purkinje fibers and the muscle fibers of the ventricles. The prolonged period decreases the frequency of heart failure.

Focus On

Amiodarone

Amiodarone is a powerful class III antidysrhythmic agent.

How does it work?

Amiodarone blocks potassium ion channels as well as sodium ion channels. This action prolongs the resting stage of the heart's contraction as well as the refractory period, which stabilizes atrial and ventricular dysrhythmias.

How is it used?

It is used to treat atrial dysrhythmias in patients with heart failure. Oral dosage forms may take several weeks to produce an effect. However, its effects can last 4–8 weeks after it is discontinued because of its extended half-life. An IV form is available, but it is usually reserved for patients with serious ventricular dysrhythmias.

What are the adverse effects?

Amiodarone has few cardiovascular adverse effects, perhaps because of its modest vasodilator action, which produces little or no left-ventricular depression. SA node activity is minimally affected. Amiodarone decreases automaticity, prolongs AV conduction, and can even block the exchange of sodium and potassium. Amiodarone is too toxic for long-term use except for serious ventricular dysrhythmias. Pulmonary fibrosis can occur in some patients treated with the drug for more than 5 years and could be fatal. Other significant potential adverse effects include changes in thyroid function—hypothyroidism or hyperthyroidism—and visual disturbances as a result of optic neuritis or corneal microdeposits. Common adverse effects that may be self-limiting include dizziness, nausea and vomiting, anorexia, bitter taste, weight loss, and numbness of the fingers and toes. Weakness can also occur.

What are the contraindications and interactions?

Amiodarone is contraindicated in patients with severe liver disease, pregnancy, children, and severe sinus bradycardia. Amiodarone interacts with many other drugs, including digoxin and phenytoin.

What are the important points patients should know?

Tell patients to notify their health-care providers immediately if shortness of breath, cough, or a change in heart rate and rhythm occurs. Also, instruct patients to immediately report any vision changes to their health-care providers. Advise patients to change positions slowly to avoid dizziness. Advise patients, especially elderly patients, to protect their skin and eyes from the sun.

SOTALOL

Sotalol has class II and III antidysrhythmic properties. Although measurable class III effects can be detected in clinical use, they are largely masked by the drug's beta-blocking properties. Sotalol is used for the treatment of documented ventricular arrhythmias that, in the judgment of the physician, are life-threatening.

DOFETILIDE

Dofetilide is a class III antidysrhythmic agent that prolongs the cardiac action potential by blocking the potassium channels. It is used for the treatment of symptomatic atrial fibrillation and flutter. Adverse effects on the body as a whole include flu-like syndrome and back pain. The most common adverse effects of dofetilide are headache, dizziness, insomnia, nausea, diarrhea, and abdominal pain.

IBUTILIDE

Ibutilide is a newly approved class III drug that differs markedly from amiodarone and sotalol. It achieves its effect by activating a slow, inward sodium current rather than by blocking outward potassium currents. Injecting ibutilide can acutely terminate atrial fibrillation and atrial flutter, particularly in patients with recent onset of dysrhythmia.

BRETYLIUM

Bretylium also has antisympathetic class III action. It may cause marked hypotension and is indicated only for the management of potentially lethal **refractory** ventricular tachyarrhythmias. The term *refractory* means the period during repolarization when cells cannot respond normally to a second stimulus. Bretylium is usually effective within 30 minutes of injection.

Class IV—Calcium Channel Blockers

Class IV drugs are termed *calcium channel blockers* because they decrease the entry of calcium into the cells of the heart and blood vessels. The SA and AV nodes require calcium for normal activity and normal sinus rhythm. Reducing calcium decreases the rate of the SA node and the conduction velocity of the AV node, and it is effective in the treatment of supraventricular tachycardia. Class IV drugs can decrease the ability of the heart to produce forceful contractions, leading to CHF. These medications also relax smooth muscle and cause vasodilation. Therefore, these agents are useful for angina and hypertension.

Focus on Geriatrics

Heart Failure and Surgery

The chance of having heart failure increases as we age. One in 15 elderly patients between the ages of 75 and 84 years is diagnosed with some type of heart failure. Men are affected more than women. CHD, heart failure, and clinically significant dysrhythmias require in-depth evaluation and control before any type of elective, noncardiac surgery is performed.

Focus On

Verapamil

Verapamil was the first calcium channel blocker approved by the FDA.

How does it work?

Verapamil acts principally on the AV node, slowing conduction. Therefore, it causes the depression of myocardial contractibility and dilation of coronary arteries. These effects lead to decreased cardiac work and cardiac energy consumption in patients with vasospastic angina. This effect increases the delivery of oxygen to myocardial cells.

How is it used?

Verapamil is used to stabilize dysrhythmias. It is also approved for use in hypertension and angina. For dysrhythmias, it is prescribed in oral forms, but sustained-release and IV forms are also available.

What are the adverse effects?

The adverse effects are dizziness, vertigo, emotional depression, sleepiness, headache, peripheral edema, hypotension, nausea, and constipation.

What are the contraindications and interactions?

Verapamil is contraindicated in patients with an allergy to this agent, hypotension, pregnancy, lactation, and CHF. Verapamil interacts with carbamazepine, lithium, cyclosporine, and calcium salts. It may also increase blood levels of digoxin.

What are the important points patients should know?

Instruct patients to take their blood pressure before taking verapamil. They should contact their health care provider if their blood pressure is below 90/60 mm Hg. Advise patients to notify their health care provider if they experience any breathing difficulty or change in heart rhythm. Also, advise patients to take verapamil with food to avoid an upset stomach and to increase their intake of fiber to avoid constipation.

Focus Point

Top 10 Prescribed Cardiovascular Drugs

1. rosuvastatin (Crestor)
2. valsartan (Diovan)
3. ezetimibe (Zetia)
4. rivaroxaban (Xarelto)
5. olmesartan (Benicar)
6. ezetimibe/simvastatin (Vytorin)
7. nebivolol (Bystolic)
8. olmesartan/hydrochlorothiazide (Benicar HCT)
9. metoprolol (Toprol-XL)
10. amlodipine/valsartan (Exforge)

DILTIAZEM

Diltiazem is less potent than verapamil in decreasing heart rate but is more potent as a vasodilator. It is used for essential hypertension, angina pectoris caused by coronary artery spasm and such dysrhythmias as atrial fibrillation, atrial flutter, and supraventricular tachycardia. Adverse effects include headache, fatigue, dizziness, nervousness, insomnia, and confusion. It may also cause edema, flushing, hypotension, nausea and vomiting, and impaired taste. Diltiazem has noted drug interactions with cyclosporine.

Focus Point

Look-Alike and Sound-Alike Drugs

Drug Name and Purpose	Looks Like/Sounds Like
amiodarone (antidysrhythmic)	amrinone (cardiac inotropic agent)
dopamine (heart stimulant)	dobutamine (sympathetic A and B agonist)
metoprolol (beta-blocker)	misoprostol (prostaglandin analog for ulcer therapy)
Lanoxin (digoxin-cardiac glycoside)	Lasix (diuretic)
pindolol (beta-blocker)	Parlodel (dopaminergic agonist inhibitor of prolactin)
Propulsid (stimulator of GI function)	propranolol (beta-blocker)

✱ Apply Your **Knowledge 27.4**

The following questions focus on what you have just learned about dysrhythmias (arrhythmias) and their therapeutic agents.

CRITICAL THINKING

1. What are the causes of dysrhythmias?
2. What is the mainstay of management for the most important dysrhythmias?
3. What are the trade names of phenytoin, esmolol, amiodarone, and diltiazem?
4. What class of antidysrhythmic can bind to sodium channels?
5. Name examples of class 1a antidysrhythmic drugs.
6. What classes of antidysrhythmics are the least toxic and most powerful drugs available?
7. What drug is a powerful class III antidysrhythmic?
8. Which drug was the first calcium channel blocker approved by the FDA?

LABELING

Answer the following drug labeling questions by using the label depicted below. You may need to use your drug guide or the *Physicians' Desk Reference* to answer some of the questions.

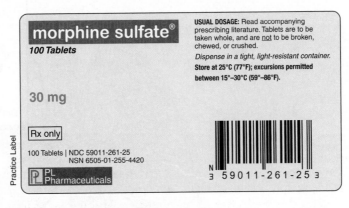

(For educational purposes only)

(continued)

Apply Your Knowledge 27.4 (*continued*)

1. Generic name: _____

2. Drug class: _____

3. Form of drug: _____

4. Drug schedule (use "Rx" if not a scheduled drug): _____

5. Adult dosage: _____

6. Typical use: _____

7. Body system that this drug targets: _____

8. Manufacturer: _____

9. Storage requirements: _____

10. Pregnancy category: _____

Congestive Heart Failure

Congestive heart failure (CHF) is a very common cardiovascular disorder in which the heart, under normal filling conditions, cannot pump adequate amounts of blood to meet the metabolic demands of the body tissues. The inability to pump blood may be caused by various abnormalities in the myocardium. This condition results in gradual congestion of both the cardiopulmonary and vascular systems. The kidneys retain salt and water. The patient experiences tiredness, shortness of breath after exertion, palpitations, weakness or dizziness, **tachypnea**, and tachycardia. As the condition progresses, fluid builds up in the interstitial spaces of the vascular system, resulting in distention of the neck veins and edema in the lower legs, ankles, and feet. There is shortness of breath while at rest, weight gain, coughing or wheezing especially while lying down, the need to urinate more at night, and feelings of bloating or nausea. CHF results in blood accumulating in the heart chambers and the stretching of the heart walls. The heart, veins, and capillaries become generally dilated with blood, and the organs receive less blood circulation. Blood volume increases as less oxygen reaches the kidneys and fluid is retained. When fluid builds up inside the abdomen, it is called **ascites**.

Underlying causes of CHF include arteriosclerotic heart disease, hypertensive heart disease, valvular heart disease, dilated cardiomyopathy, and congenital heart disease. When CHF occurs in the right side of the heart,

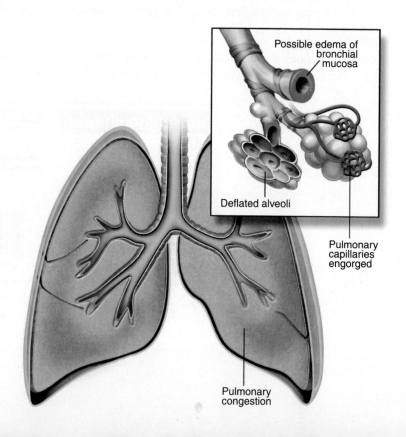

Figure 27-3 ■ Pulmonary congestion, which may result from congestive heart failure.

there is congestion of the liver and spleen, as well as peripheral edema. When CHF occurs in the left side of the heart, there is congestion and edema of the lungs (see Figure 27-3 ■). Left systolic dysfunction secondary to coronary artery disease is the most common cause of heart failure.

The therapeutic goal for CHF is to increase cardiac output. Three classes of drugs have been shown to be clinically effective in reducing symptoms and prolonging life: inotropic drugs, diuretics, and vasodilators (which include ACE inhibitors). Table 27-4 ■ lists the main classes of drugs used for CHF.

Table 27-4 ■ Main Classes of Drugs Used for Congestive Heart Failure

GENERIC NAME	TRADE NAME	AVERAGE ADULT DOSAGE	ROUTE OF ADMINISTRATION
Inotropic Drugs				
Cardiac Glycosides			
digitoxin	Crystodigin	150 mcg daily (maximum: 0.3 mg/d)	PO
digoxin	Lanoxin	10–15 mcg/kg in divided doses over 24–48 h and then 0.1–0.375 mg/d	PO
		10–15 mcg/kg in divided doses over 24 h and then 0.1–0.375 mg/d	IV
Beta-Adrenergic Antagonists			
propranolol	Inderal	40 mg bid (usually need 160–480 mg/d in divided doses)	PO
Phosphodiesterase Inhibitors			
inamrinone lactate	(Generic only)	0.75 mg/kg bolus given slowly over 2–3 min and then start infusion at 5–10 mcg/kg/min; may repeat bolus in 30 min (maximum: 10 mg/kg/d)	IV
milrinone lactate	Primacor IV	Loading dose: 50 mcg/kg over 10 min; maintenance dose: 0.375–0.75 mcg/kg/min	IV
Diuretics (see Table 28-3)			
Vasodilators (see Table 28-2)			

PO, oral; IV, intravenous; bid, twice a day.

Focus On

Inotropic Drugs

Inotropic agents increase the cardiac muscle's strength of contraction. These drugs relieve the symptoms of cardiac insufficiency but do not reverse the underlying pathologic condition. Knowledge of the physiology of heart muscle contraction is essential to an understanding of the compensatory responses evoked by the failing heart as well as the actions of drugs used to treat CHF.

Inotropic drugs act by different mechanisms; in each case, the inotropic action is the result of an increased cell calcium concentration that enhances the contractility of cardiac muscle. Inotropic drugs include cardiac glycosides and beta-adrenergic agonists (see Table 27-4). Cardiac glycosides, such as digitoxin and digoxin, are obtained from the plant leaves of *Digitalis pupurea* and *Digitalis lanata*, respectively. They are all derived from natural sources whose medicinal qualities have been recognized for centuries. The cardiac glycosides are popular and effective drugs for the treatment of patients with CHF. They act by exerting a positive inotropic action on the heart, which increases the force of myocardial contraction, thereby improving the

(continued)

Focus On (continued)

mechanical efficiency of the heart as a blood-pumping organ. This ultimately results in a reduced heart size and increased blood flow to the kidneys.

How do they work?

Cardiac glycosides act by increasing the force and velocity of myocardial systolic contraction and decreasing conduction velocity through the atrioventricular node. Cardiac glycosides inhibit the enzyme *ATPase*, which is associated with the sodium pump, and the exchange between sodium and calcium is impaired. Stores of calcium within the myocardium are released, and the membrane becomes more permeable to this ion. As a result, intracellular calcium levels are elevated. Because calcium is necessary for normal muscle contraction, the elevated calcium levels result in a stronger force of contraction.

How are they used?

Digoxin is the most commonly prescribed digitalis preparation for treating patients with CHF. It is used for rapid digitalization and maintenance therapy in CHF as well as for atrial fibrillation and flutter. Digoxin and digitoxin—the two primary cardiac glycosides—are similar in efficacy. The main difference between the two drugs is that digitoxin has a more prolonged half-life.

What are the adverse effects?

Common adverse effects of cardiac glycosides include fatigue, muscle weakness, headache, mental depression, visual disturbances, anorexia, nausea and vomiting, and diarrhea.

What are the contraindications and interactions?

Cardiac glycosides are contraindicated in patients with digitalis hypersensitivity, ventricular fibrillation, and ventricular tachycardia (unless it is caused by CHF). These drugs should be used cautiously in patients with renal insufficiency, hypokalemia, advanced heart disease, acute MI, hypothyroidism, pregnancy, and lactation and in older adults.

Antacids, cholestyramine, and colestipol decrease digoxin absorption. Diuretics, corticosteroids, amphotericin B, and laxatives may cause hypokalemia.

What are the important points patients should know?

Advise patients who are taking digoxin for atrial fibrillation to report to their physicians a pulse rate that falls below 60 or rises above 110 beats per minute. Inform patients of the occurrence of anorexia, nausea and vomiting, diarrhea, or visual disturbances because these adverse effects may be caused by toxicity. They must report these adverse effects to their physician.

Digoxin must be taken exactly as prescribed and at the same time each day; be sure to tell patients to not skip or double a dose or change dose intervals. Patients should not take OTC medications, especially those for coughs, colds, allergies, GI upset, or obesity without the approval of their physician.

Focus on Natural Products

Foxglove and Digoxin

The cardiac drug digoxin is derived from foxglove, a purple flowering plant that has been described in the medical literature for more than 200 years as a treatment for heart disease. English physician William Withering is credited with discovering in 1775 that the foxglove plant could help those with a condition of abnormal fluid buildup, which, at that time, was called *dropsy.* In 1930, the glycosides of the woolly foxglove (*Digitalis lanata*) were isolated, and the drug digoxin was born. Similar to foxglove, other plants, such as oleander and lily of the valley, also have cardiac glycoside properties. Patients must be aware of taking digoxin and these herbs together because they may receive a toxic dose. Reports of digoxin toxicity are often linked with extracts and teas containing the foxglove, oleander, and lily of the valley herbs.

Focus Point

Cardiac Glycosides and Low Pulse

If the apical pulse falls below a set parameter in a patient taking cardiac glycosides, administration of the drug should be withheld and a physician notified.

BETA-ADRENERGIC AGONISTS

Beta-adrenergic stimulation improves cardiac performance by positive inotropic effects and vasodilation (see Chapter 35 for a detailed discussion of beta-adrenergic agonists).

PHOSPHODIESTERASE INHIBITORS

Phosphodiesterase inhibitors, such as inamrinone lactate and milrinone lactate, increase the force of the heart's contraction and cause vasodilation. They work by blocking the enzyme phosphodiesterase in cardiac and smooth muscle, resulting in a positive inotropic response and vasodilation. They are commonly used for the short-term control of acute heart failure, and they have high toxicity.

DIURETICS

Diuretics relieve the pulmonary congestion and peripheral edema common in CHF. These agents are useful in reducing the symptoms of volume overload, including orthopnea and paroxysmal nocturnal dyspnea. Diuretics decrease plasma volume and subsequently decrease venous return to the heart (preload). This decreases the cardiac workload and oxygen demand. Diuretics also decrease afterload by reducing plasma volume, thus decreasing blood pressure. Diuretics are discussed in detail in Chapter 31.

✳ Apply Your Knowledge 27.5

The following questions focus on what you have just learned about CHF and its treatment.

CRITICAL THINKING

1. Describe the signs and symptoms of congestive heart failure.
2. Compare and contrast right-sided and left-sided congestive heart failure.
3. What is the mechanism of action of inotropic drugs?
4. What is the most commonly prescribed digitalis preparation for treating congestive heart failure?
5. What are the trade names of inamrinone, milrinone, digoxin, and digitoxin?

PRACTICAL SCENARIO 1

A 60-year-old man called emergency medical services, complaining of severe angina and dizziness. He told the paramedic he had been prescribed nitroglycerin for angina pectoris and was taking it as needed. He stated that he always kept a little envelope of the drug in his breast pocket and the rest in his car in case he needed more. About 2 hours earlier, he reported he had finished a large meal preceded by a cocktail and accompanied by wine. When he felt the pain begin, he slipped a nitroglycerin tablet under his tongue. When it had no effect after 10 minutes, he took another, waited, and then took another. Nothing stopped the pain, and now he was afraid he was having a heart attack. His ECG was negative for MI. The paramedic realized why the nitroglycerin did not alleviate his angina.

Michal Heron/Pearson Education/PH College

Critical Thinking Questions

1. What were the "clues" that helped the paramedic figure out why the nitroglycerin did not alleviate the man's angina?
2. Why did dizziness accompany the man's angina?
3. What important advice should be given to patients taking nitroglycerin?

PRACTICAL SCENARIO 2

A 52-year-old man was admitted to the intensive care unit with ventricular tachycardia. His physician ordered a class I antiarrhythmic agent.

Zsolt Biczo/Shutterstock

Critical Thinking Questions

1. What is another name used to describe class I antiarrhythmic agents?
2. Name all drugs that are listed as class Ia, Ib, or Ic.

Chapter Capsule

This section repeats the objectives from the beginning of the chapter and then provides a summary of the most important concepts for that objective. Use this section as a quick review and to check your knowledge.

Objective 1: Name the three layers of the heart and the four heart valves.

- Layers of the heart: endocardium, myocardium, epicardium
- Heart valves: tricuspid, pulmonary, mitral, aortic

Objective 2: Identify the electrical conduction system of the heart.

- Sinoatrial (SA) node
- Atrioventricular (AV) node
- Bundle of His
- Right and left bundle branches
- Purkinje fibers

Objective 3: Define three types of *angina pectoris*.

- Classical or stable angina: caused by a fixed obstruction in a coronary artery and brought on by exertion, emotional stress, or indigestion; usually causes chest discomfort, with pain radiating to the jaw, neck, shoulder, and left arm, which is relieved by rest or nitroglycerin; the most common form
- Variant or vasospastic angina: caused by coronary artery spasm that reduces blood flow; usually occurs at rest rather than with exertion or emotional stress
- Unstable angina: caused by significant coronary artery disease; occurs at rest for the first time and decreases in response to rest or nitroglycerin; often portends myocardial infarction

Objective 4: Name the mainstays of angina therapy.

- Beta-blockers
- Calcium channel blockers

Objective 5: Describe the action of vasodilation.

- Increases the size of blood vessels to improve the circulation of the blood

Objective 6: Explain myocardial infarction.

- Occurs when part of the myocardium experiences a prolonged restriction of oxygenated coronary blood
- Requires rapid diagnosis and treatment for a good outcome
- The leading cause of death in industrialized nations

Objective 7: Identify the classifications of antidysrhythmic drugs and explain their actions.

- Four classes (I–IV) of drugs are used to treat arrhythmias
- Class I drugs: include subtypes a, b, and c; bind to sodium channels, reducing the maximal rate of contraction of the myocardium and slowing conduction
- Class II drugs: beta-adrenergic blockers reduce the heart's oxygen demand by decreasing the heart rate and preventing the development of myocardial ischemias and angina
- Class III drugs: interfere with potassium channels to alter the repolarization phase; prolong the potential contraction duration of the Purkinje fibers and the muscle fibers of the ventricles, decreasing the frequency of heart failure
- Class IV drugs: calcium channel blockers decrease the vascular tone and cause vasodilation by interfering with the movement of calcium ions through cell membranes, thereby inhibiting the contraction of vascular smooth muscle

Objective 8: Define *calcium channel blockers*.

- Drugs that decrease vascular tone and cause vasodilation by interfering with the movement of calcium ions through cell membranes, inhibiting the contraction of vascular smooth muscle
- Can affect the heart, peripheral vasculature, or both
- Used to treat dysrhythmias, the pain of angina pectoris, vasospastic angina, and hypertension

Objective 9: Describe the newest and oldest drugs used for congestive heart failure.

- For congestive heart failure, combinations of inotropic drugs, diuretics, and vasodilators that include ACE inhibitors are the newest treatments.
- Cardiac glycosides, derived from natural plant sources, have been recognized for centuries for their medicinal qualities.

Objective 10: Explain the most common side effects of digitalis.

- Digitalis commonly causes fatigue, muscle weakness, headache, mental depression, visual disturbances, anorexia, nausea, vomiting, and diarrhea

Internet Sites of Interest

- Information on cardiovascular conditions can be found at:
  www.medicinenet.com/heart/focus.htm
- This site helps us to visualize the human cardiovascular system, including the veins, arteries, and heart: **www.innerbody.com/image/cardov.html**

■ What is coronary heart disease? Find out at: **www.nhlbi.nih.gov/health/ health-topics/topics/cad**

■ Causes and warning signs of myocardial infarction are listed here: **www.webmd.com/heart-disease/understanding-heart-attack-basics**

■ Arrhythmia is discussed at: **www.mayoclinic.org/diseases-conditions/ heart-arrhythmia/basics/definition/con-20027707**

■ The symptoms and stages of congestive heart failure are described here: **www.medicinenet.com/congestive_heart_failure_chf_overview/article.htm**

■ The Healthy Heart Handbook for Women is published at this site: **www.nhlbi.nih.gov/files/docs/public/heart/hdbk_wmn.pdf**

■ This is a good source of information about digitalis: **www.drugs.com/npp/ digitalis.html**

Chapter 28

Drugs Used to Treat Vascular Conditions

Chapter Objectives

After completing this chapter, you should be able to:

1. Explain systole and diastole.
2. Discuss the three main factors that affect blood pressure.
3. Compare the actions of baroreceptors and chemoreceptors.
4. Describe primary and secondary hypertension.
5. Identify the different types of antihypertensive agents and their actions.
6. Describe the mechanism of action and indications of beta-adrenergic blockers.
7. Compare the mechanisms of action of the centrally acting and peripherally acting adrenergic blockers.
8. Explain the effects of angiotensin-converting enzyme (ACE) inhibitors.
9. List the drugs that may interact with the angiotensin II receptor blockers.
10. Describe the mechanism of action of vasodilators.

Key Terms

blood pressure (p. 492)
blood volume (p. 492)
cardiac output (p. 492)
connective tissue (p. 492)

cutaneous flush (p. 497)
diastole (p. 492)
hypertensive crisis (p. 493)
peripheral resistance (p. 492)

primary hypertension (p. 493)
stroke volume (p. 492)
systole (p. 492)

Introduction

It is estimated that nearly 60 million people in the United States have hypertension, which is signified by a systolic blood pressure of 140 mm Hg or higher and a diastolic blood pressure of 90 mm Hg or higher. It is further subdivided into Stage I and Stage II hypertension. Additionally, *prehypertension* is classified as a systolic blood pressure of 120–139 mm Hg, or a diastolic blood pressure of 80 to 89 mm Hg. *Normal* systolic blood pressure is 119 mm Hg or less and a diastolic blood pressure of 79 mm Hg or less. Hypertension—the most common of the cardiovascular diseases (CVDs)—occurs more often in black adults than in white adults, and morbidity and mortality are greater in blacks. Men experience more hypertension than women. The actual level of pressure that can be considered hypertensive is difficult to define; it depends on a number of factors, including the patient's age, gender, race, and lifestyle.

Uncontrolled hypertension can damage small blood vessels, causing narrowing of the arteries, which can result in kidney failure, stroke, and cardiac arrest. Chronic hypertension causes the heart to work harder pumping blood to organs and tissues and can result in congestive heart failure (see Chapter 27).

The Vascular System

Circulatory pressure within the vascular system is divided into three components: (1) arterial pressure, (2) capillary pressure, and (3) venous pressure. **Blood pressure**, which commonly means arterial pressure, is created by the pumping action of the heart and varies from one vessel to another within the systemic circuit. Systemic pressures are highest in the aorta, peaking at around 120 mm Hg, and lowest at the venae cavae, averaging about 2 mm Hg. Blood pressure in large and small arteries rises and falls—rising during ventricular **systole**, when the ventricles of the heart contract and eject blood, and falling during ventricular **diastole**, when the ventricles relax and the heart stops ejecting blood.

Three main factors affect blood pressure:

1. **Cardiac output:** the volume of blood pumped per minute, which is determined by heart rate and **stroke volume**, the amount of blood pumped by a ventricle in one contraction. The higher the cardiac output, the higher the blood pressure.

2. **Peripheral resistance:** the friction in the arteries as blood flows through the vessels. The smooth muscle in artery walls can constrict, causing the inside diameter of the artery to narrow, creating more resistance and higher pressure.

3. **Blood volume:** the total amount of blood in the vascular system; more blood creates added pressure on the artery walls, increasing blood pressure.

Many of the drugs used to treat hypertension target one of these three factors.

The body regulates blood pressure through the vasomotor center, a cluster of neurons in the medulla oblongata, that signals the smooth muscle of the arteries to constrict, raising blood pressure, or relax, lowering blood pressure. Baroreceptors—one type of clusters of neurons in the aorta and internal carotid artery—sense pressure within the large vessels of the vascular system and send this information to the vasomotor center. Another type—chemoreceptors—sends information to the vasomotor center about levels of oxygen, carbon dioxide, and the acidity or pH of the blood. The vasomotor center raises or lowers blood pressure based on the information it receives.

The walls of arteries and veins contain three distinct layers (Figure 28-1 ■):

1. *Tunica interna*: the innermost layer of blood vessels, including the endothelial lining of the vessel and an underlying layer of **connective tissue** (elastic fibers)

2. *Tunica media*: the middle layer, which contains smooth muscle tissue in a framework of collagen and elastic fibers

3. *Tunica externa*: the outer layer, which is a sheath of connective tissue around the vessel

These multiple layers give arteries and veins considerable strength, and the muscular and elastic components permit controlled alterations in diameter as blood pressure or blood volume changes. Under normal circumstances, blood flow is equal to cardiac output. When cardiac output increases, so does capillary blood flow; when cardiac output declines, blood flow is reduced. Two factors—pressure and resistance—affect the flow rates of blood through the capillaries.

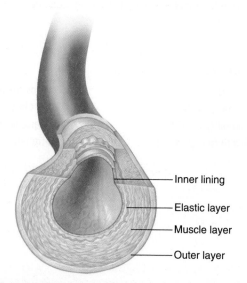

Inner lining

Elastic layer

Muscle layer

Outer layer

Figure 28-1 ■ The structure of an artery, showing the outer protective layer, muscle layer, elastic layer, and inner lining.
© Dorling Kindersley.

Hypertension

Hypertension is the most prevalent cardiovascular disorder in the United States and is the result of chronically elevated pressure throughout the vascular system. Atherosclerosis, arteriosclerosis, renal disease, and any condition that creates increased vascular pressure cause the heart to work harder as it pumps against the increased resistance. The cause of **primary hypertension**, also called *essential hypertension*, which accounts for 90% of cases, is unknown. Heredity is a predisposing factor, but the exact mechanism is unclear. Such environmental factors as dietary sodium, obesity, and stress seem to act only in genetically susceptible people. *Secondary hypertension* is associated with such renal diseases as chronic glomerulonephritis, pyelonephritis, polycystic renal disease, or endocrine disorders, which include Cushing's syndrome, pheochromocytoma, and myxedema. It may also be associated with the use of excessive alcohol, oral contraceptives, corticosteroids, and cocaine. Table 28-1 ■ summarizes the classifications of blood pressure in adults.

Hypertension is a major cause of cerebrovascular accident, cardiac disease, and renal failure. The

Table 28-1 ■ Classification of Blood Pressure in Adults

CLASSIFICATION	SYSTOLIC (mm Hg)		DIASTOLIC (mm Hg)
Normal	<120	and	<80
Prehypertension	120–139	or	80–89
Stage I hypertension	140–159	or	90–99
Stage II hypertension	≥160	or	≥100

prognosis is good if this disorder is detected early and treatment begins before complications develop. Severely elevated blood pressure, known as **hypertensive crisis**, may be fatal.

The values shown in Table 28-1 should not be considered as absolutes, but they are representative as models for treatment of hypertension. In general terms, hypertension can be defined as the level of blood pressure at which there is risk. The ultimate judgment concerning the severity of hypertension in any given patient must also include a consideration of factors other than diastolic or systolic pressure, such as age and comorbid conditions.

✳ Apply Your Knowledge 28.1

The following questions focus on what you have just learned about the vascular system and hypertension.

CRITICAL THINKING

1. What is prehypertension?
2. What are complications of uncontrolled hypertension?
3. What are lipoproteins?
4. What factors may reduce the risk of hypertension?
5. What are the three main factors affecting blood pressure?
6. What are the three walls of an artery?
7. What is the description of hypertensive crisis?
8. Which type of hypertension is the most prevalent cardiovascular disorder in the United States?

ANTIHYPERTENSIVE AGENTS

Antihypertensive agents are used to reduce blood pressure to within the normal levels. If the cause of hypertension is known, such as secondary hypertension, therapy is directed toward correction of the etiology. Unfortunately, the cause of about 90% of cases of hypertension is unknown.

Primary hypertension has no cure, but treatment can modify its course. The basic approach for antihypertensive therapy starts with changes in lifestyle. These changes include controlling weight by diet and exercise,

stopping smoking, decreasing alcohol intake, decreasing sodium intake, exercising on a regular basis, resting and avoiding stress, and taking prescribed medications. Long-term therapy is essential to prevent the morbidity and mortality associated with uncontrolled hypertension. Drug therapy used in the treatment of hypertension includes:

✳ Diuretics to reduce circulating blood volume (see Chapter 31)

✳ Beta-adrenergic blockers to slow the heartbeat and dilate vessels

✳ Vasodilators to dilate vessels

✳ Calcium channel blockers to slow the heartbeat, reduce conduction irritability, and dilate vessels

✳ Angiotensin-converting enzyme (ACE) inhibitors to produce vasodilation and increase renal blood flow.

These medications may be prescribed singly or in combination. The administration of drug therapy is designed to fit each patient's needs and response. Noncompliance is associated with poor prognosis; compliance with an individualized regimen is associated with good prognosis. Table 28-2 ■ lists the most commonly used agents for hypertension.

Table 28-2 ■ Most Commonly Prescribed Antihypertensive Agents

GENERIC NAME	TRADE NAME	AVERAGE ADULT DOSAGE	ROUTE OF ADMINISTRATION
Diuretics (see Chapter 31)			
Beta-Adrenergic Blockers (Beta-Blockers)			
acebutolol	Sectral	200–800 mg bid	PO
atenolol	Tenormin	25–100 mg/d	PO
betaxolol	Kerlone	10–20 mg/d	PO
bisoprolol	Zebeta	2.5–20 mg/d	PO
metoprolol	Lopressor	50–450 mg/d	PO
nadolol	Corgard	40–320 mg/d	PO
penbutolol	Levatol	20–80 mg/d	PO
pindolol	Visken	up to 60 mg/d	PO
propranolol	Inderal	10–240 mg/d	PO
timolol	Blocadren	20–60 mg/d	PO
Alpha-Adrenergic and Beta-Adrenergic Blockers			
labetalol	Trandate	100–400 mg PO bid (maximum: 1,200–2,400 mg/d)	PO
	(Generic only)	20 mg slowly over 2 min, with 40–80 mg q10min if needed (maximum: 300 g total dose)	IV
Centrally Acting Blockers			
clonidine	Catapres	0.1–0.8 mg bid	PO
	Catapres-TTS	Apply patch q7d	Transdermal
guanabenz	(Generic only)	4–32 mg bid	PO
guanfacine	Tenex	1–3 mg bid	PO
methyldopa	(Generic only)	250 mg bid–tid (maximum: 3 g/d in divided doses)	PO
	Methyldopate Hcl	250–500 mg q6h, increased up to 1 g q6h	IV
Peripherally Acting Blockers			
doxazosin	Cardura	1–16 mg/d	PO
guanethidine	(Generic only)	10–50 mg/d	PO

GENERIC NAME	TRADE NAME	AVERAGE ADULT DOSAGE	ROUTE OF ADMINISTRATION
prazosin	Minipress	1–20 mg/d	PO
terazosin	Hytrin	1–20 mg/d	PO
Calcium Channel Blockers			
amlodipine with benazepril	Lotrel	2.5 mg amlodipine/10 mg benazepril per day	PO
diltiazem	Cardizem	80–120 mg tid	PO
felodipine	Plendil	5–10 mg/d	PO
isradipine	DynaCirc	1.25–10 mg bid	PO
nicardipine	Cardene SR	20–40 mg tid	PO
nifedipine	Procardia, Adalat CC	10–20 mg tid	PO
nisoldipine	Sular	10–20 mg tid	PO
verapamil	Calan, Verelan	40–80 mg tid	PO
Angiotensin II Receptor Blockers			
bisoprolol	Zebeta	2.5–5 mg/d (maximum: 20 mg/d)	PO
candesartan	Atacand	8–32 mg/d	PO
eprosartan	Teveten	400–800 mg/d	PO
irbesartan	Avapro	150–300 mg/d	PO
losartan	Cozaar	25–50 mg 1–2 times/d	PO
olmesartan	Benicar	20–40 mg/d	PO
valsartan	Diovan	80–160 mg/d	PO
telmisartan	Micardis	40–80 mg/d	PO
Angiotensin-Converting Enzyme Inhibitors			
benazepril	Lotensin	4–50 mg/d	PO
captopril	Capoten	25/100 mg/d	PO
enalapril	Vasotec	5–40 mg/d	PO
fosinopril	Monopril	10–40 mg/d	PO
lisinopril	Prinivil, Zestril	10–40 mg/d	PO
moexipril	Univasc	7.5–30 mg/d	PO
perindopril	Aceon	2.5–20 mg/d	PO
quinapril	Accupril	2–8 mg/d	PO
ramipril	Altace	2.5–5 mg/d	PO
trandolapril	Mavik	1–4 mg/d	PO

(*continued*)

Table 28-2 ■ **Most Commonly Prescribed Antihypertensive Agents** (*continued*)

GENERIC NAME	TRADE NAME	AVERAGE ADULT DOSAGE	ROUTE OF ADMINISTRATION
Vasodilators			
fenoldopam	Corlopam	0.025–0.3 mcg/kg/min by continuous infusion for up to 48 h	IV
hydralazine	(Generic only)	10–50 mg qid	PO
	(Generic only)	10–40 mg q4–6h	IM
	(Generic only)	10–40 mg q4–6h	IV
minoxidil	Loniten	5 mg/d, increased q3–5d up to 40 mg/d in single or divided doses as needed (maximum: 100 mg/d)	PO
	Rogaine	1 mL/d onto scalp	Topical solution

bid, twice a day; PO, oral; IV, intravenous; tid, three times a day; qid, four times a day; IM, intramuscular.

Focus On

Beta-Adrenergic Blockers

Beta-adrenergic blockers are very popular antihypertensive drugs. They competitively antagonize the responses to catecholamines that are mediated by beta receptors. (See Chapter 24 for a detailed discussion of beta-adrenergic blockers.)

Alpha-Adrenergic and Beta-Adrenergic Blockers

Alpha-adrenergic and beta-adrenergic blockers are indicated for severe hypertension. These blockers are also known as *alpha-blockers* and *beta-blockers*. Alpha- and beta-blocking actions contribute to the blood pressure–lowering effect.

How do they work?

Alpha- and beta-blockers act as adrenergic-receptor blocking agents that combine selective alpha activity and nonselective beta-adrenergic blocking actions. Both actions contribute to blood pressure reduction.

How are they used?

Alpha- and beta-blockers, such as labetalol, are used in the treatment of mild, moderate, and severe hypertension. They may be used alone or in combination with other antihypertensive agents, especially thiazide diuretics (see Chapter 31).

What are the adverse effects?

The adverse effects include postural hypotension, dizziness, vertigo, headache, bronchospasm, and dyspnea. Alpha-receptor blockade causes vasodilation and decreased peripheral vascular resistance that is added to the beta-blocking mechanisms (see Table 28-2).

What are the contraindications and interactions?

Alpha- and beta-blockers are contraindicated in bronchial asthma, uncontrolled cardiac failure, cardiogenic shock, and severe bradycardia. Safe use during pregnancy, lactation, or in children has not been established.

Labetalol should be used cautiously in patients with impaired liver function, jaundice, and diabetes mellitus. Cimetidine may increase the effects of labetalol, and glutethimide decreases its effects.

What are the important points patients should know?

Inform patients who are taking alpha- and beta-blockers that hypotension may occur. Instruct them to make all position changes slowly and in stages, particularly from a lying to an upright position. Advise patients to avoid driving and engaging in other potentially hazardous activities until their responses to the drug are known.

Focus on Geriatrics

Alpha- and Beta-Blocker Use in Older Adults

Older adults are especially sensitive to the hypotensive effects of alpha- and beta-blockers. They must be careful not to engage in any activity that could be especially dangerous because of low blood pressure.

Focus On

Centrally Acting Adrenergic Blockers

Centrally acting adrenergic blockers, such as clonidine hydrochloride and methyldopa, are not regarded as first-line therapies in hypertension. These drugs tend to be used in cases in which the affected person has not responded to other therapies.

How do they work?

These agents are able to reduce the hyperactivity in the medulla oblongata of the brain. Sympathetic outflow from the medulla is diminished and, as a result, either systemic vascular resistance or cardiac output is decreased.

How are they used?

Centrally acting adrenergic blockers are used for the management of hypertension, especially in combination with a diuretic (see Chapter 31).

What are the adverse effects?

The adverse effects include drowsiness, sedation, headache, nightmares, anxiety, orthostatic hypotension, and congestive heart failure (see Table 28-2). Centrally-acting agents may also cause peripheral edema, tachycardia, bradycardia, **cutaneous flush**, and hepatitis.

What are the contraindications and interactions?

Centrally acting blockers are contraindicated in pregnancy, lactation, hepatitis, cirrhosis of the liver, and blood dyscrasias. These agents should be used cautiously in kidney disease, angina pectoris, and a history of mental depression.

What are the important points patients should know?

Advise patients to avoid potentially hazardous tasks, such as driving, until response to these drugs is known. Instruct them to check with their physicians before taking over-the-counter (OTC) medications. Tell women they should not breastfeed while taking these drugs without consulting their physician.

Peripherally Acting Adrenergic Blockers

Peripherally acting adrenergic blockers, such as doxazosin and phenoxybenzamine, lower blood pressure in supine or standing individuals, with the most pronounced effect on diastolic blood pressure.

How do they work?

Peripherally acting blockers are antihypertensive in that their effects depend on the inhibition of norepinephrine release and the depletion of norepinephrine from nerve terminals. These drugs reduce blood pressure by reducing vascular tone, primarily in the veins and the arteries.

How are they used?

Peripherally acting adrenergic blockers are used for severe hypertension or as adjunctive therapy with other antihypertensive agents in the more severe form of hypertension.

What are the adverse effects?

The adverse effects of these drugs are drowsiness, fatigue, headache, confusion, palpitation, dry mouth, dyspnea, and nausea and vomiting (see Table 28-2).

What are the contraindications and interactions?

Contraindications include a history of mental depression, acute peptic ulcer, and ulcerative colitis. Safe use during pregnancy and lactation and in children has not been established. Peripherally acting adrenergic blockers should be used cautiously in patients with diabetes mellitus, impaired renal or hepatic function, coronary disease

(continued)

Focus On (*continued*)

with insufficiency, and recent heart attack. Alcohol intensifies orthostatic hypotension and sedation.

What are the important points patients should know?

Inform patients about the possibility of orthostatic hypotension and advise them to have assistance getting out of bed during initial dosage adjustment. Tell them to take the drug at the same time(s) each day in relation to a daily routine activity. OTC drugs for treatment of colds, allergy, and asthma or appetite suppressants should not be used without consulting a physician or pharmacist.

Calcium Channel Blockers

Calcium channel blockers block the entry of calcium into the muscle cells of the heart and arteries. The entry of calcium is required for electrical signal conduction between muscle cells of the heart, which signals the heart to contract and pump blood. In the arteries, the entry of calcium causes contraction of arterial muscle cells, dilating (widening) the arteries.

How do they work?

By blocking the entry of calcium, calcium channel blockers reduce electrical conduction in the heart, decrease the force of contraction, and dilate arteries. Dilation of the arteries reduces blood pressure as well as the amount of effort the heart must exert in order to pump blood. This leads to a reduced requirement for oxygen by the heart. Dilation of the arteries provides more oxygen-rich blood to reach the heart, preventing angina. Calcium channel blockers also slow electrical conduction through the heart, meaning they are able to correct abnormal rapid heartbeats.

How are they used?

Calcium channel blockers are used to treat hypertension, angina, atrial fibrillation, paroxysmal supraventricular tachycardia, subarachnoid hemorrhage, pulmonary hypertension, Raynaud's phenomenon, and cardiomyopathy and to prevent migraine headaches.

What are the adverse effects?

Common adverse effects of calcium channel blockers include headache, constipation, rash, nausea, flushing, edema, drowsiness, hypotension, and dizziness. Less common adverse effects include sexual dysfunction, gingival hyperplasia, and liver dysfunction.

What are the contraindications and interactions?

Calcium channel blockers are contraindicated in advanced aortic stenosis, severe bradyarrhythmia, sick sinus syndrome, or heart block greater than the first degree (unless a functioning pacemaker is present). They should not be used in patients with hypotension, cardiogenic shock, or ventricular tachycardia. Calcium channel blockers should be used cautiously in patients with significant coronary artery disease or impaired hepatic function. Verapamil is contraindicated for the management of atrial flutter or fibrillation in patients with an accessory AV tract, in patients with severe left-ventricular dysfunction or moderate to severe symptoms of cardiac failure, and if there is any degree of ventricular dysfunction while taking a beta-adrenergic blocker.

Calcium channel blockers such as verapamil and diltiazem reduce elimination and increase blood levels of carbamazepine, simvastatin, atorvastatin, and lovastatin, which may lead to toxicity from these drugs. Diltiazem and felodipine increase the level of cyclosporine, which may lead to toxicity from this drug. Grapefruit juice may elevate serum concentrations of verapamil, felodipine, nifedipine, nicardipine, nisoldipine, and amlodipine.

What are the important points patients should know?

Patients must discuss all medical conditions with a physician before beginning calcium channel blockers, including heart or blood vessel disorders, and kidney or liver disease. All current medications must be discussed, including over-the-counter and herbal medications, because of possible interactions. Patients must avoid grapefruits or grapefruit juice, alcohol, and other blood pressure medications while taking calcium channel blockers.

Angiotensin II receptor blockers

Angiotensin II receptor blockers antagonize the effects of angiotensin II.

How do they work?

Angiotensin II receptor blockers inhibit the binding of angiotensin II to the angiotensin I receptor in vascular smooth muscle. By blocking these receptors, angiotensin II cannot raise blood pressure. This action blocks the vasoconstriction and aldosterone secretion stimulated by angiotensin II.

How are they used?

These agents have beneficial effects on patients with CHF. Angiotensin II receptor blockers have been one of the fastest-growing groups of agents for the management of hypertension. The most common angiotensin II receptor blockers are listed in Table 28-2.

What are the adverse effects?

The adverse effects of these drugs are similar to those of ACE inhibitors. One effect that is absent with these drugs but present with ACE inhibitors is a persistent cough, which can be annoying to patients.

What are the contraindications and interactions?

These drugs are contraindicated in known sensitivity to angiotensin II receptor blockers, bilateral artery stenosis, overt cardiac failure, cardiogenic shock, pregnancy, and lactation. Angiotensin II receptor blockers must be used cautiously in patients with asthma, chronic obstructive pulmonary disease, peripheral vascular disease, diabetes mellitus, hyperthyroidism, and renal or hepatic insufficiency.

Angiotensin II receptor blockers may interact with amiodarone and cause significant bradycardia. Beta-blockers may interact with angiotensin II receptor blockers and reduce glucose tolerance, inhibit insulin secretion, and produce hypertension.

What are the important points patients should know?

Advise patients to report episodes of dizziness, especially when making position changes. Inform female patients to immediately report pregnancy to their physicians. Women should not breastfeed while taking these drugs.

Angiotensin-Converting Enzyme Inhibitors

ACE inhibitors, such as enalapril maleate and ramipril, are drugs that prevent ACE from producing angiotensin II. ACE inhibitors are used to treat patients with hypertension and CHF.

How do they work?

ACE inhibitors decrease the formation of angiotensin II, which lowers blood volume and blood pressure. Renin is an enzyme that is secreted by the kidneys in response to reduced renal blood circulation or lower sodium in the blood. The renin–angiotensin system controls blood pressure and fluid balance and is one of the body's primary homeostatic mechanisms. Figure 28-2 ■ shows the renin–angiotensin system.

How are they used?

ACE inhibitors are a very popular class of drugs for the treatment of patients with severe hypertension. They are becoming the drugs of choice in the treatment of those with primary hypertension. These agents are also used to treat those with CHF.

What are the adverse effects?

Although ACE inhibitors as a group are relatively free of side effects in the majority of patients, they do occur, and some can be life-threatening. The adverse effects include loss of taste, photosensitivity, severe hypotension, hyperkalemia, renal impairment, blood dyscrasias, dizziness, and angioedema. ACE inhibitors are contraindicated in angioedema, pregnant women, renal impairment, scleroderma, and lupus erythematosus.

What are the contraindications and interactions?

ACE inhibitors are contraindicated in patients with hypersensitivity to these agents. Safety during pregnancy and lactation and in children is not established. ACE inhibitors should be used cautiously in renal impairment and renal-artery stenosis and in patients with hypovolemia, hepatic impairment, or diabetes mellitus; receiving diuretics; or undergoing dialysis.

Potassium-sparing diuretics (see Chapter 31) may increase the risk of hyperkalemia. Aspirin and other nonsteroidal anti-inflammatory drugs may antagonize hypotensive effects. ACE inhibitors may increase lithium levels and toxicity.

What are the important points patients should know?

Instruct patients who are using ACE inhibitors to consult their physicians promptly if vomiting or diarrhea occurs. OTC medications should be used only with the approval of a physician. When applicable, advise patients to inform their surgeons or dentists that they are taking ACE inhibitors.

Figure 28-2 ■ The renin–angiotensin system.

⊕ = Vasoconstriction
⊖ = Vasodilation

Focus Point

Angiotensin-Converting Enzyme Inhibitors and Diabetes

ACE inhibitors can produce hypoglycemia in patients with diabetes. Monitoring blood glucose is important during the first few weeks of therapy.

Focus On

Vasodilators

Vasodilators, listed in Table 28-2, are agents that cause blood vessels to expand, increasing blood flow and lowering blood pressure in the affected area.

How do they work?

Vasodilators produce a direct relaxation of vascular smooth muscle, and these actions result in vasodilation.

This effect is called *direct* because it does not depend on the innervation of the vascular smooth muscle and is not mediated by receptors. The vasodilators decrease total peripheral resistance and thus correct primary hypertension. Unlike many other antihypertensive agents, the vasodilators do not inhibit the activity of the sympathetic nervous system; therefore, orthostatic hypotension and impotence are not problems. In addition, most vasodilators relax the arterial smooth muscle to a greater extent than the venous smooth muscle, thereby further minimizing postural hypotension.

How are they used?

The vasodilators are generally inadequate as the sole therapy for hypertension and produce many side effects. However, the administration of beta-blockers and diuretics is more useful than vasodilators alone.

What are the adverse effects?

The main adverse effects of vasodilators include headache, dizziness, tachycardia, and nausea and vomiting. The specific adverse effects of fenoldopam, a commonly prescribed vasodilator, include insomnia, nervousness, cutaneous flush, postural hypotension, bradycardia, and heart failure.

What are the contraindications and interactions?

Vasodilators are contraindicated in patients with hypersensitivity to these agents. Fenoldopam should be avoided if beta-blockers are being used. Hydralazine is contraindicated in coronary artery disease, mitral valvular rheumatic heart disease, and myocardial infarction. Safety during pregnancy and lactation for vasodilators has not been established.

Vasodilators should be used cautiously in cerebrovascular accident, advanced renal impairment, and coronary artery disease. Drug interactions occur with epinephrine and norepinephrine, which can cause excessive cardiac stimulation. If used with guanethidine, these agents cause profound orthostatic hypotension.

What are the important points patients should know?

Instruct patients to monitor their weight, check for edema, make position changes slowly, and avoid standing still. Advise them to avoid excessive alcohol intake and driving and engaging in other potentially hazardous activities until their responses to these drugs are known. Female patients should not breastfeed while taking these drugs without consulting their physician.

✳ Apply Your **Knowledge 28.2**

The following questions focus on what you have just learned about antihypertensive agents.

CRITICAL THINKING

1. What is the role of beta-adrenergic blockers in the management of hypertension?
2. What are the trade names of nadolol, bisoprolol, clonidine, methyldopa, and doxazosin?
3. What are the 10 most commonly prescribed ACE inhibitors for hypertension?
4. What is the mechanism of action of centrally acting adrenergic blockers?
5. What are the indications of peripherally acting adrenergic blockers?
6. What are the adverse effects of ACE inhibitors?
7. What are the indications of angiotensin II receptor blockers?

PRACTICAL SCENARIO 1

The husband of an elderly woman, who had become incoherent over the past day, called emergency medical services (EMS). When they arrived at the house and asked the woman's husband for her history, he told them his wife had diabetes and hypertension for many years. Before calling EMS, he had checked her medicines and, based on the number of pills still left in the bottle, he estimated she had not been taking her antihypertensive medication for about 2 weeks. On examination, the EMS team found that she was afebrile, her pulse rate was 112 beats/min, her respirations were 24 breaths/min, and her blood pressure was 230/160 mm Hg. Primary care was started.

Michal Heron/Pearson Education/PH College

Critical Thinking Questions

1. What might be the results of this patient stopping her antihypertensive medications so abruptly?
2. What consequences could a long-term blood pressure of 230/160 mm Hg have for this patient?
3. What questions would you ask the patient and her family to help guide ongoing treatment and adherence to the medication regimen?

PRACTICAL SCENARIO 2

A 45-year-old African American man with high blood pressure and coronary artery disease was hospitalized because of angina and heart arrhythmia.

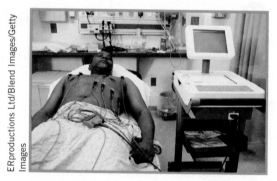

ERproductions Ltd/Blend Images/Getty Images

Critical Thinking Questions

1. What type of medication would be a good choice for this patient?
2. What should the patient avoid while taking this medication?
3. For this particular patient, which types of medications have been traditionally more effective, and which have been less effective?

Chapter Capsule

This section repeats the objectives from the beginning of the chapter and then provides a summary of the most important concepts for that objective. Use this section as a quick review and to check your knowledge.

Objective 1: Explain systole and diastole.

- Blood pressure in large and small arteries rises and falls—rising during ventricular systole, when the ventricles of the heart contract and eject blood, and falling during ventricular diastole, when the ventricles relax and the heart stops ejecting blood

Objective 2: Discuss the three main factors that affect blood pressure.

■ Cardiac output: the volume of blood pumped per minute, which is determined by heart rate and stroke volume, the amount of blood pumped by a ventricle in one contraction. The higher the cardiac output, the higher the blood pressure.

■ Peripheral resistance: the friction in the arteries as blood flows through the vessels. The smooth muscle in artery walls can constrict, causing the inside diameter of the artery to narrow, creating more resistance and higher pressure.

■ Blood volume: the total amount of blood in the vascular system; more blood creates added pressure on the artery walls, increasing blood pressure.

Objective 3: Compare the actions of baroreceptors and chemoreceptors.

■ Baroreceptors, one type of clusters of neurons in the aorta and internal carotid artery, sense pressure within the large vessels of the vascular system and send this information to the vasomotor center.

■ Chemoreceptors send information to the vasomotor center about levels of oxygen, carbon dioxide, and the acidity or pH of the blood. The vasomotor center raises or lowers blood pressure based on the information it receives.

Objective 4: Describe primary and secondary hypertension.

■ Primary (essential) hypertension: unknown etiology; heredity is a predisposing factor, but the exact mechanism is unclear; environmental and lifestyle factors (dietary sodium, obesity, stress) seem to act only in genetically susceptible people

■ Secondary hypertension: associated with such renal diseases as chronic glomerulonephritis; pyelonephritis; polycystic renal disease; or endocrine disorders, which include Cushing's syndrome, pheochromocytoma, and myxedema; may also be associated with the use of excessive alcohol, oral contraceptives, corticosteroids, and cocaine

Objective 5: Identify the different types of antihypertensive agents and their actions.

■ Diuretics (reduce circulating blood volume), discussed in Chapter 31

■ Beta-adrenergic blockers (slow the heartbeat and dilate vessels)

■ Vasodilators (dilate vessels)

■ Calcium channel blockers (slow the heartbeat, reduce conduction irritability, and dilate vessels)

■ Angiotensin-converting enzyme (ACE) inhibitors (produce vasodilation and increase renal blood flow)

Objective 6: Describe the mechanism of action and indications of beta-adrenergic blockers.

■ Beta-adrenergic blockers (as well as alpha-adrenergic blockers) act as adrenergic-receptor blocking agents that combine selective alpha activity and nonselective beta-adrenergic blocking actions. Both actions contribute to blood pressure reduction.

■ They are used in the treatment of mild, moderate, and severe hypertension. They may be used alone or in combination with other antihypertensive agents, especially thiazide diuretics.

Objective 7: **Compare the mechanisms of action of the centrally acting and peripherally acting adrenergic blockers.**

- The centrally acting adrenergic blockers are able to reduce the hyperactivity in the medulla oblongata of the brain. Sympathetic outflow from the medulla is diminished and, as a result, either systemic vascular resistance or cardiac output is decreased.

- Peripherally acting blockers are antihypertensive in that their effects depend on the inhibition of norepinephrine release and the depletion of norepinephrine from nerve terminals. These drugs reduce blood pressure by reducing vascular tone, primarily in the veins and the arteries.

Objective 8: **Explain the effects of angiotensin-converting enzyme (ACE) inhibitors.**

- ACE inhibitors decrease the formation of angiotensin II, which lowers blood volume and blood pressure.

- The renin–angiotensin system controls blood pressure and fluid balance and is one of the body's primary homeostatic mechanisms; renin is an enzyme that is secreted by the kidneys in response to reduced renal blood circulation or lower sodium in the blood.

Objective 9: **List the drugs that may interact with the angiotensin II receptor blockers.**

- Angiotensin II receptor blockers may interact with amiodarone and cause significant bradycardia. Beta-blockers may interact with angiotensin II receptor blockers and reduce glucose tolerance, inhibit insulin secretion, and produce hypertension.

Objective 10: **Describe the mechanism of action of vasodilators.**

- Vasodilators produce a direct relaxation of vascular smooth muscle, and these actions result in vasodilation. This effect is called *direct* because it does not depend on the innervation of the vascular smooth muscle and is not mediated by receptors. The vasodilators decrease total peripheral resistance and thus correct primary hypertension. Unlike many other antihypertensive agents, the vasodilators do not inhibit the activity of the sympathetic nervous system; therefore, orthostatic hypotension and impotence are not problems. In addition, most vasodilators relax the arterial smooth muscle to a greater extent than the venous smooth muscle, thereby further minimizing postural hypotension.

 Internet Sites of Interest

- Cardiovascular Physiology Concepts offers information about secondary hypertension at **www.cvphysiology.com**. Click "Hypertension" in the left column.

- Everything you have always wanted to know about hypertension is available at: **www.hypertension-facts.org**

- MedicineNet.com, a pharmacists' website, discusses ACE inhibitors at: **www.medicinenet.com/ace_inhibitors/article.htm**

- An overview of the human vascular system can be found at: **www.innerbody.com/image/cardov.html**

- The pharmacologic treatment of systemic hypertension with antihypertensive drugs is explained at: **www.cvpharmacology.com/antihypertensive/antihypertensive**

Chapter 29

Drugs Used to Treat Hyperlipidemia and Related Conditions

Chapter Objectives

After completing this chapter, you should be able to:

1. Differentiate between cholesterol, triglycerides, and phospholipids.

2. Explain how lipoproteins are metabolized.

3. Define *hyperlipidemia* and list the major plasma lipids.

4. Identify the risks of having high serum cholesterol and increased LDL.

5. Differentiate between type IIa and IIb hypercholesterolemia.

6. Explain how bile acid sequestrants lower cholesterol.

7. Define *statin drugs* (HMG-CoA reductase inhibitors).

8. Name foods that have significant interactions with the statin drug simvastatin.

9. Identify the adverse effects of niacin, including the newest information.

10. Identify the important points patients should know about fibric acid derivatives.

Key Terms

apolipoprotein B-100 (p. 506)
apolipoprotein E (p. 506)
cholesterol (p. 506)
cholesterol ester (p. 506)
chylomicrons (p. 506)

endogenous pathway (p. 506)
exogenous pathway (p. 506)
glycerol (p. 506)
hypercholesterolemia (p. 507)
lipoproteins (p. 506)

lysosomes (p. 506)
phospholipid (p. 506)
steatorrhea (p. 509)
triglyceride (p. 506)

Introduction

Hyperlipidemia is an elevation of one or more of the lipoprotein levels in the plasma. It is a strong risk factor for cardiovascular disease (CVD). The major plasma lipids are cholesterol, cholesterol ester, triglycerides, and phospholipids. The triglycerides that are bound to proteins and transported as macromolecular complexes are called *lipoproteins*. These help to form the fatty material called *plaque* that builds up in the lining of blood vessels and can cause angina, stroke, and myocardial infarction (MI). Hyperlipidemias are linked to specific genetic mutations, and most have a multifactorial basis that can respond to lifestyle changes or drug therapy.

Such lifestyle changes as the reduction of body weight; decreased intake of dietary total fat, cholesterol, saturated fatty acids, and salt; smoking cessation; increased exercise; and stress management can be effective for minor hypertension and hyperlipidemias. Pharmacologic methods combined with healthy lifestyle habits are usually necessary to treat patients with chronic hypertension and serious hyperlipidemias.

Major Plasma Lipids

The major plasma lipids consist of cholesterol, cholesterol ester, triglycerides, and phospholipids. **Cholesterol** is a steroid alcohol that is present in nearly every cell and fluid of the body. It is a precursor of bile acids and steroid hormones. Approximately two-thirds of plasm cholesterol undergoes a process in which it is esterified with fatty acids. This forms **cholesterol ester**. Fatty acids may also be esterified with **glycerol**, but in this case, the substance that is formed is known as a **triglyceride**. This lipid helps in the transfer of adipose fat and blood glucose from the liver. There are many different types of triglycerides, which may be saturated with hydrogen, or unsaturated. *Saturated fats* have a high melting point and are usually solid at room temperature, whereas *unsaturated fats* have a lower melting point and are usually liquid at room temperature. The final major plasma lipid is the **phospholipid**, which is actually a group of lipids that are the major components of cell membranes. Examples of phospholipids include *lecithin*, which is a component of the yolk of chicken eggs.

Lipoprotein Metabolism

The metabolism of **lipoproteins** in the body uses two pathways: *exogenous* and *endogenous*. Metabolism is based primarily on whether a lipoprotein is mostly composed of dietary (exogenous) lipids, or if it originated in the liver (endogenous). The **exogenous pathway** can be explained as follows: In the small intestine, epithelial cells absorb lipids from the diet, which include cholesterol, phospholipids, and triglycerides. These lipids are joined with lipoproteins to form **chylomicrons**. The chylomicrons are then secreted into the lymphatic circulation to circulate through the lymphatic vessels. They bypass the liver circulation and are drained through the thoracic duct into the bloodstream. Here, high-density lipoprotein (HDL) particles add more lipoproteins, and the chylomicrons are referred to as *mature*.

The chylomicrons then activate *lipoprotein lipase (LPL)*, which is an enzyme on endothelial cells that line the blood vessels. This enzyme catalyzes the hydrolysis of triglycerides to release glycerol and fatty acids from the chylomicrons. The glycerol and fatty acids are absorbed in the peripheral tissues, primarily muscle and adipose tissues, to be used for energy or stored. The hydrolyzed chylomicron remnants keep circulating until they interact with their receptors, which exist mostly in the liver. Via **apolipoprotein E**, the remnants undergo endocytosis, and they hydrolysis within **lysosomes**. Glycerol and fatty acids are released into the cells, to be used for energy or stored for later use.

The **endogenous pathway** is another important source of lipoproteins, primarily very-low-density lipoproteins (VLDLs). Particles of VLDLs are assembled when triglycerides and cholesterol come into contact with **apolipoprotein B-100**. The particles are released into the bloodstream, with lipoproteins acquired from HDL particles being added, resulting in mature particles. They circulate, contact LPL, and become hydrolyzed, releasing glycerol and fatty acids. These products are then absorbed in the adipose and muscle peripheral tissues primarily; at this point, the VLDL particles are called remnants or *intermediate-density lipoproteins (IDLs)*. The remnants circulate and interact with apolipoprotein E and remnant receptors, to be absorbed by the liver or additionally hydrolyzed by hepatic lipase.

The actions of hepatic lipase release glycerol and fatty acids to leave IDL remnants, called *low-density lipoproteins (LDLs)*, which have a relatively high amount of cholesterol. These lipoproteins circulate, to be absorbed by the liver and peripheral cells. The LDL binds to its target tissues via an interaction between its receptors and either apolipoprotein B-100 or apolipoprotein E. Via endocytosis, absorption occurs. The internalized particles of LDL are hydrolyzed inside lysosomes. Lipids—mostly cholesterol—are then released.

Hyperlipidemia

Hyperlipidemia is characterized by an increase in plasma cholesterol or triglycerides containing lipoprotein particles. These particles, which are key to the development of atherogenesis, are initially synthesized by the intestinal mucosa and the liver and undergo extensive metabolism in the plasma. They also play an essential role in the transport of lipids between tissues. The lipoproteins differ in density and are referred to as VLDL, LDL, HDL, and chylomicrons. Each lipoprotein includes different amounts of triglycerides and cholesterol in the core. The size of the core varies with the size of the lipoprotein. When carried as circulating lipoprotein, cholesterol is the predominant core of LDL and

HDL. Chylomicrons produced by the intestines transport dietary cholesterol and triglycerides. Triglycerides are the predominant makers of chylomicrons and the VLDL secreted by the liver.

A patient with high serum cholesterol and increased LDL is at risk for atherosclerotic coronary disease, MI, and hypertension. Disorders of hyperlipidemia are characterized by an elevation in triglycerides and an elevation of cholesterol. Elevated triglycerides can produce life-threatening pancreatitis.

RELATED DISORDERS

Although **hypercholesterolemia** or *hyperlipidemia*, is linked to specific genetic mutations, it usually has a multifactorial basis that can respond to lifestyle changes. These changes include the reduction of body weight; decreased dietary total fat, cholesterol, and saturated fatty acids; increased exercise; and stress management.

There are five different types of hypercholesterolemia. The types were traditionally classified by elevation patterns of lipids and lipoproteins. Type I is a rare, inherited condition that involves high levels of chylomicrons in the blood. It is caused by low levels of *lipoprotein lipase*, which is responsible for lowering lipoprotein levels. Cholesterol levels are usually normal, and the risk for heart disease is low. Complications from type I include premature atherosclerosis, coronary artery disease, heart attack, stroke, and premature death. Treatment involves a very low-fat diet, and is usually effective.

Type II hypercholesterolemia has two subtypes. Type IIa is associated with high levels of both cholesterol and LDL in the blood. Ischemic heart disease is common in this type. The condition may be hereditary and is then termed *familial hypercholesterolemia*. Type IIb is associated with high VLDL and LDL and, therefore, high triglycerides and cholesterol blood levels. Ischemic heart disease may result. This type may be related to high alcohol intake, obesity, diabetes mellitus, and overeating. Dietary modification is usually all that is required, but drugs may be necessary in resistant cases.

Type III hypercholesterolemia is a rare genetic condition. It involves elevated VLDL and chylomicron particles. This results in increased levels of triglycerides and cholesterol. This type is caused by an abnormality in *apolipoprotein E*, which normally allows intermediate-density lipoproteins to bind to liver cells. The outcomes of this type are the same as for type I. Dietary changes, fibrate, nicotinic acid, and statins may be used for treatment.

Type IV hypercholesterolemia is characterized by high VLDL and hypertriglyceridemia. Causes are similar to that of type IIb, but peripheral vascular disease and ischemic heart disease can be found in people with this type. The complications are the same as for the previously discussed types. The treatment is the same as for type IIb, plus the use of fibrate and nicotinic acid, and increased exercise are encouraged.

Type V hypercholesterolemia is characterized by elevated chylomicrons and VLDL, resulting in increased levels of triglycerides and cholesterol. This type is rare, and also involves reduced levels of lipoprotein lipase. Complications are the same as for the previous types. Treatments involve nicotinic acid, fibrate, diet changes and exercise.

ANTIHYPERLIPIDEMIC AGENTS

Antihyperlipidemic agents should be used if diet modification and exercise programs fail to lower LDL to normal levels. When medications are started, diet therapy must continue. Whereas some of the antihyperlipidemic drugs decrease production of the lipoprotein carriers of cholesterol and triglycerides, others increase lipoprotein degradation. Still others directly increase cholesterol removal from the body. These drugs may be used singly or in combination but are always accompanied by the requirement that dietary lipid intake be significantly low, especially cholesterol and saturated fats, and calories must be closely monitored. The major drugs for reduction of LDL cholesterol levels are bile acid sequestrants and nicotinic acid. The fibric acid derivatives, such as clofibrate, are less effective in reducing LDL cholesterol. The most effective drugs for lowering plasma LDL levels are the HMG-CoA reductase inhibitors, or statins. Antihyperlipidemic drugs are listed in Table 29-1 ■.

Table 29-1 ■ Antihyperlipidemic Drugs

GENERIC NAME	TRADE NAME	AVERAGE ADULT DOSAGE	ROUTE OF ADMINISTRATION
Bile Acid Sequestrants			
cholestyramine resin	Questran	4–6 g/d	PO
colestipol	Colestid	15–30 g/d	PO
HMG-CoA Reductase Inhibitors (Statins)			
atorvastatin	Lipitor	10–80 mg qid	PO
fluvastatin	Lescol	20–40 mg/d	PO

(continued)

Table 29-1 ■ Antihyperlipidemic Drugs *(continued)*

GENERIC NAME	TRADE NAME	AVERAGE ADULT DOSAGE	ROUTE OF ADMINISTRATION
lovastatin	Altoprev, Mevacor	20–80 mg/d	PO
pravastatin	Pravachol	10–40 mg/d	PO
rosuvastatin	Crestor	5–40 mg/d	PO
simvastatin	Zocor	10–80 mg/d	PO
simvastatin/ezetimibe	Vytorin	10/10–10/80 mg/d (ezetimibe is 10 mg)	PO
Miscellaneous Drugs			
nicotinic acid (niacin)	Niacor	1–2 g bid–tid	PO
Fibric Acid Derivatives			
clofibrate	(Generic only)	2 g/d	PO
gemfibrozil	Lopid	1,200 mg/d	PO

PO, oral; qid, four times a day; bid, twice a day; tid, three times a day.

Focus Point

PCSK-9 Inhibitors

Proprotein convertase subtilisin kexin 9 (PCSK-9) is a gene that is important for plasma cholesterol metabolism, and when it is mutated, familiar hypercholesterolemia results. In 2015, the FDA approved a new class of drugs for treating high cholesterol, which are known as the *PCSK-9 inhibitors*. These drugs work similarly to the statins and use genetic mutations that regulate the level of LDL receptors in the liver. Lower PCSK-9 means that there are more LDL receptors that can collect LDL, leaving less cholesterol in the blood. The first drug that has been approved for the United States market is alirocumab (Praluent), which is available for administration by injection. It is indicated for familial hypercholesterolemia or for patients with a history of heart disease in whom statins are not sufficiently effective. An additional drug called evolocumab is under review for approval and has been approved in Europe.

Focus Point

Alcohol and Cholesterol

Moderate alcohol intake increases HDL cholesterol (the "good" cholesterol) but does not reduce LDL cholesterol (the "bad" cholesterol).

Focus On

Bile Acid Sequestrants

Bile acid sequestrants, such as cholestyramine resin and colestipol, are drugs that chemically combine with bile acids in the intestine, causing these bile acids to be excreted from the body.

How do they work?

Bile acid sequestrants are used for their cholesterol-lowering effect. They bind with bile salts in the intestinal tract to form an insoluble complex that is excreted in the feces, thus reducing circulating cholesterol and increasing serum LDL removal rates.

How are they used?

Bile acid sequestrants are nonabsorbable drugs prescribed for decreasing serum cholesterol. Lowering the bile acid concentration causes the liver to increase the conversion of cholesterol to bile acids, resulting in a replenished supply of these compounds, which are essential components of the bile. Because the bile acids are lost in feces, LDLs and serum cholesterol are reduced. The bile acid binding resins are prescribed for primary hyperlipidemias.

What are the adverse effects?

The adverse effects of bile acid sequestrants include constipation, nausea, flatulence, and the impaired absorption of fat-soluble vitamins.

What are the contraindications and interactions?

Bile acid sequestrants should be avoided in patients with bowel obstruction, and their safety is not established for patients with dysphagia, swallowing disorders, and major gastrointestinal tract surgery. Safety during pregnancy and lactation and in children younger than 6 years of age has not been established. These agents should be used cautiously in patients with bleeding disorders, hemorrhoids, peptic ulcer, and malabsorption states, such as **steatorrhea** (elimination of large amounts of fat in the stool).

Cholestyramine resin and colestipol interfere with the intestinal absorption of many drugs—for example, tetracycline, phenobarbital, digoxin, warfarin, aspirin, and thiazide diuretics.

What are the important points patients should know?

Advise patients to report promptly to their physicians if they develop severe gastric distress with nausea and vomiting, unusual weight loss, black stools, severe hemorrhoids, and sudden back pain. A high-bulk diet with adequate fluid intake is an essential adjunct to resolve constipation.

HMG-CoA Reductase Inhibitors (Statin Drugs)

This powerful group of antihyperlipidemic agents includes the most effective drugs for reducing LDL and cholesterol levels. They share the generic name of statin and are described as "the statins."

How do they work?

Statin drugs reduce LDL and total triglyceride production. These agents are inhibitors of reductase (HMG-CoA), which is essential to hepatic production of cholesterol.

How are they used?

The statins are the most widely used drugs for lowering hyperlipidemia. Lovastatin, simvastatin, pravastatin, and fluvastatin are completely effective in inhibiting HMG-CoA reductase, which is the enzyme needed in cholesterol production. These drugs are often given in combination with other antihyperlipidemic drugs. It should be noted that despite the protection afforded by cholesterol lowering, about 25% of patients treated with these drugs still present with coronary events. Thus, such additional strategies as diet, exercise, or additional agents may be warranted.

What are the adverse effects?

Some patients may have muscle pain. A severe but rare adverse effect is life-threatening *rhabdomyolysis* (degeneration of skeletal muscle tissue, with possible renal failure). Other adverse effects may include abdominal pain, flatulence, constipation, dyspepsia, headache, and cramping. Liver function and serum transaminase levels must be measured periodically. If there is muscle pain, creatine kinase levels should be monitored to rule out rhabdomyolysis. The HMG-CoA reductase inhibitors may increase coumarin levels. Thus, it is important to evaluate prothrombin times frequently.

What are the contraindications and interactions?

Statins are contraindicated for patients who are hypersensitive to these agents and in myopathy, active liver disease, unexplained persistent transaminase elevations, and during pregnancy and lactation. Statin drugs may increase levels of digoxin, norethindrone, and the oral contraceptive ethinyl estradiol.

What are the important points patients should know?

Instruct patients they cannot interrupt, increase, decrease, or omit dosage without the advice of their physicians. They should notify their physicians promptly about muscle tenderness or pain, especially if accompanied by fever or malaise. Alcohol consumption should be avoided or reduced. Advise women that they should not breastfeed while taking these drugs without consulting their physician.

Focus on Pediatrics

Statin Drugs and Children

Statin drugs should not be prescribed for children or teenagers. The safety and effectiveness of these drugs in children and adolescents has not been established.

Focus on Natural Products

Food Interactions and Statins

Grapefruit and grapefruit juice should be avoided by patients who are taking the statin drug simvastatin. Regular consumption of the fruit or juice can lead to high levels of the drug in the blood. This is not true of other statin drugs.

MISCELLANEOUS ANTIHYPERLIPIDEMIC DRUGS

Some other antihyperlipidemic drugs lower serum lipids in primary and secondary hyperlipidemias. Nicotinic acid and the fibrates, such as clofibrate and gemfibrozil, are included in this category.

Focus On

Nicotinic Acid (Niacin)

Nicotinic acid, or niacin, has a broad lipid-lowering ability, but its clinical use is limited because of its unpleasant side effects. Derivatives of this drug, which are not available in the United States, appear to have fewer adverse effects.

How does it work?

Niacin appears to reduce the level of the VLDL, LDL, and total cholesterol. Combination drug therapy, such as nicotinic acid, bile acid binding sequestrants, and a statin, may decrease LDL cholesterol levels by 70% or more. Niacin causes a decrease in liver triglyceride synthesis, which is required for VLDL production. LDL is derived from VLDL in the plasma. Therefore, a reduction in the VLDL concentration also results in a decreased plasma LDL concentration.

How is it used?

Niacin is used in the adjuvant treatment of hypercholesterolemias in patients who do not respond adequately to diet or weight loss. It is the most potent antihyperlipidemic agent for raising plasma HDL levels.

What are the adverse effects?

The most common adverse effects of niacin therapy are an intense *cutaneous flush* (skin reddening, also referred to as *flushing*) and pruritus. The administration of aspirin before taking niacin decreases the flush. Some patients also experience nausea and abdominal pain, syncope, nervousness, and blurred vision. Hyperuricemia, gout, impaired glucose tolerance, and hepatotoxicity have also been reported.

What are the contraindications and interactions?

Niacin is contraindicated in patients with hypersensitivity to this agent. It must be avoided in hepatic impairment, severe hypotension, active peptic ulcer, pregnancy, lactation, and in children younger than 16 years of age.

Niacin should be used cautiously in patients with a history of gallbladder disease, liver disease, peptic ulcer, glaucoma, coronary artery disease, and diabetes mellitus. Niacin is able to potentiate the hypotensive effects of antihypertensive agents.

What are the important points patients should know?

Alert patients to the possibility of feeling warm and flushed in the face, neck, and ears within the first 2 hours after oral ingestion and immediately after parenteral administration. This may last for several hours. Effects are usually transient and subside as therapy continues. Instruct patients to sit or lie down, avoiding sudden posture changes if they feel weak or dizzy. These symptoms as well as persistent flushing should be reported to their physicians. Relief may be obtained by reducing the dosage, increasing subsequent doses in small increments, or changing to a sustained-release formulation. Alcohol and large doses of niacin cause increased flushing and sensations of warmth. Tell patients to avoid exposure to direct sunlight until lesions have entirely cleared if they have skin manifestations. Women should not breastfeed while taking niacin.

It must be noted, however, that more recent studies such as the one conducted by The New England Journal of Medicine in 2014, have revealed new information about niacin. These studies indicated that niacin does not reduce heart attacks or strokes, and may even be linked to an increased risk of bleeding, the development of diabetes, and death. It is possible that 1 in 200 patients taking long-acting niacin may die as a result of the therapy. This vitamin is also linked to liver problems, infections, and bleeding in areas such as the stomach, intestines, and brain. As a result of this new information, long-acting, high-dose niacin has been removed from the market. However, regular and extended-release niacin are still available.

Fibric Acid Derivatives

Gemfibrozil and clofibrate are derivatives of fibric acid that lower triglycerides and VLDL and increase HDL.

How do they work?

Both drugs cause a decrease in plasma triglyceride levels by blocking lipolysis of stored triglycerides in adipose tissue and inhibiting hepatic uptake of fatty acids. In addition to inhibiting the breakdown of fats into triglycerides, liver production of triglycerides is inhibited.

How are they used?

Fibric acid derivatives are approved for use in patients with hypertriglyceridemia who do not respond to diet—those in whom triglyceride levels can exceed 1,000 mg/dL (reference range, 10–190 mg/dL). They can also be prescribed in combination with other drugs to facilitate a reduction in triglycerides that complements the cholesterol-lowering action of the antihyperlipidemic agent. These agents are also used for severe familial hypercholesterolemia (type IIa or IIb) that develops early in childhood and has failed to respond to dietary control or to other cholesterol-lowering drugs.

What are the adverse effects?

The most common adverse effects are mild gastrointestinal disturbances, dizziness, and blurred vision. Gemfibrozil may increase cholesterol excretion into the bile, leading to gallstone formation. Treatment with clofibrate has resulted in significant occurrences of cancer. Inflammation of the skeletal muscle can occur with both drugs; thus, muscle weakness or tenderness should be evaluated.

What are the contraindications and interactions?

Fibric acid derivatives are contraindicated in patients with gallbladder disease, biliary cirrhosis, or hepatic or severe renal dysfunction and during pregnancy and lactation. Safety and efficacy in children younger than age 18 years are not established. These drugs should be used cautiously in patients with diabetes mellitus, hypothyroidism, renal impairment, and cholelithiasis (gallstones).

Fibric acid derivatives may potentiate the hypoprothrombinemic effects of oral anticoagulants. Lovastatin increases the risk of myopathy and rhabdomyolysis and may increase repaglinide levels and duration of action.

What are the important points patients should know?

Instruct patients to notify their physicians promptly if unexplained bleeding occurs. This includes easy bruising, *epistaxis* (nosebleed), and *hematuria* (blood present in the urine).

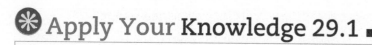

Apply Your **Knowledge 29.1**

The following questions focus on what you have just learned about hyperlipidemia, related conditions, and the medications used for their treatment.

CRITICAL THINKING

1. What are the mechanisms of action of bile acid sequestrants?
2. What are the indications of HMG-CoA reductase inhibitors?
3. What are the trade names of colestipol, cholestyramine resin, and gemfibrozil?
4. What are the generic and trade names of the HMG-CoA reductase inhibitors?
5. What is the mechanism of action of nicotinic acid?
6. What drugs are derivatives of fibric acid that lower triglycerides and increase HDL?

PRACTICAL SCENARIO 1

A 53-year-old man complains of chest pain, which is also known as angina pectoris. He has been a smoker for 30 years and has a history of diabetes mellitus. Once his physician treats his chest pain, she orders a blood test and a lipid panel.

Mangostock/Shutterstock

Critical Thinking Questions

1. Explain the four types of lipoproteins and which of these are risk factors for angina pectoris or heart attack.
2. List the most effective antihyperlipidemic agents.

PRACTICAL SCENARIO 2

A 33-year-old African American woman went to her family practitioner for a physical examination. She is overweight with a history of hypertension.

Courtesy of the author

Critical Thinking Questions

1. If her cholesterol and triglycerides are elevated, what medications could the physician order to lower her cholesterol and triglycerides?
2. List the complications of hypercholesterolemia.

Chapter Capsule

This section repeats the objectives from the beginning of the chapter and then provides a summary of the most important concepts for that objective. Use this section as a quick review and to check your knowledge.

Objective 1: Differentiate between cholesterol, triglycerides, and phospholipids.

■ *Cholesterol* is a steroid alcohol that is present in nearly every cell and fluid of the body. It is a precursor of bile acids and steroid hormones. Approximately two-thirds of plasm cholesterol undergoes a process in which it is esterified with fatty acids, forming *cholesterol ester*.

■ Fatty acids also may be esterified with *glycerol*, but in this case, the substance that is formed is known as a *triglyceride*. This lipid helps in the transfer of adipose fat and blood glucose from the liver. There are many different types of triglycerides, which may be saturated with hydrogen, or unsaturated. *Saturated fats* have a high melting point and are usually solid at room temperature, whereas *unsaturated fats* have a lower melting point and are usually liquid at room temperature.

■ The final major plasma lipid is the *phospholipid*, which is actually a group of lipids that are the major components of cell membranes. Examples of phospholipids include *lecithin*, which is a component of the yolk of chicken eggs.

Objective 2: Explain how lipoproteins are metabolized.

■ The metabolism of lipoproteins in the body uses the exogenous and endogenous pathways. Metabolism is based primarily on whether a lipoprotein is mostly composed of dietary (exogenous) lipids or if it originated in the liver (endogenous).

■ Exogenous pathway: Small intestine epithelial cells absorb lipids, which are joined with lipoproteins, form chylomicrons that are secreted into the lymphatic circulation, and drain through the thoracic duct into the bloodstream. HDL particles add more lipoproteins; the chylomicrons mature and activate *lipoprotein lipase (LPL)*. This catalyzes hydrolysis of triglycerides, releasing glycerol and fatty acids that are absorbed mostly in muscle and adipose tissues for energy or storage. Chylomicron remnants circulate until interacting with receptors, mostly in the liver. Endocytosis causes their hydrolysis within lysosomes. Glycerol and fatty acids are released into the cells for energy or storage.

■ Endogenous pathway: Important source of primarily very-low-density lipoproteins (VLDLs). The VLDL particles move into the bloodstream, lipoproteins from HDL particles are added, and mature particles result. They circulate, contact LPL, become hydrolyzed, and release glycerol and fatty acids that are absorbed primarily in adipose and muscle tissues, to be called remnants or *intermediate-density lipoproteins (IDLs)*. They circulate and are either absorbed by the liver or additionally hydrolyzed by hepatic lipase. Remnants, also called *low-density lipoproteins (LDLs)*, contain a high amount of cholesterol. The lipoproteins circulate, absorbed by the liver and peripheral cells, and the LDL binds to target tissues. Via endocytosis, absorption occurs. The LDL particles are hydrolyzed inside lysosomes. Lipids, mostly cholesterol, are released.

Objective 3: Define *hyperlipidemia* and list the major plasma lipids.

■ Hyperlipidemia is an elevation of lipoprotein levels in the plasma

■ The major plasma lipids are cholesterol, cholesterol ester, triglycerides, and phospholipids.

Objective 4: Identify the risks of having high serum cholesterol and increased LDL.

- A patient with high serum cholesterol and increased LDL is at risk for atherosclerotic coronary disease, MI, and hypertension

Objective 5: Differentiate between type IIa and IIb hypercholesterolemia.

- Type IIa is associated with high levels of both cholesterol and LDL in the blood. Ischemic heart disease is common in this type. The condition may be hereditary and is then termed *familial hypercholesterolemia*.
- Type IIb is associated with high VLDL and LDL and, therefore, high triglycerides and cholesterol blood levels. Ischemic heart disease may result. This type may be related to high alcohol intake, obesity, diabetes mellitus, and overeating. Dietary modification is usually all that is required, but drugs may be necessary in resistant cases.

Objective 6: Explain how bile acid sequestrants lower cholesterol.

- Bile acid sequestrants bind with bile salts in the intestinal tract to form an insoluble complex that is excreted in the feces, thus reducing circulating cholesterol and increasing serum LDL removal rates

Objective 7: Define *statin drugs* (HMG-CoA reductase inhibitors).

- Inhibitors of reductase (HMG-CoA), which is essential to hepatic production of cholesterol
- Most effective drugs for reducing low-density lipoprotein (LDL) and cholesterol levels
- Reduce LDL and total triglyceride production

Objective 8: Name foods that have significant interactions with the statin drug known as simvastatin.

- Grapefruit and grapefruit juice should be avoided by patients who are taking the statin drug simvastatin
- Regular consumption of the fruit or juice can lead to high levels of this drug in the blood
- This is not true of the other statins

Objective 9: Identify the adverse effects of niacin, including the newest information.

- Intense cutaneous flush and pruritus (very common)
- Nausea and abdominal pain, syncope, nervousness, and blurred vision (less common)
- Hyperuricemia, gout, impaired glucose tolerance, and hepatotoxicity (uncommon)
- More recent studies indicate that niacin may be linked to an increased risk of bleeding, the development of diabetes, and death; it is possible that 1 in 200 patients taking niacin may die as a result of the therapy with long-acting niacin; this vitamin is also linked to liver problems, infections, and bleeding in areas such as the stomach, intestines, and brain

Objective 10: Identify the important points patients should know about fibric acid derivatives.

- Instruct patients taking fibric acid derivatives to notify their physicians promptly if unexplained bleeding occurs; this includes easy bruising, epistaxis, and hematuria

Internet Sites of Interest

■ This website focuses on the causes and treatment of high triglycerides, and how to lower them: **www.webmd.com/cholesterol-management/tc/ high-triglycerides-overview**

■ An overview of lipoproteins is given at this website: **www.learn.ppdictionary.com/ exercise_and_lipoproteins5.htm**

■ A thorough explanation of hyperlipidemia can be found at: **www.beltina.org/ health-dictionary/hyperlipidemia-symptoms-treatment-definition.html**

■ The Mayo Clinic's information about hypercholesterolemia can be found at: **www.mayoclinic.org/diseases-conditions/high-blood-cholesterol/home/ ovc-20181871**

■ Antihyperlipidemic drugs are discussed at: **www.drugs.com/drug-class/ antihyperlipidemic-agents.html**

Chapter **30**

Anticoagulants

Chapter Objectives

After completing this chapter, you should be able to:

1. Explain the three events involved in hemostasis.
2. Define the terms *clotting factors* and *cascade* in relation to hemostasis.
3. Explain the role of prothrombinase in blood clotting.
4. Explain how anticoagulants work.
5. List the indications of anticoagulants.
6. Describe the mechanism of action of heparin.
7. Describe the advantages of low-molecular-weight heparin.
8. Explain the mechanism of action of warfarin.
9. Explain how antiplatelet drugs are used.
10. List the indications of thrombolytic drugs.

Key Terms

coagulation (p. 517)
embolus (p. 519)
hemostasis (p. 517)

platelet plug (p. 517)
platelets (p. 517)
serotonin (p. 517)

thrombi (p. 520)
thromboembolism (p. 522)

Introduction

The blood transports blood cells, gases, hormones, immune cells, metabolic wastes, and nutrients. Normal blood clotting protects against excessive hemorrhaging, but the development of certain clots may obstruct the flow of blood and ultimately cause a myocardial infarction (MI), stroke, or *necrosis* (death) of tissue. Hemorrhagic and thrombotic disorders may be treated with a variety of medications.

This chapter focuses on anticoagulant drug therapy, which is aimed at reducing the occurrences of thrombosis. Anticoagulants decrease the blood's ability to clot. There are two main types of anticoagulants: parenteral and oral. Often, both types are used together. Caution must be taken by health care professionals because many conditions cause an increased risk of hemorrhaging. Anticoagulants should not be used or should be used only in severely limited quantities in treating patients who have these types of conditions, such as hemophilia or *thrombocytopenia* (low platelet count).

Hemostasis

Limited intravascular coagulation of blood occurs in normal physiologic conditions. The circulatory system has to be self-sealing; otherwise, continued blood loss from even the smallest injury would be life-threatening. Bleeding usually stops spontaneously when an injury is minor. However, a more serious bleeding episode can be life-threatening and often requires medical intervention. Normally, all but the most catastrophic bleeding is rapidly stopped through a physiologic progression of several steps, known as **hemostasis** (Figure 30-1 ■).

Hemostasis involves three events:

1. *Vascular spasms.* The platelets release the neurotransmitter **serotonin**, which causes the blood vessel to go into spasms. The spasms decrease blood loss until clotting can occur.

2. *Formation of a platelet plug.* When a blood vessel is torn, the inner lining of the vessel stimulates, or activates, the **platelets**. The platelets become sticky and adhere to the inner lining of the injured vessel and to each other. By sticking together, they form a **platelet plug**. Over several minutes, the plug is invaded by activated blood-clotting factors and eventually evolves into a stable and strong blood clot.

3. *Blood clotting.* Vascular spasm and a platelet plug alone are not sufficient to prevent the bleeding caused by a larger tear in a blood vessel. With a more serious injury to the vessel wall, bleeding stops only if a blood clot forms. Blood clotting, or **coagulation**, is the third event in the process of hemostasis. A blood clot is formed by a series of chemical reactions that result in the formation of a netlike structure. The net is composed of protein fibers called *fibrin*, which seals off the opening in the injured blood vessel and stops the bleeding. The three basic steps of hemostasis are shown in Figure 30-2 ■.

HEMOSTASIS: MECHANISM OF ACTION

The mechanism of action of hemostasis is complex and involves 11 different plasma proteins called *clotting factors*. The process of blood clotting occurs in a series of sequential steps that are referred to as a *cascade*.

Normal coagulation cannot occur unless the plasma contains the necessary clotting factors. Most of the circulating clotting proteins are synthesized by the liver. The injured vessel releases a chemical called *prothrombin activator* (prothrombinase). Prothrombin activator converts the clotting factor prothrombin to an enzyme called *thrombin*. Thrombin then converts fibrinogen to fibrin. Normal blood clotting occurs in about 6 minutes. The primary steps in the coagulation cascade are shown in Figure 30-3 ■.

✳ Apply Your **Knowledge 30.1**

The following exercises focus on what you have just learned about the physiology of hemostasis.

CRITICAL THINKING

1. What are the three events of hemostasis?
2. What is serotonin and its effect on blood vessels?
3. What is fibrin and its effect on blood clotting?
4. Where is the site of formation of the circulating clotting proteins in the human body?
5. What are clotting factors?
6. How many clotting factors are involved in the mechanism of action of hemostasis?

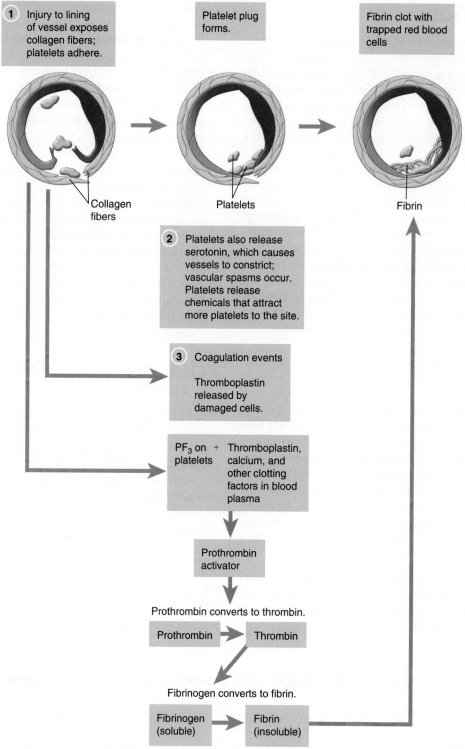

Figure 30-1 ■ Hemostasis begins when a blood vessel is damaged and ends when the fibrin threads trap blood cells, forming a clot that seals the injured vessel.

Anticoagulants

Anticoagulants are medications used to prolong bleeding time; therefore, they help to prevent harmful clots from forming in the blood vessels. These medications are sometimes called *blood thinners*, although they do not actually thin the blood. Anticoagulants do not dissolve clots that have already formed, but they may prevent the clots from becoming larger and causing more serious problems. They are often used as treatment for

Figure 30-2 ■ Basic steps of hemostasis.

Figure 30-3 ■ The steps in the coagulation cascade.

certain cardiovascular (CV) and lung conditions, such as MI, venous thrombosis, peripheral arterial **embolus** (an abnormal particle circulating in blood, such as an air bubble or blood clot), and pulmonary emboli. Anticoagulants have been used to prevent transient ischemic attacks and to reduce the risk of recurrent MI. There are two main groups of anticoagulants: (1) drugs that are administered orally and (2) drugs that are administered parenterally. Warfarin is an example of an oral anticoagulant, and heparin is an anticoagulant only given parenterally. Table 30-1 ■ lists the primary anticoagulants.

Drugs that dissolve preformed clots (thrombolytic drugs or tissue plasminogen activators), including urokinase, are not referred to as anticoagulants.

Table 30-1 ■ Anticoagulants

GENERIC NAME	TRADE NAME	AVERAGE ADULT DOSAGE	ROUTE OF ADMINISTRATION
heparin sodium*	Heparin Sodium (IV)	15,000–20,000 units bid	IV infusion
	Heparin Sodium (Subq)	5,000–40,000 units/d	SC
pentoxifylline	Trental	400 mg tid	PO
warfarin sodium	Coumadin	2–15 mg/d	PO

* For low-molecular-weight heparins, see Table 30-2.
 bid, twice a day; IV, intravenous; SC, subcutaneous; tid, three times a day; PO, oral.

Focus on Geriatrics

Anticoagulants in Elderly Patients

Older adults are more susceptible to the effects of anticoagulants. Signs of overdose include nosebleeds, blood in the stool or urine, excessive bruising, and prolonged bleeding from the gums after brushing or from cutting the face while shaving. Elderly patients especially should limit use of alcohol to only one drink per day while using anticoagulants.

Focus On

Heparin

Heparin is an anticoagulant and a protein. Two types of heparin are used clinically. The first and older of the two, standard (unfractionated) heparin, is an animal extract (from pigs). The second and newer type, called *low-molecular-weight heparin (LMWH)*, is derived from unfractionated heparin. The two classes are similar but not identical in their actions and pharmacokinetic characteristics. Standard heparin (heparin sodium) is produced by and can be released from mast cells located throughout the body. It is especially abundant in the liver, lung, and intestines.

How does it work?

Similar to other anticoagulants, heparin is a drug that increases the length of clotting time and prevents thrombi from forming or growing larger. The anticoagulation action of heparin depends on the inhibition of **thrombi**, which are blood clots that form within a blood vessel and attach to the site of formation, and clot formation by blocking the conversion of prothrombin to thrombin and fibrinogen to fibrin, which is the final step in the clotting process. Figure 30-4 ■ shows the mechanisms of action of anticoagulants.

How is it used?

Heparin is prescribed as a treatment for certain cardiovascular and lung disorders. It is also used to prevent blood clotting during open-heart surgery, coronary artery bypass graft surgery, and dialysis. Heparin is measured in International Units rather than milligrams. The dose must be determined on an individual basis. Heparin is not absorbed after oral administration and therefore must be given parenterally. Intravenous (IV) administration results in an almost immediate anticoagulant effect.

What are the adverse effects?

The major adverse effect resulting from heparin therapy is hemorrhage. Bleeding can occur in the urinary or gastrointestinal (GI) tract. Other types of hemorrhages and related conditions that may occur include *subdural hematoma* (bleeding into the areas below the dura mater, which encases the brain and central nervous system), acute hemorrhagic pancreatitis, *hemarthrosis* (blood in a joint), and *ecchymosis* (blood that has pooled in the skin). Additional adverse effects of heparin treatment include hypersensitivity reactions, fever, alopecia, osteoporosis, and ostealgia.

What are the contraindications and interactions?

Absolute contraindications include serious bleeding and intracranial bleeding. Heparin is also contraindicated in severe liver or kidney disease as well as malignant hypertension. It has not been shown to cause birth defects or bleeding problems in infants. It does not pass into breast milk.

Drugs, such as aspirin, that inhibit platelet function or produce thrombocytopenia, increase the risk of bleeding when heparin is administered. Other drugs that interact with heparin include nonsteroidal anti-inflammatory drugs (NSAIDs), anesthetics, valproic acid, sulfinpyrazone, cefamandole, cefoperazone, cefotetan, plicamycin, methimazole, propylthiouracil, probenecid, and various thrombolytics.

What are the most important points patients should know?

Teach patients how to correctly administer heparin subcutaneously if they are discharged from the hospital while on heparin. Advise patients to protect themselves from injury, such as by using an electric shaver instead of a razor. Warn patients against taking aspirin and other over-the-counter (OTC) medications. Instruct them to notify their health care provider if urine is pink, red, dark brown, or cloudy; if vomitus is red or dark brown; and/or if stools are red or black. Also, instruct patients to report bleeding gums or oral mucosa; bruising; hematoma; epistaxis; bloody sputum; chest, abdominal, lumbar, or pelvic pain; an unusual increase in menstrual flow; and severe or continuous headache, faintness, or dizziness.

Focus Point

Heparin

Overdosage of heparin can be treated by the administration of a slow infusion of 1% protamine sulfate solution. A dose of 0.5–1 mg of protamine is required to antagonize the action of each 100 units of heparin.

Figure 30-4 ■ Mechanism of action of anticoagulants.

Focus On

Low-Molecular-Weight Heparins

LMWHs are grouped as a relatively new class of anticoagulants, which have been used in Europe and are now being used more often in the United States.

How do they work?

LMWHs are derived from standard heparin. Low-molecular-weight fragments have greater *bioavailability*, the proportion of a drug's dose that is absorbed into the bloodstream, than standard heparin, a longer-lasting effect, and dose-independent clearance pharmacokinetics.

How are they used?

LMWHs are more effective than standard heparin in preventing and treating venous **thromboembolism**, which is blockage of blood vessel by a part of a thrombus that has broken away from its formation site and is circulating in the blood, such as deep venous thrombosis (DVT). The incidence of thrombocytopenia after administration of LMWHs is lower than with standard heparin. LMWHs can be given according to body weight once or twice daily without laboratory monitoring. LMWHs are superior for preventing venous thrombosis in patients undergoing hip replacement. They are administered by subcutaneous injection, and they offer the option of treatment on an outpatient basis for patients with DVT.

The clinical advantages of LMWHs include predictability, dose-dependent plasma levels, a long half-life, and less bleeding for a given antithrombotic effect. The standard treatment of DVT with IV heparin administered in a hospital offers no advantages over LMWH administered in an outpatient setting.

What are the adverse effects?

Adverse effects like those caused by standard heparin have been seen during therapy with LMWH, and overdose is treated with protamine. The most common LMWHs are shown in Table 30-2 ■.

What are the contraindications and interactions?

Although safer than regular heparin, LWMHs are contraindicated for use in children and in patients with unstable angina, allergy to heparin or pork, active bleeding, and thrombocytopenia. Drug interactions occur with oral anticoagulants, antiplatelet drugs, and thrombolytics.

What are the most important points patients should know?

The points to teach patients who are taking LMWHs are the same as those for regular heparins. See the previous section on patient teaching.

Table 30-2 ■ **Common Low-Molecular-Weight Heparins**

GENERIC NAME	TRADE NAME	PROPHYLACTIC DOSING	ROUTE OF ADMINISTRATION
dalteparin	Fragmin	2,500 International Units 1–2 h before surgery and then 2,500 International Units/d for 5–10 d	SC
enoxaparin	Lovenox	30 mg q12h or 40 mg/d for 7–10 d depending on the type of surgery; therapy should begin postoperatively	SC
tinzaparin	Innohep	175 International Units/kg/d	SC

SC, subcutaneous.

Focus Point

Low-Molecular-Weight Heparin

LMWH is associated with less bleeding and fewer episodes of heparin-induced thrombocytopenia than unfractionated heparin.

Focus On

Warfarin

Orally effective anticoagulant drugs are fat-soluble derivatives of coumarin or indandione, and they resemble vitamin K. Warfarin is the oral anticoagulant of choice. It is still among the 200 most commonly prescribed drugs in the United States. The indandione anticoagulants have greater toxicity than the coumarin drugs. Table 30-1 lists the primary anticoagulants.

How does it work?

Warfarin interferes with the hepatic synthesis of vitamin K–dependent clotting factors II [prothrombin], VII, IX, and X. This results in their eventual depletion and prolongation of clotting times. Warfarin is rapidly and almost completely absorbed after oral administration and it is bound extensively to plasma proteins. Its onset of action is from 12 hours to 3 days. Although these drugs do not cross the blood–brain barrier, they can cross the placenta and may cause *teratogenicity* (the capability of producing malformations) and hemorrhage in fetuses. Therefore, warfarin carries a strong warning against its use during pregnancy.

How is it used?

Warfarin is used on an inpatient and outpatient basis when long-term anticoagulant therapy is indicated. Warfarin is administered in conventional doses or mini-doses to reduce bleeding. The dose range is adjusted to provide the desired endpoint. The duration of action of warfarin is 2–5 days.

What are the adverse effects?

The major adverse effect of warfarin is hemorrhage that occurs at a predisposing abnormality, such as an ulcer or tumor. Prolonged therapy with the coumarin-type anticoagulants is relatively free of untoward effects. Bleeding may occur in the skin, mucous membranes, GI tract, kidneys, brain, liver, uterus, or lungs. However, close monitoring of the degree of anticoagulation is important. Practitioners are advised to keep treatment periods at a minimum to reduce risks. Rare adverse effects include diarrhea, *urticaria* (eruption of itching hives), alopecia, skin necrosis, and dermatitis.

What are the contraindications and interactions?

Oral anticoagulants are ordinarily contraindicated in the presence of active or past GI ulceration, hepatic or renal disease, malignant hypertension, bacterial endocarditis, chronic alcoholism, and pregnancy. Warfarin is an antagonist of vitamin K, a necessary element in the synthesis of clotting factors II, VII, IX, and X. Drug interactions occur with hepatic enzyme inhibitors, aspirin, NSAIDs, and thrombolytics.

What are the most important points patients should know?

Instruct patients to report signs of bleeding, including blood in the urine, red or black tarry stools, vomiting of blood, bleeding when brushing the teeth, blue or purple spots on the skin or mucous membranes, pinpoint purplish red spots, nosebleeds, and bloody sputum. Chest, abdominal, lumbar, and pelvic pain should also be reported. Advise patients to stop the drug immediately if they have signs of hepatitis or a hypersensitivity reaction. Signs of hepatitis include dark urine, itchy skin, jaundice, light stools, and abdominal pain. Instruct patients to avoid changing brands of warfarin and to take the same dose of drug at the same time each day. Advise female patients to use a barrier contraceptive to avoid pregnancy. Breast-feeding is not advised.

Focus on Natural Products

Anticoagulants and Natural Products

Dietary or supplemental intake of vitamin K can potentiate or inhibit the actions of oral anticoagulants. The top five leafy green food sources that contain vitamin K are Swiss chard, kale, parsley, Brussels sprouts, and spinach. Mineral oil and other laxatives may reduce the absorption of warfarin.

Focus Point

Warfarin

Approximately 5 days are required for the antithrombotic effects of warfarin to occur. It should not be used in patients who must undergo dental procedures.

✳ Apply Your Knowledge 30.2

The following exercises focus on what you have just learned about anticoagulant agents.

CRITICAL THINKING

1. What are three primary anticoagulants?
2. What is the major adverse effect of heparin therapy?
3. What is the treatment for an overdose of heparin?
4. What is the mechanism of action of anticoagulants?
5. What are the trade names of dalteparin and enoxaparin?
6. What is the difference between standard and low-molecular-weight heparin?
7. When long-term anticoagulant therapy is indicated, what type of anticoagulant should be used?
8. What is an antagonist of warfarin?

Focus On

Antiplatelet Drugs

Antiplatelet drugs are medications that help to prevent the formation of blood clots by keeping platelets from binding together—a process called *platelet aggregation*. Unlike the anticoagulants, which are used primarily to prevent thrombosis in veins, antiplatelet drugs are used to prevent clot formation in arteries. Antiplatelet drugs include aspirin, ticlopidine, clopidogrel, abciximab, eptifibatide, and tirofiban (Table 30-3 ■).

How do they work?

The role platelets play in blood clotting is essential when the body has been cut. Without platelets to stop the bleeding, a person would bleed to death. However, there are times when blood clotting is harmful. The size and location of blood clots may increase the person's risk of an MI or stroke. Therefore, antiplatelet drugs may be prescribed for patients with heart disease to reduce the likelihood that the platelets will aggregate and form potentially harmful blood clots.

Aspirin in low doses inhibits platelet aggregation and prolongs bleeding time. It remains the first choice in antiplatelet therapy. Aspirin is useful in preventing coronary thrombosis in patients with unstable angina, serving as an adjunct to thrombolytic therapy and reducing recurrence of thrombotic stroke.

Ticlopidine and clopidogrel are structurally related drugs that irreversibly inhibit platelet activation, leading to inhibition of platelet aggregation. Clopidogrel is preferred to ticlopidine because of its better safety profile and its lack of serious life-threatening side effects, such as leukopenia and thrombocytopenia, which can occur with ticlopidine. Clopidogrel is also more potent, is better tolerated, and can be administered as a loading dose.

Abciximab, eptifibatide, and tirofiban, which interrupt the interaction of fibrinogen with clotting factors, are capable of inhibiting the aggregation of platelets activated by a wide variety of stimuli. Abciximab is used in conjunction with angioplasty and stent procedures, and it is an adjunct to fibrinolytic therapy. Eptifibatide is approved for the treatment of acute coronary disease and for use in patients undergoing percutaneous transluminal coronary angioplasty (PTCA), commonly known as *stenting*.

How are they used?

Drugs that inhibit platelet function are administered for the relatively specific prophylaxis of arterial thrombosis and for the prophylaxis or therapeutic management of MI and stroke. The antiplatelet drugs are administered as adjuncts to thrombolytic therapy, along with heparin, to maintain *perfusion* (blood flow per unit volume of tissue) and to limit the size of MI. Recently, antiplatelet drugs have found new importance in preventing thrombosis in PCTA. The administration of an antiplatelet drug increases the risk of bleeding.

What are the adverse effects?

Antiplatelet agents may be associated with epigastric pain, heartburn, nausea, diarrhea, and major or minor bleeding events. Abciximab may also be associated with cardiac arrhythmias, abnormal thoughts, and dizziness.

What are the contraindications and interactions?

Antiplatelet drugs are generally contraindicated in patients with a history of GI ulceration, hypertension, asthma, allergies, and nasal polyps. Patients should consult their physician before taking any other medication (either prescription or OTC), nutritional supplements, and/or herbal remedies. Some of these substances can interact with antiplatelet drugs. Interactions occur with anticoagulants, platelet aggregation inhibitors, thrombolytics, dextran, abciximab, anagrelide, and dipyridamole.

What are the most important points patients should know?

Instruct patients to report nausea, diarrhea, rash, sore throat, or infection; signs of bleeding; yellow skin; dark urine; and clay-colored stools. Advise patients to not take aspirin or antacids and to keep appointments for blood tests.

Table 30-3 ■ Antiplatelet Agents

GENERIC NAME	TRADE NAME	AVERAGE ADULT DOSAGE	ROUTE OF ADMINISTRATION
abciximab	ReoPro	0.25 mg/kg initially over 5 min and then 10 mcg/min for 12 h	IV
aspirin	Ecotrin	80 mg/d–650 mg bid	PO
clopidogrel	Plavix	75 mg/d	PO
dipyridamole	Persantine	75–100 mg qid	PO
eptifibatide	Integrilin	180 mcg/kg initial bolus over 1–2 min and then 2 mcg/kg/min for 24–72 h	IV
ticlopidine	Ticlid	250 mg bid	PO
tirofiban	Aggrastat	0.4 mcg/kg/min for 30 min and then 0.1 mcg/kg/min for 12–24 h	IV

IV, intravenous; bid, twice a day; PO, oral; qid, four times a day.

Focus on Natural Products

Garlic as an Anticoagulant

Garlic has long been studied as a natural alternative to antiplatelet drugs because it has been shown to decrease platelet aggregation. Proponents of garlic claim it can reduce heart disease and the incidence of stroke. Garlic is also used by many people to treat colds, coughing, infections, bronchitis, arteriosclerosis, high blood cholesterol levels, and hypertension. It is wise to alert patients that using garlic concomitantly with anticoagulants may cause bleeding complications.

Focus Point

Antiplatelet Drugs During Pregnancy

Taking antiplatelet drugs in the last 2 weeks of pregnancy may cause bleeding problems in the baby, before and after delivery. When taken in the last 3 months of pregnancy, antiplatelet drugs may prolong the length of the pregnancy and the delivery.

✳ Apply Your Knowledge 30.3

The following exercises focus on what you have just learned about antiplatelet agents.

CRITICAL THINKING

1. What is the description of platelet aggregation?
2. What is the effect of low doses of aspirin on platelets?
3. What is the difference between ticlopidine and clopidogrel?
4. What is another name for percutaneous transluminal coronary angioplasty?
5. What are the trade names of abciximab, dipyridamole, eptifibatide, and tirofiban?

Focus On

Thrombolytic Drugs

Thrombolytic drugs (also called *thrombolytics*) are the small group of drugs used to dissolve blood clots. Four thrombolytic drugs are available: alteplase, reteplase, tenecteplase, and urokinase. Alteplase, reteplase, and tenecteplase are subclassified as recombinant tissue plasminogen activators. Urokinase is classified, uniquely, as a urokinase-type plasminogen activator. These drugs are prescribed in a hospital setting. Table 30-4 ■ lists thrombolytic drugs.

How do they work?

Thrombolytics facilitate the conversion of plasminogen to plasmin, which subsequently hydrolyzes fibrin to dissolve blood clots, or thrombi, that have already formed. Thrombolytic drugs are plasminogen activators. The ideal thrombolytic drug is one that can be administered IV to produce clot-selective fibrinolysis without activating plasminogen to plasmin in plasma. Newer thrombolytic drugs bind to fibrin and activate *fibrinolysis* (breakdown of fibrin) more than *fibrinogenolysis* (breakdown of fibrinogen).

How are they used?

Thrombolytic drugs are indicated for the management of severe pulmonary embolism, DVT, and arterial thromboembolism; they are especially important for therapy after MI and acute ischemic stroke. Thrombolysis must be accomplished quickly after MI or cerebral infarction because clots become more difficult to dissolve (or lyse) as they age. Adjunctive anticoagulant and antiplatelet drugs may contribute to bleeding during thrombolytic therapy.

What are the adverse effects?

The principal adverse effect associated with thrombolytic therapy is bleeding caused by fibrinogenolysis or fibrinolysis at the site of vascular injury. The incidence of bleeding occurs at a similar rate for all agents. Life-threatening intracranial bleeding may necessitate stopping therapy.

What are the contraindications and interactions?

The contraindications to the use of thrombolytic drugs are similar to those for anticoagulant drugs. Absolute contraindications include active bleeding, pregnancy, lactation, intracranial trauma, vascular disease, and cancer.

Anticoagulants and aspirin can cause interactions with thrombolytics and increase the risk of bleeding. Such herbs as feverfew, galling, ginger, and ginkgo may increase the risk of bleeding.

What are the most important points patients should know?

Instruct patients to immediately report signs of bleeding (blood in urine, tarry stools, or oozing from cuts) or changes in consciousness to their health care provider. Advise women to not breastfeed while taking urokinase.

Table 30-4 ■ Thrombolytic Drugs

GENERIC NAME	TRADE NAME	AVERAGE ADULT DOSAGE	ROUTE OF ADMINISTRATION
alteplase recombinant	Activase	Begin with 60 mg and then infuse 20 mg/h over next 2 h	IV
reteplase recombinant	Retavase	10 units over 2 min; repeat dose in 30 min	IV
tenecteplase recombinant	TNKase	Up to 50 mg bolus over 5 seconds based on patient weight	IV
urokinase	Kinlytic	4,400–6,000 units administered over several min to 12 h	IV

IV, intravenous.

Focus Point

Thrombocytopenia

Platelet deficiency (thrombocytopenia) is the most common cause of abnormal bleeding. The term hemophilia applies to several different hereditary bleeding disorders that result from a lack of any of the factors needed for clotting.

Focus Point

Top Five Prescribed Anticoagulants

1. enoxaparin (Lovenox)
2. rivaroxaban (Xarelto)
3. warfarin (Warfarin Sodium)
4. heparin (Heparin Sodium)
5. bivalirudin (Angiomax)

✳ Apply Your Knowledge 30.4

The following exercises focus on what you have just learned about thrombolytic drugs.

CRITICAL THINKING

1. What is the term for platelet deficiency?
2. What is the mechanism of action of thrombolytics?
3. What are the indications for thrombolytic drugs?
4. What are the top five prescribed anticoagulants?
5. What are the trade names of urokinase and tenecteplase recombinant?

PRACTICAL SCENARIO 1

A 65-year-old patient with a history of deep vein thrombosis has been admitted to the hospital with chest pain. He is having trouble breathing. His physician orders an electrocardiogram, a Doppler ultrasonography, a ventilation-perfusion scan, and a computed tomography scan. The diagnosis is a pulmonary embolus.

Critical Thinking Questions

1. What medicine will the physician likely immediately prescribe for this patient while he is hospitalized?

2. What teaching will you provide the patient and family about the reasons he is taking this medication and the precautions he needs to take during therapy?

3. Do you think the patient will be released from the hospital while taking this medication or will his medication be switched? If the medication is changed when the patient is discharged, what is a likely alternative medicine that will be prescribed?

4. What teaching will you provide the patient when he leaves the hospital, especially regarding his medication?

PRACTICAL SCENARIO 2

A 23-year-old pregnant woman underwent a caesarean section for delivery. Her physician ordered anticoagulants to prevent complications that could potentially occur.

Critical Thinking Questions

1. What is the most common complication after this type of surgery that requires the use of anticoagulants?

2. Name the common medication used after surgery for preventing clots.

Chapter Capsule

This section repeats the objectives from the beginning of the chapter and then provides a summary of the most important concepts for that objective. Use this section as a quick review and to check your knowledge.

Objective 1: Explain the three events involved in hemostasis.

- Vascular spasms: The platelets release the neurotransmitter serotonin, which causes the blood vessel to go into spasms. The spasms decrease blood loss until clotting can occur.

- Formation of a platelet plug: When a blood vessel is torn, the inner lining of the vessel stimulates, or activates, the platelets. The platelets become sticky and adhere to the inner lining of the injured vessel and to each other. By sticking together, they form a platelet plug. Over several minutes, the plug is invaded by activated blood-clotting factors and eventually evolves into a stable and strong blood clot.

- Blood clotting: Vascular spasm and a platelet plug alone are not sufficient to prevent the bleeding caused by a larger tear in a blood vessel. With a more serious injury to the vessel wall, bleeding stops only if a blood clot forms. A blood clot is formed by a series of chemical reactions that result in the formation of a netlike structure. The net is composed of protein fibers called fibrin, which seals off the opening in the injured blood vessel and stops the bleeding.

Objective 2: Define the terms *clotting factors* and *cascade* in relation to hemostasis.

- The mechanism of action of hemostasis is complex and involves 11 different plasma proteins called clotting factors.

- The process of blood clotting occurs in a series of sequential steps that are referred to as a cascade.

Objective 3: Explain the role of prothrombinase in blood clotting.

- Normal coagulation cannot occur unless the plasma contains the necessary clotting factors. Most of the circulating clotting proteins are synthesized by the liver. The injured vessel releases the chemical prothrombin activator (prothrombinase).

- Prothrombin activator converts the clotting factor prothrombin to an enzyme called thrombin. Thrombin then converts fibrinogen to fibrin. Normal blood clotting occurs in about 6 minutes.

Objective 4: Explain how anticoagulants work.

- Anticoagulants are medications used to prolong bleeding time; therefore, they help to prevent harmful clots from forming in the blood vessels.

- These medications are sometimes called blood thinners, although they do not actually thin the blood. Anticoagulants do not dissolve clots that have already formed, but they may prevent the clots from becoming larger and causing more serious problems.

Objective 5: List the indications of anticoagulants.

- Anticoagulants are often used as treatment for certain cardiovascular (CV) and lung conditions, such as MI, venous thrombosis, peripheral arterial embolus, and pulmonary emboli. Anticoagulants have been used to prevent transient ischemic attacks and to reduce the risk of recurrent MI.

Objective 6: Describe the mechanism of action of heparin.

- Heparin (a parenteral anticoagulant) increases the length of clotting time and prevents thrombi from forming or growing larger

- Its action depends on inhibition of thrombus and clot formation by blocking conversion of prothrombin to thrombin and fibrinogen to fibrin

Objective 7: Describe the advantages of low-molecular-weight heparin.

- Greater bioavailability and longer-lasting effect than standard heparins and dose-independent clearance pharmacokinetics

Objective 8: Explain the mechanism of action of warfarin.

- Warfarin interferes with the hepatic synthesis of vitamin K–dependent clotting factors II (prothrombin), VII, IX, and X. This results in their eventual depletion and prolongation of clotting times. Warfarin is rapidly and almost completely absorbed after oral administration and it is bound extensively to plasma proteins. Its onset of action is from 12 hours to 3 days. It does not cross the blood–brain barrier, but can cross the placenta and may cause teratogenicity and hemorrhage in fetuses.

Objective 9: Explain how antiplatelet drugs are used.

■ Antiplatelet drugs inhibit platelet function, and are administered for the relatively specific prophylaxis of arterial thrombosis and for the prophylaxis or therapeutic management of MI and stroke. They are administered as adjuncts to thrombolytic therapy, along with heparin, to maintain perfusion and to limit the size of MI. Recently, antiplatelet drugs have found new importance in preventing thrombosis in PCTA. The administration of an antiplatelet drug increases the risk of bleeding.

Objective 10: List the indications of thrombolytic drugs.

■ Thrombolytic drugs are indicated for the management of severe pulmonary embolism, DVT, and arterial thromboembolism; they are especially important for therapy after MI and acute ischemic stroke. Thrombolysis must be accomplished quickly after MI or cerebral infarction because clots become more difficult to dissolve (or lyse) as they age.

Internet Sites of Interest

■ An overview of anticoagulants can be found at: **www.drugs.com/drug-class/ anticoagulants.html**

■ Emboli are explained at: **www.nlm.nih.gov/medlineplus/ency/article/001102.htm**

■ An overview of heparin is given at this website: **www.webmd.com/drugs/2/ drug-3918/heparin-porcine-inj/details**

■ A focus on warfarin can be found at: **www.webmd.com/drugs/2/drug-3949/ warfarin-oral/details**

Chapter 31

Drugs Used to Treat Fluid and Electrolyte Imbalances

Chapter Objectives

After completing this chapter, you should be able to:

1. Describe the structure of a nephron.
2. Explain urea, creatinine, and uric acid.
3. Explain the processes of urine formation.
4. Discuss how water is taken into the body and how it leaves the body.
5. List the ways that electrolytes are lost from the body.
6. Describe how antidiuretic hormone and aldosterone levels influence the volume and concentration of urine.
7. Explain the indications for the use of diuretics in various conditions and disorders of the human body.
8. Classify the five major types of diuretics.
9. Describe the mechanism of action for osmotic diuretics.
10. List the major adverse effects of potassium-sparing diuretics.

Key Terms

Introduction

The primary function of the kidneys is to maintain a stable internal environment for optimal cell and tissue metabolism. The kidneys accomplish these life-sustaining tasks by balancing solute and water transport, excreting metabolic waste products, conserving nutrients, and regulating acids and bases. The kidneys also have an endocrine function and secrete the hormones **renin**, a hormone that converts angiotensinogen to angiotensin I, erythropoietin, and vitamin D_3 for the regulation of blood pressure, red blood cell (RBC) production, and calcium metabolism, respectively. The formation of urine is achieved through the process of filtration, reabsorption, and secretion by the glomeruli and tubules within the kidneys. The bladder stores the urine that is received from the kidneys by way of the ureters. Urine is then removed from the body through the urethra. Figure 31-1 ■ illustrates the urinary system.

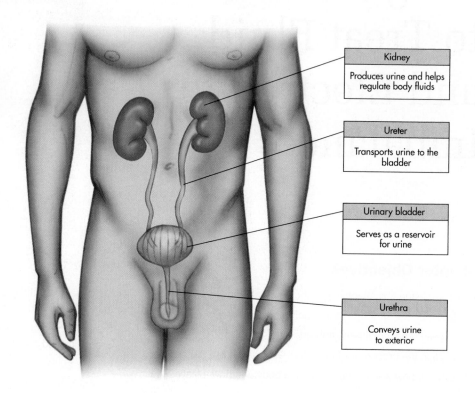

Kidney
Produces urine and helps regulate body fluids

Ureter
Transports urine to the bladder

Urinary bladder
Serves as a reservoir for urine

Urethra
Conveys urine to exterior

Figure 31-1 ■ The urinary system.

Kidney Structure and Functions

The kidneys include two distinct regions: an inner medulla and an outer cortex. The renal *cortex* is the superficial portion of the kidney. The renal *medulla* consists of 6–18 distinct triangular structures called *renal pyramids*. The base of each pyramid faces the cortex, and the tip of each pyramid—a region known as the *renal papilla*—projects into the renal sinus. The basic unit of the kidney is the nephron. The main function of the kidneys is to regulate the volume, composition, and pH of body fluids. The kidneys remove metabolic wastes from the blood and excrete them to the outside.

NEPHRONS

Each kidney contains about 1 million functional units called **nephrons**. Nephrons are located in the renal cortex. Each nephron consists of a **renal corpuscle** and a **renal tubule**. A renal corpuscle consists of a filtering unit composed of a cluster of blood capillaries called a **glomerulus** and a surrounding thin-walled, sac-like structure called a **glomerular capsule**. The renal tubule leads away from the glomerular capsule and becomes highly coiled. This coiled portion of the tubule is the *proximal convoluted tubule*. Following the proximal convoluted tubule is the *nephron loop* (**loop of Henle**). The ascending limb of this loop becomes highly coiled again and is called the *distal convoluted tubule (DCT)*. This portion of the nephron then forms a *collecting duct* (collecting tubule), which is technically not part of the nephron (Figure 31-2 ■).

PRINCIPLES OF RENAL PHYSIOLOGY

The aim of urine production is to maintain homeostasis by regulating the volume and composition of blood. This process involves the excretion of solutes—specifically, metabolic waste products. Three organic

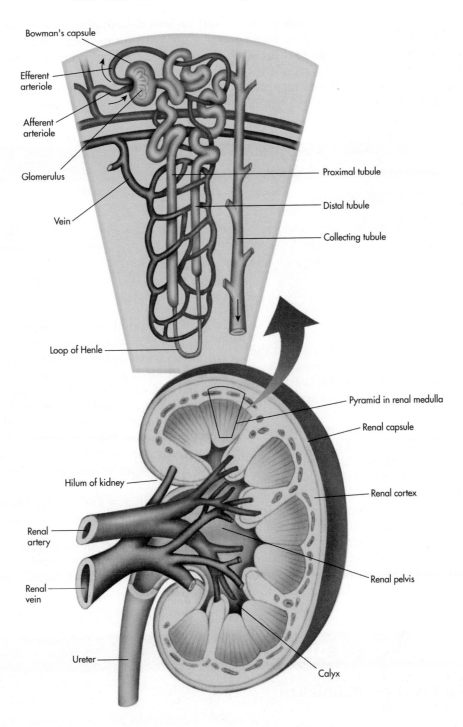

Figure 31-2 ■ The kidney with an expanded view of the nephron.

waste products are very important: urea, creatinine, and uric acid.

✳ **Urea** is the most abundant organic waste. Each person generates about 21 g of urea each day, which results in the breakdown of amino acids.

✳ **Creatinine**—a chemical waste molecule—is produced in skeletal muscle tissue by the breakdown of *creatine phosphate*, a high-energy compound that plays an important role in muscle contraction.

The body generates roughly 1.8 g of creatinine each day, and virtually all of it is excreted in urine.

✳ **Uric acid**—another type of waste molecule—is formed by recycling a nitrogenous base from RNA molecules. Humans produce approximately 480 mg of uric acid each day.

These waste products are dissolved in the bloodstream and can be eliminated only while dissolved in the bloodstream or urine. As a result, their removal is accompanied by an unavoidable water loss. The kidneys are usually capable of producing more than four times the amount of concentrated urine than plasma. If the kidneys were not able to concentrate the filtrate produced by glomerular filtration, losses of fluid would lead to fatal dehydration in a matter of hours. At the same time, the kidneys ensure that the fluid lost does not contain potentially useful organic substances that are present in blood plasma, such as sugars or amino acids. These valuable materials must be reabsorbed and retained for use by other tissues.

Focus on Geriatrics

Diuresis in Older Adults

Older adults have a decreased ability to concentrate urine and are less able to tolerate dehydration or water loads because they have fewer nephrons. In older adults, drugs eliminated by the kidneys can accumulate in the plasma, causing toxic reactions.

URINE FORMATION

The main function of the nephrons is to control the composition of the body fluids and remove wastes from the blood. The product is urine, which is excreted from the body. It contains wastes, excess water, and electrolytes.

Urine formation begins with the filtration of plasma by the glomerular capillaries—a process called **glomerular filtration**. However, glomerular filtration produces 180 L of fluid, which is more than four times the amount of **total body water (TBW)**, which is the total water content of the body, every 24 hours. Glomerular filtration could not continue for very long unless most of this filtered fluid was returned to the internal environment.

The kidneys return filtered fluid to the internal environment through **tubular reabsorption**, selectively reclaiming just the right amounts of substances that the body requires, such as water, electrolytes, and glucose. Waste products and excess substances are processed out of the body. Some substances that the body must eliminate, such as hydrogen ions and certain toxins, are removed even faster than through filtration alone by the process of **tubular secretion**. In this process, the cells of the tubules remove certain substances from the blood and deposit them into the fluid in the tubules. In other words, the following relationship determines the volume of substances excreted in the urine:

Urinary excretion = Glomerular filtration + Tubular secretion − Tubular reabsorption

The final product of these processes is urine. The kidneys contribute to homeostasis by maintaining the composition of the internal environment (see Figure 31-3 ■).

Focus on Pediatrics

Fluid Imbalances in Children

The urine of infants and children is more dilute than that of adults because of pediatric higher blood flow and shorter loops of Henle. Pediatric patients are more affected by fluid imbalances resulting from diarrhea, infection, or improper feeding because their systems have a limited ability to quickly regulate changes in pH or osmotic pressure.

CONTROL OF URINE VOLUME

Urine volume is regulated by controlling the reabsorption of water. Water is reabsorbed by osmosis in the proximal convoluted tubule and the descending limb of the loop of Henle—a long, U-shaped part of the renal tubule extending through the medulla from the end of the proximal convoluted tubule to the beginning of the DCT. The ascending limb of the loop of Henle is impermeable to water. The DCT and collecting duct are also impermeable to water, except in the presence of **antidiuretic hormone (ADH)**. ADH is a hormone that is

F = Filtration: blood to tubule
R = Reabsorption: tubule to blood
S = Secretion: blood to tubule
E = Excretion: tubule to
    external environment

Figure 31-3 ■ Sites of resorption and secretion in a nephron.

also called *vasopressin*. It is released from the posterior lobe of the pituitary gland. The higher the circulating levels of ADH, the greater water permeability of these segments of the urinary system. In the absence of ADH, water is not reabsorbed in the DCT or the collecting system. Therefore, large amounts of very dilute urine are produced, which can cause diabetes insipidus. Failure of the posterior pituitary to produce ADH, or *hypophysectomy* (removal of the pituitary gland), may cause diabetes insipidus.

Focus Point

Medications and Urine Retention

Several medications cause urine retention and require careful consideration of use in certain patients. These include:

- Anticholinergic and antispasmodic medications, such as atropine and papaverine
- Antidepressant and antipsychotic agents, such as phenothiazines and monoamine oxidase inhibitors
- Antihistamine preparations, such as pseudoephedrine
- Antihypertensives, such as hydralazine and methyldopa
- Beta-adrenergic blockers, such as propranolol
- Opioids, such as hydrocodone

Focus Point

Overactive Bladder

Overactive bladder is a condition in which the bladder forces out urine more often than normal. It is signified by urination that occurs eight or more times per day, or two or more times per night. There may be a sudden, strong urge to urinate immediately, which is sometimes followed by urine leaking from the bladder. The condition may also be signified by incontinence, which is a loss of bladder control. Overactive bladder is often of unknown cause, but may be linked to excessive fluid or caffeine consumption, as well as nerve abnormalities. Medications used for overactive bladder include anticholinergics such as darifenacin and fesoterodine, as well as a newer agent called mirabegron. These agents work by relaxing the muscles of the bladder, which helps the bladder to hold more urine.

✳ Apply Your **Knowledge 31.1**

The following questions focus on what you have just learned about urine formation and control of urine volume.

CRITICAL THINKING

1. What are the functions of renin and erythropoietin?
2. What is the process of urine formation?
3. What is meant by the terms *urea* and *creatinine*?
4. Why do older adults have fewer nephrons than younger adults?
5. What is tubular reabsorption?
6. Why is the urine of infants and children more dilute than that of adults?
7. What is another name for antidiuretic hormone?
8. What disorder may result from the absence of antidiuretic hormone?

Fluid and Electrolyte Balance

The term *balance* suggests a state of equilibrium and, in the case of water and electrolytes, it means that the quantities entering the body equal the quantities leaving it. Maintaining such a balance requires mechanisms to ensure that lost water and electrolytes are replaced and that any excesses are excreted. As a result, the levels of water and electrolytes in the body remain relatively stable at all times.

It is important to remember that water balance and electrolyte balance are interdependent because electrolytes are dissolved in the water of body fluids. Consequently, anything that alters the concentrations of the electrolytes alters the concentration of the water by adding solutes to it or by removing solutes from it. Likewise, anything that changes the concentration of the water changes the concentrations of the electrolytes by concentrating or diluting them.

Focus on Pediatrics

Threat of Dehydration in Infants

At birth, TBW represents about 75–80% of body weight and decreases to about 67% during the first year of life. Infants are particularly susceptible to significant changes in TBW because of a high metabolic rate and greater body surface area. Renal mechanisms of fluid and electrolyte conservation may not be mature enough to counter losses, thereby allowing dehydration to occur.

Focus Point

Water Deficit

Dehydration describes water deficit but is also commonly used to indicate sodium and water loss. Pure water deficits are rare because most people have access to water. Patients who are comatose or paralyzed have insensible water loss through the skin and lungs, with minimal obligatory formation of urine, and must be monitored closely for water deficit.

WATER BALANCE

Water balance exists when water intake equals water output. Homeostasis requires control of water intake and water output. Ultimately, maintenance of the internal environment depends on thirst centers in the brain to vary water intake and on the kidneys' ability to vary water output. Water balance is regulated by the secretion of ADH and the perception of thirst. Thirst stimulates water drinking and is experienced when water loss equals 2% of an individual's body weight or when there is an increase in **osmolality**, which is the concentration of particles in plasma. ADH is secreted when plasma osmolality increases or when circulating blood volume decreases and blood pressure decreases. Increased plasma osmolality occurs with **water deficit** in the body, or with sodium excess in relation to water.

Focus on Geriatrics

Fluctuating Total Body Water Content in Elderly Patients

The decline in the percentage of TBW content in elderly patients results, in part, because of increased body fat and decreased muscle as well as the kidneys' reduced ability to regulate sodium and water balance. Kidneys are less efficient in producing concentrated urine, and sodium-conserving responses are sluggish. With stress or when disease is present, this normal decrease in TBW can become life-threatening.

✳ **Water intake.** The volume of water gained each day varies among individuals (Table 31-1 ■). An average adult living in a moderate environment takes in about 2,500 mL per day. Approximately 60% is obtained from drinking water or other beverages, and another 30% comes from moist foods. The remaining 10% is a by-product of the oxidative metabolism of nutrients, which is called **water of metabolism.**

✳ **Water output.** Water normally enters the body only through the mouth, but it can be lost by a variety of routes. These include obvious losses in urine (the largest amount), feces, and sweat as well as evaporation from the skin and from the lungs during breathing (insensible water loss).

If an average adult takes in 2,500 mL of water each day, then 2,500 mL must be eliminated to maintain water balance. Of this volume, perhaps 60% is lost in urine, 6% in feces, and 6% in sweat. About 28% is lost by evaporation from the skin and lungs. These percentages vary with such environmental factors as temperature and relative humidity and with physical exercise. Therefore, the primary means of regulating water output is the control of urine production.

Table 31-1 ■ Normal Water Gains and Losses*

DAILY INTAKE	(mL)	DAILY OUTPUT	(mL)
Drinking	1,400–1,800	Urine	1,400–1,800
Water in food	700–1,000	Stool	100
Water of oxidation	300–400	Skin	300–500
		Lungs	600–800
Total	**2,400–3,200**	**Total**	**2,400–3,200**

* Based on a 70-kg adult man.

Focus Point

Maintaining Fluid and Electrolyte Balance

Remind patients of the following points to promote fluid and electrolyte balance:

- Consume six to eight glasses of water daily.
- Avoid excess amounts of foods or fluids high in salt, sugar, and caffeine.
- Eat a well-balanced diet.
- Limit alcohol intake because it has a diuretic effect.
- Increase fluid intake before, during, and after strenuous exercise.
- Maintain normal body weight.

ELECTROLYTE BALANCE

An *electrolyte* is any compound that, in solution, conducts electricity or is decomposed by it. An electrolyte balance exists when the quantities of electrolytes—molecules that release ions in water—gained and lost are equal (Figure 31-4 ■).

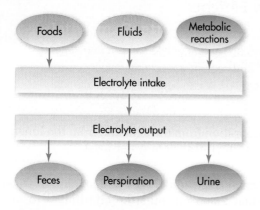

Figure 31-4 ■ Electrolyte balance. Electrolyte intake occurs through the ingestion of foods and fluids through metabolic reactions. Electrolyte output occurs through the excretion of feces, sweat, and urine.

✳ **Electrolyte intake.** The electrolytes of greatest importance to cellular functions release sodium, potassium, calcium, magnesium, chloride, sulfate, phosphate, bicarbonate, and hydrogen ions. These electrolytes are primarily obtained from foods, but they may also be found in drinking water and other beverages. In addition, some electrolytes are by-products of metabolic reactions.

✳ **Electrolyte output.** The body loses some electrolytes by perspiring. Sweat has about half the solute concentration of plasma. The quantities of lost electrolytes vary with the amount of perspiration. More electrolytes are lost in sweat on warmer days and during strenuous exercise. Varying amounts

of electrolytes are lost in the feces. The greatest electrolyte output occurs because of kidney function and urine production. The kidneys alter renal electrolyte losses to maintain the proper composition of body fluids.

The concentrations of positively charged ions—such as sodium (Na^+), potassium (K^+), and calcium (Ca^{+2})—are particularly important. For example, certain concentrations of these ions are vital for nerve impulse conduction, muscle fiber contraction, and the maintenance of cell membrane permeability. Potassium is especially important in maintaining the resting potential of nerve and cardiac muscle cells, and abnormal potassium levels may cause these cells to function abnormally.

Sodium ions account for nearly 90% of the **cations** (positively charged ions) in extracellular fluid (ECF). Primarily, the kidneys and the hormone aldosterone regulate these ions. Aldosterone, which the adrenal cortex secretes, increases sodium ion reabsorption in the DCTs and collecting ducts of the nephrons. A decrease in sodium ion concentration in the ECF stimulates aldosterone secretion.

Aldosterone also regulates potassium ions. An important stimulus for aldosterone secretion is an increasing potassium ion concentration, which directly stimulates cells of the adrenal cortex. This hormone enhances the renal tubular reabsorption of sodium ions and, at the same time, stimulates the renal tubular secretion of potassium ions.

Generally, the regulatory mechanisms that control positively charged ions secondarily control the concentrations of **anions** (negatively charged ions). For example, chloride ions (Cl^-)—the most abundant negatively charged ions in the ECF—are passively reabsorbed from the renal tubules in response to the active reabsorption of sodium ions. That is, the negatively charged chloride ions are electrically attracted to the positively charged sodium ions and accompany them as they are reabsorbed. The main electrolytes in the body are listed in Table 31-2 ■.

Table 31-2 ■ The Main Electrolytes in the Body

CATIONS	IONS	ANIONS	IONS
calcium	Ca^{++}	phosphate	PO^{4-} or HPO^{4-}
magnesium	Mg^{++}	sulfate	SO^{4-}
potassium	K^+	bicarbonate	HCO^-_3
sodium	Na^+	chloride	Cl^-

Focus on Geriatrics

Threats to Fluid and Electrolyte Imbalance in Older Adults

Certain changes related to aging cause elderly people to be at higher risk for serious problems with fluid and electrolyte imbalance if homeostatic mechanisms are compromised. Some of these changes include:

- Decreased thirst sensation
- Decreased ability of the kidneys to concentrate urine
- Decreased intracellular fluid and total body water
- Decreased response to body hormones that help regulate fluids and electrolytes
- Increased use of diuretics for hypertension and heart disease
- Decreased fluid and food intake

✳ Apply Your Knowledge 31.2

The following questions focus on what you have just learned about fluid and electrolyte balance.

CRITICAL THINKING

1. What is osmolality?
2. What is water of metabolism?
3. What are the most important electrolytes for cellular functions?
4. What are the definitions of *cations* and *anions*?
5. What is the percentage of total body water at birth?

FLUID AND ELECTROLYTE BALANCING AGENTS

Agents that are used to balance fluids and electrolytes in the body include many different varieties of diuretics. Because regulatory systems that are involved in the control of these balances are affected by normal aging, the most common patients who require diuretics are older adults. Water and sodium balances are interdependent and may be related to intake and excretion of water, thirst perception, and disordered water regulation that is linked to Alzheimer's disease.

Diuretics are a group of drugs that promote water loss from the body into the urine. Because urine formation takes place in the kidneys, it is not surprising that diuretics have their principal action at the level of the nephrons. Diuretics remove the excess ECF from the body that can result in **edema** (abnormal fluid accumulation) of the tissues, ascites, and hypertension. These conditions occur in diseases of the heart, kidneys, and liver.

Each human kidney has about 1 million nephrons. More than 120 mL of ultrafiltrate is formed per minute, but only 1 mL of urine is produced. Thus, more than

99% of ultrafiltrate is reabsorbed. Diuretics increase the rate of urine flow. Clinically useful diuretics increase the rate of excretion of sodium (Na^1) and chloride (Cl^2).

NaCl is the major determinant of the ECF volume; therefore, most clinical applications of diuretics are directed toward reducing ECF volume by decreasing total body NaCl content. Sustained positive Na^1 balance causes volume overload with pulmonary edema. Sustained negative Na^1 balance causes volume depletion and cardiovascular collapse. The five major classes of diuretics are:

1. Osmotic diuretics
2. Carbonic anhydrase inhibitors
3. Thiazide diuretics
4. Loop diuretics
5. Potassium-sparing diuretics

Focus Point

Contraindications of Diuretics in Pregnancy

Diuretics are not recommended during pregnancy because they may interfere with the normal expansion of fluid that occurs during pregnancy and disrupt neurodevelopment of the fetus. Diuretic use increases the fetus's risk of such conditions as schizophrenia, jaundice, blood problems, and potassium depletion. Most diuretics pass into breast milk and can cause dehydration in nursing babies.

Focus On

Osmotic Diuretics

The capacity of the renal tubule to reabsorb various electrolytes and nonelectrolytes is limited and varies for each ionic species. If large amounts of these substances are administered to an individual, their concentration in the body fluids and subsequently in the glomerular filtrate exceeds the reabsorption capacity of the tubules. The excess then appears in the urine, accompanied by an increased volume of water.

Generally, substances that increase urine formation in this manner are called *osmotic diuretics*. This group of diuretics (see Table 31-3 ■) includes:

✳ Osmotic electrolytes: potassium and sodium salts

✳ Osmotic nonelectrolytes: urea, glycerin, and mannitol

✳ Acid-forming salts: ammonium chloride

How do they work?

Osmotic agents may have multiple sites of action. Nevertheless, their major component is a decrease in solute content, resulting in less water reabsorption from the descending loop of Henle and collecting duct and less sodium chloride reabsorption in the proximal tubule and ascending limb of Henle.

How are they used?

Osmotic diuretics are highly effective treatments for cerebral edema and are used primarily for this purpose.

What are the adverse effects?

The major adverse effects of osmotic diuretics are related to the amount of solute administered and the effect on the volume and distribution of body fluids. They may cause headache, tremor, convulsions, dizziness, hypotension or hypertension, and thrombophlebitis. They may also produce blurred vision, dry mouth, nausea and vomiting, chills, fever, and allergic reactions.

What are the contraindications and interactions?

Osmotic diuretics are contraindicated in patients with anuria, marked pulmonary congestion or edema, severe congestive heart failure (CHF), metabolic edema, organic central nervous system disease, intracranial bleeding, shock, severe **dehydration** (excessive loss of body water), history of allergy, pregnancy, and lactation.

What are the important points patients should know?

Advise patients to report thirst, muscle cramps or weakness, paresthesia, dyspnea, and headache and to keep follow-up appointments for laboratory tests. Instruct female patients to avoid breastfeeding while taking these drugs.

Table 31-3 ■ Osmotic Diuretics

GENERIC NAME	TRADE NAME	AVERAGE ADULT DOSAGE	ROUTE OF ADMINISTRATION
glycerin	Osmoglyn	1–2 g/kg	PO
isosorbide dinitrate	Isordil	5–20 mg bid	PO
mannitol	Osmitrol	50–100 g/d	IV for edema or ascites
urea	(Generic only)	1–1.5 g/kg/d	IV

PO, oral; bid, twice a day; IV, intravenous.

Focus On

Carbonic Anhydrase Inhibitors

Carbonic anhydrase inhibitors stop the conversion of carbon dioxide to carbonic acid and bicarbonate ions. They are generally used to treat glaucoma and epilepsy and to lessen the effects of high altitudes on the body (Table 31-4 ■).

How do they work?

The enzyme carbonic anhydrase catalyzes the conversion of carbon dioxide into bicarbonate ions and vice versa according to the following equation:

$$CO_2 + H_2O \rightarrow H_2CO_3 \leftrightarrow H^+ + CO_3H^-$$

This reaction occurs in the kidneys as well as other parts of the body. In the kidneys, the reaction occurs mainly in the proximal tubule, and because it involves bicarbonate loss, it affects acid–base balance. The tubular cells are not very permeable to bicarbonate ions or carbonic acid, but they are very permeable to carbon dioxide. Under normal conditions, carbonic anhydrase in the tubular cell converts the carbonic acid into carbon dioxide and water, which are promptly reabsorbed. If the enzyme is inhibited, there will be a net loss of bicarbonate from the body, with a consequent loss of water. The drug acetazolamide is a noncompetitive inhibitor of this enzyme and has been used as a diuretic.

How are they used?

Carbonic anhydrase inhibitors are used in the treatment of absence, generalized tonic–clonic, and focal seizures. They can also be used for the reduction of intraocular pressure in glaucoma (see Chapter 37) and to treat acute high-altitude sickness.

What are the adverse effects?

The adverse effects of carbonic anhydrase inhibitors include anorexia, nausea and vomiting, weight loss, dry mouth, thirst, diarrhea, and bone marrow depression. Other adverse effects are fatigue, dizziness, drowsiness, hyperglycemia, exacerbation of gout, and hepatic dysfunction.

What are the contraindications and interactions?

Carbonic anhydrase inhibitors are contraindicated in patients with hypersensitivity to sulfonamides and derivatives such as thiazides. They should be avoided in marked renal and hepatic dysfunction, Addison's disease or other types of adrenocortical insufficiency, **hyponatremia** (abnormally low concentration of sodium ions in blood), **hypokalemia** (abnormally low concentration of potassium ions in blood), or hypochloremic acidosis. Safety during pregnancy and lactation is not established.

Carbonic anhydrase inhibitors should be used cautiously in patients with a history of hypercalciuria, diabetes mellitus, gout, obstructive pulmonary disease, and respiratory acidosis and in patients receiving digitalis. Carbonic anhydrase inhibitors, such as acetazolamide, may cause renal excretion of amphetamines, ephedrine, quinidine, and procainamide. They may decrease the effects of tricyclic antidepressants. Renal excretion of lithium is increased. Excretion of phenobarbital may be increased. Amphotericin B and corticosteroids may accelerate potassium loss.

What are the important points patients should know?

Instruct patients taking carbonic anhydrase inhibitors to avoid driving and operating heavy machinery if drowsiness or dizziness occurs.

Table 31-4 ■ Carbonic Anhydrase Inhibitors

GENERIC NAME	TRADE NAME	AVERAGE ADULT DOSAGE	ROUTE OF ADMINISTRATION
acetazolamide	Diamox Sequels	250 mg/d 1–4 times/d; 500 mg sustained release bid	PO
	(Generic only for IV use)	250–375 mg/d	IV
dichlorphenamide	Keveyis	50 mg bid	PO
methazolamide	Methazolamide	50–100 mg bid–tid	PO

bid, twice a day; PO, oral; IV, intravenous; tid, three times a day.

Focus Point

The Threat of Hypokalemia

Hypokalemia is a potentially life-threatening condition that occurs most often as a side effect of diuretic therapy or prolonged diarrhea. Hypokalemia may be caused by inappropriate or excessive use of such drugs as corticosteroids, penicillin, aminoglycosides, cardiac glycosides, laxatives, and vitamin B_{12} therapy.

Focus On

Thiazide and Thiazide-like Diuretics

Thiazides are a group of drugs that are chemically similar. The thiazide-like drugs are chemically dissimilar from the thiazides but have an identical mode of action. Thiazides are the most commonly used diuretic drugs influencing the function of the urinary tract (Table 31-5 ■).

How do they work?

The thiazide diuretics increase the urinary excretion of sodium and water by inhibiting sodium reabsorption on the DCTs and collecting ducts. They also increase the excretion of chloride, potassium, and bicarbonate ions.

How are they used?

The thiazide drugs are commonly used in the treatment of patients with hypertension and can add to the effectiveness of other antihypertensive drugs, reversing fluid retention caused by some of these agents.

Thiazide diuretics are also used as adjunctive therapy in edema associated with CHF, hepatic cirrhosis, and corticosteroids or estrogen therapy; edema caused by acute glomerulonephritis; and chronic renal failure.

What are the adverse effects?

The common adverse effects of thiazide diuretics include anorexia, gastric irritation, nausea and vomiting, cramping, diarrhea, constipation, jaundice, hypokalemia, and pancreatitis. Other adverse effects are headache, dizziness, vertigo, leukopenia, aplastic anemia, orthostatic hypotension, fever, respiratory distress, anaphylactic reactions, and hyperglycemia.

What are the contraindications and interactions?

Thiazide diuretics are contraindicated in patients with diabetes, a history of gout, severe renal disease, and impaired liver function and in elderly patients. They are not recommended for use by nursing mothers. Drug interactions may occur with corticosteroids, lithium, probenecid, and antidiabetic agents.

What are the important points patients should know?

Instruct patients with diabetes to monitor their blood glucose levels with extra care because thiazide, loop, and potassium-sparing diuretics can cause hyperglycemia.

Table 31-5 ■ Thiazides and Thiazide-like Diuretics

GENERIC NAME	TRADE NAME	AVERAGE ADULT DOSAGE	ROUTE OF ADMINISTRATION
Thiazide Diuretics			
chlorothiazide	Diuril	250–500 mg 1–2 times/d	PO
cyclothiazide	(Generic only)	2 mg/d	PO
hydrochlorothiazide	Esidrix	12.5–100 mg/d	PO
hydroflumethiazide	(Generic only)	25–100 mg 1–2 times/d	PO
methyclothiazide	Methyclothiazide	2.5–10 mg/d	PO
polythiazide	Renese	1–4 mg/d	PO
Thiazide-like Diuretics			
chlorthalidone	Thalitone	15–120 mg/d	PO
indapamide	Lozol	2.5–5 mg/d	PO

PO, oral.

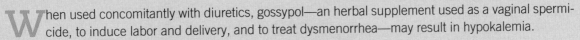

Focus on Natural Products

Gossypol and Diuretics

When used concomitantly with diuretics, gossypol—an herbal supplement used as a vaginal spermicide, to induce labor and delivery, and to treat dysmenorrhea—may result in hypokalemia.

Focus On

Loop Diuretics

The loop diuretics are sometimes referred to as high-ceiling diuretics. In high doses, loop diuretics can increase urine output astronomically, leading to severe hypovolemia (decreased blood volume) and death (Table 31-6 ■).

How do they work?

Loop diuretics act directly on the loop of Henle in the kidneys to inhibit sodium and chloride reabsorption. Potent diuretics, such as furosemide, bumetanide, and ethacrynic acid, are not thiazides but act in a similar way to increase the excretion of water, sodium, chloride, and potassium. Their action is more rapid and effective than that of thiazides with greater diuresis.

How are they used?

The loop diuretics are the drugs of choice in patients with acute pulmonary edema, resulting in CHF. Because of their rapid onset of action, the drugs are useful in emergencies, such as acute pulmonary edema. They are also useful in treating patients with hypercalcemia because they stimulate tubular calcium ion secretion. Loop diuretics are used in hypertension when other diuretics and other antihypertensives do not result in satisfactory response. In edema of nephrotic syndrome, only loop diuretics are capable of reducing edema.

What are the adverse effects?

The adverse effects of loop diuretics include abnormalities of fluid and electrolyte balance, hyponatremia, hypotension, circulatory collapse, thromboemboli, and hepatic encephalopathy. They may cause hypokalemia, which may induce cardiac dysrhythmias in patients taking glycosides, and hypocalcemia, which can lead to tetany.

Loop diuretics are toxic to the ear, particularly when used in conjunction with the aminoglycosides (antibiotics).

(continued)

Focus On (continued)

Ethacrynic acid is the most ototoxic. Irreversible damage may result with continued treatment. Furosemide and ethacrynic acid compete with uric acid for the renal and biliary secretory systems. This results in the blocking of secretions, resulting in hyperuricemia and causing gout attacks. Other adverse effects of loop diuretics may be skin rashes, photosensitivity, hypotension, shock, cardiac arrhythmias, and bone marrow depression.

What are the contraindications and interactions?

Loop diuretics are contraindicated in patients with hypersensitivity to these drugs. They are not recommended for use in infants or lactating women. They should be avoided in patients with severe diarrhea, dehydration, electrolyte imbalance, and hypotension.

Loop diuretics should be used cautiously in patients with hepatic cirrhosis, diabetes mellitus, pulmonary edema, pregnancy, and a history of gout. They may cause drug interactions with aminoglycosides, anticoagulants, lithium, propranolol, sulfonylureas, nonsteroidal anti-inflammatory drugs (NSAIDs), probenecid, and thiazide diuretics.

What are the important points patients should know?

Instruct patients to follow their physician's orders to take diuretic medications early in the morning and not at bedtime. Advise women to avoid this drug when breastfeeding.

Table 31-6 ■ Loop Diuretics

GENERIC NAME	TRADE NAME	AVERAGE ADULT DOSAGE	ROUTE OF ADMINISTRATION
bumetanide	Bumex	0.5–2 mg/d	PO
	Bumex Injection	0.5–1 mg over 1–2 min, repeated q2–3h prn (maximum: 10 mg/d)	IV, IM
ethacrynic acid	Edecrin	50–100 mg 1–2 times/day (maximum: 400 mg/d)	PO
	Sodium Edecrin	0.5–1 mg/kg	IV
furosemide	Lasix	20–80 mg/d in 1 or several divided doses (maximum: 600 mg/d)	PO
	Lasix Injection	20–40 mg in one or several divided doses, up to 600 mg/d	IM, IV
torsemide	Demadex	4–20 mg/d	PO, IV

PO, oral; IV, intravenous; IM, intramuscular.

Focus On

Potassium-Sparing Diuretics

The potassium-sparing diuretics include spironolactone, triamterene, and amiloride. The potassium-sparing diuretics are able to produce a mild diuresis without affecting blood potassium levels. The effects of these agents on urine electrolyte composition are similar in that they decrease potassium and hydrogen ion excretion. Despite this similarity, these agents actually comprise two groups with respect to mechanism of action. Spironolactone—the prototype agent of the aldosterone antagonists—is a specific competitive inhibitor of aldosterone at the receptor site level; hence, it is effective only when aldosterone is present.

The other two potassium-sparing diuretics—triamterene and amiloride—exert their effects independently of the presence or absence of aldosterone (Table 31-7 ■).

How do they work?

Spironolactone is a synthetic aldosterone antagonist that competes with aldosterone for intracellular cytoplasmic receptor sites. The spironolactone receptor complex cannot translocate into the nucleus of the target cell. Therefore, this prevents sodium reabsorption in the distal tubule.

How are they used?

The potassium-sparing agents are used in the treatment of edema associated with CHF, hepatic cirrhosis with ascites, and nephrotic syndrome. Because these diuretics have little antihypertensive action of their own, they are used mainly in combination with other drugs in the management of hypertension and to correct hypokalemia often caused by other diuretic agents. Spironolactone is also used in primary hyperaldosteronism.

What are the adverse effects?

Potassium-sparing diuretics may cause life-threatening **hyperkalemia**, which is an abnormally high amount of potassium ions in blood. The main adverse effects of these agents include hyperkalemia, acute renal failure, and kidney stones. Because spironolactone chemically resembles some of the sex steroids, it has minimal hormonal activity and may cause *gynecomastia* (increased development of the mammary glands in men and menstrual irregularities in women). At low doses,

spironolactone can be used chronically with few adverse effects. Potassium-sparing diuretics may cause nausea, lethargy, headache, and mental confusion.

What are the contraindications and interactions?

Potassium-sparing diuretics are contraindicated in patients with anuria, acute renal insufficiency, impaired renal function, or hyperkalemia. They should be used cautiously in patients with cirrhosis of the liver or who are pregnant or lactating. Potassium supplements, NSAIDs, and lithium may interact with potassium-sparing diuretics.

What are the important points patients should know?

Teach patients taking potassium-sparing diuretics about the symptoms of hypokalemia, such as muscle cramps and weakness, lethargy, anorexia, irregular pulse, and confusion. Instruct them about the symptoms of hyperkalemia, such as thirst, dry mouth, and drowsiness. Caution patients to maintain normal potassium levels while taking combination digoxin and diuretic therapy.

Table 31-7 ■ Potassium-Sparing Diuretics

GENERIC NAME	TRADE NAME	AVERAGE ADULT DOSAGE	ROUTE OF ADMINISTRATION
amiloride	(Generic only)	5–20 mg/d	PO
spironolactone	Aldactone	Up to 400 mg/d	PO
triamterene	Dyrenium	Up to 300 mg/d	PO

PO, oral.

✳ Apply Your Knowledge 31.3

The following questions focus on what you have just learned about diuretics and their effects on fluid and electrolyte balance.

CRITICAL THINKING

1. What are the major classes of diuretics?
2. What are the risks to the fetus when diuretics are used during pregnancy?
3. What are the indications for osmotic diuretics?
4. What are three examples of carbonic anhydrase inhibitors?
5. What is the mechanism of action of thiazide diuretics?
6. What are two examples of thiazide-like diuretics?
7. What are the trade names of furosemide, mannitol, polythiazide, and bumetanide?
8. What are the indications of potassium-sparing agents?
9. What are the major adverse effects of potassium-sparing diuretics?
10. Which diuretics are the drugs of choice in acute pulmonary edema, resulting in chronic heart failure?

PRACTICAL SCENARIO 1

A middle-aged man who is being treated with hydrochlorothiazide for control of mild edema presents to the physician complaining of malaise, fatigue, muscular weakness, and muscle cramps. In response to the physician's questions about how he is taking his medication, he reports that he takes the medication daily but that causes constipation. Therefore, he has been taking laxatives. The physician orders electrocardiography (ECG) and blood tests to check the patient's levels of creatinine, blood urea nitrogen, uric acid, and electrolytes.

Prentice Hall School Division

Critical Thinking Questions

1. What do you think might be the result of the man's use of diuretics and laxatives together?
2. Why do you think the physician ordered the ECG and blood tests and what is he looking for?
3. What blood test results do you expect to find?
4. When providing patient education for this man, what would you tell him?

PRACTICAL SCENARIO 2

A 58-year-old woman who had congestive heart failure was admitted to the hospital. She had a history of hypertension and liver disease.

Critical Thinking Questions

1. What type of diuretics is more appropriate for this patient?
2. If the physician prescribes potassium-sparing diuretics, what adverse effects may be caused?

forestpath/Shutterstock

Chapter Capsule

This section repeats the objectives from the beginning of the chapter and then provides a summary of the most important concepts for that objective. Use this section as a quick review and to check your knowledge.

Objective 1: Describe the structure of a nephron.

- Nephrons consist of a renal corpuscle and renal tubule.
- The renal corpuscle has a filtering unit composed of a cluster of blood capillaries called a *glomerulus* and a surrounding thin-walled, sac-like structure called a *glomerular capsule*
- The renal tubule leads away from the glomerular capsule and becomes highly coiled (the proximal convoluted tubule)
- Next is the loop of Henle, the ascending limb of which becomes highly coiled again (the distal convoluted tubule), forming a collecting duct (tubule)

Objective 2: Explain urea, creatine, and uric acid.

■ Urea is the most abundant organic waste. Each person generates about 21 g of urea each day, which results in the breakdown of amino acids.

■ Creatinine—a chemical waste molecule—is produced in skeletal muscle tissue by the breakdown of *creatine phosphate*, a high-energy compound that plays an important role in muscle contraction. The body generates roughly 1.8 g of creatinine each day, and virtually all of it is excreted in urine

■ Uric acid—another type of waste molecule—is formed by recycling a nitrogenous base from RNA molecules. Humans produce approximately 480 mg of uric acid each day.

Objective 3: Explain the processes of urine formation.

■ Urinary excretion = Glomerular filtration + Tubular secretion − Tubular reabsorption

■ Urine formation—maintains homeostasis by regulating the volume and composition of blood

■ Involves the excretion of such solutes (specifically, metabolic waste products) as urea, creatinine, and uric acid

■ Valuable materials, such as sugars or amino acids, are reabsorbed and retained for use by other tissues

Objective 4: Discuss how water is taken into the body and how it leaves the body.

■ Water intake: The volume of water gained each day varies among individuals (Table 31-1). An average adult living in a moderate environment takes in about 2,500 mL per day. Approximately 60% is obtained from drinking water or other beverages, and another 30% comes from moist foods. The remaining 10% is a by-product of the oxidative metabolism of nutrients, which is called water of metabolism.

■ Water output: Water normally enters the body only through the mouth, but it can be lost by a variety of routes. These include obvious losses in urine (the largest amount), feces, and sweat as well as evaporation from the skin and from the lungs during breathing (insensible water loss)

Objective 5: List the ways that electrolytes are lost from the body.

■ Sweat, feces, urine

Objective 6: Describe how antidiuretic hormone and aldosterone levels influence the volume and concentration of urine.

■ ADH controls water permeability; when absent, water is not reabsorbed in the distal convoluted tubules and the collecting system, producing large amounts of very dilute urine, which can cause diabetes insipidus

■ Aldosterone increases sodium ion reabsorption in the distal convoluted tubules and collecting ducts of the nephrons

Objective 7: Explain the indications for the use of diuretics in various conditions and disorders of the human body.

■ Diuretics are indicated for edema (cerebral, acute pulmonary edema or congestive heart failure), hepatic cirrhosis with or without ascites, use with corticosteroids or estrogen therapies, acute glomerulonephritis, hypercalcemia, nephrotic syndrome, and chronic renal failure), various seizures, for the reduction of intraocular pressure in glaucoma, acute high-altitude sickness, and hypertension (including the reversal of fluid retention caused by some antihypertensive drugs)

Objective 8: Classify the five major types of diuretics.

- Osmotic diuretics: affect the capacity of the renal tubule to reabsorb electrolytes and nonelectrolytes
- Carbonic anhydrase inhibitors: stop the conversion of carbon dioxide to carbonic acid and bicarbonate ions
- Thiazide and thiazide-like diuretics: inhibit sodium reabsorption on distal convoluted tubules and collecting ducts
- Loop diuretics: work on the loop of Henle to inhibit sodium and chloride reabsorption
- Potassium-sparing diuretics: decrease potassium and hydrogen ion excretion

Objective 9: Describe the mechanism of action for osmotic diuretics.

- Decrease solute content, resulting in less water reabsorption from the descending loop of Henle and collecting duct and less sodium chloride reabsorption in the proximal tubule and ascending loop of Henle

Objective 10: List the major adverse effects of potassium-sparing diuretics.

- Hyperkalemia, acute renal failure, and kidney stones

 Internet Sites of Interest

- An overview of kidney function is discussed at: **www.davita.com/kidney-disease/ vocabulary/kidney-function/e/5497**
- The process of urine formation is explained at: **www.kidneychat.com/urine-formation.html**
- A thorough review of fluid and electrolyte balance is given at: **https://mcb .berkeley.edu/courses/mcb135e/kidneyfluid.html**
- Answers to your questions about diuretics can be found at: **www.rxlist.com/ diuretics/drugs-condition.htm**
- A description of kidney diseases can be found on the National Kidney and Urologic Diseases (a service of National Institute of Diabetes and Digestive and Kidney Diseases [NIDDK]) website at: **www.niddk.nih.gov/health-information/ health-topics/kidney-disease/pages/default.aspx**
- Medical tests to determine kidney function are explained at: **www.webmd.com/ a-to-z-guides/tests-kidney-function**

Chapter 32

Drugs Used to Treat Endocrine Conditions

Chapter Objectives

After completing this chapter, you should be able to:

1. Identify the primary glands of the endocrine system.
2. List six types of hormones that are secreted from the anterior pituitary gland.
3. Explain the endocrine functions of the hypothalamus.
4. Describe conditions linked to excessive or insufficient amounts of growth hormone.
5. Explain the pharmacotherapy of diabetes insipidus.
6. Describe the role of the thyroid gland and its replacement and antithyroid drugs.
7. Explain Graves' disease and the predominant group of people it affects.
8. Identify the role of hypoglycemic medications in treating diabetes mellitus.
9. Describe the adverse effects of insulin and corticosteroids.
10. Identify the two major classes of steroids.

Key Terms

Introduction

Hormones are chemical substances secreted directly into the blood by endocrine glands—generally in response to a change in the internal condition of the body and with the goal of maintaining homeostasis. This chapter focuses on hormones that regulate growth, blood glucose, and intermediary metabolism. The synthesis and secretion of many hormones are controlled by other hormones or changes in the concentration of essential chemicals or electrolytes in the blood. The interrelationships among the peptide hormones of the hypothalamus, the trophic hormones of the anterior pituitary, and other endocrine glands are examples of elegant feedback regulation—positive feedback, in which one hormone stimulates the secretion of another, or negative feedback, in which one hormone turns off the action of the previous hormone. Drugs and diseases can modify hormone secretion as well as specific hormone effects at target organs.

Pharmacologic preparations are used to detect and treat disorders involving any of the following glands: pituitary, thyroid, adrenal cortex, pancreas, or gonads. The effects of these drugs are derived from the physiological actions of the endogenous hormones that they stimulate if they are activators (agonists) or block if they are antagonists.

Endocrine System

The endocrine system secretes hormones that control the body by maintaining its internal environment within certain narrow ranges, which is known as *homeostasis*. The maintenance of homeostasis involves growth, maturation, reproduction, metabolism, and human behavior. Responsibility for homeostasis is shared by the endocrine system and the nervous system, working in tandem in a unique partnership. The hypothalamus of the brain (a part of the nervous system) sends directions via chemical signals (the releasing of hormones) to the pituitary gland (a part of the endocrine system). It also controls the release of corticotropin-releasing hormone (CRH), growth hormone–releasing hormone (GHRH), gonadotropin-releasing hormone (GnRH), thyrotropin-releasing hormone (TRH), and anterior-pituitary hormones. The pituitary stimulates the other endocrine glands to secrete their hormones. The endocrine glands include the pituitary gland, pineal gland, thyroid gland, parathyroid glands, thymus gland, adrenal glands, **islets of Langerhans** (small clusters of cells within the pancreas), ovaries in women, and testes in men (see Figure 32-1 ■). The ovarian and testicular hormones are discussed in Chapter 33. Hormone secretion is precisely regulated by the hypothalamus, the anterior pituitary gland, and other groups of glands that respond to the hypothalamus and pituitary glands (see Figure 32-2 ■).

Pituitary Gland

The pituitary gland—sometimes called the *master gland* because of its regulatory effects on the other endocrine glands—consists of an anterior lobe (**adenohypophysis**) and a posterior lobe (**neurohypophysis**) that are under the influence of the hypothalamic hormones. The hypothalamic hormones control the secretion of specific trophic hormones; they in turn regulate other endocrine gland secretions and target tissues. Table 32-1 ■ lists the pituitary gland and other endocrine glands and their functions.

ANTERIOR PITUITARY HORMONES

The anterior lobe of the pituitary secretes at least six separate hormones: growth hormone (somatotropin, GH), adrenocorticotropin hormone (ACTH), thyroid-stimulating hormone (TSH), follicle-stimulating hormone (FSH), luteinizing hormone (LH), and prolactin (PRL). Clinically, an abnormal level of activity of the pituitary gland causes two conditions: *hyperpituitarism*—overactivity of the pituitary gland (causing gigantism or acromegaly)—and **hypopituitarism**—underactivity of the pituitary gland (causing dwarfism). The relationships between hypothalamic hormones, pituitary hormones, and target organs are shown in Table 32-2 ■.

Growth Hormone

GH causes an increase in the weight and length of the body. The increase in length is especially prominent in bone growth, but its effect is manifested in nearly all the tissues of the body. Excessive secretion of GH before puberty—usually the result of a tumor of the anterior pituitary—causes **gigantism** (a condition in which the entire body or any of its parts is abnormally large). If excessive production of GH occurs after puberty, it can result in **acromegaly** (a disorder in which the extremities, such as the hands, feet, and head, are greatly enlarged). GH insufficiency during childhood causes **dwarfism** (a condition in which the body is abnormally undersized).

Thyroid-Stimulating Hormone

TSH—another hormone of the anterior lobe of the pituitary gland—controls the secretion of the thyroid hormone and is important for the growth and function of the thyroid gland. TSH stimulates the thyroid gland to increase the uptake of iodine and increase the synthesis and release of thyroid hormones.

In the absence of TSH, the thyroid gland atrophies, producing only small amounts of thyroid hormone, which can have numerous multisystem negative effects on the body. An excess of TSH causes hypertrophy and hyperplasia of the thyroid and a severe form of hyperthyroidism called **Graves' disease** (an overactive thyroid condition characterized by numerous eye problems).

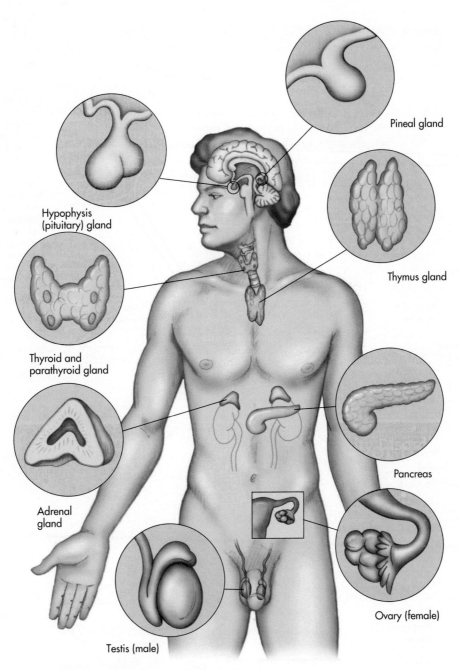

Figure 32-1 ■ Primary glands of the endocrine system.

Hypophysis (pituitary) gland

Pineal gland

Thyroid and parathyroid gland

Thymus gland

Adrenal gland

Pancreas

Testis (male)

Ovary (female)

Adrenocorticotropic Hormone

Adrenocorticotropic hormone (ACTH) is released by the anterior lobe of the pituitary gland and by the placenta during pregnancy. It stimulates the growth of the adrenal gland cortex and the secretion of corticosteroids. Hypersecretion of ACTH can cause **Cushing's syndrome**, a condition that affects the trunk of the body. This syndrome is signified by a pad of fat developing between the shoulders, producing a "buffalo hump," and the face becoming round and moon shaped. Cushing's syndrome

is called **Cushing's disease** when it is caused by a tumor in the pituitary gland.

Gonadotropic Hormones

The gonadotropic hormones include FSH and LH, which are produced by gonadotroph cells in the anterior pituitary. These two hormones affect the target gonadal tissue in men and women. The principal function of FSH is to stimulate gametogenesis and follicular development in women and spermatogenesis in men. LH is

CRH	Corticotrophin-releasing hormone
GHIH	Growth hormone-inhibiting hormone
PIH	Prolactin-inhibiting hormone
MSHIH	Melanocyte-stimulating hormone inhibiting hormone
GnRH	Gonadotrophin-releasing hormone
GHRH	Growth hormone-releasing hormone
TRH	Thyrotropin-releasing hormone
ACTH	Adrenocorticotrophic hormone
TSH	Thyroid-stimulating hormone
GH	Growth hormone
PRL	Prolactin
FSH	Follicle-stimulating hormone
LH	Luteinizing hormone
MSH	Melanocyte-stimulating hormone
ADH	Antidiuretic hormone

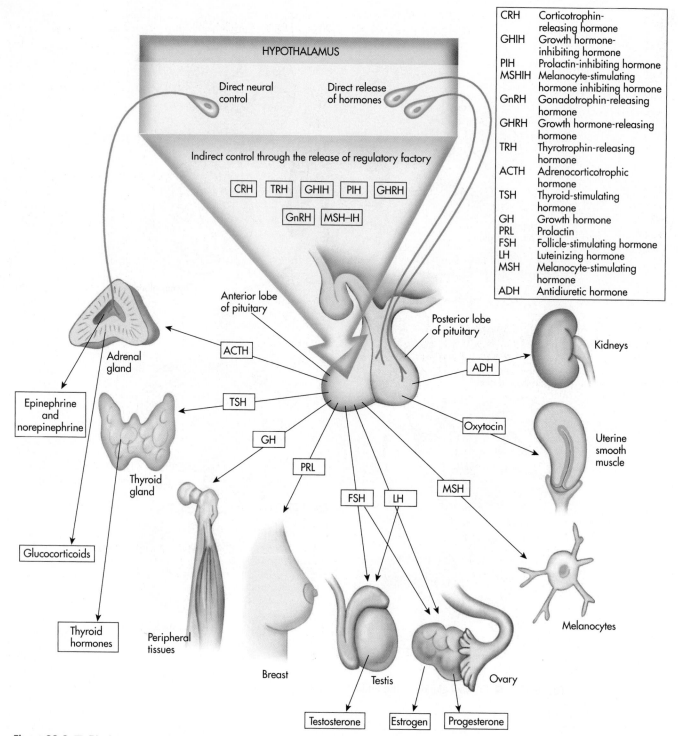

Figure 32-2 ■ Pituitary hormones and their target cells, tissues, and organs.

primarily responsible for the regulation of gonadal steroid hormone production.

Prolactin

PRL is a hormone with many different actions. By itself, PRL does not cause breast development, but by working with estrogens, progesterone, hydrocortisone, and insulin, it *is* mammotropic. In humans, it also stimulates milk secretion by the mammary glands. Other effects in humans include the increase in testicular steroidogenesis and the development of the male accessory sex organs. It is also involved in the regulation of gonadotropin release. PRL deficiency is associated with disorders of the hypothalamus or pituitary gland.

Table 32-1 ■ Endocrine Glands and Their Functions

GLAND	HORMONE	MAJOR FUNCTIONS
Anterior pituitary	Adrenocorticotropic hormone (ACTH)	Stimulates adrenal cortex to produce cortisol
	Follicle-stimulating hormone (FSH)	Stimulates follicular growth, secretion of estrogen, growth of testes; promotes development of sperm cells
	Growth hormone (GH)	Promotes growth of soft tissue and bone
	Luteinizing hormone (LH); in men, this is called *interstitial cell–stimulating hormone (ICSH)*	Causes development of corpus luteum at site of a ruptured ovarian follicle in women; can also stimulate secretion of testosterone in men
	Prolactin (PRL)	Promotes breast development in women and stimulates milk secretion
	Thyroid-stimulating hormone (TSH)	Stimulates thyroid gland to produce thyroid hormones (T3 and T4)
Posterior pituitary (hormone storage site)	Oxytocin	Increases contractility of uterus and causes milk ejection postpartum
	Vasopressin (antidiuretic hormone [ADH])	Increases reabsorption of water in kidney tubules and stimulates smooth muscle tissue in blood vessels for constriction
Thyroid	Calcitonin	Decreases plasma calcium concentrations
	Thyroid hormones (thyroxine [T4] and triiodothyronine [T3])	Increase metabolic rate; are essential for normal growth and nerve development
Parathyroid	Parathyroid hormone (PTH)	Regulates exchange of calcium between blood and bones; increases calcium level in blood
Hypothalamus	Releasing and inhibiting hormones (CRH, GHRH, GnRH, TRH)	Controls release of anterior pituitary hormones
Thymus	Thymosin	Enhances proliferation and function of T-lymphocytes

Table 32-2 ■ Relationships Among Hypothalamic, Anterior Pituitary, and Target Organ Hormones

HYPOTHALAMIC HORMONE	PITUITARY HORMONE	TARGET ORGAN (HORMONE PRODUCT)
Stimulatory Hormones		
Corticotropin-releasing hormone (CRH)	Adrenocorticotropic hormone (ACTH)	Adrenal cortex (glucocorticoids, mineralocorticoids, androgens)
Growth hormone–releasing hormone (GHRH)	Somatotropin, growth hormone (GH)	Liver (somatomedins)
Gonadotropin-releasing hormone (GnRH)	Follicle-stimulating hormone (FSH), luteinizing hormone (LH)	Gonads (estrogen, progesterone, testosterone)
Thyrotropin-releasing hormone (TRH)	Thyroid-stimulating hormone (TSH)	Thyroid (thyroxine)
Inhibitory Hormones		
Dopamine	Prolactin (PRL)	Breast (none)
Somatostatin	GH	Liver (Insulin-like growth factor)

POSTERIOR PITUITARY HORMONES

The posterior pituitary gland is also called the *neurohypophysis* and contains two peptide hormones: **vasopressin** and **oxytocin**. Neither is made in the posterior pituitary; rather, they are synthesized in neurons in the hypothalamus.

Vasopressin

Vasopressin is also called *antidiuretic hormone (ADH)*, which stimulates water reabsorption from the nephrons (collecting ducts) of the kidneys back into the bloodstream. It plays a significant role in concentrating urine to conserve water. When there is a defect in the hypothalamic–pituitary secretion of ADH, **diabetes insipidus** (chronic increased thirst and urination caused by damage of the hypothalamus) results in water diuresis. Vasopressin is used mainly for its antidiuretic effects in this disease rather than for its vasoconstrictor actions, from which the name vasopressin is derived.

Oxytocin

Oxytocin stimulates the contraction of smooth muscle in the uterus and alveoli of the lactating breast. The hormone enhances uterine contractions during labor and stimulates the release of milk during breastfeeding.

✳ Apply Your **Knowledge 32.1**

The following questions focus on what you have just learned about the endocrine system.

CRITICAL THINKING

1. What are the islets of Langerhans?
2. What are the names of the hormones of the anterior pituitary glands?
3. What is the effect of growth hormone insufficiency during childhood?
4. What is Cushing's syndrome?
5. What are the effects of hypothalamic hormones upon trophic hormones, and what do these hormones regulate?
6. When do gigantism and acromegaly occur?

Thyroid Gland

The thyroid gland lies in the neck just below the larynx and in front of the trachea. It plays a vital role in regulating the body's metabolic processes.

THYROID HORMONES

Thyroid hormone is secreted from follicular cells in the thyroid gland and includes two different hormones: thyroxine (tetraiodothyronine, or T4) and triiodothyronine (T3). Iodine is vital for the synthesis of these hormones and is provided through the dietary intake of common iodized salt. Another hormone releases from **parafollicular cells** in the thyroid gland—calcitonin—which is involved with calcium homeostasis. Calcitonin inhibits bone reabsorption and the release of calcium ions into the blood while promoting the uptake of these ions back into bone. Its effects on blood calcium levels are rapid but short-acting.

In the absence of the thyroid gland and thus thyroid hormones, the basal metabolic rate is less than half its normal rate, and growth and development are impaired. In the presence of a hyperactive gland, the metabolic rate is much higher than normal, resulting in tachycardia, nervousness, and other symptoms. An enlargement of the thyroid gland is called a *goiter*. Simple (nontoxic) goiter results from a shortage of iodine in the diet. A goiter can also be caused by constant stimulation of an underactive or nonfunctioning thyroid to release more hormones.

Focus on Geriatrics

Myxedema Coma

Myxedema coma is a medical emergency that is indicated by a diminished level of consciousness associated with severe hypothyroidism. Symptoms include hypothermia without shivering, hypoventilation, hypotension, and hypoglycemia. Older patients with severe vascular disease and moderate or untreated hypothyroidism are particularly at risk. Myxedema coma can be caused by overuse of narcotics or sedatives or, in hypothyroid patients, by an acute illness.

The two most common thyroid disorders are Graves' disease and Hashimoto's thyroiditis of the immune system, an autoimmune disease that attacks the thyroid gland, causing hypothyroidism. Graves' disease—an autoimmune disease in which antibodies overstimulate the thyroid gland—is characterized by **hyperthyroidism** (overactive thyroid), usually associated with an enlarged thyroid gland and *exophthalmos* (protrusion of the eyeballs). Graves' disease is also known as **thyrotoxicosis**.

Deficiency of thyroid hormones (hypothyroidism) during infancy causes **congenital hypothyroidism**, resulting in dwarfism and severe mental retardation. **Myxedema** is the most severe hypothyroidism, developing in older children or adults. It is characterized by swelling of the hands, feet, and face (especially around the eyes) and can lead to coma and death. In older adults, severe hypothyroidism can cause myxedema coma.

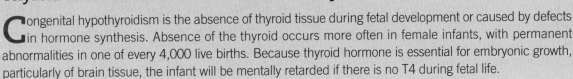

Focus on Pediatrics

Thyroid Hormone Essential to Fetal Development

Congenital hypothyroidism is the absence of thyroid tissue during fetal development or caused by defects in hormone synthesis. Absence of the thyroid occurs more often in female infants, with permanent abnormalities in one of every 4,000 live births. Because thyroid hormone is essential for embryonic growth, particularly of brain tissue, the infant will be mentally retarded if there is no T4 during fetal life.

ANTITHYROID DRUGS

Disorders of the thyroid gland are quite common, and treatment of individuals with these conditions indicates drug therapy. In the case of hyperthyroidism, a number of organic compounds inhibit the production of thyroid hormone by the thyroid gland. Iodine drugs, such as potassium iodide, radioactive iodine, and thioamide derivatives, are the drugs of choice for antithyroid therapy (see Table 32-3 ■) and are discussed here.

Table 32-3 ■ **Common Thyroid and Antithyroid Agents**

GENERIC NAME	TRADE NAME	AVERAGE ADULT DOSAGE	ROUTE OF ADMINISTRATION
Thyroid Agents			
levothyroxine	Synthroid, Levothroid, Levoxyl	100–400 mcg/d	PO (Synthroid IV is also available)
liothyronine	Cytomel	25–75 mcg/d	PO
thyroid	Armour Thyroid	15–120 mg/d	PO
Antithyroid Agents			
methimazole	Tapazole	5–15 mg/d	PO
potassium iodide	(Generic only)	0.1–1.0 mL tid	PO
propylthiouracil	Propylthiouracil	100–150 mg tid	PO
sodium iodide, i-131	Sodium Iodide I-131	0.8–150 millicurie (mCi)*	PO

PO, oral; IV, intravenous; tid, three times a day.
*Based on radiation quantity; millicurie stands for 1/1,000 of a *curie*, a measurement of radiation intensity.

Focus On

Potassium Iodide

Iodine drugs, such as potassium iodide, may be administered to inhibit thyroid hormones by saturating the thyroid gland.

How does it work?

The exact mechanism of action is not clear, but excess iodide ions cause minimal change in thyroid gland mass. Conversely, when the thyroid gland is hyperplastic, excess iodide ions temporarily inhibit the secretion of thyroid hormone.

How is it used?

Potassium iodide is used alone for hyperthyroidism or in conjunction with antithyroid drugs and propranolol in the treatment of thyrotoxic crisis. It is also prescribed for the treatment of persistent or recurring hyperthyroidism that occurs in patients with Graves' disease. Iodide can be administered as a radiation protectant.

What are the adverse effects?

Potassium iodide may cause diarrhea, nausea and vomiting, and stomach pain. Fever, joint pain, lymph node enlargement, and weakness are also seen. Iodide can produce irregular heartbeat, mental confusion, productive cough, and pulmonary edema.

What are the contraindications and interactions?

Potassium iodide is contraindicated in patients with hypersensitivity to this agent. It must be avoided in patients with hypothyroidism, *hyperkalemia* (excessive potassium in the blood), and acute bronchitis. Safety during pregnancy, lactation, and in children younger than 1 year of age is not established. Iodide must be used cautiously in patients with renal impairment, cardiac disease, pulmonary tuberculosis, and **Addison's disease** (adrenocortical insufficiency caused by an autoimmune response to the adrenal gland).

Drug interactions include antithyroid drugs; **lithium** (a drug that reduces the activity of certain neurotransmitters and is used in the treatment of bipolar disorder), which may potentiate hypothyroid and goitrogenic actions; potassium-sparing diuretics; and potassium supplements, which increase the risk of hyperkalemia.

What are the important points patients should know?

Instruct patients about the effects of iodine and its presence in shellfish, iodized salt, and certain over-the-counter cough preparations. Advise patients about the manifestations of hyperthyroidism and hypothyroidism and about the fact that each of them can occur as a result of treatment for the other. Teach patients how to monitor their pulse rate and to report any marked increase or decrease.

Focus Point

Graves' Disease

Every year, approximately 5 in 10,000 people in the United States develop Graves' disease, which is related to hyperthyroidism. There are four to eight times more female patients than male patients with Graves' disease. Most patients who develop this disease are between 20 and 45 years of age. Besides the prevalent eye problems, signs of Graves' disease also include rapid heartbeat, palpitations, nervousness, excitability, weight loss, profuse perspiration, and insomnia.

Focus On

Methimazole

Methimazole is an antithyroid drug that is approximately 10 times as potent as propylthiouracil and is faster in eliciting an antithyroid response.

How does it work?

Methimazole inhibits the synthesis of thyroid hormones as the drug accumulates in the thyroid gland. It does not affect existing T3 or T4 levels.

How is it used?

Methimazole is used for hyperthyroidism and before surgery or radiotherapy of the thyroid. It may be used cautiously to treat hyperthyroidism in pregnancy.

What are the adverse effects?

The adverse effects of methimazole include hypothyroidism, *pancytopenia* (a blood disorder), aplastic anemia, *arthralgia* (joint pain), peripheral neuropathy, drowsiness, vertigo, rash, alopecia, and pruritus.

What are the contraindications and interactions?

Methimazole is contraindicated in pregnancy and lactation. It should be used cautiously with other drugs known to cause agranulocytosis. Methimazole can reduce the anticoagulant effects of warfarin. It may increase serum levels of digoxin and alter theophylline levels. Methimazole may require decreased doses of beta-blockers.

What are the important points patients should know?

Instruct patients to take methimazole at the same time each day—preferably before breakfast. Food tends to inhibit the absorption rate.

- -

Propylthiouracil

Propylthiouracil is an antithyroid agent that has no effect on hormone release, and the antithyroid action cannot be observed until the thyroid stores of T3 and T4 become depleted.

How does it work?

Propylthiouracil belongs in the thioamide family. It interferes with the use of iodine and blocks the synthesis of T3 and T4. It does not interfere with the release and utilization of stored thyroid hormone. Therefore, antithyroid action of this drug is delayed days and weeks until preformed T3 and T4 are degraded.

How is it used?

Propylthiouracil is prescribed for hyperthyroidism, iodine-induced thyrotoxicosis, and hyperthyroidism associated with thyroiditis. It is also used to shrink the size of the thyroid before surgery.

What are the adverse effects?

Propylthiouracil may cause headache, vertigo, drowsiness, nausea and vomiting, diarrhea, loss of taste, and hepatitis. Other adverse effects include agranulocytosis, hypothyroidism, periorbital edema, puffy hands and feet, bradycardia, cool and pale skin, sleepiness, fatigue, mental depression, changes in menstrual periods, and unusual weight gain.

What are the contraindications and interactions?

Propylthiouracil is contraindicated in the last trimester of pregnancy and during lactation. It should not be concurrently administered with sulfonamides or coal tar derivatives, such as aminopyrine or antipyrine. Thyroid hormones can reverse the efficacy of amiodarone, potassium iodide, and sodium iodide.

What are the important points patients should know?

Remind patients with Graves' disease who are taking propylthiouracil about the drug's side effects. Patients taking this drug often complain about a sore throat and fever, but agranulocytosis is the most serious adverse effect of this drug. Stress the importance of reporting agranulocytosis symptoms to these patients. Instruct patients to avoid foods that can inhibit thyroid secretion, such as strawberries, peaches, pears, cabbage, turnips, radishes, peas, and spinach, and to take medication early in the day to prevent nighttime insomnia. Advise female patients to keep a record of menstruation because menstrual irregularities may occur.

THYROID DRUGS

Hypothyroidism (low or absent thyroid function) is a common disorder caused by the deficient secretion of TSH or other thyroid hormones. Replacement therapy with natural or synthetic thyroid hormone is required. Periodic testing and adjustment of the drug level may be necessary.

Focus On

Levothyroxine

Levothyroxine is a commonly prescribed synthetic form of T4.

How does it work?

The actions of levothyroxine replicate those of natural thyroid hormone, which regulates the body's basal metabolic rate.

How is it used?

Levothyroxine is used in cases of low thyroid function. It is generally taken orally, and an intravenous form is also available.

What are the adverse effects?

Too high a dose level of levothyroxine can cause symptoms resembling hyperthyroidism, including tachycardia, weight loss, insomnia, anxiety, and intolerance of heat. Women can experience menstrual irregularities, and long-term use can cause osteoporosis. Serious adverse effects include chest pain (angina) and a rapid or irregular heartbeat or pulse.

What are the contraindications and interactions?

People with allergies to povidone-iodine or tartrazine (a yellow dye in some processed foods and drugs) should inform their doctors because levothyroxine contains these ingredients.

   Patients taking amphetamines; anticoagulants such as warfarin; antidepressants or antianxiety agents; arthritis medicine; aspirin; such beta-blockers as metoprolol, propranolol, or timolol; cancer chemotherapy agents, diabetes medications, digoxin, estrogens, iron, methadone, oral contraceptives, phenytoin, steroids, or theophylline should inform their doctor. Caution should be used in prescribing the drug for women who are pregnant or may become pregnant or are breastfeeding.

What are the important points patients should know?

Instruct patients to see their physician regularly so their blood can be tested to be sure the prescribed dose is therapeutic. There is a fine line between the proper dose and one that produces adverse effects, and a periodic adjustment of the dose level may be needed. Tell patients to take levothyroxine on an empty stomach with a full glass of water (first thing in the morning is generally best) and to not eat for an hour after. Antacids, calcium carbonate, cholestyramine, colestipol, iron, sodium polystyrene sulfonate, simethicone, or sucralfate should be taken at least 4 hours before or 4 hours after taking levothyroxine. Advise patients to call their physician immediately if chest pain (angina) and rapid or irregular heartbeat or pulse are experienced.

PARATHYROID HORMONE

The four tiny parathyroid glands are located in the neck, behind the thyroid gland. Spontaneous atrophy or injury (as in thyroidectomy) of the parathyroid glands is followed by a decrease in the concentration of serum calcium and an increase in serum phosphorus. These changes can be reversed by the parenteral administration of suitably prepared extracts from the parathyroid glands of domestic animals. **Hypoparathyroidism** is a rare disorder in which the body produces little or no parathyroid hormone (PTH), resulting in an abnormally low level of blood calcium (hypocalcemia).

   Secretion of PTH is stimulated by a decrease in the free calcium ion concentration of the plasma. The hormone then acts to restore calcium concentration by:

✳ Increasing the reabsorption of calcium and the excretion of phosphate

✳ Decreasing the absorption of bicarbonate by the kidney

✳ Increasing the reabsorption of bone, with release of calcium ions

✳ Increasing the absorption of calcium and phosphate from the gastrointestinal (GI) tract

   The GI tract mediates *calcitriol* (a metabolite of vitamin D_3), which may be considered a hormone. PTH is a tropin for the renal synthesis of calcitriol. Vitamin D_2 (calciferol) can stimulate the hypercalcemic effect of PTH. Overdosage with any of these compounds can lead to dangerously high calcium concentrations in the blood, which may cause the calcification of kidneys and blood vessels.

✳ Apply Your Knowledge 32.2

The following questions focus on what you have just learned about the thyroid hormones, PTH, and antithyroid drugs.

CRITICAL THINKING

1. What are the two most common thyroid disorders?
2. What are the results of hypothyroidism during infancy and adulthood?
3. What are the indications of iodide as antithyroid drugs?
4. What is the effect of parathyroid hormone on the metabolism of calcium and vitamin D_3?
5. What are the trade names of methimazole, levothyroxine, and liothyronine?

Pancreas

The *pancreas* is found beneath the great curvature of the stomach and is connected by a duct to the duodenum of the small intestine. The pancreas is composed of clusters of glandular epithelial cells. One group of these clusters—the *islets of Langerhans*—forms the endocrine portions of the gland (and are therefore part of the endocrine system), regulating blood glucose levels and playing a vital role in metabolism.

PANCREATIC HORMONES

Some of the islets of Langerhans cells consist of alpha cells that secrete the hormone **glucagon**, which is secreted when blood glucose levels are low. The function of glucagon is to maintain adequate levels of glucose in the blood between meals. Other clusters consist of beta cells that secrete the hormone *insulin*, which is essential for the maintenance of normal blood sugar. Insulin promotes the use of glucose in cells (so it can used as fuel), thereby lowering the blood glucose level, and in the metabolism of carbohydrates, proteins, and fats. The dysregulation of beta cell function can lead to diabetes mellitus (see Figure 32-3 ■).

Diabetes mellitus is a serious endocrine disorder characterized by *hyperglycemia* (high glucose levels in the blood) and resulting from deficient insulin secretion or decreased sensitivity of insulin receptors on target cells. This condition affects approximately 17 million people in the United States. Diabetes mellitus exists in three forms: type 1, type 2, and gestational diabetes mellitus. Diabetes is more prevalent in the African American and Hispanic populations, and a genetic predisposition may increase susceptibility (especially with type 2 diabetes).

Type 1 diabetes—also called *insulin-dependent diabetes mellitus*—comprises about 10% of the diabetic population and is still sometimes referred to as *juvenile-onset diabetes* even though a significant

ALPHA CELL
Glucagon-secreting cell

BETA CELL
Insulin-secreting cell

Islet of Langerhans in the pancreas

Glucagon—raises blood glucose level
Insulin—lowers blood glucose level

A

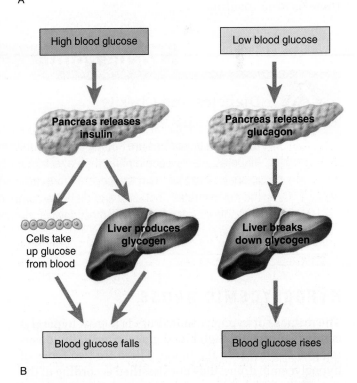

High blood glucose → Pancreas releases insulin → Cells take up glucose from blood / Liver produces glycogen → Blood glucose falls

Low blood glucose → Pancreas releases glucagon → Liver breaks down glycogen → Blood glucose rises

B

Figure 32-3 ■ (A) Diabetes mellitus can be caused by dysregulation of beta-cell function. **(B)** Interaction of blood glucose levels, insulin, and glucagon.

percentage of people are diagnosed with the disease after age 20. It results from a lack of insulin secretion by the pancreas, often occurs between the ages of 11 and 13 years, and has an abrupt onset. Within 5 to 10 years after diagnosis, the beta cells of the pancreas have been destroyed, and even minute amounts of insulin are no longer produced. The treatment of patients with type 1 diabetes involves drug therapy with insulin or other hypoglycemics—the goal being maintenance of proper blood glucose levels.

Focus on Pediatrics

Diabetes in Children

Chronic pathological conditions resulting from diabetes mellitus in children include diabetic neuropathy, retinopathy, nephropathy, stroke, coronary artery disease, and infection.

Type 2 diabetes is also called *non-insulin-dependent diabetes mellitus* and makes up approximately 90% of all cases of diabetes mellitus. It occurs mainly in adults older than 40 years of age, although the incidence has been increasing in younger patients because of physical inactivity and obesity. The onset is gradual and is often diagnosed by a routine physical examination, with the patient unaware of any signs and symptoms. Type 2 diabetics may secrete small amounts of insulin, but the greater problem is that insulin receptors in the target cells have become resistant to the hormone. Type 2 diabetes mellitus can be treated through diet and exercise (which can sometimes increase the sensitivity of the receptors) and, if needed, through the use of oral antidiabetic medications or even insulin.

Gestational diabetes mellitus develops during pregnancy, and symptoms may be similar to type 2 diabetes. Generally temporary, it ends when the pregnancy is over. The treatment is through diet and exercise. In some cases, low doses of insulin are appropriate, but oral hypoglycemics are not given.

Complications from diabetes are a leading cause of suffering, disability, and premature death. The following disorders are associated with long-term diabetes, especially with poorly controlled hyperglycemia: retinopathy, nephropathy, depressed immune function, elevated blood lipid levels, and vascular disease. The consequences of these complications are blindness, renal impairment and kidney failure, neuropathic pain, opportunistic infections, wounds and sores that do not heal, loss of limbs, atherosclerosis, hypertension, and myocardial infarction.

Focus Point

Diabetes and Obesity

Seventeen million Americans have diabetes. Forty million are obese—a major cause of type 2 diabetes. These conditions are among the top public health problems in the United States today. Usually, type 2 diabetes affects people older than age 40, but because of increased obesity in children and other young patients, more of them than ever before are being diagnosed with this condition. African Americans have the highest rates of obesity and diabetes compared with other ethnic groups. For good health, 30 minutes of moderate physical activity most days of the week is recommended, and 60 minutes is recommended to achieve significant weight loss.

HYPOGLYCEMIC DRUGS

The purpose of hypoglycemic drugs is to treat **hyperglycemia** (abnormally high blood glucose level) by lowering glucose levels in the blood. There are two types of hypoglycemic drugs; they are classified according to the manner in which they are administered: parenteral and oral. Insulin is the sole representative of the parenteral type.

Insulin Injection

Insulin is an antidiabetic hormone that lowers blood glucose levels by facilitating glucose uptake into body cells. Insulin cannot be taken orally because it is destroyed by digestive enzymes. Several types of insulin are available for subcutaneous or intramuscular injection (Table 32-4 ■). Patient participation is an essential component of comprehensive insulin care.

Table 32-4 ■ Classifications of Insulin

GENERIC NAME	TRADE NAME	AVERAGE ADULT DOSAGE	ROUTE OF ADMINISTRATION
Rapid-Acting Insulin Analogs			
lispro	Humalog	5–10 U 0–15 min ac	SC
aspart	NovoLog	0.25–0.7 U/kg/d 5–15 min ac	SC
glulisine	Apidra	Individualized doses	Inhalation
Short-Acting Insulin			
regular insulin	Humulin R, Novolin R	5–10 U 15–30 min ac and at bedtime	SC
Intermediate-Acting Insulin			
isophane insulin suspension (also known as NPH)	Humulin N, Novolin N	2–4 hours	SC

Note: Extended-acting insulins were discontinued in the United States in 2006.

SC, subcutaneous; ac, before meals.

Focus Point

Insulin Therapy

Insulin controls the level of blood glucose but does not cure diabetes. Therefore, insulin therapy is required long term.

Focus On

Rapid-Acting Insulin: Lispro

Lispro insulin is one of this class that has a rapid onset (5–10 minutes) and short duration of effect (2–4 hours). It is used to achieve glycemic control if taken immediately before or after meals, which reduces the danger of **hypoglycemia** (abnormally low blood glucose level). Rapid-acting insulins must be used in combination with longer-acting preparations.

How does it work?

Lispro—a human insulin of recombinant DNA origin—is a rapid-acting and glucose-lowering agent that increases peripheral glucose uptake, especially by skeletal muscle and fat tissue, by inhibiting the liver from changing glycogen to glucose.

How is it used?

Lispro is used in the treatment of diabetes mellitus.

What are the adverse effects?

Most adverse effects are related to hypoglycemia, which results from either an overdose of insulin or a mismatch in blood glucose levels with the appropriate dose of insulin. Lipodystrophy, allergic reactions, and insulin resistance are other complications of insulin therapy.

What are the contraindications and interactions?

Insulin is contraindicated during episodes of hypoglycemia and in patients sensitive to any ingredient in the formulation. It must be used cautiously with insulin-resistant patients, with those with hyperthyroidism or hypothyroidism, with patients with renal or hepatic impairment, with women who are lactating or pregnant, and with older adults. Safety and efficacy in children younger than 3 years old have not been established.

(*continued*)

Focus On (continued)

Alcohol, anabolic steroids, and salicylates may potentiate hypoglycemic effects. Corticosteroids, epinephrine, and dextrothyroxine may antagonize hypoglycemic effects.

What are the important points patients should know?

Instruct patients to recognize the manifestations of a hypoglycemic reaction (nervousness, sweating, tremors, rapid pulse, hunger, and weakness) as well as manifestations of a hyperglycemic reaction (thirst, sweating, a "fruity" breath odor, abdominal pain, increased urine output, and nausea and vomiting). Eating a sugary snack or taking glucose tablets followed by a food containing complex carbohydrates (milk, crackers, fruit) will reverse a hypoglycemic reaction. However, if not treated, the result can be coma and even death.

Focus on Natural Products

Garlic and Ginseng

Garlic and ginseng may potentiate the hypoglycemic effects of insulin lispro.

Focus On

Short-Acting Insulins: Regular Insulin

Regular (natural) insulin (Humulin R, Novolin R) is a short-acting insulin that is injected before a meal. The onset is 30–60 minutes, and the duration of action is 5–7 hours. Short-acting insulins are highly soluble, and their solutions have a clear appearance. Regular insulin is administered subcutaneously.

How does it work?

Regular insulin lowers blood glucose levels by increasing peripheral glucose uptake, especially by skeletal muscle and fat tissue, and by inhibiting the liver from changing glycogen to glucose.

How is it used?

Regular insulin is used in the emergency treatment of patients with diabetic ketoacidosis or coma, to initiate therapy in patients with type 1 diabetes, and in combination with intermediate-acting or long-acting insulins to provide better control of blood glucose concentrations in diabetic patients.

What are the adverse effects?

The most common adverse effects are hypoglycemic reactions, especially when diabetes is newly diagnosed, and the correct insulin dosage, which is highly individualized for each patient, has not yet been established. Symptoms of hypoglycemia include headache, hunger, weakness, sweating, tachycardia, confusion, and emotional disturbances, as well as coma and death.

What are the contraindications and interactions?

Regular insulin is contraindicated in patients with hypersensitivity to any ingredient of the product and when a patient is hypoglycemic. Insulin is used cautiously during pregnancy and in patients with kidney or liver impairments. It should be avoided during lactation. Certain drugs, such as contraceptives, corticosteroids, diuretics, epinephrine, lithium, niacin, thyroid hormones, albuterol, and dobutamine, may interact with the administration of insulin and increase or decrease blood sugar.

What are the important points patients should know?

Advise patients to drink orange juice and sugar-containing drinks and foods when a hypoglycemic reaction occurs.

Intermediate-Acting Insulins

Insulin isophane is classified as an intermediate-acting insulin. It is produced by recombinant DNA technology that uses a nonpathogenic strain of *Escherichia coli*. Insulin isophane suspension also contains protamine and zinc.

How do they work?

The mechanism of action of insulin isophane is similar to that of rapid-acting insulins. It lowers blood glucose by stimulating peripheral glucose uptake by the skeletal muscles and fat, and also by inhibiting hepatic glucose production.

How are they used?

Insulin isophane is indicated to improve glycemic control in adults and pediatric patients with diabetes mellitus.

What are the adverse effects?

The adverse effects of insulin isophane occur in fewer than 1% of patients and are similar to those of rapid-acting insulins.

What are the contraindications and interactions?

Insulin isophane is contraindicated during episodes of hypoglycemia and in patients sensitive to any ingredient in the formulation. They must be used cautiously in insulin-resistant patients, those with hyperthyroidism or hypothyroidism, patients with renal or hepatic impairment, women who are lactating or pregnant, and in older adults. Safety and efficacy in children younger than 3 years of age has not been established. Drug interactions are similar to those of rapid-acting insulins.

What are the important points patients should know?

Teach patients how to check their blood glucose levels by using a blood glucose monitoring machine. These levels should be checked about four times daily. More frequent monitoring is required if levels are not within the normal range. Stress the importance of maintaining a well-balanced diet with the dietary restrictions specified by the health care team. Delaying or missing a meal may lead to hypoglycemia. Advise patients to avoid alcohol.

Extended Insulin in Zinc Suspension

This type of suspension was discontinued in the United States in 2006 because of the development of better and more effective products derived only from human sources.

This type of insulin was obtained from the pancreases of pigs.

Focus Point

Patient Education About Diabetes

Patient education is a continuing process; regular visits are needed for reinforcement. The things that a newly diagnosed patient with diabetes needs to learn about include maintaining a positive attitude, available educational materials, dietary changes, exercise changes, glucose monitoring, following medication regimens exactly, support services, carbohydrate counting, proper responses to hypoglycemia, foot care, blood pressure monitoring, and stress relief.

COMBINATION INSULIN PRODUCTS

Combinations of different types of insulins can increase the onset of effects while maintaining a long duration of glycemic control. The following combination insulin products are examples:

* Insulin 70/30: 70% neutral protamine hagedorn (NPH) and 30% regular
* Insulin 50/50: 50% NPH and 50% regular
* Insulin 75/25: 75% insulin lispro protamine (intermediate acting) and 25% lispro

Focus Point

Hypoglycemic Reactions

Patient participation is an essential component of comprehensive diabetes care. Patients with type 1 or type 2 diabetes who are receiving insulin should be taught to be cautious about hypoglycemic reactions. Signs and symptoms include hunger, nausea, pale and cool skin, and sweating.

ORAL ANTIDIABETIC DRUGS

Patients with type 2 diabetes mellitus have a defect in insulin secretion from the pancreas, inappropriate hepatic glucose production, tissue insulin resistance, or a combination of any of these as a major cause of glucose dysregulation. Drugs that improve insulin secretion, decrease hepatic glucose production, and improve insulin sensitivity at the tissue receptors are therefore effective in treating patients with type 2 diabetes.

There are now four chemical categories of orally administered agents that act on lower blood sugar levels: sulfonylureas, biguanides, thiazolidinediones, and alpha-glucosidase inhibitors. The sulfonylureas and biguanides have been available the longest and are the traditional initial treatment choices for type 2 diabetes. Table 32-5 ■ lists common oral antidiabetic drugs.

Table 32-5 ■ Common Oral Antidiabetic Drugs

GENERIC NAME	TRADE NAME	AVERAGE ADULT DOSAGE	ROUTE OF ADMINISTRATION
First-Generation Sulfonylureas			
chlorpropamide	Diabinese	100–250 mg/d	PO
tolazamide	Tolinase	100–500 mg bid	PO
tolbutamide	(Generic only)	250–1500 mg bid	PO
Second-Generation Sulfonylureas			
glimepiride	Amaryl	1–4 mg/d	PO
glipizide	Glucotrol	2.5–20 mg bid	PO
glyburide	DiaBeta, Micronase, Glynase PresTab	1.25–5 mg/d with breakfast	PO
Biguanides			
metformin	Glucophage, Fortamet	500–850 mg tid	PO
Thiazolidinediones			
pioglitazone	Actos	15–30 mg/d	PO
rosiglitazone	Avandia	4 mg/d	PO
Alpha-Glucosidase Inhibitors			
acarbose	Precose	25–100 mg tid	PO
miglitol	Glyset	25–100 mg tid	PO

GENERIC NAME	TRADE NAME	AVERAGE ADULT DOSAGE	ROUTE OF ADMINISTRATION
Other			
pramlintide acetate	Symlin	Initially: 60 mcg before meals; insulin dose must be reduced; increase to 120 mcg as directed by physician	SC
exenatide (incretin mimetic)	Byetta	Individual dosing according to size of meal and amount of exercise	SC
sitagliptin (dipeptidyl peptidase inhibitor)	Januvia	100 mg/d in a single dose	PO

PO, oral; bid, twice a day; tid, three times a day; SC, subcutaneous.

Focus On

Sulfonylureas

The sulfonylurea drugs have been available in the United States since 1954 and have been the mainstay of oral antidiabetic therapy for many years. They are classified as either first generation—tolbutamide, tolazamide, and chlorpropamide—or second generation—glipizide, glyburide, and glimepiride—based on their pharmacokinetic profiles. Second-generation sulfonylureas tend to be prescribed more frequently because of their tolerability and dosing schedules.

How do they work?

The sulfonylureas act in three ways: (1) by stimulating the release of insulin from the pancreas, (2) by inhibiting the process of forming glucose from amino acids and fatty acids in the liver, and (3) by increasing the number of insulin receptors to target cells.

How are they used?

The sulfonylureas are used for the treatment of mild to moderately severe type 2 diabetes that cannot be controlled by diet alone and in patients who do not have complications of diabetes.

What are the adverse effects?

The adverse effects of the sulfonylureas include hypoglycemia caused by an overdosage, allergic skin reactions, fainting, confusion, blurred vision, depression of bone marrow, and GI disturbances.

What are the contraindications and interactions?

The sulfonylureas are contraindicated in hypersensitivity to these agents. They should be avoided in patients with diabetes complicated by severe infection; acidosis; and severe renal, hepatic, or thyroid insufficiency. Safe use of the sulfonylurea drugs during pregnancy, in nursing mothers, and in children has not been established. These agents should be used cautiously in older adult patients and in those with Addison's disease or hepatic porphyria.

What are the important points patients should know?

Teach patients that oral hypoglycemic drugs are not the same as insulin. They enhance the effectiveness of insulin. Instruct patients taking sulfonylureas to avoid alcohol because a disulfiram-like reaction may occur. Symptoms of this reaction include fever, chills, diarrhea, abdominal pain, and severe nausea and vomiting.

Biguanides

Metformin is a biguanide compound that keeps the blood sugar levels from increasing too high or too fast after meals. This agent does not necessarily decrease blood glucose levels.

(continued)

Focus On (continued)

How do they work?

Biguanides act by promoting glucose uptake into cells through enhanced insulin-receptor binding and by decreasing the production of glucose in the liver. They slow glucose absorption and increase glucose removal from the blood without causing hypoglycemia. They may also reduce glucagon levels.

How are they used?

Biguanides are used for type 2 diabetes when no response occurs to sulfonylureas. They may be combined with sulfonylureas, in which case dose reduction of the biguanide agent would be needed.

What are the adverse effects?

Common adverse effects of biguanides include anorexia, GI upset (such as diarrhea and nausea and vomiting), and lactic acidosis (rare).

What are the contraindications and interactions?

The biguanides are contraindicated in patients with renal disease, alcoholism, hepatic disease, and chronic cardiopulmonary dysfunction. Biguanides interact with amiloride, calcium channel blockers, cimetidine, digoxin, furosemide, morphine, procainamide, quinidine, quinine, ranitidine, trimethoprim, triamterene, and vancomycin.

What are the important points patients should know?

Instruct patients that biguanides should be taken with meals to minimize the effect of gastric irritation. Because these agents have a slow onset, glucose control may take up to 2 weeks to establish. Instruct patients to limit alcohol intake because the combination can increase the risk of lactic acidosis.

Thiazolidinediones

Two thiazolidinediones are currently available: pioglitazone and rosiglitazone. A third compound—troglitazone—was withdrawn from the market because of hepatic toxicity.

How do they work?

The thiazolidinediones improve cell sensitivity to insulin via the stimulation of a receptor in skeletal muscle, liver, and fat cells.

How are they used?

These agents are used as adjuncts to diet in the treatment of type 2 diabetes.

What are the adverse effects?

Common adverse effects include edema, anemia, headache, back pain, fatigue, weight gain, and hypoglycemia. Hepatic function needs to be closely monitored during therapy for signs of hepatic impairment.

What are the contraindications and interactions?

The thiazolidinediones are contraindicated in patients who have hypersensitivity to these agents. These drugs should be avoided in patients who have active liver impairment or during pregnancy and lactation. Safety and efficacy in children younger than age 18 have not been established. Drug interactions between insulin and the thiazolidinediones may increase risk of heart failure or edema or enhance hypoglycemia with oral antidiabetic agents. Ketoconazole and such herbs as garlic and ginseng may potentiate hypoglycemic effects.

What are the important points patients should know?

Advise patients to contact their physician if any of the following symptoms develop during thiazolidinedione therapy because these symptoms may indicate hepatic dysfunction: dark urine, jaundice, abdominal pain, nausea and vomiting, anorexia, or fatigue.

Alpha-Glucosidase Inhibitors

Dietary carbohydrates require enzymatic degradation by alpha-glucosidase to monosaccharides within the GI tract to enable absorption. Alpha-glucosidase inhibitors, such as acarbose and miglitol, make up a unique class of drugs that act on this enzyme in the small intestine.

How do they work?

Alpha-glucosidase inhibitors inhibit or delay the absorption of sugar from the GI tract.

How are they used?

Alpha-glucosidase inhibitors are used as monotherapy or in combination with a sulfonylurea in patients with type 2 diabetes mellitus.

What are the adverse effects?

Prominent adverse effects include flatulence, diarrhea, and abdominal pain; they result from the appearance of undigested carbohydrate in the colon that is then fermented into short-chain fatty acids, releasing gas. Hypoglycemia may occur with concurrent sulfonylurea treatment.

What are the contraindications and interactions?

Alpha-glucosidase inhibitors are contraindicated in patients with inflammatory bowel disease and any intestinal condition that could be worsened by gas and distention. Because miglitol and acarbose are absorbed from the gut, these medications should not be prescribed in patients with renal impairment. Acarbose has been associated with reversible hepatic enzyme elevation and should be used with caution in the presence of hepatic disease.

What are the important points patients should know?

Instruct patients that insulin might be needed instead of or to supplement oral hypoglycemic drugs in times of infection, stress, or surgery.

✳ Apply Your Knowledge 32.3

The following questions focus on what you have just learned about the pancreatic hormones and hypoglycemic drugs.

CRITICAL THINKING

1. What are the different types of diabetes mellitus?
2. What hormones are released by the islets of Langerhans cells?
3. What are the contraindications of insulin?
4. What are the three examples of combination insulin products?
5. What are the trade names of glipizide, rosiglitazone, and metformin?

Adrenal Glands

The adrenal glands sit on top of each kidney. The cortex—or outer portion of the adrenal gland—is one of the endocrine structures most vital for normal metabolic function. It is impossible for life to continue in the complete absence of adrenal cortical function.

ADRENOCORTICAL STEROIDS

The adrenal cortex secretes three types of steroid hormones: the glucocorticoids (also called adrenocortical hormones), mineralocorticoids, and gonadal corticoids.

As a group, these hormones are called *corticosteroids*. In humans, hydrocortisone (cortisol) is the main glucocorticoid and aldosterone is the main mineralocorticoid. Gonadal corticoids are a group of androgens that mostly contain testosterone, estrogen, and progesterone. They are discussed in detail in Chapter 33.

ACTH is the primary stimulus to hydrocortisone secretion. ACTH is released in response to CRH. Adrenocortical hormones (glucocorticoids) and their effects on the human body are listed in Table 32-6 ■.

Table 32-6 ■ Adrenocortical Hormones and Their Effects

HORMONE	EFFECTS
Glucocorticoids	
Cortisone, hydrocortisone	Increase blood sugar levels, stimulate protein catabolism, mobilize fats, and decrease immunity and inflammatory responses
Mineralocorticoids	
Aldosterone	Cause sodium and water retention, increase blood pressure and blood volume
Gonadal Corticoids	
Androgens	Stimulate activity of the accessory male sex organs, promote development of male sex characteristics, or prevent changes in the latter after castration

Focus On

Glucocorticoids

Glucocorticoids, such as cortisone and prednisone, have diverse effects, including alterations in carbohydrate, protein, and lipid metabolism; maintenance of fluid and electrolyte balance; and preservation of normal function of the cardiovascular system, immune system, kidneys, skeletal muscle, endocrine system, and nervous system. One of the major pharmacological uses of this class of drugs is based on their anti-inflammatory and immuno-suppressive actions. A protective role for cortisol is apparent in the physiological response to severe stress that can increase daily production more than tenfold.

The relative or complete absence of adrenocortical function, known as Addison's disease, is accompanied by a loss of sodium chloride and water, retention of potassium, lowering of blood glucose and liver glycogen levels, increased sensitivity to insulin, nitrogen retention, and lymphocytosis. The disturbances in electrolyte metabolism are the causes of morbidity and mortality in most cases of severe adrenal insufficiency. Disorders caused by adrenal insufficiency can be corrected by the administration of adrenal cortical extract or the pure adrenal cortical steroids now available. Overproduction of or overtreatment with glucocorticoids may cause Cushing's syndrome. The major adrenal corticosteroids (glucocorticoids) are listed in Table 32-7 ■.

How do they work?

The major actions of glucocorticoids are to suppress an acute inflammatory process and for immunosuppression.

How are they used?

Glucocorticoids are used for replacement therapy in adrenal insufficiency, such as Addison's disease and congenital adrenal hyperplasia. Glucocorticoids are also used to treat rheumatic, inflammatory, allergic, neoplastic, and other disorders. Glucocorticoids are of value in decreasing some cerebral edemas. Their value in the treatment of bacterial meningitis is probably caused by the decreasing of edema. Topical or systemic glucocorticoids are used to treat certain skin diseases such as pruritus, psoriasis, and eczema.

What are the adverse effects?

When the glucocorticoids are used for short periods (less than 2 weeks), serious adverse effects are unusual even with moderately large doses. However, insomnia, behavioral changes, and acute peptic ulcers are occasionally observed even after only a few days of treatment.

Most patients who are given daily doses of 100 mg of hydrocortisone or more for longer than 2 weeks undergo a series of changes that have been termed **iatrogenic** (i.e., produced inadvertently by medication or another treatment). Cushing's syndrome, acne, insomnia, and increased appetite are noted. In the treatment of dangerous or disabling disorders, these changes may not require the cessation of therapy. However, the underlying metabolic changes accompanying them can be very serious by the time they become obvious, and eventually, osteoporosis, diabetes, and aseptic necrosis of the hip bone may develop. Wound healing is also impaired under these circumstances.

What are the contraindications and interactions?

The corticosteroids are contraindicated in patients with peptic ulcer, heart disease, hypertension with heart failure, certain infectious illnesses (such as varicella and tuberculosis), psychoses, diabetes, osteoporosis, and glaucoma.

Patients receiving these drugs must be monitored carefully for the development of hypoglycemia, glycosuria, sodium retention with edema or hypertension, hypokalemia, peptic ulcer, osteoporosis, and hidden infections. Glucocorticoids decrease the hypoglycemic activity of insulin and oral hypoglycemics, so a change in dose of the antidiabetic drugs may be necessitated.

What are the important points patients should know?

Advise patients to take glucocorticoids as ordered. These drugs should not be stopped abruptly. Instead, the physician will organize the dose to be reduced over 1–2 weeks.

Warn patients that they should not have any immunizations while taking these drugs unless they have been approved by their physician. Advise patients to take oral drugs with food to prevent gastric irritation. Antacids or other antiulcer drugs may be prescribed to lessen the risk of ulceration.

Large doses of steroids may increase the patient's susceptibility to infection. Warn patients about this possibility, and instruct them to notify their physician of fever, cough, sore throat, or injuries that do not heal. They should inform other health care professionals about their use of these drugs, especially before surgery.

Table 32-7 ■ Major Adrenal Corticosteroids (Glucocorticoids)

GENERIC NAME	TRADE NAME	AVERAGE ADULT DOSAGE	ROUTE OF ADMINISTRATION
betamethasone	Celestone	0.6–7.2 mg/d	PO
cortisone	Cortone	20–300 mg/d in divided doses	PO
dexamethasone	(Generic only)	0.25–4 mg bid–qid	PO
hydrocortisone	Cortaid	0.5% cream applied daily qid	Topical
		10–320 mg tid–qid	PO
prednisolone	Prelone	5–60 mg/d qid	PO
prednisone	Rayos	5–60 mg/d qid	PO
triamcinolone	(Generic only)	4–48 mg/d qid	PO

PO, oral; bid, twice a day; qid, four times a day; tid, three times a day.

Focus Point

Glucocorticoids

A patient who is taking glucocorticoids should understand the benefits and possible side effects of long-term use and be advised to report any new side effects. The patient should also be instructed to take oral doses with meals, avoid alcohol, limit sodium intake, and increase potassium intake.

Focus On

Mineralocorticoids

Mineralocorticoids are a group of hormones secreted from the adrenal cortex. The most important mineralocorticoid in humans is aldosterone. Small amounts of desoxycorticosterone are also formed and released, although the amount is normally insignificant.

The rate of aldosterone secretion is subject to several influences. ACTH produces a moderate stimulation of its release, but this effect is not sustained for more than a few days in normal individuals.

(continued)

Focus On (continued)

How do they work?

Aldosterone and other steroids with mineralocorticoid properties regulate sodium and potassium balance in the blood by promoting the reabsorption of sodium from the distal convoluted and collecting ducts of the kidneys, which results in the excretion of potassium. Mineralocorticoids act by binding to the mineralocorticoid receptor in the cytoplasm of target cells, especially principal cells of the distal convoluted and collecting tubules.

How are they used?

Mineralocorticoids are used for replacement therapy for primary and secondary adrenocortical deficiency.

What are the adverse effects?

The adverse effects of mineralocorticoids can occur if the dosage is too high or prolonged or if withdrawal is too rapid. They can cause edema, hypertension, congestive heart failure, increased sweating, or skin rashes. They can also cause hypokalemia, muscular weakness, and headache.

What are the contraindications and interactions?

The mineralocorticoids are contraindicated in patients with hypersensitivity to these agents and those with systemic fungal infections. They must be used cautiously in patients with Addison's disease or infection and during pregnancy and lactation. Mineralocorticoids can decrease the effects of barbiturates, rifampin, and hydantoins.

What are the important points patients should know?

Advise patients to maintain a low-sodium and high-potassium diet if weight gain is an issue. Teach patients to recognize the adverse effects of these drugs, which may include edema, hypertension, congestive heart failure, increased sweating, and skin rashes.

Focus Point

Addison's Disease

Addison's disease is caused by adrenocortical insufficiency, which is characterized by an insidious onset of fatigue, weakness, lack of appetite, nausea and vomiting, weight loss, skin pigmentation, and hypotension.

✳ Apply Your Knowledge 32.4

The following questions focus on what you have just learned about adrenocortical steroids.

CRITICAL THINKING

1. What are the adrenocortical hormones and their effects?
2. What are the major actions of glucocorticoids?
3. What class of adrenocortical hormones includes aldosterone?
4. What are the trade names of prednisolone, prednisone, and hydrocortisone?
5. What is the result of adrenocortical insufficiency?

the effects of estrogen excess in the female breasts and endometrium.

How are they used?

Testosterones are given to men and women for therapeutic purposes in various conditions. Their main indications in men are to supplement low levels of testosterone to correct *hypogonadism* (abnormally decreased gonadal function that results in retarded sexual development) or *cryptorchidism* (undescended testes). Androgens are also used to increase sperm production in cases of infertility. In women, they can be used in the palliative treatment of metastatic breast cancer. Androgens are also prescribed in women for the treatment of postpartum breast engorgement, endometriosis, and fibrocystic breast disorder. These agents are able to stimulate the increased production of red blood cells, protein synthesis, and muscle mass. Therefore, athletes may use androgens to improve athletic performance.

What are the adverse effects?

The common adverse effects of androgens include insomnia, excitation, skin flushing, nausea and vomiting, anorexia, diarrhea, and jaundice. Hypercalcemia, hypercholesterolemia, sodium retention, and water retention (especially in older adults) with edema are seen. The adverse effects of testosterone may also cause renal calculi, bladder irritability, and increased libido.

What are the contraindications and interactions?

Androgens are contraindicated in patients with hypersensitivity or toxic reactions. These agents should be avoided in patients with serious cardiac, liver, or kidney diseases. Androgens must not be prescribed in male patients with known or suspected prostatic or breast cancer. Testosterone and other androgens cannot be used during pregnancy or lactation because of the possibility of *virilization* (the changes that occur as the male body develops, which are different from the development of the female body); that is, these substances would have undesired effects on women. Androgens must be used cautiously in people with cardiac, liver, and kidney diseases; prepubertal boys; older adults; and people with acute intermittent porphyria. Testosterone alters glucose tolerance tests and may increase creatinine and creatinine secretion. Androgens may suppress some clotting factors and may increase or decrease serum cholesterol.

What are the important points patients should know?

Advise patients about skin hygiene measures to reduce the severity of acne. Oral androgens should be taken with meals to reduce gastric upset. Instruct patients taking androgens to report a **priapism** (painful and prolonged erection) because the dose would need to be reduced and to also report decreased flow of urine because androgens can cause prostatic hypertrophy.

Focus on Geriatrics

Anabolic Steroids and Elderly Men

When anabolic steroids are given to elderly men, their risk of prostate cancer is increased.

✳ Apply Your Knowledge 33.1

The following questions focus on what you have just learned about the male reproductive system.

CRITICAL THINKING

1. What hormones are essential to the development and maintenance of secondary sex characteristics?
2. What are the functions of the prostate gland and seminal vesicles?
3. What are the main indications of testosterone in men and women?
4. What are four examples of anabolic steroids?
5. What are the trade names of oxandrolone, fluoxymesterone, and nandrolone?
6. What is the definition of *priapism*?

Female Reproductive System

The organs of the female reproductive system produce and maintain the female sex cells: the egg cells (or oocytes); transport these cells to the site of fertilization; provide a favorable environment for developing fetuses; propel the fetus outside the body during birth; and produce female sex hormones. A female's *primary sex organs* (gonads) are the two ovaries, which produce the female sex cells and sex hormones. The *accessory sex organs* of the female reproductive system are the internal and external reproductive organs. They include the ovaries, uterine tubes, uterus, vagina, labia majora, labia minora, clitoris, and vestibule (Figure 33-2 ■). Table 33-3 ■ summarizes the functions of the female reproductive organs.

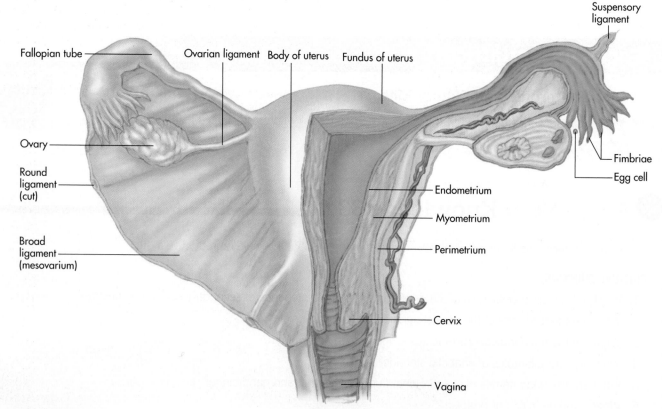

Figure 33-2 ■ The female reproductive system.

Table 33-3 ■ Functions of the Female Reproductive System

ORGAN	FUNCTION
Ovaries	Produce oocytes and female sex hormones
Uterine tubes	Convey oocytes toward the uterus and site of fertilization
Uterus	Protects and sustains the embryo during pregnancy
Vagina	Conveys uterine secretions to outside the body; receives the erect penis during sexual intercourse
Labia majora	Enclose and protect other external reproductive organs
Labia minora	Form margins of the vestibule; protect the openings of the vagina and urethra
Clitoris	Produces feelings of pleasure and sexual stimulation
Vestibule	Space between the labia minora that contains vaginal and urethral openings

FEMALE SEX HORMONES

The female body is reproductively immature until about age 10. Then, the hypothalamus begins to secrete increasing amounts of gonadotropin-releasing hormone (GnRH). GnRH, in turn, stimulates the anterior pituitary to release the gonadotropins follicle-stimulating hormone (FSH) and luteinizing hormone (LH). These hormones play primary roles in controlling female sex cell maturation and in producing female sex hormones. Several tissues, including the tissues of the ovaries, adrenal cortices, and placenta (during pregnancy), secrete female sex hormones that belong to two major groups: **estrogens** and **progesterones**. Estradiol is the most abundant of the estrogens, which also include estrone and estriol.

The ovaries are the primary source of estrogens (in nonpregnant females). At puberty, under the influence of the anterior pituitary, the ovaries secrete increasing amounts of estrogens. Estrogens stimulate enlargement of accessory organs, including the vagina, uterus, uterine tubes, ovaries, and external reproductive structures. Estrogens also develop and maintain the female secondary sex characteristics.

The ovaries are also the primary source of progesterone (in nonpregnant females). This hormone promotes changes in the uterus during the female reproductive cycle, affects the mammary glands, and helps regulate the secretion of gonadotropins from the anterior pituitary. Androgen (male sex hormone) concentrations produce certain other changes in young women at puberty. For example, increased hair growth in the pubic and axillary regions is caused by androgens secreted by the adrenal cortices. Conversely, development of the female skeletal configuration, which includes narrow shoulders and broad hips, is a response to a low androgen concentration. Estrogens support the development and maintenance of reproductive organs and the secondary sex characteristics. Table 33-4 ■ summarizes the major synthetic estrogens.

Table 33-4 ■ Major Synthetic Estrogens

GENERIC NAME	TRADE NAME	AVERAGE ADULT DOSAGE	ROUTE OF ADMINISTRATION
conjugated estrogens	Premarin	0.3–2.5 mg/d in cycles; 25 mg by injection	PO, IM, IV
estradiol	Estrace	0.45–2 mg/d in cycles	PO
estradiol hemihydrate	Vagifem	25 mcg/d for 2 wk and then 25 mcg 2 times/wk	Vaginal
estradiol transdermal system	Alora, Estraderm	0.05–0.1 mg patch 2 times/wk	Transdermal
estradiol valerate	Delestrogen	5–20 mg q2–3wk	IM

(*continued*)

Table 33-4 ■ **Major Synthetic Estrogens** (*continued*)

GENERIC NAME	TRADE NAME	AVERAGE ADULT DOSAGE	ROUTE OF ADMINISTRATION
esterified estrogens	Menest	0.3–1.25 mg/d	PO
estrone	Kestrone 5	0.1–0.5 mg 2–3 times/wk	IM
estropipate	Ogen	1–2 mg tid	PO

PO, oral; IM, intramuscular; IV, intravenous; tid, three times a day.

Focus On

Synthetic Estrogens

The most widely known synthetic estrogen is diethylstilbestrol, which possesses most of the therapeutic and untoward actions of the natural estrogenic hormones. Because nonsteroidal estrogens lose little activity after oral administration, they have advantages over the natural estrogens, but the comparative toxicities are not clear.

How do they work?

Estrogens bind to intracellular receptors that stimulate DNA and RNA to synthesize proteins responsible for the effects of these hormones.

How are they used?

The estrogens are used in both genders, including replacement estrogen therapy in women who have had their ovaries removed during the reproductive years, in older women for the prevention and treatment of osteoporosis, and as palliative therapy for breast and prostatic carcinomas in men. Estrogens are also prescribed for abnormal bleeding (hormonal imbalance) and atrophic vaginitis.

What are the adverse effects?

The adverse effects of estrogen therapy include anorexia, nausea and vomiting, stomach cramping, flatulence, headaches, changes in libido (in females), edema of the lower extremities, and breast discomfort or enlargement.

In males, feminization may occur, including changes in the fat deposit sites, atrophy of the sex organs, and loss of facial or body hair. Estrogens can cause the retention of sodium and water, resulting in weight gain, edema, and hypertension.

What are the contraindications and interactions?

The estrogens are contraindicated in women with breast cancer and those who are pregnant or lactating. Estrogens should be used with caution in patients with liver disease, gallbladder disease, endometriosis, pancreatitis, diabetes mellitus, heart failure, and kidney dysfunction.

Estrogens may interact with barbiturates, phenytoin, and rifampin, possibly causing decreased estrogen effects by increasing its metabolism. Estrogens may interfere with the effects of bromocriptine. They may also increase the levels and toxicity of cyclosporine and theophylline, and they may decrease the effectiveness of clofibrate.

What are the important points patients should know?

Advise patients to take the drug exactly as prescribed and to not omit, increase, or decrease doses without the advice of their physicians. Instruct patients about what to do when a dose is missed. Advise patients to review the package inserts to ensure the understanding of estrogen therapy. Patients should not breastfeed while taking this drug.

Focus Point

Testosterone Use During Pregnancy

The use of testosterone during pregnancy can cause the masculinization of the fetus, particularly if testosterone (androgen) therapy is provided during the first trimester of pregnancy.

Focus on Pregnancy

Estrogens During Pregnancy

Use of conjugated estrogens during the first trimester of pregnancy may increase the risk of fetal malformations, including cleft palate, heart defect, dislocated hips, absent tibiae, and *polydactylia* (the presence of more than five digits on the hands or feet).

Focus on Geriatrics

Hormonal Therapy After Menopause

In women taking an estrogen preparation on a long-term basis after menopause, a progestin should be added to estrogen preparations to prevent endometrial hyperplasia and endometrial carcinoma. This practice is not necessary for women who have had a hysterectomy.

Focus On

Progestins

Progesterone is the primary progestational substance that is naturally produced by ovarian cells of the corpus luteum. It has a physiological action that is unique and distinct from estrogen. Progestin derivatives are synthetic drugs. Table 33-5 ■ provides a summary of several progestins and combination products.

How do they work?

Progesterone transforms the endometrium from a proliferative to a secretory state; it suppresses pituitary gonadotropin secretion, thereby blocking follicular maturation and ovulation. Acting with estrogen, it promotes mammary gland development without causing lactation, and it increases body temperature 1°F at the time of ovulation. The synthetic progestins are usually preferred for clinical use because of the decreased effectiveness of progesterone when administered orally.

How are they used?

The progestins are prescribed for women with secondary amenorrhea, functional uterine bleeding, endometriosis, and premenstrual syndrome. As an intrauterine agent and in combination with estrogens, a progestin provides fertility control, largely supplanted by new progestins, which have longer action and may be taken orally.

What are the adverse effects?

Use of progestins may result in many adverse effects, and the incidence and intensity of these reactions may be varied. They may cause vaginal candidiasis, skin hyperpigmentation, cervical erosion, breakthrough bleeding, dysmenorrhea, amenorrhea, breast tenderness, edema, acne, pruritus, and mental depression. Thromboembolic disorder, pulmonary embolism, changes in vision, nausea and vomiting, and abdominal cramps are also seen.

What are the contraindications and interactions?

Progestins are contraindicated in patients who are hypersensitive to these agents. Progestins must be avoided in patients with known or suspected breast or genital malignancies. These agents are contraindicated in patients with impaired liver disease, undiagnosed vaginal bleeding, miscarriage, thrombophlebitis, and thromboembolic disorders. Progestins should be used cautiously in patients with anemia, diabetes mellitus, a history of psychic depression, previous ectopic pregnancy, presence or history of **salpingitis** (an inflammation or infection of a fallopian tube), and unresolved abnormal Pap smear result. Barbiturates, carbamazepine, phenytoin, and rifampin may alter contraceptive effectiveness. Ketoconazole may inhibit progesterone metabolism.

(continued)

Focus On (continued)

. . . .

What are the important points patients should know?

Advise patients to avoid exposure to ultraviolet light and prolonged periods of time in the sun. Tell patients to inform their physicians promptly if any of the following occurs: sudden severe headache or vomiting, dizziness or fainting, numbness in an arm or leg, and acute chest pain. Advise patients to also report an unexplained, sudden, gradual, partial, or complete loss of vision, **ptosis** (drooping eyelid), or *diplopia* (double vision). The physician should be notified if the patient becomes pregnant or suspects pregnancy. Patients should not breastfeed while taking these drugs.

Table 33-5 ■ Progestins

GENERIC NAME	TRADE NAME	AVERAGE ADULT DOSAGE	ROUTE OF ADMINISTRATION
hydroxyprogesterone caproate	Makena	250 mg (1 mL) once weekly	IM
medroxyprogesterone	Provera	2–10 mg/d × 5–10 days	PO
	Depo-Provera	150 mg q3mo or 400–1,000 mg/wk	IM
megestrol	Megace	40–30 mg 1–4 times/d in divided doses	PO
norethindrone	Ortho Micronor	0.35 mg/d	PO
Combination Products			
estrogen and androgen	Estratest	Tablets of 1.25 mg estrogen/2.5 mg androgen	PO
estrogen and androgen	(Generic only)	2 mg estrogen/50 mg/mL androgen	IM
estradiol and norethindrone	Activella	Tablets of 0.5–1 mg estradiol/0.1–0.5 mg norethindrone acetate	PO

IM, intramuscular; PO, oral.

Focus Point

Estrogen–Progestin Combinations for Postmenopausal Women

The use of estrogen–progestin combinations for postmenopausal women is very controversial. There are benefits in protection against osteoporosis and colon cancer, but there is an increased relative risk of cardiovascular disease, breast cancer, and thromboembolism.

Contraception

The contraceptive methods most commonly used in the United States are (in order of popularity) oral contraceptives (hormones), condoms, withdrawal (*coitus interruptus*), progestin injections, spermicides, diaphragms, progestin subdermal implants, and intrauterine devices. Each method has advantages and disadvantages. In this chapter, only contraceptive hormones are discussed.

Focus On

Contraceptive Hormones

Oral contraceptives usually consist of combinations of estrogen and progesterone derivatives to prevent pregnancy. Oral contraceptives are also available that contain only progesterone (progestin). Progestin-only contraceptives have a slightly higher failure rate (pregnancy) than do the combination agents. Table 33-6 ■ lists the various types of oral contraceptives.

How do they work?

Oral contraceptives provide negative feedback to the hypothalamus and inhibit GnRH. Therefore, the pituitary does not secrete FSH to stimulate ovulation. The endometrium of the uterus becomes thin, and the cervical mucus becomes thick and impervious to sperm. The mechanism of action is not fully understood.

How are they used?

Oral contraceptives are based on hormonal contraception. Combination tablets are taken every day for 3 weeks and then not taken during the fourth week to allow for withdrawal bleeding. Progestin alone is given in a small dose every day and is recommended only when estrogen is contraindicated (e.g., during breastfeeding).

What are the adverse effects?

The adverse effects of oral contraceptives include nausea, abdominal pain, gallbladder disease, hepatic adenomas, breast tenderness or pain, weight gain, thromboembolism, stroke, headache, nervousness, dizziness, hypertension, myocardial infarction, and thrombophlebitis. Oral contraceptives may also cause amenorrhea, dysmenorrhea, **menorrhagia** (abnormally heavy or prolonged menstruation), and **metrorrhagia** (uterine bleeding that occurs independent of the normal menstrual period). Other adverse effects include a decreased libido and *vaginal candidiasis* (fungal infection).

What are the contraindications and interactions?

Oral contraceptives are contraindicated in patients with hypersensitivity to any component of the products. These agents should be avoided in pregnant women; in women who suspect pregnancy; and in women with genital bleeding of unknown etiology, thrombophlebitis, or history of thrombophlebitis. Oral contraceptives must be avoided in patients with coronary artery disease; liver dysfunction; carcinoma of the endometrium, breast, or other known estrogen-dependent neoplasia; severe hypertension; and diabetes with vascular involvement. Antibiotics, barbiturates, carbamazepine, fosphenytoin, griseofulvin, modafinil, phenytoin, and rifampin may decrease contraceptive effectiveness.

What are the important points patients should know?

Instruct women who are using oral contraceptives to follow the schedule for receiving these agents and to use alternative forms of barrier contraception while taking antibiotics. Over-the-counter drugs, including vitamin C and acetaminophen, should not be used without consulting a physician. Instruct patients to report episodes of calf pain or tenderness, shortness of breath, chest pain, visual disturbances, drooping eyelids, and double vision.

Table 33-6 ■ Types of Oral Contraceptives

GENERIC NAME	TRADE NAME	AVERAGE ADULT DOSAGE
Monophasic Combinations		
estinyl estradiol/desogestrel	Desogen, Mircette	1 active tablet/d for 21 d and then none for 7 d
estinyl estradiol/ethynodiol	Demulen	1 active tablet/d for 21 d and then none for 7 d
estinyl estradiol/levonorgestrel	Alesse	30 mcg ethinyl estradiol/0.15 mg levonorgestrel in cycles
estinyl estradiol/norgestimate	Levora, Ortho-Cyclen	1 active tablet/d for 21 d and then none for 7 d
estinyl estradiol/norgestrel	Lo-Ovral	30 mcg estinyl estradiol/0.3 mg norgestrel in cycles
estrogen/progestin	Necon 1/35	1 active tablet/d for 21 d and then none for 7 d

(continued)

Table 33-6 ■ Types of Oral Contraceptives (*continued*)

GENERIC NAME	TRADE NAME	AVERAGE ADULT DOSAGE
ethinyl estradiol/drospirenone	Yasmin	1 active tablet/d for 21 d and then none for 7 d
ethinyl estradiol/norethindrone	Brevicon	35 mcg ethinyl estradiol/0.5 mg norethindrone in cycles
mestranol/norethindrone	Genora 1/50	50 mcg mestranol/1 mg norethindrone in cycles
Biphasic Combinations		
ethinyl estradiol/norethindrone	Nelova 10/11	35 mcg ethinyl estradiol/0.5 mg norethindrone (×10 tablets) or 1 mg norethindrone (×11 tablets) in cycles
Triphasic Combinations		
ethinyl estradiol/levonorgestrel	Triphasil	30 mcg ethinyl estradiol (×6 or 10 d) or 40 mcg ethinyl estradiol (×5 days)/0.05 mg levonorgestrel (×6 d) or 0.075 mg levonorgestrel (×5 d) or 0.125 mg levonorgestrel (×10 d) in cycles
ethinyl estradiol/norethindrone	Ortho-Novum 7/7/7	35 mcg ethinyl estradiol/0.5 mg norethindrone (×5 or 7 d) or 1 mg norethindrone (×9 d) in cycles
ethinyl estradiol/norgestimate	Ortho Tri-Cyclen	1 active tablet/d for 21 d and then none for 7 d
Estrophasic Combination		
ethinyl estradiol/norethindrone	Estrostep	1 active tablet/d for 21 d and then none for 7 d
Progestin-Only Medications		
norethindrone	Ortho Micronor, Nor-QD	0.35 mg/d starting on day 1 of menstrual flow, continuing indefinitely
norgestrel	Ovrette	0.075 mg/d starting on day 1 of menstrual flow, continuing indefinitely

Focus Point

Oral Contraceptives and Surgery

Oral contraceptives should be discontinued at least 4 weeks before a surgical procedure because of the risk for postoperative thromboembolic complications.

Focus Point

Combined Formulations of Injectable Contraceptives

Combined formulations are effective immediately if administered at specific times after menses.

Focus Point

Implantable Contraceptives

Contraceptive devices may be implanted either surgically or by a physician. They contain contraceptive hormones that are released regularly for 3–5 years.

✳ Apply Your Knowledge 33.2

The following questions focus on what you have just learned about the female reproductive system and female sex hormones.

CRITICAL THINKING

1. What are the functions of the ovaries?
2. What is the function of GnRH?
3. What are the actions of the gonadotropins FSH and LH on the female reproductive system?
4. How do estrogens work?
5. What are the indications of progestins?
6. What is salpingitis?
7. What are the most commonly used contraceptive methods in the United States?
8. What are the meanings of the terms *menorrhagia* and *metrorrhagia*?

Focus on Natural Products

Kelp for Menorrhagia

Kelp is seaweed found in the Atlantic and Pacific oceans that in traditional herbal medicine has been used to treat menorrhagia. It is available as a fluid or soft extract, as tablets or gel tabs, and in dried whole plant form. Until more research is done, kelp should not be used during pregnancy and lactation and should not be given to children, older adults, or persons with cardiac disorders. It may decrease the effects of thyroid hormones.

Focus Point

Smoking and Oral Contraceptives

Women must avoid smoking while using oral contraceptives. Smoking greatly increases the risk of serious cardiovascular adverse effects.

INJECTABLE CONTRACEPTIVES

Injectable contraceptives contain hormonal drugs that provide reversible contraceptive protection. They are safe and highly effective. There are two types of injectable contraceptives:

✳ *Progestogen-only formulations, which contain a progestogen hormone.* They are effective for 2–3 months. These formulations consist of depot medroxyprogesterone acetate (DMPA) or norethisterone enanthate (NET-EN). DMPA is the most widely used injectable contraceptive throughout the world. DMPA formulations are injected every 3 months. NET-EN is injected every 2 months. The most common adverse effects of the NET-EN formulations include amenorrhea, prolonged menses, spotting between periods, heavy bleeding, and weight gain. These formulations are contraindicated in women with a confirmed or suspected pregnancy, malignant disease of the breast, diabetes with vascular disease or of more than 20 years' duration, cerebrovascular or coronary artery disease, acute liver disease, liver tumors, and severe hypertension or vascular disease. Drugs that may interact with any form of injectable contraceptives include rifampicin, griseofulvin, phenytoin, carbamazepine, and barbiturates.

✱ *Combined formulations, which contain both a progestogen and an estrogen.* They are effective for 1 month. These formulations are injected once per month and contain norethisterone enanthate as well as an added estrogen. Combined formulations are administered as deep intramuscular injections into the arm or buttock. They are slowly absorbed into the bloodstream. Adverse effects of combined formulations are much less common than those caused by progestogen-only formulations. When they do occur, they include irregular or heavy bleeding, amenorrhea, prolonged bleeding, headaches, dizziness, and weight changes. Contraindications for injectable combined formulations are based on data from oral combined formulations.

Labor and Delivery

Pregnancy usually continues for 38 weeks after conception. Pregnancy ends with the birth process. A period of rapid changes and intense physical demands on the pregnant woman begins hours or days before the birth of a baby.

The declining progesterone concentration plays a major role in initiating birth. During pregnancy, progesterone suppresses uterine contractions. As the placenta ages, the progesterone concentration within the uterus declines. This stimulates the synthesis of a prostaglandin that promotes uterine contractions. At the same time, the cervix begins to thin and then open. Changes in the cervix may begin 1–2 weeks before other signs of labor occur.

Another stimulant of the birth process is the stretching of uterine and vaginal tissues late in the pregnancy. This initiates nerve impulses to the hypothalamus, which in turn signals the posterior pituitary gland to release the hormone **oxytocin**. Oxytocin stimulates powerful uterine contractions and aids labor in its later stages.

Uterine relaxants are useful in the process of preterm labor. These agents decrease uterine contraction and prolong the pregnancy to permit the fetus to develop more fully, therefore promoting neonatal survival. Oxytocic agents and uterine relaxants are listed in Table 33-7 ■.

Table 33-7 ■ Effects of Drugs on Labor and Delivery

GENERIC NAME	TRADE NAME	AVERAGE ADULT DOSAGE	ROUTE OF ADMINISTRATION
Oxytocics			
ergonovine	Ergotrate	0.2 mg q2–4h	IM, IV
methylergonovine	Methergine	0.2–0.4 mg q6–12h until the danger of atony passes (2–7 d)	PO
		0.2 mg q2–4h (maximum: 5 doses)	IM, IV
oxytocin	Pitocin	Antepartum: 1 mU/min; increase by 1 mU/min q15min (maximum: 20 mU/min)	IV
		Postpartum: infuse a total of 10 U at a rate of 20–40 mU/min after delivery	IM, IV
Uterine Relaxants			
terbutaline	Terbutaline Sulfate	10 mcg/min q10min to 80 mcg/min	IV
		250 mg/h until contractions stop	SC
		2.5 mg q4–6h until delivery	PO

IM, intramuscular; IV, intravenous; PO, oral; SC, subcutaneous.

Focus On

Oxytocic Agents

Oxytocic drugs are able to induce uterine contractions before birth in normal labor. These agents are desirable in early vaginal delivery to stimulate the uterus.

How do they work?

Oxytocic drugs are identical pharmacologically to the oxytocic principle of the posterior pituitary gland. By direct action on uterine muscle, this produces phasic contractions characteristic of normal delivery. These agents also promote the milk ejection (letdown) reflex in nursing mothers, thereby increasing the flow of milk. Uterine sensitivity to oxytocin increases during the gestation period and peaks sharply before birth.

How are they used?

Oxytocic drugs are used to initiate or improve uterine contractions at term only in carefully selected patients, only after the cervix is dilated, and after presentation of the fetus has occurred. These drugs are also used to stimulate the letdown reflex in nursing mothers and to relieve pain from breast engorgement. Oxytocic drugs are prescribed for the management of inevitable, incomplete, or missed abortion; the control of postpartum hemorrhage; and the promotion of postpartum uterine involution. Oxytocic drugs are also used to induce labor in cases of maternal diabetes and preeclampsia or eclampsia.

What are the adverse effects?

The adverse effects of oxytocic drugs are varied. Generally, they cause nausea and vomiting, maternal cardiac arrhythmias, hypertensive episodes, chest pain, dizziness, headache, and intracranial (within the cranium) hemorrhage. Allergic reactions may also occur.

What are the contraindications and interactions?

The oxytocic preparations are contraindicated in hypersensitive patients. Ergonovine and methylergonovine must be avoided in patients with hypertension and preeclampsia. They are not to be used to induce labor or before delivery of the placenta. Oxytocin injection is contraindicated in patients with significant *cephalopelvic disproportion* (the fetal head is too large to pass through the mother's pelvis), an unfavorable fetal position or presentation (undeliverable without conversion before delivery), obstetric emergencies in which the benefit-to-risk ratio for mother or fetus favors surgical intervention, and fetal distress in which delivery is not imminent. Oxytocin should be avoided in placenta previa and in women with previous cesarean section.

Oxytocic drugs may interact with vasoconstrictor drugs, causing severe hypertension. They may also interact with cyclopropane anesthesia, causing hypotension, maternal bradycardia, and arrhythmias. Some herbal supplements, such as ephedra and ma huang, may cause hypertension.

What are the important points patients should know?

Instruct patients to report severe cramping, increased bleeding, cold or numb fingers or toes, nausea and vomiting, chest pain, and sudden, severe headache immediately to their health care providers. Advise patients to avoid breastfeeding while taking ergonovine or methylergonovine.

Uterine Relaxants

Uterine relaxants are beta$_2$-adrenergic agonists that are prescribed as uterine relaxants in the management of preterm (premature) labor. Terbutaline is the currently used uterine relaxant in the United States. The drug known as ritodrine (Yutopar) was removed from the U.S. market due to significant adverse effects.

How do they work?

Beta$_2$-adrenergic agonists are clinically effective in preventing or delaying preterm labor because of their tocolytic effect. Uterine contractions decrease in frequency and intensity during treatment.

How are they used?

Beta$_2$-adrenergic agonists are used to manage premature labor in selected patients.

What are the adverse effects?

Terbutaline alters maternal and fetal heart rates and maternal blood pressure (dose related). It can also cause chest pain, palpitations, arrhythmias, and pulmonary edema. Additional common adverse effects of beta$_2$-adrenergic agonists include headache, nausea and vomiting, nervousness, restlessness, sweating, and emotional upset.

(continued)

Focus On (*continued*)

What are the contraindications and interactions?

Terbutaline is contraindicated in patients with severe cardiac disorders, digital toxicity, and hypertension. It is given cautiously in patients with cardiac disease, hyperthyroidism, seizure disorders, and migraine headaches. Epinephrine and other sympathomimetic bronchodilators may increase the effects of terbutaline.

What are the important points patients should know?

Advise patients about the potential adverse effects and drug interactions of these agents. Instruct women to avoid breastfeeding while taking beta$_2$-adrenergic agonist drugs. Patients must be instructed to review instructions for the use of inhalators and how to take their own pulses.

✳ Apply Your Knowledge 33.3

The following questions focus on what you have just learned about labor and delivery and the drugs that affect labor and delivery.

CRITICAL THINKING

1. What are three examples of oxytocic drugs?
2. What are the indications of oxytocic agents?
3. What are the names of two uterine relaxants?
4. What medications are used to manage premature labor in selected patients?
5. What are the trade names of ergonovine and terbutaline?

PRACTICAL SCENARIO 1

A 34-year-old mother of three children has just been prescribed a combination oral contraceptive because she wants to avoid having any more children. She has never taken oral contraceptives before. Her physician told her about the possible side effects of the hormones and what symptoms she should report immediately. She is now talking with you and says that she works in a bar on the weekends, and her coworkers smoke. She says that her husband hates the smell of smoke on her clothes when she gets home from work. She also starts rummaging through her purse, looking for her car keys. She says that she can be very forgetful and loses everything, but she just attributes that to her crazy schedule and the kids.

Monkey Business/Fotolia

Critical Thinking Questions

1. What are some key areas of concern to raise in your discussion with this patient?
2. What teaching should you provide to her?

PRACTICAL SCENARIO 2

A 25-year-old pregnant woman in her first pregnancy went into labor. She had only 1 cm dilation of the cervix after 8 hours.

Paul Hakimata/Fotolia

Critical Thinking Questions

1. What are the most common drugs given intravenously to induce delivery?
2. What are the most common adverse effects of these drugs?

Chapter Capsule

This section repeats the objectives from the beginning of the chapter and then provides a summary of the most important concepts for that objective. Use this section as a quick review and to check your knowledge.

Objective 1: Describe the male and female reproductive structures.

- Male: testes, epididymis, vas deferens, seminal vesicle, prostate gland, bulbourethral (Cowper's) glands, scrotum, penis

- Female: ovaries, uterine tubes, uterus, vagina, labia majora, labia minora, clitoris, and vestibule

Objective 2: Discuss the male and female sex hormones and their effects on the reproductive system.

- Male sex hormones—androgens

- Testosterone—most abundant

- Between 13 and 15 years of age, a young man's androgen production usually increases rapidly as he reaches puberty

- After puberty, testosterone secretion continues throughout the life of a man

- Female sex hormones: estrogen and progesterone

- Several tissues, including the tissues of the ovaries, adrenal cortices, and placenta (during pregnancy), secrete female sex hormones

- Estradiol—most abundant estrogen

- At puberty, under the influence of the anterior pituitary, the ovaries secrete increasing amounts of estrogens, which stimulate the enlargement of accessory organs, including the vagina, uterus, uterine tubes, ovaries, and external reproductive structures

- Estrogens—develop and maintain female secondary sex characteristics

- Progesterone promotes changes in the uterus during the female reproductive cycle, affects the mammary glands, and helps regulate the secretion of gonadotropins from the anterior pituitary

Objective 3: Explain the contraindications of estrogens.

■ Contraindicated in women with breast cancer or who are pregnant or lactating

■ Used with caution in women with liver disease, gallbladder disease, endometriosis, pancreatitis, diabetes mellitus, heart failure, and kidney dysfunction

Objective 4: Describe how oral contraceptives work to prevent pregnancy.

■ Provide negative feedback to the hypothalamus and inhibit gonadotropin-releasing hormone

■ Pituitary does not secrete follicle-stimulating hormone to stimulate ovulation; the endometrium of the uterus becomes thin; cervical mucus becomes thick and impervious to sperm

Objective 5: Discuss menopause and hormone therapy.

■ Postmenopausal patients who are on long-term estrogen therapy should also be given progestin, to prevent endometrial hyperplasia and endometrial carcinoma

■ Progestin is not given to women who have had a hysterectomy

Objective 6: Provide information about androgens and anabolic steroids.

■ Chief drugs that affect the male reproductive system

■ Synthetic steroids that compound with androgenic and anabolic activity to control the development and maintenance of secondary sexual characteristics

■ Androgenic activity: responsible for the growth spurt of adolescents and the growth termination by epiphyseal closure

■ Anabolic activity: increases protein metabolism and decreases its catabolism; large doses suppress spermatogenesis, thereby causing testicular atrophy

■ Androgens: antagonize effects of estrogen excess in the female breasts and endometrium

Objective 7: Explain the indications of androgens.

■ Main indications in men: to supplement low levels of testosterone to correct hypogonadism or cryptorchidism

■ Also used to increase sperm production in cases of infertility

■ Indications in women: palliative treatment of metastatic breast cancer; for treatment of postpartum breast engorgement, endometriosis, and fibrocystic breast disorder

■ Able to stimulate increased production of red blood cells, protein synthesis, and muscle mass; athletes may use androgens to improve athletic performance

Objective 8: Discuss the major adverse effects of progestins.

■ Vaginal candidiasis, skin hyperpigmentation, cervical erosion, breakthrough bleeding, dysmenorrhea, amenorrhea, breast tenderness, edema, acne, pruritus, and mental depression

■ Thromboembolic disorder, pulmonary embolism, changes in vision, nausea and vomiting, and abdominal cramps also seen

Objective 9: Describe the contraindications of oral contraceptives.

- Hypersensitivity of any component of the products; should be avoided in pregnant women, women who suspect pregnancy, women with genital bleeding of unknown etiology, thrombophlebitis, or a history of thrombophlebitis

- Must be avoided in patients with coronary artery disease; liver dysfunction; carcinoma of the endometrium, breast, or another known estrogen-dependent neoplasia; severe hypertension; and diabetes with vascular involvement

Objective 10: Explain the mechanism of action for oxytocic drugs.

- Identical pharmacologically to the oxytocic principle of posterior pituitary

- By direct action on uterine muscle, they produce phasic contractions characteristic of normal delivery

- They also promote a milk ejection (letdown) reflex in nursing mothers, thereby increasing the flow of milk

- Uterine sensitivity to oxytocin (Pitocin) increases during the gestation period and peaks sharply before birth

 ## Sites of Interest

- Further information about contraceptive options can be found at: **www.verywell.com/womens-health-pregnancy-4014318**

- Personal stories of menopause and hormone therapy are available at: **www.womenshealth.gov/Menopause**

- Visit the National Institute on Drug Abuse at: **www.drugabuse.gov/drugs-abuse/steroids-anabolic**

- The effectiveness of various methods of birth control is discussed at: **www.cdc.gov/reproductivehealth/unintendedpregnancy/contraception.htm**

- The male and female reproductive systems are explained at: **www.fao.org/docrep/005/y4359e/y4359e07.htm**

Chapter 34

Drugs Used to Treat Gastrointestinal Conditions

Chapter Objectives

After completing this chapter, you should be able to:

1. Describe the major parts of the digestive system.
2. Explain how medications are absorbed from the gastrointestinal tract and metabolized.
3. Describe the use of histamine-2 (H$_2$) receptor antagonists in the treatment of peptic ulcers.
4. Describe the use of antacids for the treatment of peptic ulcers.
5. Explain the effects of prostaglandins on the digestive tract.
6. List generic names and trade names for proton pump inhibitors.
7. Describe the drug treatment for diarrhea.
8. Explain the problems associated with laxative use.
9. Describe the mechanism of action for bulk-forming laxatives, osmotic laxatives, and laxative stimulants.
10. Identify causes of vomiting and the main neurotransmitters that produce nausea and vomiting.

Key Terms

Introduction

Growth of the body depends on the consumption, absorption, and metabolism of food. The gastrointestinal (GI) tract is involved in the first essential components of these processes and is subject to many disease conditions, some of which are very common. It is not surprising that a number of drugs are used to treat these varying conditions. Because of the number of drugs available, it is helpful for discussion to divide the GI tract into two parts: the upper part (from the mouth to the stomach) and the lower part (from the duodenum to the anus). Some problems of the GI tract, specifically nausea and vomiting, are sometimes associated with the central nervous system (CNS).

The Digestive System

The digestive system consists of the alimentary canal, which extends about 8 m from the mouth to the anus, and several accessory organs that secrete substances used in the process of digestion into the canal. The **alimentary canal** includes the mouth, pharynx, esophagus, stomach, small intestine, large intestine, rectum, and anus; the accessory organs include the salivary glands, liver, gallbladder, and pancreas (Figure 34-1 ■). Overall, the

Organ	Primary Functions
Salivary Glands	Provide lubrication; produce buffers and the enzymes that begin digestion
Pharynx	Passageway connected to the esophagus
Esophagus	Delivers food to the stomach
Stomach	Secretes acids and enzymes
Small Intestine	Secretes digestive enzymes; absorbs nutrients
Liver	Secretes bile; regulates blood chemistry
Gallbladder	Stores bile for release into the small intestine
Pancreas	Secretes digestive enzymes and buffers; contains endocrine cells
Large Intestine	Removes water from fecal material; stores waste

Figure 34-1 ■ The digestive system.

digestive system is a tube, open at both ends, that has a surface area of 186 m². It supplies nutrients for body cells. Therefore, digestion changes food into its simpler constituents before absorption.

Primary digestion occurs in the mouth. When food is ingested in the mouth, it is chewed and mixed with saliva that is excreted from the three major pairs of salivary glands: the parotid, submandibular, and sublingual glands. Saliva contains the digestive enzyme **amylase**. The three processes—digestion, absorption, and metabolism—begin here in the mouth.

The 25-cm-long esophagus is a straight tube through which food passes from the pharynx to the stomach. When food enters the stomach from the mouth and esophagus, it is mixed with stomach juices that include hydrochloric acid and some enzymes, such as pepsin, which breaks it into much smaller, digestible pieces. The final stages of chemical digestion occur in the small intestine, where almost all nutrients from the ingested food are absorbed. Excessive secretions of hydrochloric acid, under certain conditions, may break down the gastric surface and cause sores or **ulcers** (breaks in mucous membranes with loss of surface tissue, disintegration, and necrosis). The term *gastric ulcer* is used interchangeably with *peptic ulcer* for this condition. Peptic ulcer disease (PUD) is the most common disorder of the stomach.

Focus Point

Gastric Juice

The 40 million cells that line the stomach's interior can secrete 2–3 qt (about 2–3 L) of gastric juice per day. No wonder peptic ulcer disease is so common!

The liver is the center of metabolic activity in the body, playing a very important role in the digestion and absorption of nutrients as well as metabolic activities. The *detoxification* (removal of toxins from the blood) and secretion of bile are the key functions of the liver. The pancreas secretes pancreatic juice, which contains such digestive enzymes as amylase, lipase, and nucleases, to aid in digestion.

The small intestine is a tubular organ that extends from the pyloric sphincter of the stomach to the beginning of the large intestine. The small intestine receives secretions from the pancreas and liver. It also completes the digestion of nutrients and absorbs the products of digestion. The small intestine transports residue to the large intestine. The large intestine absorbs water and electrolytes. It also forms and stores feces.

Peptic Ulcers

The problems associated with hyperacidity and excessive pepsin activity—some of which may be related to lifestyle choices—may eventually lead to the formation of a gastric or duodenal ulcer. Alcohol and caffeine have been linked to irritation of the mucosal lining of the esophagus and stomach. Smoking has been linked to greater volume and concentration of gastric acid. Upper GI radiography is usually performed to diagnose PUD or gastroesophageal reflux disease (GERD).

Several groups of drugs have revolutionized the pharmacologic treatment of ulcers. Three receptors in the stomach wall need to be stimulated to cause the production of hydrochloric acid. These are the histamine-2 (H$_2$) receptors, muscarinic cholinergic receptors, and gastrin receptors. Gastric ulcers are caused mainly by a defect in mucus production, and duodenal ulcers usually result from an increase in acid production. This makes the treatment of each somewhat different.

Many cases of gastric ulcer or *gastritis* (inflammation of the stomach) are caused by the bacterium *Helicobacter pylori*. In bacteria-related peptic ulcers, successful treatment usually includes a combination of such antibacterials as metronidazole, amoxicillin, or tetracyclines with such agents as colloidal bismuth or omeprazole. Colloidal bismuth in combination with two antibacterials is sometimes referred to as "triple therapy." Table 34-1 ■ summarizes drugs commonly used to treat patients with peptic ulcers.

Table 34-1 ■ Drugs Commonly Used in Peptic Ulcer Disease

GENERIC NAME	TRADE NAME	AVERAGE ADULT DOSAGE	ROUTE OF ADMINISTRATION
Antacids			
aluminum hydroxide	Amphojel	600 mg tid–qid	PO
calcium carbonate	Titralac, Tums	1–2 g bid–tid	PO
calcium carbonate with magnesium hydroxide	Mylanta Gelcaps, Rolaids	2–4 capsules or tablets prn (maximum: 12 tablets/d)	PO
magaldrate	Riopan	480–1,080 mg (5–10 mL suspension or 1–2 tablets) 4 times/d (maximum: 20 tablets or 100 mL/d)	PO
magnesium hydroxide	Milk of Magnesia	2.4–4.8 g (30–60 mL)/d in one or more divided doses	PO
magnesium hydroxide/ aluminum hydroxide with simethicone	Maalox Plus	10–20 mL prn (maximum: 120 mL/d) or 2–4 tablets prn (maximum: 24 tablets/d)	PO
sodium bicarbonate	Alka-Seltzer, and various trade names of baking soda	0.3–2 g 1–4 times/d or ½ tsp of powder in a glass of water	PO
H$_2$-Receptor Antagonists			
cimetidine	Tagamet	800 mg/d in divided doses	PO
		300 mg q6–8h	IM, IV
famotidine	Pepcid	20–40 mg/d in divided doses	PO
		20 mg q12h	PO
nizatidine	(Generic only)	300 mg at bedtime or in two divided doses	PO
ranitidine	Zantac	300 mg/d in two divided doses	PO
		50 mg q6–8h; 150–300 mg/24 h by continuous infusion	IV
Proton Pump Inhibitors			
esomeprazole	Nexium	20–40 mg/d	PO
lansoprazole	Prevacid	15–30 mg/d	PO
omeprazole	Prilosec	20–40 mg/d	PO
pantoprazole	Protonix	40 mg/d for 8–16 wk	PO
		40 mg/d for 7–10 d	IV
rabeprazole	AcipHex	20 mg/d	PO
Combination Medications			
bismuth-tetracycline-metronidazole	(Generic only)	1 blister pack/d for 14 d	PO
bismuth-ranitidine	Tritec	1 blister pack/d for 14 d	PO
Prostaglandins			
misoprostol	Cytotec	100–200 mcg qid with food	PO

tid, three times a day; qid, four times a day; PO, oral; bid, twice a day; IM, intramuscular; IV, intravenous.

Focus On

Antacids

Antacids are alkaline compounds that may be used to neutralize hydrochloric acid in the stomach, thereby relieving the pain of hyperacidity or even peptic ulcer.

How do they work?

The antacids are weak bases that readily combine with and neutralize hydrochloric acid. The combination of an antacid with digestive acid produces water and carbon dioxide gas.

How are they used?

The bases used in antacid preparations are usually basic compounds of aluminum, magnesium, sodium, calcium, and potassium. Of these, the most common are **aluminum hydroxide** and **magnesium carbonate**—usually used in combination. Antacids counteract hyperacidity of the stomach, protect from peptic ulcers, and promote ulcer healing.

What are the adverse effects?

Depending on the type of antacid, the most common adverse effects may be diarrhea or constipation. For example, the magnesium- and sodium-containing antacids may cause diarrhea. Calcium- and aluminum-containing products can produce constipation. The other adverse effects that are less common but more serious include anorexia, weakness, bone pain, and tremors (aluminum-containing antacids). Hypermagnesemia may produce nausea and vomiting, confusion, renal calculi, metabolic alkalosis, and headache. Neurologic disorders sometimes occur with the use of calcium-containing antacids.

What are the contraindications and interactions?

The contraindications of antacids depend on their compounds; for example, calcium carbonate (Tums) should not be used in hypercalcemia and hyperparathyroidism, vitamin D overdosage, and decalcifying tumors. Calcium carbonate is also contraindicated in patients with severe renal disease, renal calculi, ventricular fibrillation, and pregnancy. Magnesium-containing antacids are contraindicated in patients with hypermagnesemia and pregnant women.

Antacids should be used cautiously in patients with impaired kidney function, lactation, and dialysis of the kidneys. Calcium carbonate should be used with caution in older adults and in lactating patients. Some antacids may interact with digoxin. Calcium-containing antacids may decrease the absorption of tetracyclines and ciprofloxacin.

What are the important points patients should know?

Instruct patients to take antacids 1–3 hours after meals and at bedtime. Patients must avoid taking antacids within 1 to 2 hours of other oral medications. Advise them to increase fluid intake to about 3,000 mL per day to prevent kidney stones. Instruct those with heart disease and those on sodium-restricted diets to avoid antacids high in sodium content. Teach patients to alternate an aluminum or calcium salt antacid with a magnesium salt antacid to prevent diarrhea or constipation. Remind patients that antacids should be used only for symptomatic relief and that they should notify their physician if relief does not occur in 1 or 2 days.

Focus on Geriatrics

Cautious Use of Tums in Older Adults

Calcium carbonate (Tums) should be used with caution in older adults because it is contraindicated in a wide variety of diseases and conditions that affect elderly people, including calcium loss caused by immobilization, renal disease, renal calculi, ventricular fibrillation, and cardiac disease.

Focus On

H₂-Receptor Antagonists

The H₂-receptor antagonists, of which cimetidine is the prototype, were a huge discovery in the treatment of patients with PUD and GERD.

How do they work?

Acid secretion is stimulated by H₂-receptor activation. H₂-receptor antagonists reduce the secretion of gastric acid from stomach cells by blocking these receptors.

How are they used?

H₂-receptor antagonists are used in short-term treatment of active duodenal ulcer and prevention of ulcer recurrence (at reduced dosage). They are also used for the short-term treatment of active benign gastric ulcer, pathologic hypersecretory conditions such as Zollinger-Ellison syndrome, and heartburn.

What are the adverse effects?

The most common adverse effects are GI disturbances, headache, drowsiness, confusion, agitation, hallucinations, and reversible impotence. H₂-receptor antagonists may also cause cardiac arrhythmias and cardiac arrest after a rapid intravenous bolus dose.

What are the contraindications and interactions?

These medications are contraindicated in patients with known hypersensitivity to cimetidine or other H₂-receptor antagonists. They must not be used in lactating or pregnant patients or in children younger than 16 years.

What are the important points patients should know?

Warn patients to avoid smoking and drinking alcohol while taking H₂-receptor antagonists because these substances can impede the effectiveness of the drug.

Proton Pump Inhibitors

Several compounds have been investigated because of their ability to block hydrochloric acid production.

How do they work?

The formation of hydrochloric acid depends on the production of hydrogen ions (protons) in the parietal cells, and proton pump inhibitors (PPIs) block the enzyme in the stomach wall that produces this acid.

How are they used?

PPIs are used to heal stomach and duodenal ulcers and to relieve symptoms of GERD and esophagitis.

What are the adverse effects?

Common adverse effects of PPIs include headache, dizziness, fatigue, diarrhea, abdominal pain, nausea, skin rash, and, rarely, hematuria.

What are the contraindications and interactions?

Long-term use of PPIs for GERD or duodenal ulcers is contraindicated. These drugs should not be used in hypersensitive patients or in children younger than 18 years. PPIs should be avoided in pregnancy and in patients with GI bleeding.

What are the important points patients should know?

Advise patients that treatment with PPIs is for a short course of therapy only. Treatment is usually limited to about 4–8 weeks.

Focus on Pediatrics

Use Care in Choosing Over-the-Counter Medications for Children

Over-the-counter (OTC) formulations of omeprazole must not be used in children younger than 18 years of age. Omeprazole has not been significantly tested in children.

Focus On

Prostaglandins

The prostaglandins are perhaps the most versatile and powerful substances used to treat patients with GI disorders. They affect GI motility and gastric acid secretions.

How do they work?

Prostaglandins produce a variety of actions on the body. The effects of these substances (related to the stomach) include the inhibition of gastric acid and gastrin production, the stimulation of mucus, and the secretion of bicarbonate. The prostaglandin analogue misoprostol is most commonly used and, although not as effective as the H_2-receptor antagonists, it has been effective in some cases when treatment with the latter has not been effective.

How are they used?

Prostaglandins tend to be antagonistic to ulcer formation in the stomach and the duodenum. This avenue seems to offer a promising new approach to ulcer therapeutics in certain cases. Prostaglandins are used to prevent complications of gastric ulcers that result from nonsteroidal anti-inflammatory drugs (NSAIDs), especially in patients at high risk for complications from a gastric ulcer (e.g., older adults and patients with a concomitant debilitating disease or a history of ulcers). These drugs are taken for the duration of NSAID therapy and do not interfere with the efficacy of the NSAID.

What are the adverse effects?

Prostaglandins, such as misoprostol, can cause diarrhea in some patients, which is usually mild and of short duration. The only other significant adverse effect is menorrhagia in women.

What are the contraindications and interactions?

Prostaglandins should not be used in pregnant women because they may induce premature labor by increasing uterine tone and contractility. Prostaglandins are contraindicated in lactation and in a history of allergies to prostaglandins.

What are the important points patients should know?

Ask female patients if they are or might be pregnant because prostaglandins are contraindicated in pregnant women. Tell female patients that these agents may cause women of childbearing age to experience spontaneous abortion, so they should use reliable contraception. Advise patients that diarrhea may occur with these drugs but will disappear after the first month of therapy.

✳ Apply Your Knowledge 34.1

The following questions focus on what you have just learned about the digestive system, peptic ulcers, and related medications.

CRITICAL THINKING

1. Where do the processes of digestion, absorption, and metabolism begin?
2. Which organ of the GI tract receives secretions from the liver and pancreas?
3. What are the generic names of proton pump inhibitors?
4. What are the generic and trade names of H_2-receptor antagonists?
5. What is the mechanism of action of the prostaglandins in treating GI disorders?
6. Identify combination medications used to treat peptic ulcers.
7. What is the treatment of gastric ulcers when caused by *H. pylori*?
8. What is the mechanism of action of PPIs?

Diarrhea

Diarrhea is defined as an increase in the volume, fluidity, or frequency of bowel movements relative to a particular individual's usual pattern. The causes of this condition are numerous and, consequently, the treatments are varied. In many instances, drug intervention is not required. For example, antidiarrheals are not used in the case of infective gastroenteritis, in which the diarrhea is a protective mechanism used by the body to flush out the offending pathogen. Clearly, the use of drugs to slow down GI motility in such circumstances would be inadvisable. Similarly, the use of antibiotics in diarrhea-causing bacterial infections of the GI tract may kill the offending pathogen but also kill off some normal bacterial flora. Indeed, the World Health Organization recommends that the first-line emergency treatment for diarrhea should be rehydration and electrolyte replacement therapy. Diarrhea is usually self-limiting and resolves without further effects. The antidiarrheal drugs may be classified as opioids, synthetic opioid medications, and adsorbents (Table 34-2 ■).

Table 34-2 ■ Classifications of Antidiarrheal Drugs

GENERIC NAME	TRADE NAME	TYPE	COMMENTS
bismuth subsalicylate	Pepto-Bismol	Adsorbent	OTC
camphorated opium tincture (paregoric)	(Generic only)	Opioid	Schedule III
difenoxin hydrochloride with atropine sulfate	(Generic only)	Opioid	Schedule IV
diphenoxylate hydrochloride with atropine sulfate	Lomotil	Opioid	Schedule V
loperamide	Imodium, Maalox Anti-Diarrheal	Opioid	OTC (abuse is very low, and it is not classified as a controlled substance)

Note: Formerly, kaolin with pectin was a combination medication used as an adsorbent, but this combination is no longer available in the United States.

OTC, over the counter.

Focus Point

Acute Diarrhea in Adults

Acute diarrhea in adults is usually self-limiting. Treatment with an antidiarrheal agent is usually unnecessary. However, symptomatic control may help some adults.

Focus On

Opioid and Synthetic Opioid Drugs

These drugs require a prescription and are controlled substances. Opioid antidiarrheals are the most effective drugs for controlling diarrhea.

How do they work?

Most of the narcotic analgesics can act on opioid receptors in the GI tract and are actually stimulants at these receptors. The stimulus increases the segmentation or mixing movements of the gut and simultaneously decreases the peristaltic movements. These effects in turn slow down forward movement and at the same time reabsorption.

How are they used?

The most commonly used opioid antidiarrheal drug is camphorated opium tincture (paregoric; generic only). This is a Schedule III drug and requires a prescription. When paregoric is combined with another drug, the medication becomes a Schedule V product (i.e., if the

(continued)

Focus On (continued)

. . . .

combination contains less than 25 mL of paregoric per 100 mL of preparation).

What are the adverse effects?

The main adverse effect of these drugs is a reversal in the movement of the bowels that results in constipation. Other possible adverse effects include nausea and vomiting, agitation, drowsiness, tachycardia, and numbness of the hands and feet.

What are the contraindications and interactions?

Opioid preparations are contraindicated in patients with intestinal obstruction and should be avoided in children younger than 6 years. In patients who have chronic diarrhea, treatment with opioids is not recommended.

What are the important points patients should know?

Encourage patients to keep a record of bowel movements while they are taking these medications to determine its effectiveness and possible constipating effect. Advise patients to ingest a clear fluid diet for a few days, avoid fruit juices, and maintain fluid intake of about 3,000 mL per day. Patients should avoid the use of alcohol because it promotes diuresis.

Focus on Geriatrics

Elderly Patients and Opioid Antidiarrheals

Vital signs should be monitored regularly in older patients taking opioid antidiarrheals. These drugs may cause respiratory depression and decreased blood pressure in older adults.

Focus On

Adsorbents

The other class of antidiarrheals is adsorbents. These preparations are still used in some parts of the world because they are inexpensive and relatively effective.

How do they work?

Adsorbents act by coating the walls of the GI tract and adsorbing the toxins that might be implicated in causing diarrhea.

How are they used?

These medications are usually taken after each loose bowel movement until the diarrhea is controlled.

What are the adverse effects?

Adsorbents may cause constipation, which is usually mild and transient.

What are the contraindications and interactions?

The contraindications of adsorbents include a suspected obstructive bowel lesion, pseudomembranous colitis, diarrhea (associated with bacterial toxins), and the presence of fever. They should not be used for more than 48 hours without medical direction. Safety during pregnancy or lactation is not established. Adsorbents may interact with chloroquine, digoxin, penicillamine, tetracycline, ciprofloxacin, and many other drugs.

What are the important points patients should know?

Instruct patients not to exceed prescribed dosages and to notify their physicians if diarrhea is not controlled within 48 hours or if fever develops. Women taking these drugs should not breastfeed without consulting their physicians.

✳ Apply Your Knowledge 34.2

The following questions focus on what you have just learned about antidiarrheals.

CRITICAL THINKING

1. Which antidiarrheals are the most effective drugs for controlling diarrhea?
2. What are the trade names for bismuth subsalicylate, diphenoxylate hydrochloride with atropine sulfate, and loperamide?
3. What are the contraindications of opioid antidiarrheals?
4. What is the significant adverse effect of absorbents?

Constipation

Many people misunderstand the meaning of the word *constipation* and therefore resort to the use of laxatives in cases of what could be termed as "perceived" constipation—that is, slow gut transit time. A common cause of constipation is dehydration caused by inadequate liquid ingestion, especially in hot weather and among older adults. Nondietary constipation can be caused by **paralytic ileus** (no peristaltic movements in the intestines), which can occur after abdominal surgery.

Many drugs, particularly those with antimuscarinic activity, can slow down peristalsis and lead to constipation.

Laxatives, which are used to combat constipation, are among the most misused drugs because of misperceptions about constipation. Individuals tend to self-treat with easily available OTC drugs. Overuse of laxatives can in turn cause constipation. Laxatives are classified into several different categories depending on their mechanism of action: osmotic (saline) laxatives, stool softeners, stimulants, and bulk-forming laxatives. Table 34-3 ■ presents the characteristics of different laxative categories.

Table 34-3 ■ Categories of Laxatives

GENERIC NAME	TRADE NAME	AVERAGE ADULT DOSAGE	ROUTE OF ADMINISTRATION
Osmotic Laxatives			
lactulose	Cephulac	30–60 mL/d prn	PO
magnesium citrate	Citrate of Magnesia, Citroma	240 mL/d in 8 oz of water	PO
magnesium hydroxide	Milk of Magnesia	2.4–4.8 g (30–60 mL)/d in 1 or more divided doses	PO
magnesium sulfate	Epsom Salt	10–15 g/d in 8 oz of water	PO
Stool Softeners			
docusate calcium	Surfak	50–500 mg/d	PO
docusate potassium	Dialose	50–500 mg/d	PO
docusate sodium	Colace	50–500 mg/d	PO
		50–100 mg added to enema fluid	Rectal
glycerin	Glycerol, Osmoglyn	Insert 1 suppository of 5–15 mL of enema high into rectum and retain for 15 min	Rectal

(continued)

Table 34-3 ■ **Categories of Laxatives** (*continued*)

GENERIC NAME	TRADE NAME	AVERAGE ADULT DOSAGE	ROUTE OF ADMINISTRATION
Stimulant Laxatives			
bisacodyl	Apo-Bisacodyl, Dulcolax	5–15 mg prn (maximum: 30 mg for special procedures)	PO
		10 mg prn	Rectal
cascara sagrada	Cascara Sagrada Aromatic Fluid-extract, Cascara Sagrada Fluidextract	Tablets: 325–1,000 mg/d Aromatic Fluidextract: 2–6 mL/d; Fluidextract: 0.5–1.5 mL/d	PO
senna (sennosides)	Black-Draught, Senokot	Standard concentrate: 1–2 tablets or ½–1 tsp at bedtime (maximum: 4 tablets or 2 tsp bid); syrup: 10–15 mL at bedtime	PO
Bulk-Forming Laxatives			
calcium polycarbophil	FiberCon, Mitrolan	1 g qid prn (maximum: 6 g/d)	PO
psyllium hydrophilic mucilloid	Metamucil	1–2 rounded tsp or 1 packet 1–3 times/d prn	PO

PO, oral; bid, twice a day; qid, four times a day.

Focus On

Osmotic Laxatives

Osmotic (or saline) laxatives are a mixture of sodium and magnesium salts.

How do they work?

These drugs work via **osmosis**, in which sodium and magnesium ions attract water into the bowel, causing a more liquid stool to be formed. The contents are hypertonic, causing water to be retained, and if the osmotic pressure is great enough, it can pull water from the bowel's capillaries back into the bowel lumen. This results in an increase in pressure and volume in the colon and rectum, leading to stimulation of the defecation reflex.

How are they used?

Osmotic laxatives are used for the short-term treatment of occasional constipation. They have also been used in the treatment of poisoning by mineral acids and arsenic or as mouthwash to neutralize acidity.

What are the adverse effects?

Common adverse effects include nausea and vomiting, abdominal cramps, diarrhea, weakness, lethargy, and electrolyte imbalance. In severe cases, they may cause hypotension, bradycardia, mental depression, and coma.

What are the contraindications and interactions?

The use of osmotic laxatives is contraindicated in patients with renal impairment and hypertension because sodium ions can be absorbed and accumulate in the blood.

What are the important points patients should know?

Instruct patients that the action of osmotic laxatives does not occur until the drugs reach the colon; therefore, about 24–48 hours are needed before an effect results. Advise patients not to self-medicate with another laxative while waiting for the onset of action. Patients should notify their physician if diarrhea (more than two to three soft stools per day) persists more than 24–48 hours after taking a laxative. Diarrhea is a sign of overdosage. Dose adjustment may be indicated. Women should not breastfeed while taking these drugs without consulting their physician.

Focus Point

Laxative Abuse

The potential abuse of laxatives should be evaluated in patients suspected of having bulimia nervosa or anorexia nervosa. Elderly patients, whose diets and changing digestive systems may cause them to perceive constipation, may also overuse laxatives. Be alert for volume depletion, which causes serious electrolyte imbalances, especially among older adults.

Focus On

Stool Softeners

Stool softeners are sometimes known as emollients or surfactants. Few of these compounds are in common use. One of them is docusate sodium.

How do they work?

Docusate sodium has detergent-like properties and seems to act mainly by holding water molecules in the fecal material, thus rendering them softer and easier to pass. Because the main mechanism of action is the softening process, these laxatives do not work quickly. Their effect usually takes several days to become apparent.

How are they used?

Stool softeners are used to ease bowel movements in constipated patients. They are used prophylactically in patients who should avoid straining during defecation and for the treatment of constipation associated with hard and dry stools.

What are the adverse effects?

Stool softeners may cause mild abdominal cramps, diarrhea, nausea, and a bitter taste.

What are the contraindications and interactions?

Stool softeners are contraindicated in patients with atonic constipation, nausea and vomiting, abdominal pain, and intestinal obstruction or perforation. These drugs should be used cautiously in patients with a history of congestive heart failure, edema, and diabetes mellitus. Docusate may interact with and increase the systemic absorption of mineral oil, which is also commonly used as a lubricant to treat constipation.

What are the important points patients should know?

Instruct patients to take sufficient liquids with each dose and increase fluid intake during the day. Advise them that docusate should not be taken for prolonged dietary management.

Focus Point

Diabetes and Laxatives

The blood glucose levels of patients with diabetes must be carefully monitored while taking laxatives that contain high amounts of lactose and galactose.

Focus On

Laxative Stimulants

Laxative stimulants include cascara sagrada and senna.

How do they work?

Laxative stimulants are true purgatives in that they directly affect the walls of either the small or large intestine. They cause an increase in peristaltic movements, leading to defecation.

How are they used?

Laxative stimulants are used for the temporary relief of constipation in various disease conditions and to prevent straining during defecation. Laxative stimulants are sometimes used with magnesium hydroxide.

What are the adverse effects?

Common adverse effects of laxative stimulants include anorexia, nausea, gripping, abnormally loose stools, constipation rebound, and **melanosis** (abnormal dark pigmentation) of the colon. They may cause the discoloration of urine and hypokalemia.

What are the contraindications and interactions?

Laxative stimulants are contraindicated in patients with abdominal pain, fecal impaction, GI bleeding, ulcerations, appendicitis, and intestinal obstruction. They should not be used during pregnancy or in patients with congestive heart failure. Laxative stimulants should be used cautiously in lactating women and patients with renal impairment, diabetes, or rectal bleeding. They may interact with oral anticoagulants and decrease their effect.

What are the important points patients should know?

Instruct patients that the frequent or prolonged use of irritant cathartics disrupts normal reflex activity of the colon and rectum, leading to drug dependence for evacuation.

Bulk-Forming Laxatives

The proper functioning of the bowel depends on the presence of adequate amounts of liquids as well as dietary fiber. Dietary fiber consists of such plant products as cellulose, hemicellulose, and lignin, which are all found in high quantities in the outer coating of seeds and grains. Many vegetables and fruits also contain high amounts of fiber. These substances are not digestible (to any great extent) in humans and therefore add bulk to the colonic contents, which stimulates forward-propulsive movements and the defecation reflex. Examples of bulk-forming laxatives are psyllium hydrophilic mucilloid and polycarbophil.

How do they work?

Bulk-forming laxatives absorb free water in the intestinal tract and oppose the dehydrating forces of the bowel by forming a gelatinous mass.

How are they used?

Bulk-forming laxatives are used in chronic atonic or spastic constipation and constipation associated with rectal disorders or anorectal surgery.

What are the adverse effects?

Common adverse effects include nausea and vomiting, diarrhea (with excessive use), and abdominal cramps.

What are the contraindications and interactions?

Bulk-forming laxatives are contraindicated in patients with esophageal and intestinal obstruction, nausea and vomiting, fecal impaction, undiagnosed abdominal pain, and appendicitis and in children younger than age 2 years. They should be used cautiously in patients with diabetes, pregnant women, and during lactation. Bulk-forming laxatives may decrease absorption and clinical effects of antibiotics, warfarin, digoxin, nitrofurantoin, and salicylates.

What are the important points patients should know?

Instruct patients who are on a low-sodium or low-calorie diet to note the sugar and sodium content of these preparations. Some of them contain natural sugars, but others contain artificial sweeteners. Be sure that patients understand that these drugs work to relieve both diarrhea and constipation by restoring a more normal moisture level to the stool. These drugs may reduce appetite if taken before meals. Women should not breastfeed while taking these drugs without consulting their physician.

✳ Apply Your Knowledge 34.3

The following questions focus on what you have just learned about laxatives.

CRITICAL THINKING

1. What are the classifications of laxatives?
2. What are the adverse effects of stool softeners?
3. What are two examples of laxative stimulants?
4. What is the mechanism of action for bulk-forming laxatives?
5. What is the mechanism of action for osmotic laxatives?

Vomiting

Vomiting is an act of disgorging the contents of the stomach through the mouth. It is also called *emesis*. Infectious diseases can directly irritate vomiting centers to inhibit impulses going to the stomach. Certain drugs, radiation, and chemotherapy may irritate the GI tract or stimulate the chemoreceptor trigger zone and vomiting center in the brain (medulla). After surgery, particularly abdominal surgery, nausea and vomiting are common. The main neurotransmitters that produce nausea and vomiting include dopamine, serotonin, and acetylcholine.

Focus On

Emetics

Emetic drugs can induce vomiting. Vomiting is a reflex primarily controlled by the medulla oblongata of the brain (often affected by such drugs as morphine and digitalis).

How do they work?

Ipecac syrup has central and peripheral emetic actions, but after oral administration, the peripheral action is predominant. Vomiting is triggered by intense irritation of the mucosal layer of the intestinal wall. Not surprisingly, the central action comprises the stimulation of the vomiting center via the chemoreceptor trigger zone in the medulla.

How are they used?

Ipecac syrup is used as an emergency emetic to remove unabsorbed ingested poisons. The use of ipecac syrup as an emetic is controversial and in decline. In some regions, its use has been completely abandoned in the clinical setting, and it is not recommended for the treatment of poisoning in the home.

What are the adverse effects?

The adverse effects of ipecac syrup may include stiff muscles, severe myopathy, convulsions, and coma. Cardiac arrhythmias, chest pain, dyspnea, hypotension, and fatal myocarditis may also occur. Diarrhea and mild GI upset are seen in some cases.

What are the contraindications and interactions?

Ipecac syrup is contraindicated in comatose, semi-comatose, or deeply sedated patients. It should not be used in patients who are in shock or having seizures or in patients with impaired cardiac function. Ipecac syrup must be used cautiously during pregnancy and lactation and in infants younger than 6 months old.

What are the important points patients should know?

Instruct patients or their families to call an emergency department, poison control center, or physician before using ipecac syrup. Patients should not breastfeed after using this drug without consulting their physician.

Focus Point

Ipecac Toxicity

The misuse of ipecac has occurred in persons with eating disorders, such as bulimia, and may result in ipecac toxicity. Patients must immediately report to their physician if vomiting persists longer than 2–3 hours after ipecac syrup is given.

Focus On

Antiemetics

Antiemetics are agents used to prevent or relieve nausea and vomiting that may be caused by many different disorders. Table 34-4 ■ shows the most commonly used antiemetics.

How do they work?

The mechanism of action of antiemetics is largely unknown except that they help to relax the portion of the brain controlling the muscles that cause vomiting.

How are they used?

The antiemetics are used for the prevention or treatment of patients with nausea and vomiting, especially to treat those with motion sickness and radiation or postchemotherapy vomiting.

What are the adverse effects?

Drowsiness is a common adverse effect of antiemetics. Additional adverse effects include confusion, dry mouth, headache, hypotension, hypersensitivity reactions, and blurred vision.

What are the contraindications and interactions?

Antiemetic drugs should be avoided in patients with known hypersensitivity to these medications, coma, and severe CNS depression. Antiemetics are contraindicated during pregnancy or lactation, especially during the first trimester. Antiemetics are also contraindicated if there is nausea and vomiting with an undiagnosed condition. This is especially true in patients with suspected appendicitis, intestinal obstruction, brain tumors, or drug toxicity. Different types of antiemetics may have different drug interactions. For example, whereas serotonin antagonists usually have no drug interactions, the effects of dopamine are altered by antiemetics.

What are the important points patients should know?

Advise patients who are taking antiemetics to avoid driving a car and operating heavy machinery. Instruct them to avoid alcohol because it intensifies the sedative effects of antiemetics. Pregnant women should avoid antiemetics during the first trimester; nonpharmacological measures for nausea are safer and more appropriate, which include small, frequent meals; dry biscuits; and a quiet environment. Advise patients with motion sickness to take antiemetics 30 minutes before travel.

Table 34-4 ■ The Most Commonly Used Antiemetics

GENERIC NAME	TRADE NAME	AVERAGE ADULT DOSAGE	ROUTE OF ADMINISTRATION
Dopamine Antagonists			
haloperidol	Haldol	1–2 mg q12h	PO
chlorpromazine	Thorazine	10–25 mg q4–6h	PO, IM, IV
perphenazine	Perphenazine Tablets	8–16 mg/d	PO
prochlorperazine	Compazine	5–10 mg tid–qid	PO, IM, IV, rectal
promethazine	Phenergan	25 mg q4–6h	PO, IM, IV, rectal

GENERIC NAME	TRADE NAME	AVERAGE ADULT DOSAGE	ROUTE OF ADMINISTRATION
thiethylperazine	Torecan	10 mg 1–3 times/d	PO, IM, rectal
Miscellaneous Agent			
metoclopramide	Reglan	1–2 mg/kg 30 min before chemotherapy and q2–4h prn	IV
Serotonin Antagonists			
granisetron	Kytril	1 mg 1 h before chemotherapy	PO, IV
ondansetron	Zofran	4–8 mg tid	PO, IV
Antihistamines			
dimenhydrinate	Dramamine	50–100 mg q4–6h prn	PO, IM, IV
diphenhydramine	Benadryl	10–50 mg q4–6h prn	PO, IM, IV
hydroxyzine	Atarax, Vistaril	25–100 mg q6h prn	PO, IM
meclizine	Antivert	25–50 mg/d	PO
Anticholinergics			
scopolamine	Transderm-Scop	0.5 mg q72h	Transdermal
trimethobenzamide	Tigan	250 mg tid–qid	PO, rectal

PO, oral; IM, intramuscular; IV, intravenous; tid, three times a day; qid, four times a day.

Focus on Natural Products

Ginger for Nausea

For thousands of years, the Chinese have used ginger medicinally to treat people with nausea and vomiting, morning sickness, and motion sickness. Studies have shown ginger to be about as effective as OTC medications sold for these purposes. It is also said to have anti-inflammatory properties and is given to patients who have arthritis. Ginger is also used to soothe coughing or for fever. Because ginger may affect blood clotting, it should be avoided by patients who are taking anticoagulants.

✳ Apply Your Knowledge 34.4

The following questions focus on what you have just learned about vomiting, emetics, and antiemetics.

CRITICAL THINKING

1. Where is the vomiting center in the human body?
2. What are the causes of vomiting?
3. What is the mechanism of action of ipecac syrup?
4. What are the indications of antiemetics?
5. What are the contraindications of ipecac syrup?
6. What are the trade names of chlorpromazine, promethazine, and dimenhydrinate?

PRACTICAL SCENARIO 1

A 26-year-old woman in graduate school visits the family physician because for the past 3–4 months she has been experiencing gnawing pains in her upper-middle abdomen. When you ask her what seems to precipitate the pain, she is unable to say for sure. She says she feels the best in the early morning before eating. As the day progresses, she usually feels worse and takes Mylanta or Milk of Magnesia to relieve the pain. Sometimes, her pain is accompanied by severe diarrhea, and she has been tired, weak, and nauseous. In response to your question about stress, she tells you she is under extreme stress because she is preparing to defend her thesis for her Ph.D. She has been smoking more cigarettes than usual and drinking 6–8 cups of coffee each morning. In the evening, she often has a few glasses of wine to help her relax.

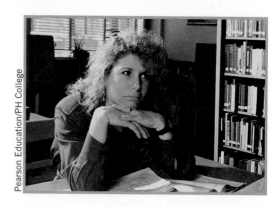

Pearson Education/PH College

Critical Thinking Questions

1. Based on this patient's complaints, lifestyle, and use of OTC medications, what do you expect may be the cause of her initial complaint of upper-middle abdomen pain and her symptoms of fatigue, weakness, and nausea?
2. What diagnostic tests do you anticipate the physician ordering and for what possible diagnoses?
3. Instead of OTC antacids, what are the other choices for this patient to relieve her symptoms? Is there a class of medications you think might be the better choice for her? If so, what and why?

PRACTICAL SCENARIO 2

A 75-year-old man complained about constipation, telling the physician assistant that he only had a bowel movement every 4 or 5 days. The physician assistant gave him laxatives.

gwimages/Fotolia

Critical Thinking Questions

1. Explain the classifications of laxatives.
2. Explain the mechanism of action of stimulant laxatives.

Chapter Capsule

This section repeats the objectives from the beginning of the chapter and then provides a summary of the most important concepts for that objective. Use this section as a quick review and to check your knowledge.

Objective 1: Describe the major parts of the digestive system.

- Alimentary canal, including the mouth, pharynx, esophagus, stomach, small intestine, large intestine, rectum, and anus
- Accessory organs, including the salivary glands, liver, gallbladder, and pancreas

Objective 2: Explain how medications are absorbed in the gastrointestinal tract and metabolized.

- Stomach juices mix with a substance and break it down for absorption

- Chemical digestion occurs in the small intestine

- The liver is the center of metabolic activity and is very important in digestion, absorption, and metabolic activities

Objective 3: Describe the use of histamine-2 (H_2) receptor antagonists in the treatment of peptic ulcers.

- Short-term treatment of active duodenal ulcer and the prevention of ulcer recurrence (at reduced dosage) after it is healed

- Short-term treatment of active benign gastric ulcer, pathologic hypersecretory conditions such as Zollinger-Ellison syndrome, and heartburn

Objective 4: Describe the use of antacids for the treatment of peptic ulcers.

- For hyperacidity of the stomach, to protect from peptic ulcers, and to promote peptic ulcer healing

Objective 5: Explain the effects of prostaglandins on the digestive tract.

- Most versatile and powerful substances used to treat gastrointestinal (GI) disorders

- Involved in GI motility and gastric acid secretions

- Inhibit gastric acid and gastrin production, mucus production, and bicarbonate secretion

- Prostaglandin analogue misoprostol (Cytotec) is most commonly used

Objective 6: List generic names and trade names for proton pump inhibitors.

- esomeprazole (Nexium)

- lansoprazole (Prevacid)

- omeprazole (Prilosec)

- pantoprazole (Protonix)

- rabeprazole (AcipHex)

Objective 7: Describe the drug treatment for diarrhea.

- Opioid and synthetic opioid drugs: most effective

- Absorbents: inexpensive and, to a certain extent, effective

Objective 8: Explain the problems associated with laxative use.

- Nausea and vomiting, abdominal cramps, diarrhea, weakness, reduced appetite, lethargy, bitter taste, anorexia, gripping, constipation rebound, melanosis of the colon, discoloration of urine, hypokalemia, and electrolyte imbalance

- In severe cases, hypotension, bradycardia, mental depression, and coma

- Contraindicated in patients with renal impairment, atonic constipation, nausea and vomiting, abdominal pain, fecal impaction, esophageal obstruction, intestinal obstruction, intestinal perforation, GI bleeding, ulcerations, appendicitis, hypertension, and in patients younger than 2 years

- Cautious use in patients with a history of congestive heart failure, edema, rectal bleeding, and diabetes mellitus

Objective 9: Describe the mechanism of action for bulk-forming laxatives, osmotic laxatives, and laxative stimulants.

- Bulk-forming laxatives absorb free water in the intestinal tract and oppose the dehydrating forces of the bowel by forming a gelatinous mass

- Osmotic laxatives use the ions of sodium and magnesium to attract water (osmosis), which causes a more liquid stool to be formed. Hypertonic contents cause water to be retained and to be pulled from the bowel's capillaries back into the bowel lumen, resulting in an increase in pressure and volume in the colon and rectum, leading to the stimulation of the defecation reflex.

- Laxative stimulants are true purgatives that cause an increase in peristaltic movements and lead to defecation

Objective 10: Identify causes of vomiting and the main neurotransmitters that produce nausea and vomiting.

- Infectious diseases can directly irritate vomiting centers to inhibit impulses going to the stomach. Certain drugs, radiation, and chemotherapy may irritate the GI tract or stimulate the chemoreceptor trigger zone and vomiting center in the brain (medulla). After surgery, particularly abdominal surgery, nausea and vomiting are common.

- The main neurotransmitters that produce nausea and vomiting include dopamine, serotonin, and acetylcholine

 Internet Sites of Interest

- The National Institute of Diabetes and Digestive and Kidney Diseases (NIDDK) at **http://digestive.niddk.nih.gov** presents information on how the digestive system works. The information is appropriate for patient teaching. Search for "digestive system."

- Good information about peptic ulcer disease is found at: **www.webmd.com/ digestive-disorders/digestive-diseases-peptic-ulcer-disease**

- The Family Doctor website offers information on the use of OTC laxatives at: **http://familydoctor.org/familydoctor/en.html**. Search for "laxatives."

- For information on the use of laxatives, see Medical News Today at: **www.medicalnewstoday.com**. Search for "laxative use."

Chapter 35

Drugs Used to Treat Respiratory Conditions

Chapter Objectives

After completing this chapter, you should be able to:

1. Describe the upper and lower respiratory tracts.
2. Explain asthma, including its classifications and symptoms.
3. List the most commonly used medications for asthma.
4. Explain xanthine derivatives in the treatment of asthma.
5. Identify how corticosteroids are used to treat asthma and other conditions for which they are used.
6. Describe the mechanism of action of leukotriene inhibitors.
7. Explain the contraindications of mast cell stabilizers.
8. Describe the use of opioid cough suppressants.
9. Define *expectorants* and *mucolytic agents*.
10. Explain the mechanism of action for decongestants.

Key Terms

alveolar duct (p. 611)
alveolar sacs (p. 611)
alveoli (p. 611)
antitussives (p. 621)
asthma (p. 611)
atelectasis (p. 622)
bronchioles (p. 611)

bronchitis (p. 616)
bronchodilators (p. 616)
bronchospasm (p. 616)
cystic fibrosis (p. 622)
decongestants (p. 623)
emphysema (p. 617)
expectorants (p. 622)

leukotriene inhibitors (p. 619)
mast cells (p. 619)
mucolytics (p. 622)
nebulizer (p. 617)
nonproductive cough (p. 621)
productive cough (p. 622)
xanthine derivatives (p. 617)

Introduction

All cells of the body require oxygen to break down nutrients and thereby release and produce energy (adenosine triphosphate [ATP]). The cells must also excrete the carbon dioxide that results from the process. Obtaining oxygen and removing carbon dioxide are the primary functions of the respiratory system, which includes tubes that filter incoming air and transport air into and out of the lungs as well as microscopic air sacs where gases are exchanged. The respiratory organs also entrap particles from incoming air, help control the temperature and water content of the air, produce vocal sounds, and participate in the sense of smell and the regulation of blood pH.

Organs of the Respiratory System

The organs of the respiratory system can be divided into two groups, or tracts. Those in the *upper respiratory tract* include the nose, nasal cavity, paranasal sinuses,

and pharynx. Those in the *lower respiratory tract* include the larynx, trachea, bronchial tree, and lungs (Figure 35-1 ■).

The lower respiratory tract is essential for the exchange of oxygen and carbon dioxide. As the bronchi enter the lungs, they subdivide into bronchial tubes and small **bronchioles** (which are 1 mm or less in diameter and have abundant smooth muscle and elastic fibers). At the end of each bronchiole is an **alveolar duct**. These ducts lead to thin-walled outpouchings called **alveolar sacs**. Alveolar sacs lead to smaller microscopic air sacs called **alveoli**, which lie within capillary networks (Figure 35-2 ■).

Asthma

Asthma is a chronic disease caused by the increased reactivity of the tracheobronchial tree to various stimuli. It is a leading cause of chronic illness and school absenteeism in children (Figure 35-3 ■). Asthma is also one of the most common chronic conditions in the United States, affecting about 23 million Americans, 7 million of which are children.

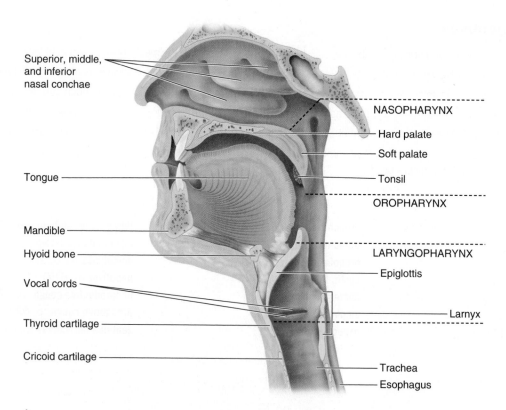

A

Figure 35-1 ■ The upper (**A**) and lower (**B**) respiratory tracts.

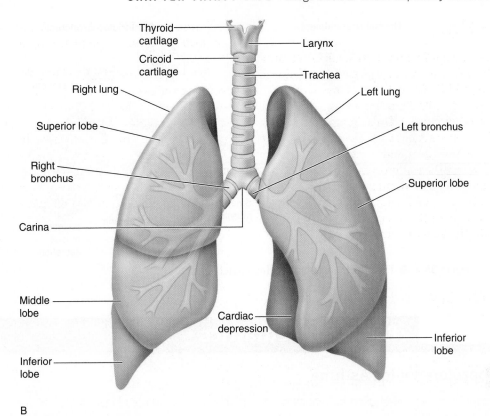

B

Figure 35-1 ■ (*continued*)

Figure 35-2 ■ Bronchioles and alveoli.

Normal Bronchiole

Constricted Bronchiole

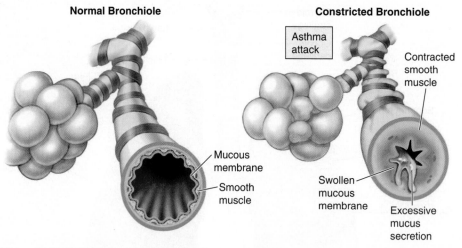

Figure 35-3 ■ The effects of asthma on the bronchioles.

Focus on Pediatrics

Isoproterenol for Asthma

Isoproterenol is often used to treat status asthmaticus in children even though such use is not a labeled indication. Parents should tell their children that saliva and sputum may appear pink after inhalation treatment and that this is normal.

Asthma is frequently classified according to its cause: allergy, exercise induced, or infections of the respiratory tract. Symptoms include breathlessness, cough, wheezing, and chest tightness. The airway becomes inflamed with *edema* (abnormal accumulation of fluid) and mucous plugs; hyperactivity of the bronchial tree adds to the symptoms. During asthmatic attacks, when bronchiole constriction and increased secretions are present, bronchodilators are used for relief. Classifications of the most common medications that are used for asthma are listed in Table 35-1 ■.

Table 35-1 ■ The Most Common Antiasthma Drugs

GENERIC NAME	TRADE NAME	AVERAGE ADULT DOSAGE	ROUTE OF ADMINISTRATION
Beta₂-Adrenergic Agonists			
albuterol	Proventil, Ventolin	2–4 mg tid	PO
		1–2 inhalations q4–6h; 2 inhalations before exercise	Inhalation
epinephrine	EpiPen	Individualized: solution 1:1,000, 0.3–0.5 Ml	SC, IM
formoterol	Foradil	One 12-mg capsule q12h	Inhalation (aerolizer inhaler)
ipratropium	Atrovent, Atrovent HFA	2 inhalations qid at 4-h intervals (maximum: 12 inhalations in 24 h)	Inhalation (MDI)
		500 mcg (1 unit-dose vial) q6–8h	Inhalation (nebulizer)
		Intranasal: 2 sprays of 0.06% in each nostril tid–qid up to 4 d	Nasal spray

GENERIC NAME	TRADE NAME	AVERAGE ADULT DOSAGE	ROUTE OF ADMINISTRATION
isoetharine	(Generic only)	3–7 inhalations 1:3 dilution	Inhalation
isoproterenol	Isuprel	Inhalations 4–6 times/d (maximum: 6 inhalations in any hour during 24-h period)	Inhalation (MDI)
		Solution: 0.5 mL of 0.5% solution diluted to 2–2.5 mL with water or saline over 10–20 min, up to 5 times/d	IPPB
levalbuterol	Xopenex	0.63 mg tid q6–8h; may increase to 1.25 mg tid prn	Inhalation (nebulizer)
metaproterenol	Alupent	20 mg q6–8h	PO
		2–3 inhalations q3–4h (maximum: 12 inhalation/d)	Inhalation (MDI)
		5–10 inhalations of undiluted 5% solution	Inhalation (nebulizer)
		2.5 mL of 0.4–0.6% solution q4–6h	IPPB
pirbuterol	Maxair	2 inhalations (0.4 mg) q6h (maximum: 12 inhalations/d)	Inhalation
salmeterol	Serevent	2 inhalations of aerosol (42 mcg) or 1 powder diskus (50 mcg) bid, 12h apart	Inhalation (various)
terbutaline	Terbutaline Sulfate (tablets)	5 mg tid at 6-h intervals during waking hours	PO
	Terbutaline Sulfate (injection)	0.25 mg q15–30min, up to 0.5 mg in 4 h	SC
	Brethaire (inhalation)	2 inhalations separated by 60 sec q4–6h	Inhalation
Xanthine Derivatives			
aminophylline	(Generic only)	Loading dose: 6 mg/kg over 30 min; maintenance dose: 0.25–0.75 mg/kg/h	IV
		0.6 mg/kg/h qid	PO
dyphylline	Lufyllin	Up to 15 mg/kg q6h	PO
oxtriphylline	(Generic only)	200–800 mg q6h up to 15 mg/kg	PO
theophylline	Theolair	300-600 mg/day, divided q6–8h	PO
Corticosteroids			
beclomethasone	Beconase*, QVAR	2 inhalations tid–qid, up to 20 inhalations/d	Inhalation, nasal
budesonide	Pulmicort, Rhinocort	Maintenance: 1–2 inhalations (200 mcg/inhalation 1–2 times/d)	Inhalation
dexamethasone	Decadron	Up to 3 inhalations tid–qid (maximum: 800 mcg bid)	Inhalation
flunisolide	AeroBid, Nasalide	2 sprays orally or intranasally in each nostril bid; may increase to tid if needed	PO, nasal

(continued)

Table 35-1 ■ **The Most Common Antiasthma Drugs** (*continued*)

GENERIC NAME	TRADE NAME	AVERAGE ADULT DOSAGE	ROUTE OF ADMINISTRATION
fluticasone	Flonase, Flovent	100 mcg (1 inhalation in each nostril 1–2 times/d (maximum: 4 times/d)	Nasal
		1–2 inhalations bid	Inhalation
hydrocortisone	Cortaid	10–320 mg/d in 3–4 divided doses (maximum: 2 g/d)	PO
mometasone furoate monohydrate	Nasonex	2 sprays (50 mcg each) in each nostril/d	Nasal
prednisolone	Prelone	5–60 mg/d in single or divided doses	PO
prednisone	Deltasone	40 mg q12h for 3–5 d	PO
triamcinolone	Azmacort	2 puffs 3–4 times/d or 4 puffs bid	Inhalation
		2 spray/nostril once daily (maximum: 8 sprays/d)	Nasal
Leukotriene Inhibitors			
montelukast	Singulair	10 mg at bedtime	PO
zafirlukast	Accolate	20 mg bid	PO
zileuton	Zyflo	600 mg qid	PO
Mast Cell Stabilizers			
cromolyn	Intal, NasalCrom	1 spray or 1 capsule inhaled qid	MDI
		1 spray in each nostril 3–6 times/d at regular intervals	Nasal
nedocromil	Alocril, Tilade	2 inhalations qid at regular intervals (*not* for acute asthma attacks)	Inhalation
Combination Drugs			
fluticasone with salmeterol	Advair Diskus, Advair HFA	1 puff bid approx, 12h apart	Inhalation
budesonide with formoterol	Symbicort	2 inhalations per dose, q12h	Inhalation

*Beconase AQ is a nasal spray and is also available as an inhalation aerosol.

tid, three times a day; PO, oral; SC, subcutaneous; IM, intramuscular; qid, four times a day; MDI, metered-dose inhaler; IPPB, intermittent positive-pressure breathing; bid, twice a day; IV, intravenous;

Focus Point

Severe Asthma

Severe forms of asthma are associated with frequent attacks of wheezing dyspnea, especially at night, and chronic limitation of activity. Asthma causes the contraction of the airway smooth muscle, mucosal thickening, and abnormally thick plugs of mucus.

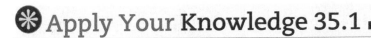

✳ Apply Your Knowledge 35.1

The following questions focus on what you have just learned about organs of the respiratory system and the effects of drugs on asthma.

CRITICAL THINKING

1. What are the primary functions of the respiratory system?
2. What organs are included in the lower respiratory tract?
3. What are the symptoms of asthma?
4. What are the classifications of antiasthma drugs?
5. What are the trade names of cromolyn, montelukast, and terbutaline?

BRONCHODILATORS

Bronchodilators are agents that widen the diameter of the bronchial tubes. They include beta$_2$-adrenergic agonists, such as salmeterol, and xanthines, such as theophylline and aminophylline.

Focus On

Beta$_2$-Adrenergic Agonists

Beta$_2$-adrenergic agonists are the drugs of choice in the treatment of acute bronchoconstriction, and they have replaced some of the older agents, such as epinephrine, because they cause fewer cardiac adverse effects. Some of these drugs, such as isoproterenol, produce therapeutic effects immediately but last for 2–3 hours, but other drugs, such as salmeterol, provide 12 hours of therapy.

How do they work?

Beta$_2$-adrenergic agonists produce bronchodilation by relaxing smooth muscles of the bronchial tree. This effect decreases airway resistance, facilitates mucus drainage, and increases vital capacity.

How are they used?

Beta$_2$-adrenergic agonists are used to relieve **bronchospasm** (the contraction of smooth muscle in the walls of the bronchi and bronchioles) associated with acute or chronic asthma, **bronchitis** (inflammation of the mucous membrane of the bronchial tubes), or other reversible obstructive airway diseases. Some of them are also used to prevent exercise-induced bronchospasm. Many of these types of agents are inhaled by using a **nebulizer** (a device that disperses a fine-particle mist of medication into the deeper parts of the respiratory tract).

What are the adverse effects?

Adverse effects of such beta$_2$-adrenergic drugs as epinephrine and isoproterenol may cause restlessness, headache, dizziness, palpitations, tachycardia, insomnia, nausea and vomiting, and anorexia.

What are the contraindications and interactions?

Contraindications are hypersensitivity to sympathomimetic amines, narrow-angle glaucoma, and hemorrhagic and traumatic or cardiogenic shock. Safety during pregnancy or lactation is not established. Beta$_2$-adrenergic drugs should be used cautiously in older adults and debilitated patients and in those with prostatic hypertrophy, hypertension, diabetes mellitus, hyperthyroidism, Parkinson's disease, tuberculosis, and psychoneurosis. No significant drug interactions with beta$_2$-adrenergic agents have been reported.

What are the important points patients should know?

Instruct patients not to exceed the recommended dosage. They should use caution if driving or performing tasks that require alertness. Advise patients to eat small, frequent meals to avoid nausea and vomiting and a change in taste. Instruct patients to immediately report chest pain, dizziness, insomnia, weakness, tremors, an irregular heartbeat, difficulty breathing, a productive cough, or a lack of therapeutic effects to their physicians.

Focus on Geriatrics

Cautious Use of Beta₂-Adrenergic Drugs in Elderly Patients

Care must be taken when using Beta₂-adrenergic drugs, such as epinephrine, in older adults. These drugs are contraindicated in numerous conditions that affect elderly patients, including hypertension, Parkinson's disease, heart disease, glaucoma, and arteriosclerosis.

Focus On

Xanthine Derivatives

Xanthine derivatives are a group of drugs chemically related to caffeine that dilate bronchioles in the lungs. Xanthines are most often used to treat asthma and are administered by the oral or intravenous route. Examples of xanthenes include aminophylline and theophylline.

How do they work?

Xanthine derivatives relax smooth muscle by direct action on the bronchi and pulmonary vessels. They stimulate the medullary respiratory center, resulting in an increase in the vital capacity of the lungs. Methylxanthines (such as caffeine) are bases of xanthine derivatives, which must be converted to theophylline. Theophylline has a narrow therapeutic range and is not used as commonly today.

How are they used?

Xanthine derivatives are used for prophylaxis and the symptomatic relief of bronchial asthma as well as bronchospasm associated with chronic bronchitis and **emphysema** (a condition in which the walls between the alveoli lose their elasticity; the alveoli become weakened and break; air is trapped in the alveoli; and the exchange of oxygen and carbon dioxide is reduced).

What are the adverse effects?

The common adverse effects of xanthine derivatives include palpitations, tachycardia, flushing, hypotension, insomnia, nervousness, nausea and vomiting, diarrhea, tachypnea, and respiratory arrest.

What are the contraindications and interactions?

Xanthine derivatives are contraindicated in hypersensitivity to these agents. Xanthine preparations should not be given to patients who have coronary artery disease, a history of angina pectoris, or severe renal or liver impairment. Safety during pregnancy or lactation is not established. Xanthine derivatives should be used cautiously in children and older adults and in those with hyperthyroidism, hypertension, peptic ulcer, prostatic hypertrophy, glaucoma, and diabetes mellitus. The xanthine drugs may produce drug interactions with antibiotics, rifampin, phenobarbital, phenytoin, cimetidine, and caffeine.

What are the important points patients should know?

Advise patients to take these medications at the same time every day. They should avoid charbroiled food (or food cooked using charcoal), which may increase theophylline elimination and reduce the half-life as much as 50%. Instruct patients to limit caffeine intake because it may increase the incidence of adverse effects. Instruct them to avoid cigarette smoking, which may significantly lower the plasma concentration of xanthine drugs. Women should not breastfeed while taking these drugs without consulting a physician.

Focus on Geriatrics

Cautious Use of Xanthines

Xanthine derivatives must be used cautiously in older adults because their adverse effects include severe hypotension and cardiac arrest, which have higher fatality rates in this group of patients.

Focus On

Corticosteroids

Corticosteroids, such as prednisone, are steroid hormones used to treat a wide variety of inflammatory diseases. Inhaled corticosteroids help prevent asthmatic attacks. Oral corticosteroids are used for the short-term management of acute severe asthma.

How do they work?

The precise mechanism of action of corticosteroids is not known. It is thought that they diminish the activation of inflammatory cells and increase the production of anti-inflammatory mediators, which in turn reduces mucus production and edema and decreases airway obstruction.

How are they used?

Corticosteroids are used to treat respiratory conditions, such as nasal congestion, and allergic conditions, such as rhinitis and asthma.

What are the adverse effects?

The adverse effects of corticosteroids include the irritation of mucous membranes, headache, pharyngitis, epistaxis, nausea and vomiting, asthma-like symptoms, and coughing. Less common adverse effects include blood in the nasal mucus, runny nose, abdominal pain, diarrhea, fever, flu-like symptoms, body aches, dizziness, and bronchitis.

What are the contraindications and interactions?

Corticosteroids are contraindicated in patients with known hypersensitivity to these types of drugs. They should not be used if symptoms of hypercorticism (such as Cushing's syndrome) are present. They must be used with caution in patients with immune system infections, tuberculosis, herpes simplex, ulcers, nasal surgery, and nasal trauma and in women who are pregnant or lactating. They should not be used in children younger than age 4 years. Corticosteroids may interact with ritonavir, ketoconazole, other cytochrome P450 inhibitors, and other inhaled corticosteroids.

What are the important points patients should know?

Advise patients to avoid exposure to chickenpox or measles while taking corticosteroids and to contact their physician if exposure occurs. Women who are pregnant or lactating should not use corticosteroids without their physician's approval.

Focus on Pediatrics

Growth Retardation and Corticosteroids

Growth retardation is of particular concern when corticosteroids are used in children. Guidelines for use of corticosteroids with certain age groups must be followed closely.

Focus On

Leukotriene Inhibitors

Leukotriene inhibitors, such as zafirlukast, are bronchodilator and leukotriene-receptor antagonists. Leukotrienes are metabolized from arachidonic acid, which is also responsible for forming prostaglandins. Leukotrienes cause inflammation and allergic reactions. They increase edema, vascular permeability, and mucus in bronchioles.

How do they work?

A leukotriene inhibitor blocks either the synthesis of or the body's inflammatory responses to leukotrienes. Blocking the receptors also blocks the tissue's inflammatory response. Thus, leukotriene inhibitors control asthmatic attacks.

How are they used?

Leukotriene inhibitors are used in the prophylaxis and treatment of chronic asthma or allergic rhinitis.

What are the adverse effects?

Adverse effects of leukotriene inhibitors include arrhythmias, dizziness, lightheadedness, anxiety, headache, and euphoria. Common adverse effects are nausea, diarrhea, dry mouth, and abdominal discomfort.

What are the contraindications and interactions?

Leukotriene inhibitors are contraindicated in hypersensitive patients and in those with severe asthma attacks, bronchoconstriction caused by asthma or nonsteroidal anti-inflammatory drugs, and status asthmaticus. They should not be used by lactating women and should be used cautiously in patients with severe liver disease, pregnant patients, and children younger than 12 months. No significant drug interactions with leukotriene inhibitor agents have been reported.

What are the important points patients should know?

Instruct patients not to use these drugs for the reversal of an acute asthmatic attack and instead to inform their physician if they need short-acting inhaled bronchodilators more often than leukotriene inhibitors.

Focus Point

Oral Administration Advantage

The principal advantage of leukotriene inhibitors is that they are taken orally. Some patients (especially children) do not comply well with inhaled medications.

Focus On

Mast Cell Stabilizers

Mast cells are large cells found in connective tissue that contain a wide variety of biochemicals, including histamine. Mast cells are involved in inflammation secondary to injuries and infections, and they are sometimes implicated in allergic reactions. A mast cell stabilizer is able to stabilize mast cell membranes against rupture caused by antigenic substances. As a result, less histamine and other inflammatory substances are released in airway tissue. Examples of mast cell stabilizers include cromolyn and nedocromil.

How do they work?

Mast cell stabilizers are synthetic asthma-prophylactic agents with unique action. They inhibit the release of bronchoconstrictors, such as histamine, from sensitized pulmonary mast cells, thereby suppressing an allergic response.

How are they used?

Cromolyn sodium is used primarily for the prophylaxis of mild to moderate seasonal and perennial bronchial asthma and allergic rhinitis. It is also used for the prevention of exercise-related bronchospasm and the prevention of acute bronchospasm induced by known pollutants or antigens. Nedocromil sodium is used as maintenance therapy for patients with mild to moderate asthma.

What are the adverse effects?

Common adverse effects include nausea and vomiting, dry mouth, throat irritation, cough, hoarseness, slightly bitter aftertaste, headache, dizziness, urticaria, and rash.

What are the contraindications and interactions?

Mast cell stabilizers are contraindicated in patients with coronary artery disease or a history of arrhythmias,

dyspnea, acute asthma, and status asthmaticus. These agents should not be used during pregnancy or in children younger than age 6 years. Cromolyn sodium should be given cautiously in patients with renal or hepatic dysfunction. No clinically significant interactions with cromolyn sodium or nedocromil sodium have been established.

What are the important points patients should know?

Advise patients that throat irritation, cough, and hoarseness can be minimized by gargling with water, drinking a few swallows of water, or sucking on a lozenge after each treatment. Women should not breastfeed while taking these drugs.

Focus on Geriatrics

Contraindications of Mast Cell Stabilizers

Mast cell stabilizers, such as cromolyn, are contraindicated in patients with coronary artery disease, a history of arrhythmias, and renal or hepatic dysfunction—all conditions with higher rates of occurrence in older adults.

✳ Apply Your Knowledge 35.2

The following questions focus on what you have just learned about the various types of drugs used for respiratory disorders.

CRITICAL THINKING

1. What are the four examples of xanthine derivatives?
2. What are the three examples of leukotriene inhibitors?
3. What are the three examples of bronchodilators?
4. What are the mechanisms of action of beta$_2$-adrenergic agonists on asthma patients?
5. What are the indications of xanthine derivatives?
6. What are mast cells and their involvement in asthma?
7. What are the contraindications of cromolyn?
8. What are the indications of leukotriene inhibitors?
9. Why must xanthine derivatives be used cautiously in older adults?

Focus On

Antitussives

Antitussives are agents that reduce coughing. They are also called *cough suppressants*. The initial stimulus for a cough probably arises in the bronchial mucosa, where irritation results in bronchoconstriction. *Coughing* is a sudden expulsion of air from the lungs and through the mouth. A cough is often described as productive or nonproductive. A **productive cough** brings up fluid or mucus from the lungs. A **nonproductive cough** is a sudden ejection of air from the lungs and through the mouth that does not expel or produce mucus or fluid from the throat or lungs. Antitussives are classified into two major groups: opioid and nonopioid. Various cough suppression agents are summarized in Table 35-2 ■.

How do they work?

The opioid cough suppressants cause respiratory depression similar to that of morphine. An antitussive action occurs at doses that are lower than those required for analgesia. Examples of opioid cough suppressants are codeine, hydrocodone, and chlorpheniramine and hydrocodone.

Nonopioid cough suppressants, such as dextromethorphan, do not suppress respiration. These drugs reduce the activity of peripheral cough receptors and appear to increase the threshold of the central cough center.

How are they used?

The opioid cough suppressants are used to suppress nonproductive cough, but they have limited use because of unwanted side effects. Codeine and hydrocodone are not generally effective but are used because they elevate the cough threshold.

Nonopioid cough suppressants are indicated for temporary relief of cough spasms in nonproductive coughs caused by colds, pertussis, and influenza. The major nonopioid cough suppressants are over-the-counter (OTC) medications.

What are the adverse effects?

The adverse effects of antitussives may include difficulty breathing, drowsiness, skin rash, itching, dizziness, constipation, nausea, nervousness, and restlessness.

What are the contraindications and interactions?

Antitussives are contraindicated in patients with known hypersensitivity, asthma, emphysema, diabetes, heart disease, seizure conditions, thyroid conditions, chronic bronchitis, and liver disease. They should be used only if directed by a physician in women who are pregnant or lactating. Antitussives interact with monoamine oxidase inhibitors (MAOIs), alcohol, sedatives and hypnotics, cold and allergy medications, muscle relaxants, and analgesics.

What are the important points patients should know?

Advise patients to call their physician if their coughing does not improve or if it lasts longer than 1 week, worsens, or produces yellow-colored mucus. They should also contact their physician if symptoms of fever, rash, sore throat, vomiting, or continuing headache occur.

Table 35-2 ■ Major Types of Cough Suppressants

GENERIC NAME	TRADE NAME	AVERAGE ADULT DOSAGE	ROUTE OF ADMINISTRATION
Opioids			
chlorpheniramine and hydrocodone	Tussionex	5 mL bid	PO
hydrocodone and homatropine	Hycodan	5–10 mg q4–6h prn (maximum: 15 mg/dose)	PO
codeine	(Generic only)	10–20 mg q4–6h prn (maximum: 120 mg/d)	PO

GENERIC NAME	TRADE NAME	AVERAGE ADULT DOSAGE	ROUTE OF ADMINISTRATION
Nonopioids			
benzonatate	Tessalon	100–200 mg tid (maximum: 600 mg/d)	PO
dextromethorphan	Robitussin	10–20 mg q4h or 30 mg q6–8h (maximum: 120 mg/d) or 60 mg of sustained-action liquid bid	PO
diphenhydramine	Benadryl	25 mg q4–6h (maximum: 100 mg/d)	PO

bid, twice a day; PO, oral; tid, three times a day.

Focus on Natural Products

Natural Expectorant

Wild cherry bark acts as an expectorant and as a mild sedative. It is available in syrup and tincture forms. It is good for coughs, colds, bronchitis, and asthma. However, wild cherry bark should not be used during pregnancy.

Focus Point

Opioids for Cough

Opioid analgesics are among the most effective drugs used as cough suppressants. Their effect is often achieved at doses below those required to produce analgesia. For example, 15 mg of codeine is usually sufficient to relieve coughing.

Focus On

Expectorants and Mucolytics

Expectorants and **mucolytics** are medications that are capable of dissolving or promoting liquefaction of mucus in the lungs. They also facilitate the elimination of mucus through coughing. These medications (Table 35-3 ■) are available OTC and by prescription. Expectorants and mucolytics include acetylcysteine, guaifenesin, and dornase alfa.

How do they work?

Acetylcysteine lowers viscosity and facilitates the removal of secretions. Guaifenesin enhances reflex outflow of respiratory tract fluids by the irritation of gastric mucosa.

How are they used?

These agents are used as adjuvant therapy in patients with abnormal, sticky, or thickened mucous secretions in acute and chronic bronchopulmonary disease and in pulmonary complications of **cystic fibrosis** (a disorder marked by abnormal secretions of the exocrine glands causing obstruction of bronchial pathways), tracheostomy, and **atelectasis** (absence of gas from the lungs).

What are the adverse effects?

The adverse effects of these expectorants and mucolytics are not significant. A low incidence of nausea and drowsiness is reported.

(continued)

Focus On (continued)

What are the contraindications and interactions?

Expectorants and mucolytics are contraindicated in patients with hypersensitivity to these agents. They should be avoided in pregnancy and lactation. Guaifenesin may interact with heparin therapy by inhibiting platelet function and increasing the risk of hemorrhage.

What are the important points patients should know?

Instruct patients to increase fluid intake to help loosen mucus and drink at least eight glasses of fluids daily. They should contact their physician if cough persists beyond 1 week. Advise women to avoid breastfeeding while taking these drugs without their physician's approval.

Table 35-3 ■ Expectorants and Mucolytics

GENERIC NAME	TRADE NAME	AVERAGE ADULT DOSAGE	ROUTE OF ADMINISTRATION
acetylcysteine	Mucomyst	10 mL of 20% solution or 2–20 mL of 10% solution q2–6h	Inhalation
dornase alfa	Pulmozyme	2.5 mg/d inhaled through a nebulizer	Inhalation
guaifenesin	Organidin NR	1–2 tablets (200–400 mg) q4h, not to exceed 2400 mg in 24h	PO
potassium iodide	(Generic only)	300–1,000 mg after meals, bid–tid up to 1.5 g tid	PO

PO, oral; bid, twice a day; tid, three times a day.

Focus On

Decongestants

Decongestants are a class of drugs that reverse excessive blood flow (congestion) into an area. These agents are available in oral and nasal preparations. Table 35-4 ■ shows the most commonly used decongestants, such as pseudoephedrine.

How do they work?

Decongestants are vasoconstricting agents that shrink the swollen mucous membranes of the nasal airway passage of the upper respiratory tract. Most oral agents are adrenergic medications or medications that mimic the effects of the sympathetic nervous system.

How are they used?

The most common uses for decongestants are for the relief of nasal congestion caused by the common cold, upper respiratory allergies, and sinusitis.

What are the adverse effects?

All patients may experience nervousness, insomnia, restlessness, dizziness, headaches, and irritability. Decongestants may also cause tachycardia, blurred vision, and nausea and vomiting.

What are the contraindications and interactions?

Decongestants should not be used by patients who are taking other sympathomimetic drugs. They are also contraindicated in patients with diabetes, heart disease, uncontrolled hypertension, hyperthyroidism, and prostatic hypertrophy.

Nasal decongestants may cause severe hypertension with certain MAOIs. They may also decrease the vasopressor response with reserpine, methyldopa, and urine acidifiers. Nasal decongestants increase the duration of action of urine alkalinizers (sodium citrate, lactate, and sodium bicarbonate). They decrease the antihypertensive effects of methyldopa.

What are the important points patients should know?

Instruct patients to avoid taking oral decongestants within 2 hours of bedtime because pseudoephedrine may act as a stimulant. Advise patients to discontinue the medication and consult their physician if extreme restlessness or signs of sensitivity occur. Women should not breastfeed while taking decongestants without consulting their physician.

Table 35-4 ■ The Most Commonly Used Decongestants

GENERIC NAME	TRADE NAME	AVERAGE ADULT DOSAGE	ROUTE OF ADMINISTRATION
Oral Decongestants			
Pseudoephedrine	Sudafed	60 mg q4–6h or 120 mg sustained-release q12h	PO
Combination Decongestants/Antihistamines			
cetirizine-pseudoephedrine	Zyrtec-D	5–10 mg once daily	PO
clemastine fumarate	Tavist	1.34 mg bid; may increase to 8.04 mg/d	PO
fexofenadine-pseudoephedrine	Allegra D	60 mg tid	PO
loratadine-pseudoephedrine	Claritin-D	10 mg/d on empty stomach	PO
naproxen-pseudoephedrine	Aleve Cold and Sinus	275–1,100 mg/d	PO
Nasal Decongestants			
oxymetazoline 0.05%	Afrin	2–3 drops in each nostril bid, up to 3–5 d	Nasal
phenylephrine 1%	Neo-Synephrine, Sinex	1–2 drops in each nostril q3–4h	Nasal
tetrahydrozoline 0.1%	Tyzine	2–4 drops in each nostril q3h prn	Nasal

PO, oral; bid, twice a day; tid, three times a day.

❋ Apply Your Knowledge 35.3

The following questions focus on what you have just learned about antitussives and decongestants.

CRITICAL THINKING

1. What is another name for antitussives?
2. What are the classifications of antitussives?
3. How do codeine and hydrocodone affect the cough threshold?
4. What are the trade names of dornase alfa and acetylcysteine?
5. What are the conditions known as cystic fibrosis and atelectasis?
6. What are the adverse effects of decongestants?
7. What are the trade names of pseudoephedrine, fexofenadine-pseudoephedrine, and phenylephrine?
8. What are decongestants, and how do they work?

PRACTICAL SCENARIO 1

A 60-year-old man with a history of depression and hypertension visited his local pharmacy to buy a decongestant and cough suppressant for a bad chest cold. He asked the pharmacist to recommend a brand. The pharmacist recommended pseudoephedrine for his congestion and dextromethorphan for his cough. At home, the man took the recommended dose of each medicine. Within 1 hour, he began having palpitations, chest pains, and severe headache. He was sweating, and his heart rate was 120 beats per minute. His wife called emergency medical services (EMS). The EMS team obtained an electrocardiogram and asked the man's medical history. The man reported taking phenelzine for depression and atenolol for hypertension. His wife stated that he had just taken pseudoephedrine and dextromethorphan for his cold and cough. The EMS team stabilized his heart rate and transferred him to the hospital for observation.

Michal Heron/Pearson Education/PH College

Critical Thinking Questions

1. What is the significance of the man's use of phenelzine, atenolol, and the OTC cold and cough medications?
2. What mistake did the pharmacist make in helping the man choose OTC cough and cold preparations?
3. What patient teaching would you provide this patient if he was seen in your office for a routine check-up and review of his prescriptions?

PRACTICAL SCENARIO 2

A 7-year-old girl was brought to the emergency department with a severe asthma attack.

Vladislav Gajic/Fotolia

Critical Thinking Questions

1. What is the drug of choice in the treatment of acute bronchoconstriction?
2. List all medications used for asthma.

Chapter Capsule

This section repeats the objectives from the beginning of the chapter and then provides a summary of the most important concepts for that objective. Use this section as a quick review and to check your knowledge.

Objective 1: Describe the upper and lower respiratory tracts.

- Upper respiratory tract: nose, nasal cavity, paranasal sinuses, and pharynx
- Lower respiratory tract: larynx, trachea, bronchial tree, and lungs

Objective 2: Explain asthma, including its classifications and symptoms.

- Asthma is a chronic disease caused by the increased reactivity of the tracheobronchial tree to various stimuli. It is one of the most common chronic conditions in the United States
- Asthma is frequently classified according to its cause: allergy, exercise induced, or infections of the respiratory tract
- Symptoms include breathlessness, cough, wheezing, and chest tightness

Objective 3: List the most commonly used medications for asthma.

- Asthma is most commonly treated with bronchodilators, xanthine derivatives, leukotriene inhibitors, corticosteroids, and mast cell stabilizers

Objective 4: Explain xanthine derivatives in the treatment of asthma.

- Xanthine derivatives treat asthma by relaxing smooth muscle via direct action on the bronchi and pulmonary vessels

Objective 5: Identify how corticosteroids are used to treat asthma and other conditions for which they are used.

- Inhaled corticosteroids help prevent asthmatic attacks. Oral corticosteroids are used for the short-term management of acute severe asthma.
- Corticosteroids are used to treat other respiratory conditions such as nasal congestion and allergic conditions such as rhinitis.

Objective 6: Describe the mechanism of action for leukotriene inhibitors.

- Leukotriene inhibitors—block either the synthesis of leukotrienes or the body's inflammatory responses to leukotrienes

Objective 7: Explain the contraindications of mast cell stabilizers.

- Mast cell stabilizers are contraindicated in patients with coronary artery disease, history of arrhythmias, dyspnea, acute asthma, status asthmaticus, during pregnancy, and in children younger than age 6; cromolyn sodium should be used cautiously in patients with renal or hepatic dysfunction

Objective 8: Describe the use of opioid cough suppressants.

- Opioid cough suppressants—used to suppress nonproductive cough but have limited use because of unwanted side effects; codeine and hydrocodone are not as effective but are used to elevate the cough threshold

Objective 9: Define *expectorants* and *mucolytic agents*.

- Expectorants and mucolytics are medications capable of dissolving or promoting the liquefying of mucus in the lungs and facilitating the elimination of mucus through coughing

Objective 10: Explain the mechanism of action of decongestants.

- Decongestants are vasoconstricting agents that shrink the swollen mucous membranes of the nasal airway passage of the upper respiratory tract; most oral agents are adrenergic medications or medications that mimic the effects of the sympathetic nervous system

 Internet Sites of Interest

- Information on various asthma topics and guidelines are available on the National Heart Lung and Blood Institute website at: **www.nhlbi.nih.gov**. Search for "asthma."
- The Family Doctor offers useful information on OTC decongestants at: **http://familydoctor.org**. Search for "over the counter decongestants."
- Various lung disorders, including asthma and cough, are discussed in detail on the American Lung Association website at: **www.lung.org**
- The Asthma and Allergy Foundation of America provides information, advocacy, and research on asthma at: **www.aafa.org**
- A wealth of information about asthma and its treatments (including alternative therapies), screening tools, and prevention tips are found at MedlinePlus at: **www.nlm.nih.gov/medlineplus/asthma.html**

Chapter 36

Drugs Used to Treat Musculoskeletal Conditions

Chapter Objectives

After completing this chapter, you should be able to:

1. Describe the major functions of the skeletal system.
2. Identify the most common bisphosphonate agents used for osteoporosis.
3. Define *rheumatoid arthritis*.
4. List the major drugs used for rheumatoid arthritis.
5. Describe the major indications of methotrexate.
6. Explain gouty arthritis and the cause of gout.
7. Describe the mechanism of action for colchicine.
8. Explain the indications of allopurinol.
9. Name three disorders that may cause spasticity.
10. List commonly used central skeletal muscle relaxants.

Key Terms

dysphagia (p. 632)
flatulence (p. 632)
hyperuricemia (p. 638)

nephrotic syndrome (p. 640)
oligospermia (p. 638)
osteopenia (p. 631)

osteoporosis (p. 631)
spasticity (p. 641)

Introduction

Disorders of the musculoskeletal system are very common in people of all ages. Musculoskeletal conditions include osteoarthritis, muscle spasms, gout, bursitis, tendonitis, and rheumatoid arthritis (RA). Medications used to treat these conditions include skeletal muscle relaxants, nonsteroidal anti-inflammatory drugs (NSAIDs), aspirin, and gold salts.

Musculoskeletal System

The musculoskeletal system consists of two body systems: (1) the muscular system and (2) the skeletal system. The muscular system includes three types of muscle tissues: (1) skeletal, (2) cardiac, and (3) smooth.

Skeletal muscle, which is discussed in this chapter, contains connective tissues, nerves, and blood vessels. Skeletal muscles produce movement, maintain posture and body position, support soft tissue, and maintain body temperature.

The skeletal system includes the bones of the skeleton and the cartilages, ligaments, and other connective tissues that stabilize or connect the bones. The five primary functions of the skeletal system are (1) support, (2) storage of minerals and lipids, (3) blood cell production, (4) protection, and (5) leverage (Figure 36-1 ■).

Calcium is the most abundant mineral in the human body. Its proper balance and interaction with other minerals and hormones are essential to optimal functioning of several body systems, particularly the musculoskeletal system. A typical human body contains 1–2 kg of

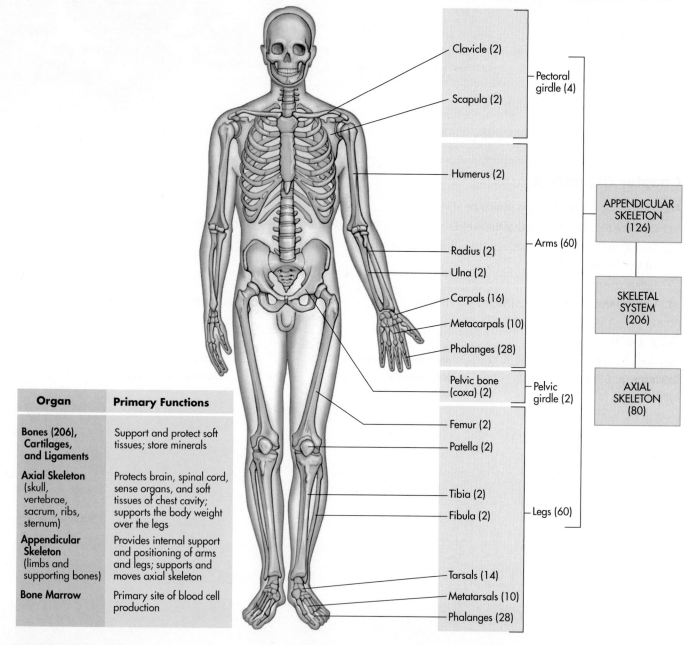

Organ	Primary Functions
Bones (206), Cartilages, and Ligaments	Support and protect soft tissues; store minerals
Axial Skeleton (skull, vertebrae, sacrum, ribs, sternum)	Protects brain, spinal cord, sense organs, and soft tissues of chest cavity; supports the body weight over the legs
Appendicular Skeleton (limbs and supporting bones)	Provides internal support and positioning of arms and legs; supports and moves axial skeleton
Bone Marrow	Primary site of blood cell production

Clavicle (2) — Pectoral girdle (4)
Scapula (2)

Humerus (2)

Radius (2) — Arms (60)
Ulna (2)
Carpals (16)
Metacarpals (10)
Phalanges (28)

Pelvic bone (coxa) (2) — Pelvic girdle (2)

Femur (2)
Patella (2)

Tibia (2) — Legs (60)
Fibula (2)

Tarsals (14)
Metatarsals (10)
Phalanges (28)

APPENDICULAR SKELETON (126)

SKELETAL SYSTEM (206)

AXIAL SKELETON (80)

Figure 36-1 ■ The skeletal system and its functions.

calcium, with roughly 99% of it deposited in the skeleton. Calcium ion homeostasis is maintained by a negative feedback system involving a pair of hormones with opposing effects. These hormones—parathyroid hormone and calcitonin—coordinate the storage, absorption, and excretion of calcium ions. Three target sites are involved: (1) bones (storage), (2) digestive tract (absorption), and (3) kidneys (excretion).

Osteoporosis

The bones of the skeleton become thinner and weaker as a normal part of the aging process. Inadequate *ossification* (the process of bone formation) is called **osteopenia**, and most people become slightly osteopenic as they age. This reduction in bone mass begins between the ages of 30 and 40.

When the reduction in bone mass is sufficient to compromise normal function, the condition is known as **osteoporosis**. As bones become more fragile, they are likely to break when exposed to stresses that younger individuals could easily tolerate. For example, a hip fracture can occur when a woman in her 90s simply tries to stand. Any fractures that do occur lead to loss of independence and immobility that further weakens the skeleton.

With its loss of normal bone density, osteoporosis literally leads to porous bone that can be described as being compressible like a sponge rather than dense like a brick. It occurs more often in women than in men, especially in postmenopausal women, whose levels of the hormone estrogen are greatly decreased. Osteoporosis can cause permanent disability if not arrested, and the treatment varies depending on the cause.

AGENTS AFFECTING POSTMENOPAUSAL OSTEOPOROSIS

The treatment of postmenopausal osteoporosis is an important area of new drug development because estrogen replacement therapy (ERT) and hormone replacement therapy (HRT)—once popular forms of treatment for several postmenopausal conditions, including osteoporosis—have been associated with increased cardiovascular problems as well as a potential increased risk of endometrial and breast cancer in some patients (Table 36-1 ■). New drug developments include the selective estrogen-receptor modulators (SERMs), such as raloxifene, plus new-generation bisphosphonates.

For patients who are unable to take ERT or bisphosphonates, such hormonal agents as calcitonin and raloxifene are often prescribed.

Table 36-1 ■ Drugs Used to Treat Osteoporosis

GENERIC NAME	TRADE NAME	AVERAGE ADULT DOSAGE	ROUTE OF ADMINISTRATION
Bisphosphonates			
alendronate sodium	Fosamax	5–10 mg/d 70 mg once a wk	PO
risedronate sodium	Actonel	5 mg/d	PO
Hormonal Agents			
calcitonin salmon	Calcimar, Miacalcin	1 spray/d	Intranasal spray
raloxifene	Evista	60 mg/d	PO
sodium fluoride	(Generic only)	In cycles	PO
PO, oral.			

Focus On

Bisphosphonates

The first bisphosphonate available for clinical use was etidronate, but several new analogues are now available, including pamidronate, alendronate, tiludronate, and risedronate. For the treatment of osteoporosis, only alendronate and risedronate are used. Alendronate was the first oral bisphosphonate to be approved for the treatment and prevention of osteoporosis in postmenopausal women.

How do they work?

Alendronate is a highly selective inhibitor of bone demineralization and *resorption* (breakdown). It appears to
(*continued*)

Focus On (continued)

increase bone mineral density. The mechanism of action of risedronate is not fully understood.

How are they used?

Only alendronate and risedronate have been approved for the treatment of osteoporosis, but other bisphosphonates are used for other purposes. For example, etidronate, pamidronate, and tiludronate are used for Paget's disease, a disorder similar to osteoporosis in that bones become very weak and brittle but are characterized by constant bone resorption and formation, resulting in enlarged and abnormal bones. Pamidronate is also indicated for hypercalcemia of malignancy. Ibandronate sodium is a once-monthly medication for postmenopausal osteoarthritis used to build bone mass and maintain bone density.

What are the adverse effects?

Several gastrointestinal (GI) adverse effects may occur that include **flatulence** (presence of excess gas in the stomach and intestines), acid regurgitation, **dysphagia** (difficulty in swallowing), and gastritis. Other effects include headache, musculoskeletal pain, and rash.

What are the contraindications and interactions?

Alendronate and risedronate are contraindicated in hypersensitivity to these agents, severe renal impairment, hypocalcemia, lactation, and pregnancy. These agents should be used cautiously in patients with renal impairment, congestive heart failure, hyperphosphatemia, liver disease, fever or infection, and peptic ulcer. Calcium and food (especially dairy products) reduce alendronate absorption.

What are the important points patients should know?

Review with patients the correct administration of these medications and advise them to report fever, especially when accompanied by arthralgia and myalgia. Instruct patients to take the drugs at least 30 minutes before food, beverages, or other medications. Women should not breastfeed while taking these drugs.

Calcitonin

Calcitonin is secreted by the parafollicular cells of the thyroid glands of mammals. Calcitonin is a natural product obtained from salmon. Human calcitonin is also available but is not as potent or long lasting.

How does it work?

The principal effects of calcitonin are to lower serum calcium and phosphate by action on the bones and kidneys. Calcitonin inhibits bone resorption and lowers serum calcium. Thus, calcitonin increases bone density and reduces the risk of vertebral fractures.

How is it used?

Calcitonin is approved for the treatment of osteoporosis in postmenopausal women, hypercalcemia, and symptomatic Paget's disease.

What are the adverse effects?

The adverse effects of calcitonin include headache, eye pain, hypersensitivity reactions, and anaphylaxis (reported for human calcitonin only). Urination frequency, chills, chest pressure, weakness, dizziness, nasal congestion, and shortness of breath are other adverse effects of calcitonin.

What are the contraindications and interactions?

Calcitonin is contraindicated in patients with hypersensitivity to fish proteins or to synthetic calcitonin. It should be avoided in patients with a history of allergy. Safe use in children and during pregnancy and lactation is not established. Calcitonin should be used cautiously in patients with renal impairment and pernicious anemia. Calcitonin may interact with and may decrease serum lithium levels.

What are the important points patients should know?

Advise patients to watch for redness, warmth, or swelling at the injection site and to report any of these effects to their physician because they may indicate an inflammatory reaction. Instruct patients to consult their physician before using such over-the-counter (OTC) preparations as some supervitamins, hematinics (which improve the condition of the blood), and antacids containing calcium and vitamin D.

Focus on Natural Products

Dimethyl Sulfoxide

Dimethyl sulfoxide (DMSO) has a long history as a topical agent that can help reduce pain and inflammation in various musculoskeletal disorders, such as tendonitis. DMSO should only be used under the guidance of a qualified health care professional.

Focus On

Raloxifene Hydrochloride

Raloxifene is one of the SERMs and is considered to be an estrogen antagonist.

How does it work?

Raloxifene acts by combining with estrogen receptors. It decreases bone resorption and increases bone mass and density by acting through the estrogen receptor. Raloxifene has not been associated with endometrial proliferation or the increased risk of uterine or breast cancers.

How is it used?

Raloxifene is used primarily to prevent and treat osteoporosis in postmenopausal women. It is also used to reduce the risk of breast cancer in postmenopausal women. This agent is able to reduce total serum cholesterol and low-density lipoprotein.

What are the adverse effects?

The adverse effects of raloxifene include hot flashes, migraines, headache, flu-like symptoms, uterine disorders, vaginal bleeding, urinary tract disorders, and breast pain. Other adverse effects are depression, insomnia, and dizziness.

What are the contraindications and interactions?

Raloxifene is contraindicated in women who are or who might become pregnant and in those with active (or a history of) venous thromboembolic events (e.g., pulmonary embolism or retinal vein thrombosis). It is also contraindicated with the concurrent use of a systemic ERT. Raloxifene should be used cautiously with diazepam, lidocaine, and diazoxide. It can interact with cholestyramine and warfarin.

What are the important points patients should know?

Advise patients to contact their physician immediately if unexplained calf pain or tenderness occurs. They should avoid prolonged restriction of movement during travel. Be sure patients are aware that raloxifene can induce hot flashes. Patients should not breastfeed while taking this drug.

Focus Point

Raloxifene

Raloxifene is the first of the SERMs to be approved for the prevention of osteoporosis.

✳ Apply Your Knowledge 36.1

The following questions focus on what you have just learned about the musculoskeletal system, osteoporosis, and related medications.

CRITICAL THINKING

1. What is osteoporosis?
2. What are the primary functions of the skeletal system?
3. What hormones coordinate the storage, absorption, and excretion of calcium ions?
4. What drugs are used to treat or prevent osteoporosis?
5. What is the mechanism of action of calcitonin?
6. What are the indicators of raloxifene?

Rheumatoid Arthritis

Rheumatoid arthritis (RA) is a systemic autoimmune disease that involves the inflammation of the membranes lining the joints and often affects internal organs. Most patients exhibit a chronic fluctuating course of disease that can result in progressive joint destruction, deformity, and disability. It occurs two to three times more often in women, and the peak onset occurs between the fourth and sixth decades of life.

Most commonly, the joints first affected by RA include the metacarpophalangeal joints of the hands, metatarsophalangeal joints of the feet, and the wrists. Other areas affected by this disease include the spine, shoulders, ankles, and hips. RA involves not only joint capsules but also tendons, ligaments, and skeletal muscles. The goals in the management of RA are to:

✳ Prevent or control joint damage

✳ Prevent loss of function

✳ Decrease pain

✳ Maintain the patient's quality of life

✳ Avoid or minimize adverse effects of the treatment

ANTIRHEUMATIC DRUGS

Drug therapy for RA involves the treatment of symptoms and the use of disease-modifying agents. Drugs with anti-inflammatory activity are the agents of choice for the symptomatic relief of RA. Salicylates, NSAIDs, and cyclooxygenase 2 (COX-2) inhibitors (as discussed in Chapter 21) reduce joint pain and swelling, but they do not alter the course of the disease or prevent joint destruction. Corticosteroids have excellent anti-inflammatory activity and are immunosuppressants. Disease-modifying antirheumatic drugs (DMARDs) reduce or prevent joint damage and preserve joint function. DMARDs are listed in Table 36-2 ■. Penicillamine is a metabolite of penicillin and is rarely used today because of toxicity. Therefore, it is not discussed here for the treatment of RA.

Table 36-2 ■ Disease-Modifying Drugs for Rheumatoid Arthritis

GENERIC NAME	TRADE NAME	AVERAGE ADULT DOSAGE	ROUTE OF ADMINISTRATION
Gold Compounds			
auranofin	Ridaura	3–6 mg/d; may increase up to 3 mg tid after 6 mo	PO
aurothioglucose	Solganal	10–50 mg; initially, 10 mg and then increased weekly until 1 g is reached	IM
gold sodium thiomalate	Myochrysine	Dose may be continued at 25–50 mg every other wk for 2–20 wk	IM

GENERIC NAME	TRADE NAME	AVERAGE ADULT DOSAGE	ROUTE OF ADMINISTRATION
Miscellaneous Agents			
adalimumab	Humira	40 mg every other wk (may use 40 mg/wk if not on concomitant methotrexate)	SC
etanercept	Enbrel	25 mg twice weekly or 0.08 mg/kg (or 50 mg) once weekly	SC
hydroxychloroquine sulfate	Plaquenil	200–600 mg/d	PO
methotrexate	Trexall	Single dose of 7.5 mg weekly, or divided doses of 2.5 mg q12h, for 3 doses, given once weekly	PO
sulfasalazine	Azulfidine	250–500 mg/d (maximum: 8 g/d)	PO

tid, three times a day; PO, oral;. IM, intramuscular; SC, subcutaneous.

Focus On

Gold Compounds

Gold compounds, such as auranofin, aurothioglucose, and gold sodium thiomalate, were first proved to be effective in a large group of patients in 1960. Because of their toxicity, they are used infrequently today.

How do they work?

The mechanism of anti-inflammatory action of gold compounds is not clearly understood. Gold uptake by macrophages with subsequent inhibition of migration and phagocytic action occurs, thereby suppressing immune responsiveness, which may be the principal mechanism of action.

How are they used?

Gold compounds are effective for active RA. They are generally used when adequate trials with salicylates or other NSAIDs have not been satisfactory.

What are the adverse effects?

The adverse effects of gold compounds include hypersensitivity, syncope, bradycardia, thickening of the tongue, and a metallic taste in the mouth. Hematologic abnormalities are thrombocytopenia, leukopenia, and aplastic anemia.

What are the contraindications and interactions?

These agents are contraindicated in patients with a gold allergy or a history of severe toxicity from previous therapy with gold or other heavy metals. Gold compounds should not be used in patients with uncontrolled diabetes mellitus, renal or hepatic insufficiency, or a history of hepatitis. Gold compounds may increase the risk of blood dyscrasias if they are used with antimalarials, immunosuppressants, and penicillamine, another DMARD.

What are the important points patients should know?

Be sure that patients are aware of possible adverse effects and know to report them to their physicians. If therapy is interrupted at the onset of gold toxicity, serious reactions can be avoided. Advise patients to report any unusual color or odor of their urine and to avoid contact with anyone who has a cold, has had a recent vaccination, or has been recently exposed to a communicable disease.

Focus Point

Gold Compounds

Adverse reactions to gold compounds are most likely to occur during the second and third months of therapy. However, reactions may appear at any time during therapy or even several months after treatment has been discontinued.

Focus On

Hydroxychloroquine

Hydroxychloroquine sulfate is classified as an anti-infective and an antimalarial. This agent is used mainly to treat malaria.

How does it work?

The mechanism of the anti-inflammatory action of this drug in rheumatic diseases is unclear.

How is it used?

Hydroxychloroquine is approved for RA but is not considered one of the most efficacious DMARDs. Hydroxychloroquine is often used for the treatment of lupus erythematosus.

What are the adverse effects?

The adverse effects of hydroxychloroquine are fatigue, headache, mood or mental changes, anxiety, retinopathy, blurred vision, and difficulty focusing. Other adverse effects include anorexia, nausea and vomiting, diarrhea, and abdominal cramps.

What are the contraindications and interactions?

Hydroxychloroquine is contraindicated in patients with known hypersensitivity to this agent. Safe use in pregnancy and lactation is not established. Hydroxychloroquine must be used cautiously in patients with hepatic disease, alcoholism, and impaired renal function.

Antacids and laxatives that contain aluminum or magnesium decrease hydroxychloroquine absorption. This agent may interfere with the response to rabies vaccine.

What are the important points patients should know?

Teach patients about the adverse effects and symptoms of prolonged therapy with this drug. Advise them to follow the drug regimen exactly as prescribed by their physician and to make sure to keep this drug out of the reach of children. Because this drug may cause damage to the eyes, advise patients to get regular eye examinations. Instruct patients to avoid breastfeeding while taking this drug without consulting their physician.

Focus on Pediatrics

Hydroxychloroquine

Hydroxychloroquine has not been established for safe use in juvenile arthritis. It should not be used during pregnancy (because it crosses the placental barrier) nor during lactation.

Focus On

Methotrexate

Formerly called amethopterin, methotrexate was once considered the DMARD of first choice in the treatment of patients with RA. However, newer DMARDs, such as adalimumab and etanercept, are becoming first-choice agents (see Table 36-2).

How does it work?

Methotrexate is a folic acid blocker and immunosuppressant that affects lymphocyte and macrophage function.

How is it used?

Methotrexate is principally used in combination regimens to maintain induced remissions in patients with neoplastic diseases. Methotrexate is also used to treat those with severe psoriasis, psoriatic arthritis, and RA.

What are the adverse effects?

The most common toxicity of methotrexate is dose-related bone marrow suppression. Infertility with *azoospermia* (absence of living spermatozoa in the semen) and amenorrhea also occur. GI upset and mouth sores are less serious common adverse effects.

What are the contraindications and interactions?

Methotrexate is contraindicated in pregnancy and lactation, in men and women of childbearing age, hepatic and renal insufficiency, and preexisting blood dyscrasias. Methotrexate should be used cautiously in patients with infections, peptic ulcer, ulcerative colitis, cancer patients with preexisting bone marrow impairment, and poor nutritional status.

Alcohol, azathioprine, and sulfasalazine increase the risk of hepatotoxicity if used with methotrexate. Chloramphenicol, sulfonamides, salicylates, NSAIDs, phenytoin, tetracyclines, and probenecid may increase methotrexate levels with increased toxicity.

What are the important points patients should know?

Be sure patients are aware of the dangers of this drug and know to promptly report any abnormal symptoms to their physician. They should know that the most common adverse affects are stomach upset, mouth sores, headache, and drowsiness. Alcohol ingestion increases the incidence and severity of methotrexate hepatotoxicity. Instruct patients that they should not self-medicate with vitamins or OTC compounds that include folic acid, which alters methotrexate response. They should avoid exposure to sunlight and ultraviolet light and wear sunglasses and sunscreen.

Focus Point

Methotrexate

P rolonged treatment with small frequent doses of methotrexate may lead to hepatotoxicity, which is best diagnosed by liver biopsy.

Focus On

Sulfasalazine

Sulfasalazine is a GI and anti-inflammatory agent.

How does it work?

Sulfasalazine is a locally acting sulfonamide that is believed to be converted by intestinal microflora to sulfapyridine, providing antibacterial action, and to 5-aminosalicylic acid or mesalamine, which may exert an anti-inflammatory effect. It may also inhibit prostaglandins that are known to cause diarrhea and affect mucosal transport as well as interfere with the absorption of fluids and electrolytes from the colon.

(continued)

Focus On (continued)

How is it used?

Sulfasalazine is effective in RA and reduces the rate of appearance of new joint damage. It has been used in juvenile chronic arthritis and ankylosing spondylitis.

What are the adverse effects?

Approximately 30% of patients using sulfasalazine discontinue the drug because of toxicity. Common adverse effects include nausea and vomiting, headache, and rash. Other adverse effects include anemia, **oligospermia** (a subnormal concentration of spermatozoa in the ejaculate), blood dyscrasias, liver injury, and allergic reactions.

What are the contraindications and interactions?

Sulfasalazine is contraindicated in patients with sensitivity to this agent or other sulfonamides and salicylates.

It should not be used in patients with agranulocytosis, intestinal and urinary tract obstruction, or porphyria. Sulfasalazine is contraindicated in pregnancy and in children younger than 2 years of age. It should be used cautiously in patients with severe allergy or bronchial asthma, hepatic or renal impairment, and in children younger than age 6. Antibiotics may alter the absorption of sulfasalazine.

What are the important points patients should know?

Instruct patients that this drug may color the urine and skin orange-yellow. Women should not breastfeed while taking sulfasalazine without consulting their physician.

✳ Apply Your Knowledge 36.2

The following questions focus on what you have just learned about RA and antirheumatic drugs.

CRITICAL THINKING

1. What is the definition of *RA*?
2. What are the drugs of choice for the symptomatic relief of RA?
3. What are three generic names of gold compounds for RA?
4. What are the adverse effects of gold compounds?
5. What are DMARDs?
6. What is the mechanism of action of methotrexate?
7. What are the indications of sulfasalazine?
8. What are the contraindications of gold compounds?

Gout and Gouty Arthritis

Several distinct diseases are characterized by crystal deposition in and around joint spaces. This deposition can lead to acute inflammation of the joint. Gout is a metabolic disorder of sodium urate deposition (which involves uric acid crystals) in which uric acid accumulates in the bloodstream or joint cavities, causing inflammation and pain. Gout is classified as primary, secondary, or gouty arthritis. Primary gout is a disease primarily found in men, with a peak incidence in the fifth decade of life.

The cause of gout is either the overproduction or underexcretion of uric acid. Primary gout is generally caused by the overproduction of uric acid and may be caused by enzyme deficiencies in the metabolic pathway for purines or genetic dysfunction. Secondary gout, characterized by underexcretion of uric acid, may be caused by diminished renal function, interaction with various medications, or unknown causes.

Primary gout has three manifestations: (1) asymptomatic **hyperuricemia** (elevated uric acid blood level), (2) acute gouty arthritis, and (3) chronic gouty arthritis. In acute gouty arthritis, the onset of the attack is abrupt and typically occurs at night or early in the morning as synovial fluid is reabsorbed. In acute gouty arthritis, immobilization of the affected joints—most often the big toes, heels, ankles, wrists, fingers, elbows, or knees—is very important.

ANTIGOUT DRUGS

Anti-inflammatory drug therapy should begin immediately, and urate-lowering drugs should not be given until the acute attack has been controlled. Specific drugs include colchicine, allopurinol, NSAIDs, and corticosteroids (Table 36-3 ■).

Table 36-3 ■ Antigout Medications

GENERIC NAME	TRADE NAME	AVERAGE ADULT DOSAGE	ROUTE OF ADMINISTRATION
allopurinol	Aloprim, Zyloprim	200–800 mg/d	PO, IV
colchicine	Colchicine	0.5–0.6 mg/d prophylactically; 0.5–1.2 mg q1–2h for acute attack	PO
probenecid	Benemid	250–500 mg bid	PO
sulfinpyrazone	Anturane	100–400 mg/d	PO

PO, oral; IV, intravenous; bid, twice a day.

Focus On

Colchicine

Colchicine is an anti-inflammatory agent specifically used for gout and is ineffective for any other disease. Colchicine is not an analgesic, so it does not relieve the symptoms of any condition but gout.

How does it work?

Colchicine acts by inhibiting the formation of white blood cells, which decreases joint inflammation.

How is it used

Colchicine may be used to treat acute gouty attacks or to reduce the incidence of attacks in chronic gout.

What are the adverse effects?

The most common adverse effects are GI disturbances, such as nausea and vomiting, diarrhea, and abdominal pain. Colchicine may decrease the intestinal absorption of vitamin B_{12}.

What are the contraindications and interactions?

Colchicine is contraindicated in blood dyscrasias, severe GI conditions, severe renal conditions, severe hepatic conditions, and severe cardiac disease. The use of IV colchicine is contraindicated in patients with renal and hepatic dysfunction. Severe local irritation can result from subcutaneous or intramuscular use. It is also contraindicated during pregnancy, and its safe use in children has not been established.

What are the important points patients should know?

Instruct patients taking colchicine at home to withhold the drug and to report to their physicians any onset of GI symptoms or signs of bone marrow depression (nausea, sore throat, bleeding gums, sore mouth, fever, fatigue, malaise, and unusual bleeding or bruising). Advise patients to keep colchicine on hand at all times to start therapy or to increase dosage—if a physician directs—at the first suggestion of an acute attack. Advise patients to avoid beer, ale, and wine because they may precipitate gouty attack. Women taking colchicine should not breast-feed without consulting their physician.

Focus on Geriatrics

Colchicine Use in Elderly Patients

Colchicine should be used with care in older adults because of the dangers of cardiac, renal, hepatic, and GI diseases.

Focus On

Allopurinol

Allopurinol is known as an antigout agent because it improves the solubility of uric acid. It is used for chronic gout and will not relieve an attack already started. The drug must be taken regularly for a few months to be effective.

How does it work?

Allopurinol reduces endogenous uric acid by selectively inhibiting the action of xanthine oxidase, the enzyme responsible for converting xanthine derivatives to uric acid (the end product of purine catabolism). Allopurinol has no analgesic, anti-inflammatory, or *uricosuric* (increasing excretion of uric acid) actions.

How is it used?

Allopurinol is used to control primary hyperuricemia that accompanies severe gout and to prevent possibilities of acute gouty attack.

What are the adverse effects?

Allopurinol may cause drowsiness, headache, dizziness, nausea and vomiting, diarrhea, and abdominal pain. In some cases, this agent may cause hepatotoxicity and renal insufficiency. Allopurinol can produce pruritus and skin rash.

What are the contraindications and interactions?

Allopurinol is contraindicated in patients with hypersensitivity to this agent. Allopurinol is also contraindicated as an initial treatment for acute gouty attacks. This medication should be avoided in children (except in those with hyperuricemia secondary to cancer and chemotherapy). Safety during pregnancy and lactation is not established. Allopurinol should be used cautiously in patients with impaired hepatic or renal function, a history of peptic ulcer, lower GI tract disease, and bone marrow depression.

Drug interaction of allopurinol with alcohol, caffeine, and thiazide diuretics may increase the uric acid level; it may also increase the risk of skin rash if used with ampicillin and amoxicillin. Allopurinol enhances the anticoagulant effect of warfarin.

What are the important points patients should know?

Advise patients to drink enough fluid (at least 3,000 mL, or 3 quarts, per day) to produce a urine output of at least 2,000 mL, or 2 quarts, per day. Instruct patients to report diminishing urine output, cloudy urine, an unusual color or odor of urine, pain or discomfort on urination, and the onset of itching or rash. Tell patients to stop taking allopurinol if a skin rash appears even after 5 or more weeks of therapy. Patients should minimize exposure to ultraviolet light or sunlight and not drive or engage in potentially hazardous activities until their response to this drug is known. This drug should only be taken under constant medical supervision, and women taking allopurinol should not breastfeed without consulting their physician.

Uricosuric Agents

Probenecid and sulfinpyrazone are uricosuric drugs that are used to decrease the amount of urate in patients with increasingly frequent gouty attacks.

How do they work?

These agents work by competitively inhibiting the renal tubular reabsorption of uric acid, thereby promoting its excretion and reducing serum urate levels.

How are they used?

Uricosuric therapy should be initiated if several acute attacks of gouty arthritis have occurred or when plasma levels of uric acid in patients with gout are so high that tissue damage is almost inevitable.

What are the adverse effects?

Adverse effects of uricosuric agents do not provide a basis for preferring one or the other. Both of these organic acids cause GI irritation, but sulfinpyrazone is more active in this regard. Probenecid is more likely to cause allergic dermatitis, but a rash may appear after the use of either compound. Another adverse effect of using probenecid is **nephrotic syndrome** (a clinical state characterized by edema, various abnormal substances present in the urine, decreased plasma albumin, and usually increased blood cholesterol).

What are the contraindications and interactions?

Uricosuric therapy is contraindicated in patients with blood dyscrasias and uric acid kidney stones. Safety during pregnancy, lactation, and in children younger than 2 years of age has not been established. These agents should be used cautiously in patients with a history of peptic ulcer.

Salicylates may decrease uricosuric activity and methotrexate elimination. There is an increased risk of nitrofurantoin toxicity if used with probenecid or sulfinpyrazone.

What are the important points patients should know?

Advise patients to drink fluids liberally (approximately 3,000 mL per day) to maintain daily urine output of at least 2,000 mL or more. Physicians may advise the restriction of high-purine foods during early therapy until uric acid levels stabilize. Foods high in purine include organ meats (sweetbreads, liver, kidneys), meat extracts, meat soups, and gravy. Instruct patients to avoid alcohol because it may increase serum urate levels. They should be instructed not to stop taking these drugs or to take aspirin or other OTC medications without first consulting their physician.

Focus Point

Uricosuric Therapy

Urate-lowering drugs should not be started until after the acute attack has completely resolved—a process that takes 2–3 weeks.

✳ Apply Your Knowledge 36.3

The following questions focus on what you have just learned about gouty arthritis and its drug therapy.

CRITICAL THINKING

1. What are the definitions of *gout* and *gouty arthritis*?
2. How many types of gout are known?
3. What are the trade names of probenecid, allopurinol, and sulfinpyrazone?
4. What drug is specifically used for gout and what are the most common adverse effects of this agent?
5. What is the mechanism of action of allopurinol?
6. What are examples of uricosuric agents?

Muscle Spasms and Pain

Muscular spasms and pain are often associated with traumatic injuries and **spasticity** (an inability of opposing muscle groups to move in a coordinated manner) from such chronic debilitating disorders as cerebral palsy, stroke, or head and spinal cord injuries. Muscle spasms can also be caused by an overmedication of antipsychotic drugs, epilepsy, and hypocalcemia.

The transmission of impulses from motor nerves to muscle cells occurs across spaces known as *neuromuscular junctions*. These spaces are sensitive to chemical changes in their immediate environment. Therefore, somatic motor nerve impulses cannot be generated, which may also decrease the availability of calcium ions to the myofibrillar contractile system.

There are two types of muscle spasms: tonic and clonic. Whereas a single, prolonged contraction is called a *tonic spasm*, multiple, rapidly repeated contractions are known as *clonic spasms*. Most muscle spasms and strains are self-limited and respond to rest, physical therapy, and the short-term use of aspirin and other analgesics.

SKELETAL MUSCLE RELAXANTS

The treatment of muscle spasms may be nonpharmacologic and pharmacologic (muscle relaxants). Nonpharmacologic treatments include the immobilization of the affected muscle, the application of heat or cold, ultrasonography, hydrotherapy, and massage. Local anesthesia may also effect the relaxation of limited muscle groups, and the local anesthetic block of efferent somatic motor outflow is sometimes used to relieve localized skeletal muscle spasms.

Spasticity results from increased muscle tone caused by hyperexcitable neurons or a lack of inhibition in the spinal cord (or at the skeletal muscles). Many neurologic disorders that cause spasticity require the long-term use of muscle relaxants. The skeletal muscles are voluntary muscles under control of the central nervous system (CNS). Skeletal muscle relaxants work by blocking somatic motor nerve impulses through the depression of specific neurons within the CNS.

Focus On

Centrally Acting Muscle Relaxants

These agents, such as baclofen, cyclobenzaprine, and lorazepam, relieve symptoms of muscular stiffness and rigidity. Centrally acting muscle relaxants improve the mobility of the part of the body that is affected. Pharmacotherapy for muscle spasms can be a combination of analgesics, anti-inflammatory medications, and centrally acting skeletal muscle relaxants. The centrally acting muscle relaxants are listed in Table 36-4 ■.

How do they work?

The exact mechanism of action of these agents is unknown, but they may affect the brain or spinal cord to inhibit upper motor neuron activity.

How are they used?

Skeletal muscle relaxants are used to treat local spasms to reduce pain and increase range of motion. Baclofen is often a drug of first choice because of its wide safety margin.

What are the adverse effects?

All the centrally acting agents can cause sedation. Common adverse effects include drowsiness, dizziness, weakness, and fatigue. Tizanidine and other centrally acting agents may cause hallucinations or *ataxia* (loss of coordination, such as that caused by benzodiazepines).

What are the contraindications and interactions?

Baclofen is contraindicated in patients with *bacteremia* (the presence of viable bacteria in circulating blood) and clotting disorders. Carisoprodol should be avoided in patients with acute intermittent porphyria and in children younger than age 5 years. Clonazepam is contraindicated in patients with liver disease and glaucoma. None of the centrally acting muscle relaxants should be used during pregnancy and lactation.

Centrally acting muscle relaxants, such as baclofen, should not be used with alcohol and other CNS depressants, monoamine oxidase inhibitors, and antihistamines. Baclofen may increase blood glucose levels, making it necessary to increase the dosages of sulfonylureas and insulin.

What are the important points patients should know?

Instruct patients to avoid consuming alcoholic beverages and other CNS depressants because this combination will potentiate CNS depression. Incidence of CNS symptoms are reportedly high in patients older than 40 years. Advise patients with diabetes to closely monitor their blood glucose for loss of glycemic control. Patients should avoid driving and using heavy machinery until the effect is stabilized because these drugs are prone to cause drowsiness and dizziness. Tell patients to report all adverse reactions to their physician. Instruct patients not to self-dose with OTC drugs without their physician's approval. These drugs should not be stopped abruptly, and the stopping of these drugs should be directed by a physician. Instruct female patients that these drugs should not be taken during pregnancy or while breastfeeding.

Table 36-4 ■ Centrally Acting Muscle Relaxants

GENERIC NAME	TRADE NAME	AVERAGE ADULT DOSAGE	ROUTE OF ADMINISTRATION
baclofen	Baclofen	15–80 mg/d in divided doses	PO
carisoprodol	Soma	350 mg tid–qid	PO
chlorzoxazone	Parafon Forte	250–750 mg tid–qid	PO
clonazepam	Klonopin	0.5–20 mg tid	PO
cyclobenzaprine	Flexeril	10–60 mg/d in divided doses	PO
dantrolene	Dantrium	Initially, 25 mg/d and then 50–400 mg/d in divided doses	PO
diazepam	Valium	2–10 mg bid–qid	PO
		2–10 mg	IM, IV
lorazepam	Ativan	1–10 mg bid–tid	PO
methocarbamol	Robaxin	1.5 g qid for 2–3 d and then 4–4.5 g/d in 3–6 divided doses	PO
		0.5–1 g q8h	IM
		1–3 g/d in divided doses (maximum: rate of 300 mg/min)	IV
orphenadrine citrate	Norflex	100 mg bid	PO
		60 mg bid	IM, IV

PO, oral; tid, three times a day; qid, four times a day; bid, twice a day; IM, intramuscular; IV, intravenous.

Focus Point

Baclofen

Baclofen is at least as effective as diazepam in reducing spasticity and produces much less sedation.

✱ Apply Your Knowledge 36.4

The following questions focus on what you have just learned about skeletal muscle relaxants and centrally acting muscle relaxants.

CRITICAL THINKING

1. What are neuromuscular junctions?
2. How many types of muscle spasms are known?
3. What are the nonpharmacologic treatments for muscle relaxants?
4. What is the drug of first choice of the centrally acting muscle relaxants?
5. What are the trade names of lorazepam, methocarbamol, and dantrolene?

PRACTICAL SCENARIO 1

Leonora, a slightly built 73-year-old woman, visits her long-time family physician complaining of low-grade but constant back pain. The nurse's examination finds that her weight has remained consistent over time but that she has lost almost 2 inches in height in the past 10 years. Reviewing her chart, the doctor notes that Leonora has been postmenopausal for more than 25 years, declined to take hormone replacement therapy, and broke her ankle 2 years ago after stepping off a curb into the street. Physical examination shows *kyphosis* (humpback or hunchback). The physician orders a dual-emission X-ray absorptiometry scan to measure bone density but tells Leonora that even without the results of the scan, she is quite sure that the osteopenia most people experience as they get older has, in this case, degenerated into osteoporosis.

Bill Aron/PhotoEdit

Critical Thinking Questions

1. What is the significance of the fact that Leonora has been postmenopausal for many years?
2. What is the difference between osteopenia and osteoporosis and why does one lead to a reduction in height in patients?
3. Would drug therapy or lifestyle changes work best for Leonora in managing her osteoporosis?

PRACTICAL SCENARIO 2

A 56-year-old postmenopausal woman was diagnosed with osteoporosis. Her physician prescribed bisphosphonates.

Alexander Raths/Shutterstock

Critical Thinking Questions

1. Explain several new bisphosphonate analogs that are now available.
2. Explain the common adverse effects of bisphosphonates.

Chapter Capsule

This section repeats the objectives from the beginning of the chapter and then provides the most important concept for that objective. Use this section as a quick review and to check your knowledge.

Objective 1: Describe the major functions of the skeletal system.

■   Support, storage of minerals and lipids, blood cell production, protection, and leverage

Objective 2: Identify the most common bisphosphonate agents used for osteoporosis.

- Alendronate: first oral bisphosphonate approved for treatment and prevention of osteoporosis in postmenopausal women

- Risedronate

Objective 3: Define *rheumatoid arthritis*.

- Systemic autoimmune disease; involves inflammation of the membranes lining the joints; often affects internal organs

- A chronic fluctuating course of disease that can result in progressive joint destruction, deformity, and disability

- Occurs two to three times more often in women; peak onset is between the fourth and sixth decades of life

Objective 4: List the major drugs used for rheumatoid arthritis.

- Treatment of symptoms: drugs with anti-inflammatory activity, such as salicylates, nonsteroidal anti-inflammatory drugs (NSAIDs), and cyclooxygenase 2 (COX-2) inhibitors; corticosteroids have excellent anti-inflammatory activity and are immunosuppressants

- Treatment to prevent joint damage and preserve joint function: disease-modifying antirheumatic drugs (DMARDs), such as methotrexate, sulfasalazine, etanercept, and adalimumab

Objective 5: Describe the major indications of methotrexate.

- Principally used in combination regimens to maintain induced remissions in neoplastic diseases; also used to treat severe psoriasis, psoriatic arthritis, and rheumatoid arthritis

Objective 6: Explain gouty arthritis and the cause of gout.

- Disorder of sodium urate deposition (which involves uric acid crystals) characterized by crystal deposition in and about joint spaces, which can lead to acute inflammation of the joint

- Primarily a disease found in men, with a peak incidence in the fifth decade of life

- Caused by either an overproduction or underexcretion of uric acid

- Primary gout has three manifestations: asymptomatic hyperuricemia, acute gouty arthritis, and chronic gouty arthritis

- The onset of acute gouty arthritis is abrupt, typically occurring at night or early in the morning as synovial fluid is reabsorbed

Objective 7: Describe the mechanism of action for colchicine.

- Inhibits the formation of white blood cells to decrease joint inflammation

Objective 8: Explain the indications of allopurinol.

- Used to control primary hyperuricemia (high levels of uric acid in the blood circulation) that accompanies severe gout and to prevent acute gouty attack

Objective 9: Name three disorders that may cause spasticity.

- Cerebral palsy

- Stroke

- Head or spinal cord injuries

Objective 10: List commonly used central skeletal muscle relaxants.

- baclofen (Baclofen)

- carisoprodol (Soma)

- chlorzoxazone (Parafon Forte)

- clonazepam (Klonopin)

- cyclobenzaprine (Flexeril)

- dantrolene (Dantrium)

- diazepam (Valium)

- lorazepam (Ativan)

- methocarbamol (Robaxin)

- orphenadrine citrate (Norflex)

 Internet Sites of Interest

- The National Institute of Neurological Disorders and Stroke, a division of the NIH, provides information about spasticity and its treatments at: **www.ninds.nih.gov**. Search for "spasticity."

- MedicineNet.com provides an in-depth look at rheumatoid arthritis at: **www.medicinenet.com**. Search for "rheumatoid arthritis."

- Johns Hopkins University's Division of Rheumatology offers a comprehensive discussion about treatments for rheumatoid arthritis at: **www.hopkinsmedicine.org**. Search for "rheumatology."

- For more information about the rheumatoid arthritis drug methotrexate, visit: **www.rxlist.com/trexall-drug.htm**.

Chapter 37

Drugs Used to Treat Eye Conditions

Chapter Objectives

After completing this chapter, you should be able to:

1. Describe the structure and function of the eye.
2. Define the terms *cataract* and *retinopathy*.
3. Explain glaucoma and the types of glaucoma.
4. Identify the drugs of first choice for intraocular hypertension and chronic open-angle glaucoma, and explain how they work.
5. State the rationale for the use and the mechanism of action for carbonic anhydrase inhibitors in the treatment of glaucoma.
6. Identify direct-acting miotics (cholinergic drugs) and list two generic and trade names.
7. Discuss the adverse effects of indirect-acting miotics (cholinesterase inhibitors).
8. How do sympathomimetic agents and prostaglandin agonists work?
9. Explain mydriatic agents and their indications.
10. State the mechanism of action of antimuscarinics.

Key Terms

accommodation (p. 648)
aqueous humor (p. 648)
blepharitis (p. 656)
cataract (p. 649)
choroid layer (p. 648)
ciliary body (p. 648)
ciliary muscle (p. 648)

cornea (p. 648)
glaucoma (p. 649)
iris (p. 648)
lens (p. 648)
optic nerve (p. 648)
photoreceptors (p. 649)

pupil (p. 648)
retina (p. 649)
retinal detachment (p. 653)
retinopathy (p. 649)
sclera (p. 648)
vitreous humor (p. 649)

Introduction

A number of the key drug groups mentioned elsewhere in the text are used in ophthalmology. Such drug groups as antimicrobials, corticosteroids, adrenergic drugs, muscarinic drugs, and nonsteroidal anti-inflammatory drugs (NSAIDs) have ophthalmic indications. In this chapter, the effects of these drugs on the eye are emphasized.

Structure and Function of the Eye

The eye is a hollow, spherical structure about 2.5 cm in diameter. Its wall has three distinct layers. These layers consist of an outer layer (**sclera**), a middle layer (**choroid layer** or "coat"), and an inner layer (retina). The spaces within the eye are filled with fluids that support its wall and internal parts.

The anterior of the sclera bulges forward as the transparent **cornea**—the window of the eye—and helps to focus entering light rays. Along the circumference, the cornea is continuous with the sclera (the white portion of the eye). In the back of the eye, the **optic nerve** and certain blood vessels pierce the sclera.

The middle layer includes the choroid layer, ciliary body, and iris (Figure 37-1 ■). The choroid layer contains many pigment-producing melanocytes. The melanin that these cells produce absorbs excess light and helps to keep the inside of the eye dark.

The **ciliary body**, which is the thickest part of the middle layer, extends forward from the choroid layer and forms an internal ring around the front of the eye, which constitutes the **ciliary muscle**. Many strong but delicate fibers, called *suspensory ligaments*, extend inward from the ciliary processes and hold the transparent **lens** in position. The distal ends of these fibers attach along the margin of a thin capsule that surrounds the lens. The ciliary muscles and suspensory ligaments, along with the structure of the lens itself, enable the lens to adjust its shape to facilitate focusing—a phenomenon called **accommodation**. The functions of the ciliary body are controlled by the parasympathetic nervous system. The uveal tract of the eye consists of the iris, ciliary body, and choroid.

The **iris** is a thin diaphragm composed mostly of connective tissue and smooth muscle fibers. From the outside, the iris is the colored portion of the eye. The ciliary body secretes a watery fluid called **aqueous humor** into the posterior chamber. The iris extends forward from the periphery of the ciliary body and lies between the cornea and lens (see Figure 37-1). The fluid circulates from this chamber through the **pupil**—a circular opening in the center of the iris—and into the anterior chamber. Aqueous humor fills the space between the cornea and lens, helps nourish these parts, and aids in maintaining the shape of the front of the eye. It subsequently leaves the anterior chamber through veins and a special drainage canal—the scleral venous sinus (Schlemm canal)—located in its wall at the junction of the cornea and the sclera. The iris consists of circular and radially arranged bands of smooth muscle, innervated by the autonomic nervous system, that control the size of the pupil. The autonomic nervous system plays an important part in the regulation of eye functions.

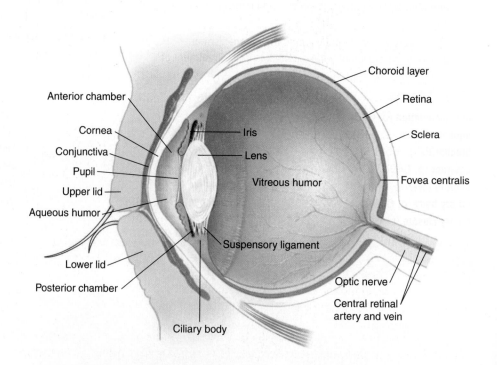

Figure 37-1 ■ Anatomy of the eye.

Table 37-1 ■ Effects of Autonomic Nervous System on the Eye

PARTS OF THE EYE	EFFECTS OF SYMPATHETIC STIMULATION	EFFECTS OF PARASYMPATHETIC STIMULATION
Ciliary muscle	Relaxation (for far vision)	Accommodation
Ciliary processes	Vasoconstriction of ciliary processes increases aqueous humor production	Increased outflow of aqueous humor and vasodilation
Iris	Contraction of the radial muscle: pupil dilation (mydriasis)	Contraction of the circular muscle: pupil constriction (miosis)
Conjunctival vasculature	Vasoconstriction	Vasodilation
Lacrimal apparatus	Vasoconstriction	Increased secretion and vasodilation

Such structures as the iris, ciliary body, lens, lacrimal glands, and ocular vasculature receive autonomic innervation. The effects of this stimulation are summarized in Table 37-1 ■.

The inner layer consists of the **retina**, which contains the visual receptor cells (**photoreceptors**). This layer is continuous with the optic nerve in the back of the eye and extends forward on the inner layer of the eyeball.

The space bounded by the lens, ciliary body, and retina is the largest compartment of the eye and is called the *posterior cavity*. It is filled with a transparent, jelly-like fluid called **vitreous humor**. The vitreous body supports the internal parts of the eye and helps maintain its shape.

Disorders of the Eye

The eyes are subject to various disorders, some of which are serious. These disorders may include inflammation, infections, injuries, glaucoma, **cataract** (an opacity of the lens of the eye), and diabetic **retinopathy** (degeneration of the blood vessels of the retina). One of the most common and serious disorders of the eye is glaucoma, for which treatment usually begins with medication. Therefore, in this chapter, most emphasis will be on drugs used in treatment of glaucoma. The other disorders or conditions of the eye that are initially treated with lasers or surgery are not discussed here. Anti-inflammatory drugs and antibiotics are explained in other chapters.

Focus on Pediatrics

Congenital Cataracts

Congenital cataracts may result from chromosomal abnormalities and maternal diseases during pregnancy. If the cataracts are dense and obscure the view of the optic disk, an ophthalmologist must determine the possible long-term effects on the infant's vision and surgery may be recommended.

GLAUCOMA

Glaucoma damages the optic nerve and is often caused by elevated intraocular pressure (IOP). This elevation of the IOP results from excessive production of aqueous humor or diminished ocular fluid outflow. When the pressure is persistently high, blindness may occur secondary to optic nerve damage. Glaucoma is the second-most common cause of blindness in the United States (cataract is number one). Normal IOP ranges from 11 to 21 mm Hg; however, this level may not necessarily be healthy for all people. Some people with normal

pressure develop optic nerve injury. In contrast, many patients have IOP of more than 21 mm Hg without any optic nerve injury (ocular hypertension). The two types of glaucoma are acute angle-closure and chronic open-angle glaucoma. Figure 37-2 ■ shows the normal condition of the eye as well as open-angle and angle-closure glaucoma.

Open-angle glaucoma is by far the more common form, accounting for about 90% of cases. Risk factors for primary open-angle glaucoma are listed in Table 37-2 ■. This type of glaucoma is generally responsive to drug therapy. Other treatments for open-angle glaucoma may

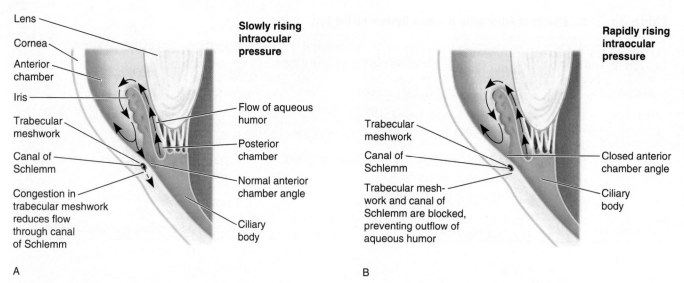

Figure 37-2 ■ The pathophysiology of glaucoma: (**A**) slowing rising intraocular pressure (IOP) and (**B**) rapidly rising IOP.

Table 37-2 ■ **Risk Factors for Primary Open-Angle Glaucoma**

Elevated intraocular pressure	Diabetes
Old age	Hypertension
Family history	Myopia
Black race	Use of corticosteroids

include lasers or surgery. Most of the drugs used in the treatment of open-angle glaucoma are also used in the acute management of narrow-angle glaucoma before surgery.

Angle-closure glaucoma accounts for 10% of all cases of glaucoma in the United States. Angle-closure glaucoma can be primarily caused by pupillary block. It is most common among Eskimos and Asians. Primary open-angle closure is more common in women, older adults, and those with a family history of angle-closure glaucoma.

Focus on Geriatrics

Glaucoma in Older Adults

Although glaucoma can occur in any age group, it is six times more common in persons older than 60 years of age.

✳ Apply Your Knowledge 37.1

The following questions focus on what you have just learned about the structure and function of the eye.

CRITICAL THINKING

1. What are the three layers of the eye?
2. Which layer of the eye contains the ciliary body?
3. What is the meaning of accommodation?
4. What are the iris and pupil?
5. Where is the location of the photoreceptors in the eye?
6. What is diabetic retinopathy?
7. How many types of glaucoma exist and which type is more common in women and older adults?
8. What are the risk factors for primary open-angle glaucoma?

Ophthalmic Preparations to Treat Glaucoma

Drug therapy is directed toward reducing the raised IOP. In general, the medications used either reduce the formation of aqueous humor or enhance the drainage of aqueous humor from the eye. Some drugs, such as adrenaline, possess both these actions. The drugs used for the treatment of glaucoma include beta-adrenergic blockers, cholinergic direct-acting agents (miotics), cholinesterase inhibitors, sympathomimetics, carbonic anhydrase inhibitors, and prostaglandin inhibitors (Table 37-3 ■).

Osmotic diuretic drugs are commonly used in patients needing eye surgery or for acute closed-angle glaucoma. These agents include glycerin anhydrous, isosorbide, and mannitol. The osmotic diuretics are discussed in Chapter 31.

Table 37-3 ■ Drug Therapies in Glaucoma that Decrease Formation of Aqueous Humor

GENERIC NAME	TRADE NAME	AVERAGE ADULT DOSAGE	ROUTE OF ADMINISTRATION
Beta-Adrenergic Blocking Agents			
betaxolol	Betoptic, Kerlone	1 drop 0.5% solution bid	Topical
carteolol	Carteolol Hydrochloride	1 drop 1% solution bid	Topical
levobunolol	Betagan	1–2 drops 0.25–0.5% solution 1–2 times/d	Topical
metipranolol	OptiPranolol	1 drop 0.3% solution bid	Topical
timolol	Betimol, Timoptic	1–2 drops of 0.25–0.5% solution 1–2 times/d	Topical
Alpha$_2$–Adrenergic Blocking Agents			
apraclonidine	Lopidine	1 drop 0.5% solution bid	Topical
brimonidine tartrate	Alphagan P	1 drop 0.2% solution bid	Topical
Carbonic Anhydrase Inhibitors			
acetazolamide	Diamox	250 mg 1–4 times/d	PO
dorzolamide hydrochloride	Trusopt	1 drop 2% solution tid	PO
methazolamide	Neptazane	50–100 mg bid–tid	PO
Osmotic Diuretics			
glycerine anhydrous (ophthalmic)	Ophthalgan	1–1.8 g/kg 1–1.5 h before ocular surgery; may repeat q5h	PO
isosorbide	Ismotic	1–3 g/kg bid–qid	PO
mannitol	Osmitrol	1.5–2 mg/kg as a 15–25% solution over 30–60 min	IV

bid, twice a day; PO, oral; tid, three times a day; qid, four times a day; IV, intravenous.

Focus On

Beta-Adrenergic Blockers

Beta-blocker agents are relatively safe, highly efficacious, act longer than the cholinergic agonists, and have no effects on pupil size or accommodation.

How do they work?

Beta-blockers lower the cyclic adenosine monophosphate (cAMP) levels within the ciliary body necessary for aqueous humor production. This reduces elevated IOP in chronic open-angle glaucoma by reducing the formation of aqueous humor.

How are they used?

The beta-blockers are considered the drugs of first choice in the treatment of intraocular hypertension and chronic open-angle glaucoma.

What are the adverse effects?

The most common adverse effects are local, mild ocular stinging; dry eyes; tearing; blurred vision; and eye irritation. Beta-adrenergic blockers may also have the adverse effects of systemic beta-blockers. These agents may mask symptoms of acute hypoglycemia in patients with diabetes (tachycardia and tremor but not sweating).

Beta-adrenergic blockers may precipitate thyrotoxic crisis in patients with hyperthyroidism.

What are the contraindications and interactions?

Beta-adrenergic blockers are contraindicated in patients with angle-closure glaucoma (unless used with a miotic), sinus bradycardia, and cardiogenic shock. Safety during pregnancy and in children younger than 18 years of age is not established. These drugs should be used cautiously in patients with heart failure or diabetes mellitus, in those who have evidence of airflow obstruction, and during lactation.

Reserpine may interact with beta-blockers and cause addictive hypotensive effects or bradycardia. Verapamil may cause addictive heart block.

What are the important points patients should know?

Advise patients to report unusual or significant changes in pulse rate to their physician, according to the parameters provided. Instruct patients to follow their dosing regimen exactly as prescribed. They should not stop these drugs abruptly. Instruct patients to report difficulty in breathing promptly to their physician because the drug may need to be withdrawn.

Carbonic Anhydrase Inhibitors

Carbonic anhydrase inhibitors are diuretic agents, but they are also available as eye preparations.

How do they work?

Carbonic anhydrase inhibitors act on the enzyme responsible for the conversion of carbon dioxide to bicarbonate and hydrogen ions. The mechanism of action of this group (in glaucoma) is different from that described for the kidneys in Chapter 31. In the eye, carbonic anhydrase plays a significant role in aqueous humor formation by the ciliary body cells. In the ciliary bodies, carbonic anhydrase facilitates the secretion of bicarbonate ions in the aqueous humor. Carbonic anhydrase inhibitors therefore decrease the formation of aqueous humor.

How are they used?

Glaucoma has become the main clinical indication for the carbonic anhydrase inhibitors. Most of these drugs must be administered systemically. Dorzolamide is available in a topical preparation.

What are the adverse effects?

The carbonic anhydrase inhibitors are closely related to the sulfanilamide antibacterial agents. As such, they produce a similar profile of adverse effects, including skin rashes, kidney stones, and aplastic anemia. Other adverse effects associated with this group are depression, anorexia, and electrolyte imbalances (especially potassium).

What are the contraindications and interactions?

Carbonic anhydrase inhibitors are contraindicated in patients with chronic noncongestive angle-closure glaucoma. These drugs should be avoided in patients with hypersensitivity and marked renal or hepatic dysfunction. Safety during pregnancy or lactation is not established. Carbonic anhydrase inhibitors should be used cautiously in patients with a history of hypercalciuria, diabetes mellitus, gout, and asthma. These drugs may interact with amphetamines, ephedrine, and procainamide to decrease renal excretion.

What are the important points patients should know?

Instruct patients to avoid touching the eye with the tip of the drug dispenser. Tell them to discontinue the drug and report to their physician if ocular irritations, infections, or systemic hypersensitivity occurs. Be sure to advise patients that some of these drugs may cause drowsiness and that they should avoid hazardous activities until the response to drugs is known. If patients are using oral medications such as acetazolamide, they should report any numbness, tingling, burning, drowsiness, visual problems, sore throat, fever, or renal problems. Advise them to eat potassium-rich foods and take potassium supplements while taking acetazolamide in high doses or for prolonged periods.

Focus on Natural Products

Bilberry for Eye Health

The berries, roots, and leaves of the bilberry plant have been used to improve night vision; to prevent cataracts, macular degeneration, and glaucoma; and to prevent and treat diabetic retinopathy and myopia. However, bilberry should be avoided during pregnancy and lactation and may cause constipation if large amounts of the dried fruit are consumed. Higher-than-recommended doses of this herb for extended periods will result in toxicity and may even result in death.

Focus On

Direct-Acting Miotics (Cholinergic Agents)

Miotic muscarine agonists (Table 37-4 ■) are agents that constrict the pupils. Miotics are often used to treat glaucoma.

How do they work?

Miotic agents act primarily to increase the drainage of aqueous humor out of the anterior cavity through the canal of Schlemm. They achieve this effect through *miosis* (pupil constriction) and contraction of the ciliary muscles responsible for accommodation. These effects are mediated by the parasympathetic nervous system.

How are they used?

The muscarinic agonists are used in open-angle and angle-closure glaucoma. Examples of muscarinics include acetylcholine chloride, pilocarpine, and carbachol.

What are the adverse effects?

Systemic adverse effects of topical muscarinic agonists are few, with headache being the most common. The most common adverse effect of the muscarinic agonists on the eye is pupil constriction.

What are the contraindications and interactions?

Cholinergic agents (miotics) are contraindicated in patients with hypersensitivity, contact allergy, cataract, **retinal detachment** (separation of the retina from the corneal layer), and depression. Cholinergic drugs may interact with monoamine oxidase inhibitors (MAOIs) and cause an increased risk of hypertensive emergency. They may increase the effects of beta-blockers and other antihypertensives on blood pressure and heart rate.

What are the important points patients should know?

Advise patients to use caution during nighttime driving and in performing hazardous activities in poor light. Instruct them to report to their physician if any sensitivity or severe adverse drug reactions occur.

Table 37-4 ■ **Drug Therapy in Glaucoma That Increases the Outflow of Aqueous Humor**

GENERIC NAME	TRADE NAME	AVERAGE ADULT DOSAGE	ROUTE OF ADMINISTRATION
Direct-Acting Miotics (Cholinergic Agents)			
carbachol	Miostat	1–2 drops 0.75%–3% solution q4h tid	Topical
pilocarpine hydrochloride	Isopto Carpine	1 drop of 1% solution in affected eye	Topical
Indirect-Acting Miotics (Cholinesterase Inhibitors)			
demecarium bromide	Humorsol	1–2 drops of 0.125–0.25% solution 2 times/wk	Topical
physostigmine salicylate	Antilirium	1 drop of 0.25–0.5% solution 1–4 times/d	Topical
Sympathomimetics			
dipivefrin hydrochloride	Propine	1 drop in eye q12h	Topical
epinephrine borate	(Generic only)	1–2 drops as needed	Topical
phenylephrine hydrochloride	Neo-Synephrine	1 drop of 2.5% or 10% solution before examination	Topical
Prostaglandins and Prostamides			
bimatoprost	Lumigan	1 drop of 0.03% solution daily in the evening	Topical
latanoprost	Xalatan	1 drop of 1.5-mg solution daily in the evening	Topical
travoprost	Travatan	1 drop in affected eye(s) once daily in the evening	Topical
unoprostone	Rescula	1 drop of 0.15% solution bid	Topical

tid, three times a day; bid, twice a day.

Focus On

Indirect-Acting Miotics (Cholinesterase Inhibitors)

The cholinesterase inhibitors are more potent and longer-acting than the direct-acting miotic agents.

How do they work?

The cholinesterase inhibitors produce severe miosis and muscle contractions. These actions cause a decreased resistance to aqueous outflow.

How are they used?

The cholinesterase inhibitors are used to treat open-angle glaucoma. Examples of this group include demecarium and physostigmine.

What are the adverse effects?

Ophthalmic-related adverse effects of cholinesterase inhibitors include lacrimation, burning conjunctivitis, retinal detachment, and conjunctival thickening. Systematic adverse effects are nausea and vomiting, diarrhea, abdominal cramps, difficulty breathing, urinary incontinence, salivation, and fainting.

What are the contraindications and interactions?

Cholinesterase inhibitors are contraindicated in patients with hypersensitivity to these agents. The drugs are also contraindicated in patients with any acute inflammatory disorders of the eye and during pregnancy and lactation. The cholinesterase inhibitors should be used cautiously in patients with chronic angle-closure glaucoma and in patients with myasthenia gravis. Drug interactions occur with carbachol, beta-blockers, atropine, ipratropium, and echothiophate.

What are the important points patients should know?

Instruct patients that aching around the eyebrows or temporary burning or stinging may occur initially but usually disappears as the body adjusts to the medication. Vision may be temporarily blurred or unstable after applying eye drops. Advise patients to use caution if driving and performing duties requiring clear vision. Because the medication may cause sensitivity to bright light, instruct patients to wear sunglasses. Advise patients to inform their physicians about changes in vision, eye pain, sweating, nausea and vomiting, diarrhea, difficulty breathing, increased urination or salivation, or irregular heartbeat.

Focus Point

Eye Protection and Insecticides and Pesticides

Individuals working with insecticides or pesticides that contain organophosphate or carbonate and who are using cholinesterase inhibitors must wear respiratory masks, change their clothes frequently, and wash exposed clothes thoroughly.

Focus On

Sympathomimetic Agents

Sympathomimetics have both alpha- and beta-adrenergic activity (see Chapter 24). Apraclonidine and brimonidine are relatively selective alpha$_2$ agonists. Dipivefrin and phenylephrine are beta-adrenergic agonists.

How do they work?

The sympathomimetics can decrease the formation of aqueous humor and increase its outflow by activating adrenoreceptors associated with the ciliary body.

How are they used?

The sympathomimetic drugs we have listed can be used in the management of glaucoma.

What are the adverse effects?

Common adverse effects of dipivefrine and phenylephrine include headache, blurred vision, a stinging sensation during instillation, and increased sensitivity to light. *Rebound nasal congestion* (hyperemia and edema of mucosa), nasal burning, and sneezing may also occur. Other adverse effects of sympathomimetics include palpitation, tachycardia, bradycardia (overdosage), extrasytole, hypertension, sweating, sleeplessness, anxiety, and dizziness.

What are the contraindications and interactions?

Sympathomimetic agents are contraindicated in patients with hypersensitivity to these drugs and in patients with severe coronary disease, severe hypertension, angle-closure glaucoma (ophthalmic preparations), pregnancy, and lactation. Ophthalmic solution (10%) of dipivefrin and phenylephrine should be used cautiously in cardiovascular disease, diabetes mellitus, hyperthyroidism, hypertension, pregnancy, older adults, and infants. Epinephrine should not be used while wearing soft lenses because discoloration of the lenses may occur. There are no known drug interactions with ophthalmic preparations. Dobutamine may increase the risk of hypertension when it is given along with beta-adrenergic blockers. The effects of dopamine may be increased when given with a tricyclic antidepressant (TCA) or MAOI. Epinephrine may interact with a TCA and cause an increased risk of sympathomimetic effects. Excessive hypertension may occur when epinephrine is used with propranolol.

What are the important points patients should know?

Patients should be aware that the instillation of 2.5–10% strength ophthalmic solution can cause burning and stinging. Instruct them to not exceed the recommended dosage regardless of formulation. Tell patients that systemic absorption from nasal and conjunctival membranes could occur. Instruct patients to discontinue the drug and report to their physicians if adverse effects occur and to wear sunglasses in bright light because the pupils will be large and the eyes may be more sensitive to light than usual. Advise patients that some ophthalmic solutions may stain contact lenses.

Focus Point

Eye Drops and Contact Lenses

Patients with contact lenses must remove them and leave them out for at least 15 minutes after the administration of eye drop preparations.

Focus On

Prostaglandin Agonists

Research has shown that prostaglandins also have a role in the movement of aqueous humor through the eye.

How do they work?

Prostaglandin agonist agents increase aqueous humor outflow by reducing congestion in the trabecular meshwork, resulting in lowered IOP.

How are they used?

Prostaglandin agonists are used in the treatment of open-angle glaucoma and intraocular hypertension to lower IOP. Travoprost can be used as first-line monotherapy or in combination with timolol.

What are the adverse effects?

The ocular adverse effects of prostaglandin agonists include ocular dryness, visual disturbance, ocular burning, foreign body sensation, eye pain, pigmentation of the periocular skin, **blepharitis** (inflammation of one or both eyes), cataract, ocular irritation, eye discharge, tearing, increased pigmentation of the iris, and photophobia.

What are the contraindications and interactions?

Prostaglandin agonists should be avoided in patients with hypersensitivity and during pregnancy. These agents are to be used cautiously in patients with active intraocular inflammation, those wearing contact lenses, and in lactating women. These agents may interact with thimerosal and other topical ophthalmic drugs.

What are the important points patients should know?

Instruct patients, especially those with green eyes, of a possible change in iris pigmentation, which is an irreversible condition.

Focus Point

Allergic Blepharoconjunctivitis

Apraclonidine should be used only for the short term for lowering IOP because, with chronic use, it is associated with allergic blepharoconjunctivitis.

✳ Apply Your Knowledge 37.2

The following questions focus on what you have just learned about the treatment of glaucoma.

CRITICAL THINKING

1. What are the trade names of acetazolamide, methazolamide, mannitol, carteolol, and apraclonidine?
2. Why are beta-blockers better than cholinergic agonists?
3. When are osmotic diuretics commonly used for eye disorders?
4. What are examples of muscarinic agonists?
5. What is the mechanism of action of cholinesterase inhibitors?
6. What are the trade names of sympathomimetics used in glaucoma?
7. What are the indications of prostaglandin agonists?
8. What are the trade names of bimatoprost, pilocarpine, and phenylephrine?

Drug Therapy for Minor Eye Conditions

There is a broad range of agents indicated for eye examinations, minor irritations, and injury. These drugs include antimicrobials, local anesthetics, and anti-inflammatories. Antimicrobials and anti-inflammatory drugs were discussed previously. Some drugs, including mydriatic drugs and cycloplegic agents, are used for ophthalmic examinations.

MYDRIATIC AGENTS

Mydriatic drugs are agents that dilate the pupil of the eye. These drugs are commonly used during eye examinations to permit examination of the retina. Examples of mydriatics or sympathomimetics include hydroxyamphetamine and phenylephrine hydrochloride, which are used to dilate pupils in angle-closure glaucoma. These drugs were discussed previously in this chapter.

Focus On

Cycloplegics (Anticholinergic) Agents

Cycloplegic drugs (Table 37-5 ■) cause paralysis of ciliary muscles, resulting in pupillary dilation.

How do they work?

Such antimuscarinic agents as atropine, homatropine, and cyclopentolate act by blocking all muscarinic responses to acetylcholine. The mechanism of action for anticholinergic agents includes mydriasis (pupillary dilation) and cycloplegia (paralysis of ciliary muscles).

How are they used?

Anticholinergic drugs are used locally by inserting drops in the eyes for eye examinations and preoperatively for eye surgery; however, they can also aggravate glaucoma-producing mydriasis and cycloplegia.

What are the adverse effects?

Antimuscarinic drugs may cause mydriasis, blurred vision, photophobia, increased IOP, cycloplegia, eye dryness, and local redness.

What are the contraindications and interactions?

Contraindications include hypersensitivity to antimuscarinic drugs, angle-closure glaucoma, urinary bladder neck obstruction caused by prostatic hypertrophy, intestinal atony, severe ulcerative colitis, tachycardia secondary to cardiac insufficiency, acute bleeding, and myasthenia gravis. Safety during pregnancy or lactation is not established.

Antimuscarinic agents should be used cautiously in elderly patients and in patients with brain damage (in children), hyperthyroidism, asthma, and hepatic or renal disease. Antimuscarinic drugs may interact with the ocular antihypertensive effects of carbachol, pilocarpine, and physostigmine.

What are the important points patients should know?

Instruct patients to use caution when driving or engaging in other potentially hazardous activities because these drugs may cause blurred vision. Patients should be advised to avoid touching the dropper to any skin or eye surface. Advise patients to not wear soft contact lenses when eye drops are being inserted and to immediately report difficulty breathing; swelling of the lips, tongue, or face; hives; palpitations; and unusual behavior.

Table 37-5 ■ Cycloplegics (Anticholinergic Drugs)

GENERIC NAME	TRADE NAME	AVERAGE ADULT DOSAGE	ROUTE OF ADMINISTRATION
atropine sulfate	Atropine Ophthalmic	Solution: 1–2 drops in affected eye(s) up to 4 times/day; Ointment: 0.3–0.5 cm in conjunctival sac(s) 1–3 times/day	Topical
cyclopentolate	Cyclogyl	1–2 drops of 0.5–2% solution 40–50 min before surgery	Topical
homatropine	Isopto Hyoscine	1–2 drops of 2% or 5% solution before eye examination	Topical

PRACTICAL SCENARIO 1

A 72-year-old African American man with a history of hypertension, coronary artery disease, and diabetes mellitus presents with the inability to clearly see objects at a distance and visual field loss. He also states that 2 days ago, he missed some stairs as he was walking up to the second floor of his home. The physician conducts an eye examination and determines that the patient's IOP is 25 mm Hg, there is no hemorrhage in the retina, and his right eye has a mild cataract. The physician diagnoses this patient as having glaucoma.

MBI/Alamy Stock Photo

Critical Thinking Questions

1. After the physician leaves the room, the patient asks the medical assistant about this condition. How should the medical assistant explain the diagnosis to this patient, including its complications and possible relationship to his other disorders?
2. What available treatment options would you tell the patient about?
3. What would you tell the patient about his lifestyle that may be helpful with regard to this diagnosis?

PRACTICAL SCENARIO 2

A 72-year-old man went for an annual eye check-up. A medical assistant administered two different types of eye drops to dilate his pupils before the physician examined his eyes.

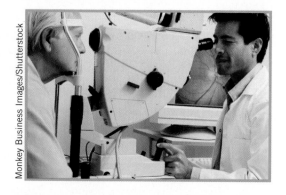

Monkey Business Images/Shutterstock

Critical Thinking Questions

1. What are the most common mydriatic drugs used to dilate the eyes?
2. If the patient has had a history of diabetes mellitus, what condition is likely to be present?

Chapter Capsule

This section repeats the objectives from the beginning of the chapter and then provides a summary of the most important concepts for that objective. Use this section as a quick review and to check your knowledge.

Objective 1: Describe the structure and function of the eye.

- A hollow, spherical structure about 2.5 cm in diameter with three distinct layers in its walls: an outer layer (sclera), a middle layer (choroid layer or "coat"), and an inner layer (retina)
- Spaces within the eye—filled with fluids that support its wall and internal parts
- Structures—the iris, ciliary body, lens, lacrimal glands, and ocular vasculature receive autonomic innervation

Objective 2: Define the terms *cataract* and *retinopathy*.

- Cataracts and retinopathy are both serious eye conditions
- A cataract is an opacity of the lens of the eye
- Retinopathy is degeneration of the blood vessels of the retina

Objective 3: Explain glaucoma and the types of glaucoma.

- Damage to the optic nerve, often caused by elevated IOP
- Results from excessive production of aqueous humor or diminished ocular fluid outflow
- Can cause blindness secondary to optic nerve damage
- Two types of glaucoma: acute angle closure and chronic open angle

Objective 4: Identify the drugs of first choice for intraocular hypertension and chronic open-angle glaucoma, and explain how they work.

- The beta-blockers are considered the drugs of first choice in the treatment of intraocular hypertension and chronic open-angle glaucoma
- They lower the cyclic adenosine monophosphate (cAMP) levels within the ciliary body necessary for aqueous humor production. This reduces elevated IOP in chronic open-angle glaucoma by reducing the formation of aqueous humor.

Objective 5: State the rationale for the use and the mechanism of action for carbonic anhydrase inhibitors in the treatment of glaucoma.

- Plays a significant role in aqueous humor formation by the ciliary body cells of the eye
- Facilitates the secretion of bicarbonate ions in the aqueous humor, decreasing the formation of aqueous humor
- Main clinical indication: glaucoma
- Most administered systemically

Objective 6: Identify direct-acting miotics (cholinergic drugs) and list two generic and trade names.

- Agents that constrict the pupil, often used to treat glaucoma
- Carbachol (Miostat)
- Pilocarpine hydrochloride (Isopto Carpine)

Objective 7: Discuss the adverse effects of indirect-acting miotics (cholinesterase inhibitors).

- Ophthalmic-related adverse effects of indirect-acting miotics (cholinesterase inhibitors) include lacrimation, burning conjunctivitis, retinal detachment, and conjunctival thickening
- Systemic adverse effects are nausea and vomiting, diarrhea, abdominal cramps, difficulty breathing, urinary incontinence, salivation, and fainting

Objective 8: How do sympathomimetic agents and prostaglandin agonists work?

- Sympathomimetic agents can decrease formation of aqueous humor and increase its outflow by activating adrenoreceptors associated with the ciliary body
- Prostaglandin agonists increase aqueous humor outflow by reducing congestion in the trabecular meshwork, resulting in lowered intraocular pressure (IOP)

Objective 9: Explain mydriatic agents and their indications.

- Agents that dilate the pupil of the eye; commonly used during eye examinations to permit examination of the retina

- Used locally by inserting drops in the eyes for eye examinations and preoperatively for eye surgery; however, can aggravate glaucoma-producing mydriasis and cycloplegia

Objective 10: State the mechanism of action of antimuscarinics.

- Act by blocking all muscarinic responses to acetylcholine

- Mechanism of action of antimuscarinic agents is mydriasis (pupillary dilation) and cycloplegia (paralysis of ciliary muscles)

Internet Sites of Interest

- Learn more about glaucoma at the Glaucoma Research Foundation website at: **www.glaucoma.org**.

- More information about carbonic anhydrase inhibitors can be found on the Mayo Clinic website at: **www.mayoclinic.com**. Search for "carbonic anhydrase inhibitors."

- The Eye Foundation of America's official website is: **www.eyefoundationofamerica.org**

- The National Eye Institute promotes eye health at: **https://nei/nih.gov**

Checkpoint Review 4

MULTIPLE CHOICE

Select the best answer for the following questions.

1. Which of the following neurotransmitters is released by the preganglionic sympathetic neuron?

   a. Norepinephrine
   b. Acetylcholine
   c. Dopamine
   d. Serotonin

2. Which of the following neurotransmitters is released by the parasympathetic postganglionic neurons?

   a. Serotonin
   b. Norepinephrine
   c. Dopamine
   d. Acetylcholine

3. Sympathomimetics are also called:

   a. Cholinergic antagonists
   b. Cholinergic agonists
   c. Adrenergic agonists
   d. Adrenergic antagonists

4. The "pacemaker," or SA node, is located in which of the following chambers of the heart?

   a. Left atrium
   b. Right atrium
   c. Right ventricle
   d. Left ventricle

5. Which of the following are class I antidysrhythmic drugs?

   a. Beta-adrenergic blockers
   b. Drugs that bind to sodium channels
   c. Drugs that interfere with potassium outflow
   d. Calcium channel blockers

6. Which of the following drugs has antisympathetic class III action?

   a. Bretylium (Bretylium)
   b. Verapamil (Calan)
   c. Propranolol (Inderal)
   d. Lidocaine (Xylocaine)

7. Alpha$_2$-receptor agonists are used to treat:

   a. Hypertension
   b. Hypotension
   c. Hepatitis
   d. Impotence

8. Sublingual nitroglycerin is rapidly effective and lasts for about:

   a. 15 minutes
   b. 30 minutes
   c. 1 hour
   d. 3 hours

9. Which of the following describes stage 2 of anesthesia?

   a. Surgical
   b. Analgesia
   c. Medullary paralysis
   d. Excitement

10. Beta$_2$-receptor agonists are used in patients with:

    a. Cardiac arrhythmias associated with digitalis intoxication
    b. Chronic obstructive airway disease
    c. Hypertension
    d. Thyrotoxicosis

11. The most common adverse effects of phenytoin (Dilantin) include which of the following?

    a. Nosebleed
    b. Asthma
    c. Bloody urine
    d. Gingival hyperplasia

12. Specialized cells in the epidermis called *melanocytes* produce:

    a. Melatonin
    b. Melanin
    c. Melanogen
    d. Melanotropin

13. Beta-receptor antagonists are used in the management of:

    a. Hypertension and weight reduction
    b. Cardiac arrhythmias
    c. Angina pectoris
    d. All of the above

14. Which of the following stages of anesthesia is called an *anesthetic accident*?

    a. Medullary paralysis
    b. Excitement
    c. Surgical anesthesia
    d. Analgesia

15. Pilocarpine is used most commonly in which of the following?

    a. Gynecology
    b. Ophthalmology
    c. Dermatology
    d. Cardiology

16. Cholinergic blockers are also called:

    a. Sympatholytics
    b. Sympathomimetics
    c. Parasympatholytics
    d. Parasympathomimetics

17. Which of the following is the cause of primary (essential) hypertension?

    a. Obesity
    b. Chronic glomerulonephritis
    c. Excessive alcohol
    d. Unknown

18. Discontinuation of nitroglycerin should take place over time because the length of action of these drug preparations can cause:

    a. Hypertension
    b. Vasospasms
    c. Bradycardia
    d. Vomiting

19. Which of the following is/are the mechanism(s) of action for quinidine?

    a. Slowing of the heart rate
    b. Decreasing the contractile force of the heart
    c. Depressing the myocardium and the conduction system
    d. All of the above

20. General anesthetics are contraindicated in patients who have received monoamine oxidase inhibitors within how many days?

    a. 2
    b. 4
    c. 7
    d. 14

21. Which of the following must patients do when taking nitroglycerin?

    a. Avoid food or liquids.
    b. Avoid alcoholic beverages.
    c. Avoid coffee and tea.
    d. Discard unused tablets after 5 minutes.

22. Which of the following is the mainstay of treatment for acute or chronic inflammatory disorders of the skin and may be topical or oral?

    a. Emollients (skin-softening agents)
    b. Keratolytic agents
    c. Antibiotics
    d. Corticosteroids

23. Which of the following drugs are mainstays of hypertensive therapy?

    a. Diuretics
    b. Statin drugs
    c. Beta-adrenergic blockers
    d. Centrally acting adrenergic blockers

24. **Rhabdomyolysis** (degeneration of skeletal muscle tissue) is a rare but life-threatening adverse effect of:

    a. Diuretics
    b. Angiotensin II receptor blockers
    c. Statins
    d. Fat-soluble vitamins

25. Parasympathomimetics (or cholinergic agonists) produce symptoms of:

    a. Fight or flight
    b. Rest and digest
    c. Fight and rest
    d. Speed and rest

26. Acne vulgaris is an inflammatory disorder of which of the following glands?

    a. Sweat
    b. Sebaceous
    c. Bartholin
    d. Mammary

27. Dopamine is released from which of the following?

    a. Kidneys
    b. GI tract
    c. Brain
    d. All of the above

28. Which of the following is an example of a beta-adrenergic blocker?

    a. Verapamil
    b. Diltiazem
    c. Inderal
    d. Amiodarone

29. A chemical compound containing nitrogen that is derived from the amino acid tyrosine is called:

    a. Catecholamine
    b. Melanin
    c. Melatonin
    d. Cardiolipin

30. Which of the following agents are used in the treatment of corns, calluses, and plantar warts?

    a. Topical antibiotics
    b. Topical corticosteroids
    c. Keratolytics
    d. Emollients

31. Peripherally acting blockers are antihypertensive in that their effects depend on the inhibition of:

    a. Renin release
    b. Norepinephrine release
    c. Acetylcholine release
    d. Serotonin release

32. Beta$_1$-receptor agonists are used to treat which of the following?

    a. Cardiac arrest
    b. Circulatory shock
    c. Hypotension
    d. All of the above

33. Atropine acts by selectively blocking all muscarinic responses to:

    a. Dopamine
    b. Acetylcholine
    c. Norepinephrine
    d. Serotonin

34. Which of the following agents is a popular choice for infiltration anesthesia?

    a. Lidocaine
    b. Nitrous oxide
    c. Sevoflurane
    d. Cocaine

35. Which of the following is the trade name of lidocaine?

    a. Marcaine
    b. Carbocaine
    c. Novocain
    d. Xylocaine

36. The primary use of bethanechol, which is a cholinergic agonist used in the cardiovascular field, is in the diagnosis of:

    a. Prolapse of the mitral valve
    b. Atrial tachycardia
    c. Myocardial infarction
    d. Hypertensive crises

37. During spinal anesthesia, the anesthetic agent is injected into which of the following spaces or parts of the spinal column?

    a. Pia mater
    b. Arachnoid
    c. Subarachnoid
    d. Epidural

38. Which of the following is the most commonly used route to administer local anesthetics?

    a. Local infiltration
    b. Topical anesthesia
    c. Spinal anesthesia
    d. Epidural anesthesia

39. Which of the following is the most frequent adverse effect associated with barbiturates?

    a. Blurred vision
    b. Thrombocytopenia
    c. Sedation
    d. Aplastic anemia

40. Stage 3 (surgical anesthesia) is characterized by progressive:

    a. Muscular contraction
    b. Circulatory collapse
    c. Muscular relaxation
    d. Dysfunction of the respiratory system, which can cause sudden death

41. Valproic acid is classified as an:

    a. Antipyretic
    b. Anticonvulsant
    c. Anticoagulant
    d. Antineoplastic

42. The trade name of ethosuximide is:

    a. Celontin
    b. Dilantin
    c. Ativan
    d. Zarontin

43. Cholinergic drugs exhibit effects similar to which of the following substances?

    a. Monoamine oxidase inhibitors
    b. Methotrimeprazine
    c. Acetylcholine
    d. Amphetamines

44. Stimulation of beta$_2$ receptors results in which of the following?

    a. Postural hypotension
    b. Nasal congestion
    c. Bronchoconstriction
    d. Bronchodilation

45. Which of the following is a cholinergic drug?

    a. Noradrenaline

    b. Dopamine

    c. Acetylcholine

    d. Any calcium channel blocker

46. Which of the following properties of general anesthetics is essential for the drug to cross the blood–brain barrier?

    a. Lipophilic

    b. Hydrophilic

    c. Proteinphilic

    d. None of the above

47. All the following inhaled anesthetics are commonly used in the United States except:

    a. Nitrous oxide

    b. Sevoflurane

    c. Diethyl ether

    d. Isoflurane

48. Which of the following drugs is in the group of ester-type local anesthetics?

    a. Bupivacaine

    b. Etidocaine

    c. Ropivacaine

    d. Benzocaine

49. Which of the following drugs is used to treat ophthalmic disorders and in preoperative situations?

    a. Niacin

    b. Atropine

    c. Alcohol

    d. Amantadine

50. Beta$_2$-receptor agonists are used in patients with all the following except:

    a. Premature labor

    b. Circulatory shock

    c. Anaphylactic shock

    d. Chronic obstructive airway disease

51. An opacity of the eye's lens is called:

    a. Glaucoma

    b. Cataract

    c. Retinopathy

    d. Choroiditis

52. Gold sodium thiomalate (Myochrysine) is effective in which of the following disorders?

    a. Bronchitis

    b. Hepatitis

    c. Acute glomerulonephritis

    d. Active rheumatoid arthritis

53. All the following are adverse effects of estrogen replacement therapy in the treatment of postmenopausal osteoporosis except:

    a. Breast cancer

    b. Lung cancer

    c. Endometrial cancer

    d. Cardiovascular problems

54. Carbonic anhydrase inhibitors act on the enzyme responsible for the conversion of carbon dioxide to which of the following?

    a. Bicarbonate and calcium ions

    b. Bicarbonate and sodium ions

    c. Bicarbonate and hydrogen ions

    d. None of the above

55. Colchicine is used for which of the following conditions or diseases?

    a. Peptic ulcer

    b. Gout

    c. Severe hepatic conditions

    d. Severe cardiac disease

56. Which of the following is an example of a new drug that is a selective estrogen-receptor modulator for the treatment of postmenopausal osteoporosis?

    a. carisoprodol (Soma)

    b. lorazepam (Ativan)

    c. acetazolamide (Diamox)

    d. raloxifene (Evista)

57. Baclofen is at least as effective as which of the following drugs?

    a. lorazepam (Ativan)

    b. dorzolamide (Trusopt)

    c. diazepam (Valium)

    d. levobunolol (Betagan)

58. Even when applied directly to the eye, several drugs may have systemic effects. This is because the drug enters via which of the following routes?

    a. The lungs

    b. The nasolacrimal ducts

    c. The mouth and nasopharyngeal ducts

    d. All of the above

59. The anterior of the sclera of the eye that bulges forward is called the:

    a. Retina

    b. Pupil

    c. Iris

    d. Cornea

60. All the following are primary functions of the skeletal system except:

a. Blood cell production
b. Storage of minerals
c. Production of heat and energy
d. Protection of other organs

61. Which of the following is the generic name of Fosamax?

a. risedronate sodium
b. alendronate sodium
c. raloxifene
d. calcitonin salmon

62. The ciliary body is the thickest part of which layer of the eye?

a. Inner
b. Middle
c. Outer
d. Inner and middle

63. Pigment-producing melanocytes are located in which of the following organs?

a. Mouth
b. Liver
c. Spleen
d. Eye

64. Photoreceptors are located in which of the following portions of the eyes?

a. Pupils
b. Retina
c. Aqueous humor
d. Choroid

65. Which of the following is a systemic autoimmune disease?

a. Osteoporosis
b. Osteomyelitis
c. Rheumatoid arthritis
d. Rheumatoid fever

66. When the lenses of the eyes adjust shape and facilitate focusing, it is known as:

a. Presbyopia
b. Diplopia
c. Amblyopia
d. Accommodation

67. All the following are risk factors for primary open-angle glaucoma except:

a. Myopia
b. Diabetes
c. Peptic ulcer
d. Black race

68. When benzodiazepines are combined with other central nervous system depressants, which of the following adverse effects can occur?

a. Coma and renal failure
b. Coma and respiratory depression
c. Hypertension
d. Hyperthermia

69. Which of the following is one of the most common and serious disorders of the eye?

a. Retinal detachment
b. Conjunctivitis
c. Glaucoma
d. Cataract

70. Adverse effects of acetazolamide (Diamox) include:

a. Blurred vision, urinary retention
b. Dry mouth, thirst
c. Paresthesias, drowsiness, nausea
d. Congestive heart failure

71. Auranofin (Ridaura) is used in the treatment of:

a. Rheumatoid arthritis
b. Multiple sclerosis
c. Ear infections
d. Ulcerative colitis

72. Which of the following hormones is secreted by the kidneys?

a. Vasopressin
b. Oxytocin
c. Luteinizing
d. Erythropoietin

73. Following the proximal convoluted tubule is the:

a. Distal convoluted tubule
b. Loop of Henle
c. Glomerular capsule
d. Collecting duct

74. Which of the following is a major adverse effect of potassium-sparing diuretics?

a. Hyperkalemia
b. Hypercalcemia
c. Hypokalemia
d. Hypocalcemia

75. Antidiuretic hormone is also called:

a. Oxytocin
b. Adrenocorticotropic hormone
c. Vasopressin
d. Prolactin

76. Graves' disease is characterized by:

    a. Hypothyroidism
    b. Hyperthyroidism
    c. Myxedema
    d. Congenital hypothyroidism

77. Iodide is used alone for which of the following disorders or conditions?

    a. Hyperkalemia
    b. Hyperthyroidism
    c. Acute bronchitis
    d. Asthma

78. Propylthiouracil is classified as a(n):

    a. Diuretic drug
    b. Antihistamine
    c. Antithyroid agent
    d. Antihypertensive agent

79. Glucagon hormone is secreted by which of the following glands?

    a. Pancreas
    b. Thymus
    c. Thyroid
    d. Adrenal gland

80. The sulfonylureas are categorized as:

    a. Oral hypoglycemics
    b. Oral contraceptives
    c. Oral anticoagulants
    d. Loop diuretics

81. The alpha cells of the islets of the pancreas secrete:

    a. Insulin
    b. Thymosin
    c. Heparin
    d. Glucagon

82. Which of the following agents is used for nasal congestion and asthma?

    a. Furosemide
    b. Corticosteroids
    c. Potassium iodide
    d. Regular insulin

83. Loop diuretics are toxic to which of the following organs of the body?

    a. Ears
    b. Eyes
    c. Lungs
    d. Ovaries

84. Which of the following chronic conditions of the lungs is the most common in the United States?

    a. Nasal polyps
    b. Pneumonia
    c. Asthma
    d. Pulmonary edema

85. Bronchodilators that widen the diameter of the bronchial tubes include which of the following agents?

    a. Corticosteroids
    b. Narrow-spectrum antibiotics
    c. Beta$_2$-adrenergic agonists
    d. Alpha$_2$-adrenergic agonists

86. Gestational diabetes develops during:

    a. Childhood
    b. The neonatal period
    c. Lactation
    d. Pregnancy

87. The antacids are all:

    a. Weak acids
    b. Weak alkalines
    c. Strong acids
    d. Strong alkalines

88. Which of the following are among the most misused drugs?

    a. Opioid analgesics
    b. Antidiarrheals
    c. Laxatives
    d. Antacids

89. All the following are indications of androgens in women except:

    a. Postpartum breast engorgement
    b. Fibrocystic breast disorders
    c. Breast cancer
    d. Endometriosis

90. Which of the following portions of the body secretes gonadotropin-releasing hormone?

    a. The hypothalamus
    b. The anterior pituitary
    c. The posterior pituitary
    d. The ovaries

91. A patient who is receiving insulin should be taught to be cautious about which of the following adverse effects?

    a. Malignant hyperthermia
    b. Severe hypotension
    c. Hypoglycemic reaction
    d. Malignant hypertension

92. Which of the following are the most effective drugs for controlling diarrhea?

    a. Osmotics
    b. Electrolytes
    c. Adsorbents
    d. Opioid antidiarrheals

93. A 70/30 combination of insulin means:

    a. NPH 70% and regular insulin 30%
    b. NPH 30% and regular insulin 70%
    c. NPH 30% and Novolin 70%
    d. NPH 70% and Novolin 30%

94. Stool softeners are sometimes called:

    a. Laxatives
    b. Osmotics
    c. Adsorbents
    d. Emollients

95. Which of the following is the best-known synthetic estrogen?

    a. Norethindrone
    b. Diethylstilbestrol
    c. Megestrol
    d. Norgestrel

96. Which of the following is the trade name of insulin glargine (long-acting)?

    a. Novolin
    b. Lantus
    c. Humalog
    d. Humulin U

97. Which of the following chemical substances increases sodium ion reabsorption in the distal convoluted tubules and collecting ducts of the nephrons?

    a. Erythropoietin
    b. Insulin
    c. Glucagon
    d. Aldosterone

98. Water balance is regulated by the secretion of which of the following hormones?

    a. Vasopressin
    b. Thyroxin
    c. Erythropoietin
    d. Growth hormone

99. Exophthalmos (protrusion of the eyeball) is seen in which of the following conditions or disorders?

    a. Hyperparathyroidism
    b. Hyperthyroidism
    c. Hypertension
    d. Myxedema

100. Laxative stimulants are contraindicated in all the following conditions except:

    a. Fecal impaction
    b. Abdominal pain
    c. Pregnancy
    d. Constipation

101. Which of the following diuretics are used primarily for cerebral edema?

    a. Osmotic agents
    b. Carbonic anhydrase inhibitors
    c. Thiazide agents
    d. Loop diuretics

102. Which of the following portions of the male reproductive system stores sperm cells?

    a. Vas deferens
    b. Prostate gland
    c. Scrotum
    d. Epididymis

103. Which of the following agents stimulates powerful uterine contractions?

    a. Prolactin
    b. Progesterone
    c. Oxytocin
    d. Estrogen

104. Which of the following is the trade name of spironolactone?

    a. Dyrenium
    b. Aldactone
    c. Midamor
    d. Lasix

105. Which of the following drugs is an antiemetic?

    a. Ipecac
    b. Chlorpromazine
    c. Magnesium hydroxide
    d. Senna

106. Uterine relaxants include which of the following agents?

    a. Beta$_2$-adrenergic agonists
    b. Alpha$_2$-adrenergic agonists
    c. Cholinergic agonists
    d. Oxytocin hormone

107. Estrogen therapy in older women is used to prevent or treat which of the following disorders or conditions?

    a. Breast cancer
    b. Pregnancy
    c. Endometriosis
    d. Osteoporosis

108. Stoppage of blood flow is known as:
    a. Hemopoiesis
    b. Hemostasis
    c. Hemosiderosis
    d. Hemolysis

109. Which of the following chemical substances is released from the platelets?
    a. Serotonin
    b. Heparin
    c. Histamine
    d. Fibrinogen

110. Tagamet and Zantac are known as which of the following?
    a. Histamine agonists
    b. Histamine antagonists
    c. Antispasmodics
    d. Antacids

111. Which of the following is an example of an oral anticoagulant?
    a. Heparin
    b. Urokinase
    c. Streptokinase
    d. Coumadin

112. Allergic rhinitis is also known as:
    a. Rhinovirus
    b. Coryza
    c. Hives
    d. Hay fever

113. Which of the following anticoagulants should not be used during pregnancy?
    a. Warfarin
    b. Heparin
    c. Enoxaparin
    d. Ardeparin

114. The adrenal medulla synthesizes, stores, and secretes which of the following?
    a. Epinephrine and norepinephrine
    b. Androgen and glucocorticoids
    c. Parathormone
    d. Thyroxine

115. All the following leafy green foods contain vitamin K except:
    a. Parsley
    b. Swiss chard
    c. Spinach
    d. Sweet potatoes

116. Patients should be instructed to avoid exposure to UV light while taking which of the following drugs?
    a. Coumarin derivatives
    b. Thrombolytics
    c. Xanthine derivatives
    d. Progestins

117. Xanthine derivatives are used for prophylaxis and the symptomatic relief of which of the following conditions or disorders?
    a. Bronchial asthma
    b. Osteoporosis
    c. Dementia
    d. Pancreatitis

118. The process of blood clotting occurs in a series of sequential steps that are referred to as a:
    a. Prothrombin activator
    b. Cascade
    c. Thrombus
    d. Low-molecular-weight heparin

119. Most of the circulating clotting proteins are synthesized by which of the following organs in the human body?
    a. Lungs
    b. Liver
    c. Bones
    d. Brain

120. Conjugated estrogens (during the first trimester) may increase the risk for which of the following?
    a. Dysrhythmia in the fetus
    b. Heart failure in the fetus and infant
    c. Malabsorption in the infant
    d. Malformations in the fetus and infant

121. Which of the following is an example of antiplatelet agents?
    a. Heparin
    b. Abciximab
    c. Abbokinase
    d. Warfarin

MATCHING 1

For questions 122–126, match the lettered drug class to the numbered description.

DESCRIPTION	DRUG CLASS
122. _____ Converted to theophylline	a. Leukotriene inhibitors
123. _____ Causes masculinization of the fetus	b. Oxytocic agents
124. _____ Used to treat gastrointestinal disorders	c. Prostaglandins
125. _____ Metabolized from arachidonic acid	d. Androgen derivatives
126. _____ Produces phasic contractions characteristic of normal delivery	e. Xanthine derivatives

MATCHING 2

For questions 127–131, match the lettered drug trade name to the numbered drug generic name.

GENERIC NAME	TRADE NAME
127. _____ dalteparin	a. Lovenox
128. _____ pentoxifylline	b. Innohep
129. _____ warfarin sodium	c. Coumadin
130. _____ enoxaparin	d. Fragmin
131. _____ tinzaparin	e. Trental

FILL IN THE BLANK

Select terms from your reading to fill in the blanks.

132. The space between each synapse is bridged by chemicals called _____.

133. Intraorbital block is often used for _____ surgery.

134. Atropine is a classic anticholinergic or _____ antagonist drug.

135. Neurons that release acetylcholine are termed _____.

136. Cryoanesthesia involves the reduction of nerve conduction by localized _____.

137. Alpha-receptor antagonists can be reversible or _____.

138. There are two types of cholinergic receptors: muscarinic and _____.

139. Beta-blockers competitively antagonize the responses to _____ that are mediated by beta receptors.

140. Cholinergic blockers are also called _____.

141. Volatile anesthetics are combined with intravenous agents in regimens of so-called _____ anesthesia.

142. Oral androgens should be taken with meals to reduce _____.

143. The testes secrete _____.

144. The best-known synthetic _____ is diethylstilbestrol.

145. The ovaries are the primary source of progesterones and _____.

146. Primary digestion occurs in the _____.

147. H_2-receptor antagonists are used for the short-term treatment of active _____.

148. The prostaglandins are involved in gastrointestinal _____ and gastric acid secretions.

149. Bronchodilators include _____ adrenergic agonists and _____.

150. Leukotriene inhibitors are bronchodilators and leukotriene receptor _____.

151. The pancreas is an accessory organ of the _____.

UNIT 5

Special Populations

" Health professionals must ensure that drugs are administered safely and effectively to patients of all ages. "

Chapter 38

Drugs Used to Treat Geriatric Patients

Chapter Objectives

After completing this chapter, you should be able to:

1. Discuss the process of aging.
2. Identify factors influencing drug dosages for elderly patients.
3. Explain the leading causes of diseases and death in older adults.
4. Identify the factors that influence drug absorption in older adults.
5. Discuss creatinine clearance in elderly patients and use the measurement formula.
6. Identify polypharmacy and its effects on older adults.
7. List common cardiovascular disorders in elderly individuals.
8. Identify conditions that contribute to a high incidence of digitalis-induced arrhythmias in elderly patients.
9. Discuss the effects of sedatives and hypnotics on elderly patients.
10. List six principles that are important in treating older adults.

Key Terms

Alzheimer's disease (p. 678)
cognitive (p. 673)
creatinine clearance (p. 674)

glycoprotein (p. 674)
polypharmacy (p. 675)

stroke (p. 673)
thiazides (p. 676)

Introduction

The process of aging is complex and includes biological, psychological, sociological, and behavioral changes. *Biologically*, the body gradually loses the ability to renew itself. Various body functions begin to slow down and the vital senses become less acute. *Psychologically*, aging persons experience changing sensory processes; perception, motor skills, problem-solving abilities, and emotions are frequently altered. *Sociologically*, they must cope with the changing roles and definitions of self that society imposes on older adults. *Behaviorally*, aging individuals may move more slowly and have less dexterity.

Major changes that are not physiological also occur during the aging process and impact health, including **cognitive** (intellectual processes, such as thinking, reasoning, and remembering) changes, such as forgetting to take daily medications; economic changes caused by decreased income, increased health expenses, and other factors; and unforeseen changes, including the death of a spouse.

Geriatric Drug Therapy

Older adults require increased health care attention. In the United States, the elderly population grew more than tenfold during the twentieth century. In 1900, there were just over 3 million Americans age 65 or older. In 2011, the same group numbered nearly 42 million. Drug therapy for geriatric patients requires specific knowledge of their physiology, pathology, and other age-related factors. Drug dosages must be adjusted according to an elderly patient's weight, amount of body fat, laboratory results (e.g., blood urea nitrogen, creatinine, serum protein, liver enzymes, electrolytes), and current health conditions.

Significant changes in common responses to certain drugs can occur in older people. Other drugs may affect elderly patients in only slightly differing ways. As people age, their drug usage patterns change—generally increasing—because the incidence of disease or multiple diseases increases with age. In addition, many older adults experience problems with nutrition and finances that may decrease dosing compliance in prescribed drugs. Health care practitioners who deal with elderly patients must be aware of these issues and understand how to deal with them. Equally important, it is essential for health care personnel to be aware of the leading causes of death in older adults.

Disease and Death in Older Adults

Heart disease and cancer have been the two leading causes of death among people age 65 and older for the past two decades. More than one-third (35%) of all deaths are caused by heart disease, including heart attacks and chronic ischemic heart disease. Cancer accounts for about one-fifth (22%) of all deaths.

Other important chronic diseases among persons age 65 and older include **stroke** (cerebrovascular disease), chronic obstructive pulmonary disease, diabetes, pneumonia, and influenza. Alzheimer's disease and several important renal diseases (such as chronic nephritis and nephrotic syndrome) have gained significance as causes of death among the elderly population during the past two decades. Alzheimer's disease is now among the 10 leading causes of death for older white people but not for other racial groups.

Physiologic Changes in Older Adults

Most organ systems show a decline that begins during young adulthood and continues as people age. Individuals age differently, and older adults accumulate physiologic deficiencies with the passage of time in varying amounts. The most important decline appears to be in renal function. The physiologic changes in older adults are shown in Table 38-1 ■.

Table 38-1 ■ Physiologic Changes in Geriatric Patients

ORGANS	PHYSIOLOGIC CHANGES
Heart	Cardiac output and blood flow decrease
Liver	Function of enzymes and blood flow decrease
Kidneys	Blood flow, glomerular filtration, and nephron function decrease
Stomach	Gastric secretions decrease
Intestines	Peristalsis and motility decrease; first-pass effect decreases

Changes in Pharmacokinetics

Pharmacokinetics deal with the absorption, distribution, metabolism, and elimination of drugs as well as the amount of time each of these processes requires. In many cases, pharmacokinetics can explain why different people react differently to a drug.

ABSORPTION

Although drug absorption is not altered in any major way with age, the rate at which some drugs are absorbed does change. Conditions that influence drug absorption in older adults include slower gastric emptying, altered nutritional habits, and greater use of over-the-counter (OTC) medications.

DISTRIBUTION

Elderly people tend to have increased body fat but reduced lean body mass and reduced total body water (Table 38-2 ■).

Serum albumin, which binds to many drugs, especially weak acids, is usually decreased. There may be a concurrent increase in alpha-1 acid **glycoprotein**—a specific serum protein that binds to many basic drugs. Changes such as these may alter a drug's appropriate loading dose. Because of a decreased volume of distribution, the loading dose of a drug, such as digoxin, should be reduced (if it is used at all) in an older person with heart failure. Because of reduced drug clearance, maintenance doses also may have to be reduced.

Table 38-2 ■ **Pharmacokinetic Changes Due to Aging**

TYPE OF CHANGE	YOUNG ADULTS (BEGINNING AT AGE 20)	OLDER ADULTS (BEGINNING AT AGE 60)
Body fat	18–20% of body weight (men)	36–38% of body weight (men)
	26–33% of body weight (women)	38–45% of body weight (women)
Body water	61% of body weight	53% of body weight
Hepatic blood flow	100% in a young adult	55–60% in an older adult
Kidney weight	100% in a young adult	80% in an older adult
Lean body mass	19% of body weight	12% of body weight
Serum albumin	4.7 g/d	3.8 g/d

Focus Point

Age Affects the Pharmacokinetic Process

The efficiency of pharmacokinetic processes varies across one's lifespan. In very young and very old people, the manner in which their bodies handle drugs can be significantly different from that of young or middle-aged adults.

METABOLISM

The liver's capacity to metabolize drugs does not appear to consistently decline as age increases. This is true for all drugs. However, as we age, the liver's ability to heal from an injury (such as from viral hepatitis or alcohol use) declines. The health care professional should realize that a history of recent liver disease in an elderly patient should lead to caution when administering drugs that are mostly cleared by the liver. This is true even after the patient has apparently completely recovered from hepatic damage. Also in elderly people, heart failure and other diseases that affect liver function (such as malnutrition) are more common. Heart failure may alter liver metabolism and reduce hepatic blood flow. Impaired hepatic function may also result from severe nutritional deficiencies.

ELIMINATION

Because of decreased cardiac output and blood flow in the circulatory system, the liver and kidneys are affected. By age 65, nephron function may decline by

35%, and after age 70, blood flow to the kidneys may decrease 40%.

Creatinine clearance is an indicator of the glomerular filtration rate. Evaluating renal function based on serum creatinine alone may not be accurate for older adults because of the decrease in muscle mass. Creatinine is a by-product of the muscle breakdown of stored proteins. However, creatinine is primarily excreted by the kidneys. A decrease in muscle mass can cause a decrease in serum creatinine. In elderly patients, serum creatinine may be within normal values because of a lack of muscle mass, but there could still be a decrease in renal function. In young or middle-aged adults, serum creatinine would be increased with a decrease in renal function.

The serum creatinine level may be measured by the 24-hour creatinine clearance test to evaluate renal function. Creatinine clearance can also be calculated by this formula:

Creatine clearance mL/min

$$= \frac{(140 - \text{age}) \times (\text{weight in kg})}{72 \times \text{serum creatinine in mg/dL}}$$

The normal creatinine clearance value for an adult is 80–130 mL/min.

With liver and kidney dysfunction, the efficacy of a drug dose is usually decreased. If several drugs are being taken, drug effects may be intensified in elderly patients. If the efficiency of the hepatic and renal systems is decreased, the half-life of the drug is prolonged, resulting in drug toxicity. Special medications must be administered in reduced dosages in older patients (Table 38-3 ■).

Table 38-3 ■ Medications Administered in Elderly Patients That Require Reduced Dosages

DRUG OR CLASS OF DRUG	ADVERSE EFFECTS
aminoglycosides	Ototoxicity, nephrotoxicity
carbamazepine (Carbatrol)	Ataxia, drowsiness
cimetidine (Tagamet)	Confusion
digoxin (Lanoxin)	Overdose toxicity
levodopa (Dopar)	Hypotension
morphine (Avinza)	Respiratory depression
thioridazine (Mellaril)	Confusion
thyroxine	Myocardial infarction
vitamin D (Calcijex)	Renal toxicity
warfarin (Coumadin)	Bleeding

Changes in Pharmacodynamics

The term *pharmacodynamics* refers to how drugs interact at target organs or receptor sites. Pharmacodynamics examines the way drugs bind with receptors, the concentration required to elicit a response, and the time required for each of these events. Because there is a lack of affinity to receptor sites throughout an older adult's body, the pharmacodynamic response may be changed.

Many changes in pharmacodynamics in elderly individuals result from altered pharmacokinetics or diminished homeostatic responses. There may be changes with age in the characteristics or numbers of some receptors. The elderly patient may be more or less sensitive to drug action because of age-related changes in the central nervous system (CNS), changes in the number of drug receptors, and changes in the affinity of receptors to drugs. If the patient is more sensitive to the drug's action, the dose may need to be lowered and vice versa. Changes in organ functions are important to consider in drug dosing. Most studies show that older adults experience a decrease in responsiveness to beta-adrenoceptor stimulants.

In the cardiovascular system of older adults who do not have obvious cardiac disease, the increment of cardiac output required by mild to moderate exercise is successfully provided until at least age 75. However, the increased output results mostly from increased stroke volume in the elderly (in young adults, it results from tachycardia). Average blood pressure and symptomatic orthostatic hypotension increase with age. An elderly patient should be checked for orthostatic hypotension during every physician visit. Other physiologic changes in older adults include increased blood sugar, impaired temperature regulation, and poor tolerance to hypothermia.

Focus on Natural Products

Yohimbe

Yohimbe is a natural supplement widely taken to treat erectile dysfunction. However, in the absence of standardization in dietary supplement labeling in the United States, there is no reliable way to determine the amount of the drug yohimbine that is contained in the supplement. Yohimbe is not recommended for patients with hypertension or hepatic, renal, or peptic ulcer diseases—all common conditions affecting older adults.

POLYPHARMACY

The practice of prescribing multiple medicines to a single patient simultaneously is called **polypharmacy**. In general, it is better to use as few medicines as possible. Polypharmacy increases the patient's costs for treatment as well as increases the chances for multiple adverse effects and drug interactions. Administration of many drugs together is more common in the elderly population because of their need for different medical specialists and the use of OTC drugs and herbal therapies.

Polypharmacy may cause liver dysfunction, malnutrition, confusion, and falls. Liver dysfunction contributes to delirium or an acute confusional state. Confusion and disturbances of perception (including misinterpretations of information) are commonly seen.

Herbal preparations must also be considered drugs, and their use with prescribed medications contributes to polypharmacy.

Focus on Geriatrics

Polypharmacy

Multiple drug therapies may cause confusion in elderly patients and lead to medication errors and further drug interactions.

✳ Apply Your Knowledge 38.1

The following questions focus on what you have just learned about disease, death, and physiologic changes in older adults.

CRITICAL THINKING

1. What are the major changes during the aging process that impact health?
2. What are the two leading causes of death among older adults?
3. What is the most important physiologic decline in elderly individuals?
4. What factors may influence medication absorption in older adults?
5. What is an indicator of the glomerular filtration rate?
6. What are the adverse effects of morphine, thyroxine, warfarin, and aminoglycosides?
7. What are the contraindications of yohimbe?
8. What is polypharmacy?

Changes in the Effects of Drugs on Elderly Patients

Antihypertensives, cardiac glycosides, antiarrhythmics, CNS drugs (sedative–hypnotics, opioid analgesics, antidepressants, and antipsychotics as well as medications used for Alzheimer's disease), anti-inflammatory drugs, antimicrobial drugs, and gastrointestinal (GI) drugs (antiulcer drugs and laxatives) all have different effects on elderly patients. Drug selection for this group of patients is extremely important. Drugs with longer half-lives may accumulate and cause toxicity.

CARDIOVASCULAR DRUGS

Such cardiovascular disorders as hypertension, congestive heart failure, myocardial infarction, and stroke are very common in older adults. Almost one-third of all deaths in Western countries are attributed to heart disease. Many drugs can be used for these disorders, and some of them must be used cautiously in elderly individuals.

Antihypertensive Drugs

In the United States, blood pressure increases with age, especially in elderly women. It is clear that uncontrolled hypertension leads to serious health problems and, especially in older adults, should be treated very seriously.

Weight reduction and salt restriction are indicated before drug therapy, which usually begins with **thiazides**, the most commonly prescribed class of diuretics. These agents often cause hyperglycemia, hyperuricemia, and hypokalemia in elderly patients because of their higher incidence of arrhythmias, type II diabetes, and gout. It is important that antihypertensives be used in lowered doses. If the patient also has atherosclerotic angina, calcium channel blockers are effective and safe when their use is controlled. Beta-blockers are prescribed less often because of their effects on patients with obstructive airway disease, although they are important if heart failure is present. Angiotensin-converting enzyme (ACE) inhibitors are less useful unless diabetes or heart failure is present.

Alpha$_1$-blockers, such as prazosin and terazosin, and centrally acting alpha$_2$-agonists, such as methyldopa, clonidine, guanabenz, and guanfacine, are infrequently used for elderly patients because of their adverse effects.

Focus on Geriatrics

Antihypertensives and Elderly Patients

All older adults who receive antihypertensive drugs should be regularly monitored for orthostatic hypotension to avoid cerebral ischemia and falls.

Cardiac Glycosides

Physicians often overuse cardiac glycosides, partially because of their fear of heart failure in elderly patients. Because older patients are more susceptible to arrhythmias, the toxic effects of cardiac glycosides are particularly dangerous and the long-term use of these drugs should be carefully monitored because of their narrow therapeutic range. The half-life of digoxin may be increased by 50% or more in elderly patients, and renal function must be considered when a dosing regimen is being contemplated. In geriatric patients, coronary atherosclerosis, hypokalemia, hypomagnesemia, and hypoxemia all contribute to a high incidence of digitalis-induced arrhythmias. Other, less common digitalis toxicities, including delirium, endocrine abnormalities, and visual changes, are also seen in elderly patients. With close monitoring of serum digoxin levels, creatinine clearance tests, and vital signs (the pulse should not be less than 60 beats/min), digoxin is considered safe for older adults.

Antiarrhythmic Drugs

Treating elderly patients who have dysrhythmias (also called *arrhythmias*) is challenging. Whereas clearances of quinidine and procainamide decrease, their half-lives increase in aging patients. Older people exhibit changes in hemodynamic reserve, an incidence of severe coronary disease, and different frequencies of electrolyte disturbances—all of which contribute to arrhythmias. Disopyramide should be avoided because of its major toxicities. The half-life of lidocaine is increased in elderly patients, and its loading dose should be reduced to avoid toxicity.

However, patients with atrial fibrillation do as well with simple control of their ventricular rate as they do with conversion to normal sinus rhythm. For safety, measures should still be taken to reduce possible thromboembolism in chronic atrial fibrillation (such as with anticoagulant drugs or aspirin therapy).

Anticoagulants

Bleeding may occur with the chronic use of anticoagulants in elderly patients. Warfarin is 99% protein-bound and, with a decrease in serum albumin, which is common among older adults, there is an increase in free, unbound circulating warfarin. There is a significant risk for bleeding as a result. Regular testing to determine the level of warfarin in the blood and to regulate anticoagulant drug therapy is essential for everyone taking the drug, particularly older adults.

Focus Point

Prothrombin Time

Elderly patients who are taking anticoagulants must undergo periodic monitoring of prothrombin time or international normalized ratio to determine the level of anticoagulant in the blood and to regulate anticoagulant drug therapy.

CENTRAL NERVOUS SYSTEM DRUGS

Numerous drugs influence the action of chemical mediators and affect neurotransmitter release and reception. These drugs may act by blocking receptors, preventing the transmitters from binding to them. CNS drugs for geriatric patients—sedative–hypnotics, narcotic analgesics, antidepressants, antipsychotics, and drugs used for Alzheimer's disease—are discussed in this section.

Sedatives and Hypnotics

Insomnia is a common problem for older adults. Sedatives and hypnotics are the second-most common group of drugs prescribed for or taken OTC by elderly patients. In those who are 60–70 years old, the half-lives of many barbiturates and benzodiazepines show their greatest age-related increase. These agents are eliminated more slowly if the patient has reduced renal function or liver disease. It is generally believed that elderly patients have more variances in their sensitivity to sedative and hypnotic drugs on a pharmacodynamic basis. To avoid injuries and accidents, ataxia and other motor impairments should be especially watched for in older individuals taking these drugs.

Narcotic Analgesics

Narcotics may cause dose-related adverse effects when taken by elderly patients. Geriatric patients are often more sensitive to the respiratory effects of narcotic analgesics because of the way respiratory function changes with increased age. Patients should be evaluated regarding their sensitivity to these agents before administration, and caution should be continually used. Hypotension may also result from narcotic use. However, for conditions requiring strong analgesia (such as cancer), opioids are frequently underutilized for this group of patients. Good pain management plans are easily obtained, and the underutilization of narcotic analgesics is generally unjustified.

Antidepressants and Antipsychotics

Phenothiazines, such as promazine and perphenazine, and phenothiazine-like drugs, such as haloperidol, have sometimes been overused in managing psychiatric diseases in elderly patients. These agents are effective in treating schizophrenia, delirium, dementia, aggressiveness, and paranoia but are not fully satisfactory for geriatric patients. These drugs do not appear to be effective in dementia caused by Alzheimer's disease. When an antipsychotic drug that has sedative effects is required in elderly patients, a phenothiazine, such as thioridazine, is adequate except in patients with a preexisting extrapyramidal disease. Older drugs, such as chlorpromazine, should be avoided in elderly patients because of their orthostatic hypotension-inducing effects. Drug doses should be gradually increased according to the patient's tolerance and the desired therapeutic effect. There should be close monitoring for possible adverse effects.

The half-lives of some phenothiazines are increased in the geriatric population, and dosages should be started at just a fraction of the amounts used for young adults. Lithium must be dosage-adjusted because of its clearance by the kidneys, and thiazide diuretics should not be used with lithium because it further reduces renal clearance.

Older adults are more likely to experience toxic effects of antidepressants, but they are just as responsive to them as other adults. Senile dementia and major depression must be carefully diagnosed because they may resemble each other. If a tricyclic antidepressant is to be used, nortriptyline and desipramine are good choices because of their reduced antimuscarinic effects.

Focus Point

Depression and Suicide

The suicide rate among people older than age 65 is more than twice the national average, and psychiatric depression—a leading cause of suicide—is often undertreated in elderly patients.

Medications Used for Alzheimer's Disease

Alzheimer's disease is characterized by progressive memory and cognitive function impairment, which may lead to a completely vegetative state and, ultimately, death. The biochemical defects responsible for Alzheimer's disease have not been identified. It is believed that abnormal neuronal lipoprotein processing, together with changes in choline acetyltransferase, brain glutamate, dopamine, norepinephrine, serotonin, and somatostatin, are causative factors.

Cholinomimetic drugs are usually the focus of treatment for Alzheimer's patients. Cerebral vasodilators have been deemed ineffective. A cholinesterase inhibitor called tacrine enters the CNS quickly and has a duration

of 6–8 hours. This drug apparently increases the release of acetylcholine from cholinergic nerve endings and may inhibit monoamine oxidase; decreases the release of gamma-aminobutyric acid; and increases the release of norepinephrine, dopamine, and serotonin from nerve endings. However, it has significant toxic effects, including nausea and vomiting and liver toxicity.

Donepezil, rivastigmine, and galantamine have been shown to improve cognitive activity in some patients with Alzheimer's disease. They may even reduce morbidity from other diseases and slightly prolong the life of the patient. These agents should be used with caution in patients receiving other cytochrome P450 enzyme inhibitors, such as ketoconazole and quinidine.

Focus on Geriatrics

Central Nervous System Drug Toxicities

Alzheimer's patients are often very sensitive to CNS toxicities of drugs that have antimuscarinic effects.

ANTI-INFLAMMATORY DRUGS

For osteoarthritis and rheumatoid arthritis, nonsteroidal anti-inflammatory drugs (NSAIDs), such as naproxen and ibuprofen, must be used with special care because of toxicity. Although aspirin causes GI irritation and bleeding, newer NSAIDs may cause irreversible kidney damage. They accumulate more rapidly in geriatric patients, especially in those with renal disease. Elderly patients receiving large doses of NSAIDs must be carefully monitored for changes in renal function.

For those who cannot tolerate full NSAID doses, corticosteroids, such as hydrocortisone and prednisone, are very useful. However, these agents can cause osteoporosis that is related to the dose and duration of corticosteroid therapy. Increased calcium and vitamin D intake may reduce these effects. Frequent exercise should also be encouraged during corticosteroid therapy.

GASTROINTESTINAL AGENTS

Histamine-2 (H_2) receptor blockers are safer drugs than other antiulcer agents for the treatment of peptic ulcers. Ranitidine, famotidine, and nizatidine may be used for elderly patients. Cimetidine is not suggested for older adults because of its side effects and multiple potential drug interactions.

Laxatives are commonly taken by elderly patients. In long-term facilities, such as nursing homes, 75% of older adult patients use laxatives on a daily basis. Fluid and electrolyte imbalances may occur with excessive use. Increased GI motility with laxative use may decrease the absorption of other drugs.

ANTIMICROBIAL DRUGS

Older adults appear to have reduced host defenses due to alterations in their T-lymphocyte function. As a result, they are more susceptible to serious infections and diseases, such as cancer. Antimicrobial drugs have been used since 1940 to compensate for this deterioration of natural body defenses. Important changes in the half-lives of antimicrobial drugs may be expected because of decreased renal function. This is very important in the case of aminoglycosides owing to their toxicities to the kidneys and other organs. For example, the half-lives of gentamicin, kanamycin, and netilmicin are more than doubled in elderly patients.

Penicillins, such as amoxicillin; cephalosporins, such as cefotaxime; sulfonamides, such as sulfadiazine; and tetracyclines, such as tetracycline HCI, are considered safe for elderly patients. If the patient has a decrease in renal drug clearance and the drug has a prolonged half-life, the drug dose should be reduced.

✳ Apply Your Knowledge 38.2

The following questions focus on what you have just learned about changes in the effects of drugs on the elderly population.

CRITICAL THINKING

1. Why should all elderly patients who receive antihypertensive drugs be regularly monitored?
2. Which psychiatric disorder is a leading cause of suicide in older adults?
3. Why is cimetidine not suggested for older adults?
4. What are two factors that indicate drug doses for elderly patients should be reduced?
5. What group of patients is often very sensitive to CNS toxicities of drugs with antimuscarinic effects?

Special Considerations

Inadequate health care and prescription coverage often force older patients to avoid taking required medications that are important for their quality of life. For example, newer NSAID therapies for arthritis treatment may cost more than $100 a month.

Noncompliance because of forgetfulness may result in patients not staying on a regular drug regimen, thereby greatly reducing effectiveness. Deliberate noncompliance may also occur based on prior poor experience with a drug. Other noncompliance in taking drugs may be caused by physical disabilities or difficulty in using spoons, syringes, and other equipment. Enlisting the elderly patient as an educated, willing participant in drug therapies is vital. Labels should be large enough for patients to read, and any other impediments to sticking to a drug regimen should be noted and efforts should be made to overcome them.

Health care practitioners should adhere to the following principles when treating elderly patients:

* Take drug histories carefully
* Prescribe drugs only for specific, rational indications
* Define the goal of drug therapy
* Start with small doses, adjust slowly, and check blood levels when necessary
* Maintain suspicion regarding drug reactions and interactions by knowing what other drugs the patient is taking
* Keep the drug regimen as simple as possible. Try to use drugs that may be taken at the same time every day and use the smallest number of drugs possible.

Focus Point

More Drugs Prescribed for the Elderly Population

People older than 65 account for more than 33% of the drugs prescribed in the United States, even though they represent only about 13% of the total population.

PRACTICAL SCENARIO 1

An 82-year-old man arrives at the hospital complaining of chest pains. An electrocardiogram reveals congestive heart failure, and he is treated with various drugs, including a diuretic and an ACE inhibitor. His condition stabilizes, and he is discharged. Seven days later, he experiences nausea and confusion. His doctor treats the nausea but does not treat the confusion, assuming it is related to senility. The patient develops a tremor in his hands, which is an adverse effect of the drug prescribed for his nausea. He is given benztropine, which then causes constipation. The doctor gives him docusate tablets for the constipation, but the patient's confusion increases until he is extremely anxious.

Kupicoo/E+/Getty Images

Next, the doctor prescribes an antipsychotic, which calms the patient down but results in depression. The doctor prescribes an antidepressant, but the patient soon dies from ventricular tachycardia.

Critical Thinking Questions

1. What action by the physician may have led to this patient's death?
2. What are the principles that might have helped the physician make different drug therapy decisions for the patient?
3. What assumptions did the physician make early in the course of therapy that may have been unwarranted or incorrect?

PRACTICAL SCENARIO 2

A 73-year-old woman has insomnia. Her physician prescribes a benzodiazepine. This patient also has cirrhosis of the liver.

Critical Thinking Questions

1. What is the most important caution that her physician should consider when prescribing a benzodiazepine for this patient?
2. What is the half-life of a benzodiazepine in an elderly patient?

Chapter Capsule

This section repeats the objectives from the beginning of the chapter and then provides a summary of the most important concepts for that objective. Use this section as a quick review and to check your knowledge.

Objective 1: Discuss the process of aging.

- Physiologic changes: decreased cardiac output and blood flow, function of liver enzymes and blood flow, kidney blood flow, glomerular filtration, nephron function, gastric secretions, peristalsis and motility, first-pass effect, body water, hepatic blood flow, kidney weight, lean body mass, serum albumin, and increased body fat

- Biological, psychological, sociological, and behavioral changes; changes in sensory processes and in roles and self-definitions; slowdown of physical movement; decreased dexterity

Objective 2: Identify factors influencing drug dosages for elderly patients.

- Drug dosages must be adjusted according to an elderly patient's weight, amount of body fat, laboratory results (e.g., blood urea nitrogen, creatinine, serum protein, liver enzymes, electrolytes), and current health conditions

Objective 3: Explain the leading causes of diseases and death in older adults.

- Heart disease, including heart attacks and chronic ischemic heart disease: 35% of deaths among elderly individuals

- Cancer: about 22% percent of deaths in older adults

- Chronic diseases: stroke, chronic obstructive pulmonary disease, diabetes, pneumonia, and influenza

- Alzheimer's disease and several serious renal diseases: have increased over the past two decades as causes of death in elderly individuals

Objective 4: Identify the factors that influence drug absorption in older adults.

- Slower gastric emptying
- Altered nutritional habits
- Greater use of OTC medications

Objective 5: Discuss creatinine clearance in elderly patients and use the measurement formula.

- Creatinine clearance is an indicator of the glomerular filtration rate; creatinine is a by-product of the muscle breakdown of stored proteins but is excreted primarily by the kidneys; serum creatinine level can be measured by the 24-hour creatinine clearance test to evaluate renal function

- Creatinine clearance can also be calculated by this formula:

$$\text{Creatinine clearance in mL/min} = \frac{(140 - \text{age}) \times (\text{weight in kg})}{72 \times \text{serum creatinine in mg/dL}}$$

Objective 6: Identify polypharmacy and its effects on older adults.

- Polypharmacy: prescribing multiple medicines to a single patient simultaneously by one or more physicians; taking herbal drugs in addition to prescribed drugs

- Effects: increased costs of treatment; increased chances for side effects and drug interactions; possible liver dysfunction, malnutrition, confusion, and falls

Objective 7: List common cardiovascular disorders in elderly individuals.

- Hypertension

- Congestive heart failure

- Myocardial infarction

- Stroke

Objective 8: Identify conditions that contribute to a high incidence of digitalis-induced arrhythmias in elderly patients.

- In geriatric patients, coronary atherosclerosis, hypokalemia, hypomagnesemia, and hypoxemia all contribute to a high incidence of digitalis-induced arrhythmias

Objective 9: Discuss the effects of sedatives and hypnotics on elderly patients.

- The half-lives of many sedatives and hypnotics increase in patients ages 60–70

- The reduced elimination of the drugs occurs if the patient has impaired renal function or a liver disease

- Elderly patients often have more variances in their sensitivity to these drugs

- Ataxia and other motor impairments can occur

Objective 10: List six principles that are important in treating older adults.

- Take drug histories carefully

- Prescribe drugs only for specific, rational indications

- Define the goal of drug therapy

- Start with small doses, adjust slowly, and check blood levels

- Know what other drugs the patient is taking

- Keep the drug regimen as simple as possible

Internet Sites of Interest

- For a review of renally excreted drug dosing, visit: **www.rxkinetics.com/renal.html**

- WebMD presents an article on the prescribing of sedatives for older adults with insomnia based on material from the *British Medical Journal* at: **www.webmd.com**. Search for "sedatives elderly."

- PharmacyTimes.com offers "Understanding and Managing Polypharmacy in the Elderly": **www.pharmacytimes.com**. Search for "polypharmacy in the elderly."

- Reducing polypharmacy in older adults is an important issue today. Read information on this topic at: **www.ncbi.nlm.nih.gov/pmc/articles/pmc3785**, and search for "reducing polypharmacy in the elderly."

Chapter 39

Drugs Used to Treat Pediatric Patients

Chapter Objectives

After completing this chapter, you should be able to:

1. Give examples of drugs that may be dangerous because of changes in peripheral blood circulation of infants.

2. Explain peristalsis in neonates, its relationship to drug absorption, and factors that can delay gastric emptying.

3. Describe drug toxicities in neonates from percutaneous absorption.

4. List three example drugs that should not be used in neonates because of their lowered protein binding.

5. Explain the factors that affect pharmacokinetics in children.

6. Discuss the differences between the glomerular filtration rates of newborns, older children, and adults.

7. Describe the means by which adult doses must be adjusted for pediatric drug administration.

8. Discuss pharmacodynamics in newborns, infants, and children.

9. List five drugs that produce pharmacological effects in nursing infants.

10. Explain the effects of radioactive substances in breast milk.

Key Terms

elixirs (p. 686)
gestation (p. 686)
infants (p. 685)

kernicterus (p. 686)
neonates (p. 685)
peripheral blood circulation (p. 685)

peristalsis (p. 685)
suspensions (p. 686)
toddlers (p. 685)

Introduction

Lack of knowledge and understanding of the clinical pharmacology of specific drugs in pediatric patients, particularly in newborns, can result in many problems in drug therapy. The problem of establishing efficacy and dosing guidelines for infants is further complicated by the fact that the pharmacokinetics of many drugs change greatly as an infant ages from birth to several months after birth. The dose–response relationships of some drugs may change markedly during the first few weeks after birth. Then, during the first few months of life, physiologic processes and their resulting pharmacokinetic variables change significantly. This is why it is vital to pay special attention to the pharmacokinetics of pediatric patients. The differences between younger patients and other groups have not been greatly researched.

Neonates refer to newborns from birth to 28 days old, **infants** are from 29 days old to walking age (typically 1 year), and **toddlers** are children from approximately 1 year to 3 years.

Pharmacokinetics

The basic pharmacologic principles that apply to adults (see Chapter 1) also apply to neonates, infants, and younger children. Only the ways in which they differ in neonates and infants are discussed in this chapter.

DRUG ABSORPTION

In infants and children, the drug absorption process is similar to that of adults. Factors such as blood flow at the site of administration and gastrointestinal (GI) function influence drug absorption. These factors change rapidly soon after birth.

Physiologic conditions that can reduce the rate of blood flow to the site of administration include heart failure, cardiovascular shock, and vasoconstriction. For example, there is very little muscle mass in a preterm infant who is sick. Drugs may remain in the muscles and be absorbed more slowly than anticipated. If **peripheral blood circulation** (the circulation in the body's extremities) improves, a sudden increase of circulating drugs may result in potentially toxic drug concentrations. Drugs that can be especially dangerous in these situations include aminoglycoside antibiotics, anticonvulsants, and cardiac glycosides.

Because of rapidly changing biochemical and physiologic changes that occur in the GI tract of infants, drugs that are inactivated by the low pH of gastric contents should not be given orally. **Peristalsis** (the rhythmic movement of the intestines) in neonates is irregular and may be slower than anticipated. Great care must be taken in administering drugs to neonates because of the unpredictability of their rates of absorption.

The rate of gastric emptying is an important determinant of the overall rate and extent of drug absorption. It is variable during the neonatal period and is affected by gestational maturity, postnatal age, and type of feeding. Gastroesophageal reflux, respiratory distress syndrome, and congenital heart disease in neonates can delay gastric emptying.

Chemical agents applied to the skin of a premature infant may result in inadvertent poisoning. For example, drug toxicities in neonates are reported for percutaneous absorption of such agents as hexachlorophene, laundry detergents with pentachlorophenol, hydrocortisone, and disinfectant solutions with aniline.

DRUG DISTRIBUTION

Neonates have higher percentages of water than adults. Extracellular water makes up 40% of body weight in neonates, compared with 20% in adults. Most neonates experience diuresis in the first 2 days of life. It is important, especially for water-soluble drugs, to determine the concentration of a drug at receptor sites.

The amount of body fat in full-term neonates is about 15%. Organs that accumulate high concentrations of lipid-soluble drugs in older children may accumulate smaller amounts of these types of agents in younger infants. Another important factor is drug binding to plasma proteins. Albumin's affinity for acidic drugs and the total plasma protein concentration increase during the time from birth into early infancy. These do not reach normal adult values until 10–12 months of age. Usually, protein binding of drugs is lowered in neonates. This has been seen with local anesthetic drugs, diazepam, phenobarbital, ampicillin, and phenytoin. Therefore, the concentration of free (unbound) drug in plasma is increased. This results in greater drug effect or toxicity.

Focus on Pediatrics

Physiologic Impacts on Pharmacokinetics

The physiologic processes that influence pharmacokinetics in children include GI function, tissue blood flow, body fluid levels, plasma protein concentrations, liver function, and renal function.

Certain drugs compete with serum bilirubin in binding to albumin. Drugs given to a neonate with jaundice can displace bilirubin from albumin, and because of the greater permeability of a neonate's blood–brain barrier, large amounts of bilirubin may enter the brain and cause **kernicterus**, which is a serious form of jaundice in newborns.

DRUG METABOLISM

Most drugs are metabolized in the liver. Drug-metabolizing oxidases and conjugating enzymes exhibit substantially lower activity in neonates. Because of these lower metabolic activities, many drugs have slow clearance rates and longer half-life elimination times. Drug doses and dosing schedules must be altered appropriately. If not, the neonate may experience adverse effects from drugs that are metabolized in the liver.

The limited knowledge and understanding of the clinical pharmacology of specific drugs in pediatric patients predispose this population to problems in the course of drug treatment, particularly in newborns and infants. There are no FDA requirements for pediatric studies, which means that determining appropriate efficacy and dosage guidelines for the therapeutic use of drugs in children must rely extensively on pharmacologic data derived primarily from adults. The problem of establishing efficacy and dosage guidelines for infants is further complicated by the fact that the pharmacokinetics of many drugs

change appreciably as an infant ages from birth (which is sometimes premature) to several months after birth. The dose–response relationships of some drugs may change markedly during the first few weeks after birth.

Pharmacokinetics and organ responsiveness also change dramatically during development from the embryonic and fetal periods to adulthood. Prematurely born neonates at gestations as short as 24 weeks are now surviving (a full-term **gestation**, or the period of fetal development from conception until birth, is 40 weeks).

DRUG EXCRETION

The glomerular filtration rate (GFR) is much lower in newborns than in older children and adults. Based on body surface area, a neonate's GFR is only 30–40% that of an adult. Premature babies show an even lower GFR. However, GFRs do improve greatly during the first week after birth. By the end of the third week, glomerular filtration is 50–60% of an adult's. Adult values are reached by the time an infant is 6–12 months old. Drugs that require renal function for elimination are removed from the body very slowly during the first weeks of life.

Toddlers may have shorter elimination half-lives of drugs than older children and adults, probably as a result of higher renal elimination and metabolism. One example concerns the drug digoxin. The dose per kilogram of this drug is much higher for toddlers than for adults, which is a fact that is still not fully understood.

✳ Apply Your Knowledge 39.1

The following questions focus on what you have just learned about pediatric pharmacokinetics.

CRITICAL THINKING

1. What physiologic processes may influence pharmacokinetics in children?
2. What are the definitions of the terms *neonate*, *infant*, and *toddler*?
3. What is the cause of kernicterus?
4. What is the result of lower metabolic activities in neonates?
5. Compare the GFR of newborns to older children and adults.

Pediatric Dosage Forms and Compliance

Actual pediatric dosages are determined by taking into account the form of the drug and how a parent or caregiver will dispense it to the child. Elixirs and suspensions are popular forms for pediatric administration. **Elixirs** are alcoholic solutions that offer consistent dissolution and distribution of the drugs they contain. **Suspensions** are dosage forms that contain undissolved

drug particles and must be shaken to evenly distribute them. This is essential because if a suspension drug form is not adequately shaken, it will cause dangerous variations in dosages. For example, an uneven distribution of drug is a potential cause of inefficacy or toxicity in children taking phenytoin suspensions. The prescriber must provide proper instructions to the pharmacist and the child's parents or caregivers.

Major dosing errors may result from incorrect calculations because many pediatric doses are calculated by using body weight. A common but potentially fatal mistake is that 10 times the amount of medication is administered because a decimal point was placed incorrectly. A good rule to use in avoiding decimal point errors is to always use a zero to the left of a decimal point for doses that are less than 1 (Figure 39-1 ■). Also, zeros should not be used after decimal points if they are not needed.

Focus Point

Pediatric Doses

Pediatric doses can be based on body surface area, age, and body weight.

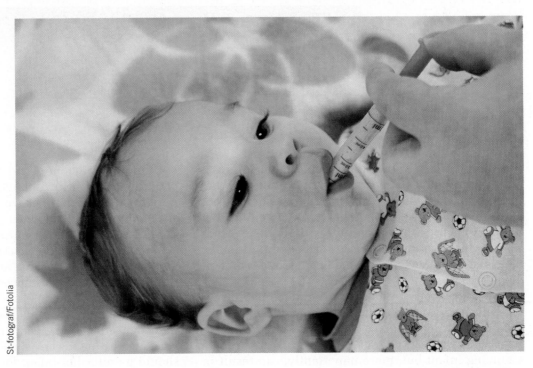

Figure 39-1 ■ Using the measuring device provided by the pharmacy or physician is important for giving the correct dose to children.

St-fotograf/Fotolia

Pharmacodynamics

The mechanisms of action of drugs in newborns, infants, and children involve a complex sequence of events. An inadequate response to an effective concentration of a drug may result from the presence or absence of receptors, inadequate drug–receptor binding, or the inability of the organ or tissue to respond to the postreceptor signal. One particular drug may have a specific affinity for a special cell. Some drugs may act by affecting the enzyme functions of the body.

Each of these events progresses at different rates during development—beginning with growth to biochemical maturation and eventually to structural maturation, at which point the organ can respond fully to the events initiated by a drug.

Certain drugs pose particular difficulties when used in neonates because of the unique character of their distribution or elimination in patients in this age group or because of the unusual side effects they may cause. These drugs include antibiotics, digoxin, indomethacin, and methylxanthines.

Focus Point

Pediatric Pharmacokinetic Differences

The differences in pharmacokinetics can lead to stronger or weaker drug effects in children compared with those in young adults.

Drug Administration During Lactation

Many women avoid breastfeeding because they incorrectly believe that drugs they may be taking are in sufficient quantities to cause great risk to their infants. In actuality, more babies die because of problems from baby formula than from the milk of their mothers.

Still, it is important to realize that most drugs taken by lactating women do pass through to the breast milk. Drug concentration in breast milk is usually low. In a 1-day period, the amount of drug an infant receives from nursing is much less than what would be considered a "therapeutic dose." If a drug is prescribed as safe for a mother to take while she is breastfeeding, she should take it 1–2 hours before breastfeeding or 3–4 hours after breastfeeding to minimize the effect on the infant. Most over-the-counter (OTC) medications provide information on the label about their safety during lactation. Nursing mothers should avoid OTC products that contain multiple ingredients, such as cold remedies, as well as those containing more than 20% alcohol. Nursing mothers should not take more than the dosage listed on the product label.

Focus on Pediatrics

Drug Safety During Lactation

If data are not available about a certain drug and its effects on breastfeeding, the mother should not take it.

Many antibiotics are highly detectable in breast milk. Tetracyclines appear at about 70% of maternal serum concentrations and can stain the developing teeth of an infant. Isoniazid can quickly reach equilibrium between maternal blood and breast milk. Its concentrations in breast milk can cause signs of pyridoxine deficiency in the infant if the mother does not take pyridoxine supplements.

Sedatives and hypnotics can produce pharmacologic effects in nursing infants. Barbiturates can produce sedation and poor sucking reflexes; sedation can also be caused by chloral hydrate. Diazepam can also sedate a nursing infant but, more importantly, can result in significant drug accumulation.

Heroin, methadone, and morphine can cause narcotic dependence in infants, and these infants may have to be tapered off, as would their mothers. Excessive amounts of alcohol can produce alcoholic effects in infants. Lithium enters breast milk in concentrations equal to those in maternal serum, and the baby may be exposed to relatively large amounts of this drug as a result. Radioactive substances can increase the risk of thyroid cancer in infants, and chemotherapeutic, cytotoxic, or immune-modulating agents are also potentially dangerous to the pediatric population. No matter what medication the breastfeeding mother is taking, she should monitor her infant for any signs of drug effect and report this to the infant's health care provider.

Focus on Natural Products

Lobelia Dangers

Lobelia is found in dietary supplements that are marketed for use by children and infants as well as pregnant women. Lobelia may be very dangerous to use because it contains alkaloids with pharmacologic actions that are similar to nicotine. It can cause autonomic nervous system depression or stimulation, bronchial dilation, increased respiratory rate, respiratory depression, sweating, rapid heart rate, hypotension, and even coma or death.

Pediatric Drug Dosages

It is not always safe to proportionally reduce adult doses to determine safe pediatric doses. Patients or their parents should always follow their physician's instructions about pediatric dosages and double-check them with the drug manufacturer's product inserts and labels. The FDA is moving toward more stringent demands on the testing and thorough labeling of new drug products for children. The recommended pediatric dose—usually stated as milligrams per kilogram or milligrams per pound—should always be followed.

✳ Apply Your **Knowledge 39.2**

The following questions focus on what you have just learned about pediatric dosage forms.

CRITICAL THINKING

1. What pediatric dosage forms are more popular for drug administration?
2. Which pediatric dosage form must be shaken before administration to an infant?
3. What factor is the major cause of dosing errors?
4. What is the effect of heroin in nursing infants?
5. What is the result of the difference in pharmacokinetics in children compared with those in young adults?

PRACTICAL SCENARIO 1

Alice, age 32, is breastfeeding her newborn. Alice has developed a cold and says she is not sleeping at night because of her symptoms. She wants to take an OTC decongestant and cough suppressant. But Alice's health care provider instructed her that she cannot take any medication while breastfeeding without first checking with her physician. Alice is confused and questions you about this.

Ruth Jenkinson/DK Images

Critical Thinking Questions

1. How would you address Alice's concerns?
2. Is it safe for Alice to take an OTC product for her cold symptoms while she is breastfeeding?
3. How can Alice help to minimize any effect on her infant from taking a medication?

PRACTICAL SCENARIO 2

A newborn baby was in the neonatal care ward with seizures. Her pediatrician prescribed a barbiturate medication for intramuscular injection.

Evok20/Shutterstock

Critical Thinking Questions

1. Describe the four stages of pharmacokinetics.
2. Because an infant's kidneys do not develop fully until 6 months of age, what important consideration should the pediatrician remember before administering any medications?

Chapter Capsule

This section repeats the objectives from the beginning of the chapter and then provides a summary of the most important concepts for that objective. Use this section as a quick review and to check your knowledge.

Objective 1: Give examples of drugs that may be dangerous because of changes in peripheral blood circulation of infants.

- Drugs that can be especially dangerous to newborns or infants include aminoglycoside antibiotics, anticonvulsants, and cardiac glycosides

Objective 2: Explain peristalsis in neonates, its relationship to drug absorption, and factors that can delay gastric emptying.

- Peristalsis (the rhythmic movement of the intestines) in neonates is irregular and may be slower than anticipated

- Great care must be taken in administering drugs to neonates because of the unpredictability of their rates of absorption

- Gastroesophageal reflux, respiratory distress syndrome, and congenital heart disease in neonates can delay gastric emptying

Objective 3: Describe drug toxicities in neonates from percutaneous absorption.

- Agents that may result in inadvertent poisoning in neonates include hexachlorophene, pentachlorophenol-containing laundry detergents, hydrocortisone, and aniline-containing disinfectant solutions

Objective 4: List three example drugs that should not be used in neonates because of their lowered protein binding.

- Local anesthetic drugs

- Diazepam

- Phenobarbital

Objective 5: Explain the factors that affect pharmacokinetics in children.

- Drug absorption: physiologic conditions that can reduce the rate of blood flow to the site of administration include heart failure, cardiovascular shock, and vasoconstriction; if peripheral blood circulation improves, a sudden increase of circulating drugs may result in potentially toxic drug concentrations; rate of gastric emptying

- Drug distribution: neonates have higher percentages of water than do adults; their amount of body fat is about 15%; another important factor is drug binding to plasma proteins; protein binding of drugs is lowered in neonates

- Drug metabolism: neonates exhibit substantially lower drug-metabolizing activities of oxidases and conjugating enzymes; the dose–response relationships of some drugs may change markedly during the first few weeks after birth

- Drug excretion: in newborns, the glomerular filtration rate is much lower than in older children or adults; drugs that require renal function for elimination are removed from the body very slowly during the first weeks of life

Objective 6: Discuss the differences between the glomerular filtration rates of newborns, older children, and adults.

- The glomerular filtration rate (GFR) is much lower in newborns than in older children and adults. Based on body surface area, a neonate's GFR is only 30–40% that of an adult. Premature babies show an even lower GFR. However, GFRs do improve greatly during the first week after birth. By the end of the third week, glomerular filtration is 50–60% of an adult's. Adult values are reached by the time an infant is 6–12 months old.

Objective 7: Describe the means by which adult doses must be adjusted for pediatric drug administration.

- Pediatric drug dosages are based on proportionally reduced adult doses
- They can be based on body surface area, age, and body weight

Objective 8: Discuss pharmacodynamics in newborns, infants, and children.

- An inadequate response to an effective concentration of a drug may result from the presence or absence of receptors or inadequate drug–receptor binding
- A particular drug has a specific affinity for a special cell
- Some drugs may act by affecting the enzyme functions of the body
- Certain drugs pose particular difficulties when used in neonates because of the unique character of their distribution or elimination in patients in this age group or because of the unusual side effects they may cause

Objective 9: List five drugs that produce pharmacological effects in nursing infants.

- Antibiotics
- Sedatives and hypnotics
- Heroin
- Alcohol
- Lithium

Objective 10: Explain the effects of radioactive substances in breast milk.

- These substances can increase the risk of thyroid cancer in infants, and chemotherapeutic, cytotoxic, and immune-modulating agents are also potentially dangerous to babies

 Internet Sites of Interest

- Pediatric pharmacotherapy: **www.medscape.com/viewpublication/87**
- The site **www.mapharm.com/med_calc_pedi.htm** provides information about medical assisting pharmacology with calculation examples.
- Pediatric medication handbook is available at: **www.chkd.org/uploadedfiles/ documents/medical_professionals/pedmedhandbook.pdf**
- Pediatric dosage calculations are explained in this website: **www.drugguide.com/ ddo/ub/view/davis-drug-guide/109514/0/pediatric_dosage_calculations**
- Medications for babies and toddlers are featured at: **www.babycenter.com/303_ medications-for-babies-toddlers_10402250.bc**
- Medications for children and adolescents are described at: **www.drugwatch.com/ children/**

Chapter 40

Drugs Used to Treat Pregnant Patients

Chapter Objectives

After reading this chapter, you should be able to:

1. Describe various stages of reproduction that may potentially be affected by drug toxicity.

2. Identify at least one example drug for each pregnancy risk category.

3. Define the terms *reproductive toxicology, developmental toxicity,* and *embryo toxicity* and *fetotoxicity.*

4. Explain the four principles concerning a drug's potential to induce developmental disorders.

5. Define *pharmacokinetics* in pregnant women.

6. Discuss the possible outcomes if toxic agents contact a developing embryo or fetus during embryogenesis or organogenesis.

7. Describe which drugs used during lactation can cause disruption to the infant's normal sleeping patterns.

8. Define the term *teratology.*

9. Discuss immunizations during pregnancy.

10. Identify which vaccine may be administered during pregnancy without any harm to the mother or baby.

Key Terms

cohort (p. 697)
developmental toxicity (p. 698)
dysmorphology (p. 699)
embryotoxicity or fetotoxicity (p. 698)
epidemiological (p. 697)
fetal (p. 693)

fetotoxic (p. 697)
metabolites (p. 696)
oogonia (p. 693)
perinatal (p. 693)
phenylketonuria (p. 698)
reproductive toxicology (p. 698)

teratogenicity (p. 698)
teratogens (p. 696)
teratology (p. 698)
tidal volume (p. 694)
transplacental (p. 693)

Introduction

Pregnancy begins with conception and ends with the delivery of the baby. During the lifespan, organs and body systems undergo physiological changes that affect the absorption, metabolism, distribution, and elimination of medications. Health professionals must understand these changes to ensure that drugs are administered safely and effectively to patients of all ages. It is important to understand the effects of medications before becoming pregnant, during the entire time a fetus is carried, and throughout early life.

Drugs can affect all stages of pre- and postnatal development. During embryonic life, the majority of organs and systems are forming. Drugs and other substances, including radiation, may be particularly harmful during the first trimester of pregnancy. Pregnant women must be educated about the use of medications when attempting to become pregnant because their effects on an embryo may be severe. The study of drug effects on pregnant patients is not as advanced as the study of other areas of pharmacology, although advances are being made. Drugs used during pregnancy have the potential to cause **fetal** malformations, restricted growth, functional defects, and death.

Health and Development

Although most normal pregnancies require only minimal medical intervention, high-risk pregnancies may require intensive care and medications. When a pregnant woman is ill, the treatment or lack of treatment of her condition may be harmful to the developing fetus. It is widely known that cigarette smoking and alcohol use are damaging to fetuses, but many prescription and over-the-counter (OTC) drugs also have harmful effects. Herbal supplements must also be carefully used, and proper nutrition during pregnancy is essential. The effects of improper nutrition and the use of certain medications have been linked to diseases later in the life of the fetus, including fertility disorders, metabolic imbalances, diabetes, cardiovascular conditions, and even schizophrenia.

STAGES OF REPRODUCTION

Each developmental stage has its own sensitivities to toxic agents. The following list details specific potential outcomes of use of toxic agents and poor nutrition at each stage of development.

✳ Germ cell formation: sterility, damage to sperm or egg cells, chromosomal defects, menstrual and menopausal defects, hormone imbalances

✳ Fertilization: impotence, sterility, chromosomal defects, reduced sperm function

✳ Implantation: spontaneous abortion, low birth weight, stillbirth

✳ Embryogenesis: spontaneous abortion, birth defects, chromosomal defects, low birth weight, stillbirth

✳ Organogenesis: spontaneous abortion, birth defects, retarded development, functional disorders (such as autism), **transplacental** carcinogenesis

✳ **Perinatal** period: premature birth, birth defects (usually nervous system related), stillbirth, neonatal death, toxicity, withdrawal symptoms

✳ Postnatal period: mental retardation, infant death, retarded development, metabolic and functional disorders, developmental disabilities (such as epilepsy or cerebral palsy)

About 1 month after the first day of the last menstrual period, primordial germ cells are present in an embryo. These cells differentiate into **oogonia** and oocytes or into spermatogonia. During a female's lifespan, nearly 400 oocytes undergo ovulation. In males, the onset of meiosis begins at puberty, and spermatogenesis continues throughout the reproductive life. Therefore, prenatal and postnatal drug exposure may be toxic during any stage of development. Each sex reacts differently to various toxic agents.

✳ Apply Your Knowledge 40.1 ▬▬▬

The following questions focus on what you have just learned about health and development.

CRITICAL THINKING

1. Why are many medications prohibited during the first trimester of pregnancy?

2. What are the potential outcomes when toxic agents are used during organogenesis?

3. How can fetal toxicity from drugs be best prevented?

DRUG ADMINISTRATION DURING PREGNANCY AND LACTATION

Great caution should be taken when administering drugs during pregnancy and lactation. When possible, it should be avoided completely or nonpharmacologic methods should be undertaken. However, for specific, serious conditions, pharmacotherapy is required. If epilepsy, hypertension, or psychiatric disorders exist before pregnancy, drug therapy should not be discontinued during pregnancy or lactation. Conditions that occur during pregnancy, such as gestational diabetes and hypertension, must be treated to maintain the health of the growing fetus. Because such infections as acute urinary tract infections and sexually transmitted diseases may harm fetuses, antibiotics may be indicated. Regardless of the condition, health care practitioners must determine whether the therapeutic benefits of drug administration outweigh potential adverse effects.

PHARMACOTHERAPY IN THE PREGNANT PATIENT

The effects of a drug on the mother and the fetus must be considered before it can be administered. Certain substances easily pass from the mother to the fetus through the semipermeable placenta. Other substances are blocked from this passage. The membranes of the fetus detoxify some substances, such as insulin, as they cross the membrane. Drugs that are bound to plasma proteins, ionized, or water soluble are not as likely to cross the placenta.

Major physiological and anatomic changes occur in pregnant women. Some of these changes alter drug pharmacokinetics and pharmacodynamics. Changes in hormone levels as well as pressure exerted on the blood supply by the expanding uterus may affect the absorption of drugs. Progesterone slows the transit time for food and drugs in the gastrointestinal (GI) tract. This allows for a longer time for absorption of drugs taken orally. Gastric emptying also slows, and gastric acidity is decreased. Inhaled drugs may be absorbed more readily because increased **tidal volume** and pulmonary vasodilation occur in pregnant women.

Cardiac output, plasma volume, and regional blood flow may be increased, causing dilution of drugs and decreased plasma protein concentration. Lipid-level alterations may affect drug transport and distribution (primarily during the third trimester). Drug metabolism increases may cause higher doses of certain drugs to be used (primarily anticonvulsants). Because fat-soluble drugs are distributed into breast milk (which is rich in lipids), they may be passed to the lactating infant.

Blood flow through the mother's kidneys increases between 40 and 50% by the third trimester. This affects glomerular filtration rate, renal plasma flow, and renal tubular absorption. Drug excretion is then affected, including the onset of action and dosage timing.

Pregnancy Drug Categories and Registries

Only a small number of prescription drugs have been verified as being teratogenic or are strongly suspected as teratogens. Alternative drugs can be safely used instead. Newer or infrequently used drugs should be avoided in pregnant women until their outcomes are better understood. The FDA has created drug pregnancy categories, as shown in Table 40-1 ■.

Illicit drugs, such as cocaine, also affect fetuses. Although testing drugs in human subjects for teratogenicity is unethical and legally prohibited, animal testing is regularly undertaken. However, these studies do not provide identical outcomes because human placentas (and other components) are structurally different from those of animals. The following rule must be remembered: No prescription drug, OTC medication, herbal product, or dietary supplement should be taken during pregnancy unless a physician verifies that the therapeutic benefits to the mother clearly outweigh the potential risks for the unborn.

Unfortunately, the current pregnancy drug labeling system does not give specific clinical information to help understand the true safety of medications. It does not indicate how doses should be adjusted during pregnancy. Most drugs are ranked as Category C for pregnancy because high doses produce teratogenicity in animals. All drugs in Category D or Category X must be avoided during pregnancy because of potentially severe birth defects. Women of childbearing age must be asked about their intentions of becoming pregnant before being prescribed any drugs that are potentially harmful to the fetus.

Pregnancy Registries

Pregnancy registries gather information from women who have taken certain medications during pregnancy to determine those that are safe for use by others when they become pregnant. By comparing women who did not take a specific medication while pregnant with those who did, data are compiled on fetal outcomes. Pregnancy registries are maintained by drug companies, governmental agencies, and special interest groups.

Table 40-1 ■ **Food and Drug Administration Pregnancy Drug Categories**

RISK CATEGORY	DESCRIPTION	EXAMPLES
A	Well-controlled studies of pregnant women with no demonstrated increased risk of fetal abnormalities in any trimester	Folic acid, insulin, prenatal multivitamins, thyroxine
B	Either animal reproduction studies have not demonstrated a fetal risk but there are no controlled studies in pregnant women, or animal reproduction studies have shown an adverse effect that was not confirmed in controlled studies in women in the first trimester	Acetaminophen, azithromycin, cephalosporins, penicillins, ibuprofen in the first and second trimesters
C	Either studies in animals have revealed adverse effects on the fetus and there are no controlled studies in women, or studies in women and animals are not available. Drugs should be given only if the potential benefit justifies the potential risk to the fetus.	Most prescription medications, most antihypertensives, antimicrobials (such as clarithromycin, co-trimoxazole, and fluoroquinolones), corticosteroids, SSRIs
D	Well-controlled studies of pregnant women have demonstrated fetal risk, but benefits of therapy may outweigh the risk, especially in life-threatening situations or serious diseases that cannot be effectively treated with safer drugs	ACE inhibitors and ARBs in the second and third trimesters; alcohol, gentamicin, ibuprofen in the third trimester; nicotine; conjugated estrogens; tetracyclines
X	Well-controlled or observational animal studies have shown positive risk of fetal abnormalities; use of these products is contraindicated in pregnant women and those who may become pregnant. *There is no indication for use in pregnancy.*	Isotretinoin, misoprostol, thalidomide

SSRI, selective serotonin reuptake inhibitor; ACE, angiotensin-converting enzyme; ARB, angiotensin receptor blocker.

Focus Point

Examples of Pregnancy Registries

Here is a list of some pregnancy registries:

- MotherToBaby—http://mothertobaby.org
- The Antiretroviral Pregnancy Registry—www.apregistry.com
- MotheRisk—www.motherisk.org/women/index.jsp
- Massachusetts General Hospital Antiepileptic Drug Pregnancy Registry—www2.massgeneral.org/aed/

Also, the FDA's list of pregnancy registries is located at: www.fda.gov/ScienceResearch/SpecialTopics/WomensHealthResearch/ucm134848.htm

❋ Apply Your Knowledge 40.2

The following questions focus on what you have just learned about drug administration during pregnancy and lactation.

CRITICAL THINKING

1. Why must drug therapy be continued during pregnancy when the patient has hypertension?
2. How can physiological and anatomic changes in pregnant women alter drug pharmacokinetics and pharmacodynamics?
3. Why may increases in metabolism require higher doses of anticonvulsants?
4. Which federal agency has created drug pregnancy categories and why?
5. Which category of pregnancy drugs is contraindicated in pregnant women? List three examples.

Toxic Effects and Responses

Developmental toxicity may cause many different conditions, including chromosomal and genetic disorders, infertility, intrauterine death, spontaneous abortion, low birth weight, prematurity, functional disorders, and birth defects. Toxic effects may occur at different times and be highly unpredictable. Many structural malformations occur during the period of organogenesis (between 20 and 70 days after the first day of last menstrual period). They can also occur from 1 week before the missed period until the woman is 44 days past due. Exposure to radiographs may also

have unpredictable timed effects. Also, **teratogens** may be **metabolites** and not the actual administered compounds.

During fetal development, common responses to toxic agents include restricted growth, structural malformations, functional impairment, fetal death, and transplacental carcinogenesis. Because organ and system maturation occurs beyond organogenesis and the prenatal period, responses may occur over a much longer period of time. This may lead to behavioral, reproductive, immunologic, and other responses, including those related to endocrine, metabolic, and intelligence functions. Also, carcinogenic effects of certain agents are increased because fetal tissues are more vulnerable to their effects.

Focus Point

Radiographs

The primary manifestations of intrauterine radiation effects on humans are growth retardation and central nervous system defects.

Pharmacokinetics

During pregnancy, metabolism and kinetics of drugs are more complicated. Influences include uptake, distribution, metabolism, and excretion by the mother. Other factors involve the passage and metabolism of agents through the yolk sac and placenta. Embryos and fetuses distribute, metabolize, and excrete agents differently than in the postnatal period, with reabsorption and swallowing of substances from the amniotic fluid being unique to fetal development.

During pregnancy, GI motility and distribution to plasma proteins is decreased compared with other times during life. However, nearly all other resorptive, distributive, metabolic, and excretive processes are

increased. These include lung function, skin–blood circulation, distribution to plasma volume, distribution to body water, distribution to fat deposition, and the glomerular filtration rate. However, metabolic liver activity in developing fetuses may be increased or decreased depending on many factors.

Because total body water may be increased up to 81% during pregnancy, drugs can be distributed in a greatly increased volume. Because albumin is decreased in concentration, the binding of acidic drugs, such as aspirin or phenytoin, is likewise decreased. Increased female hormones due to pregnancy may inactivate certain medications and environmental agents. During the last trimester, greatly increased renal plasma flow causes a more rapid elimination of drugs without being changed by the kidneys.

✳ Apply Your Knowledge 40.3

The following questions focus on what you have just learned about toxic effects and responses.

CRITICAL THINKING

1. What are the common responses to toxic agents during fetal development?
2. Why are drugs with shorter half-lives preferable during lactation?
3. Why do many structural malformations occur during the first trimester?
4. Why is distribution of plasma protein decreased during pregnancy?
5. Why does more rapid elimination of drugs occur during the last trimester?
6. Why should radiographs not be used during the first trimester of pregnancy?

Drug Effects on the Newborn

The passage of drugs to fetuses and the way that fetal kinetics work are of primary concern with long-term drug therapy. The placenta allows oral medications to pass between the maternal and fetal circulation. Drugs cross the placenta by passive diffusion. It should be understood that basically any drug will reach the fetus. The only drugs that are not able to cross the placenta are conjugated steroid and peptide hormones, such as growth hormone and insulin. Others, such as modified immunoglobulins (such as abciximab), are instead metabolized by the placenta itself.

By the third month of pregnancy, the liver of the fetus can activate or inactivate chemical substances by the process of oxidation. Accumulation of biologically active substances can take place in the fetal compartment. At this stage, fetuses have not yet developed the blood–brain barrier, making many chemicals **fetotoxic**. Penicillins, cephalosporins, and antiretrovirals concentrate in the fetal compartment. Fetuses can also swallow excreted substances in the amniotic fluid.

RISKS OF TOXICITY

Risks of toxicity concerning embryos and fetuses are assessed using a variety of methods. These include animal experimentation, **epidemiological** studies, case studies, and other methods. Drugs that have been proven to have significant toxicity to embryos and fetuses include:

* Angiotensin-converting enzyme inhibitors and angiotensin II receptor antagonists
* Alcohol
* Androgens
* Antimetabolites
* Benzodiazepines
* Carbamazepine
* Cocaine
* Coumarin anticoagulants
* Diethylstilbestrol
* Ionizing radiation
* Iodine overdose
* Lead
* Lithium
* Methyl mercury
* Misoprostol
* Penicillamine
* Phenobarbital and primidone in anticonvulsive doses
* Phenytoin
* Polychlorinated biphenyls
* Retinoids
* Tetracycline after week 15
* Thalidomide
* Trimethadione
* Valproic acid
* Vitamin A (over 25,000 International Units per day)

Ideally, every pregnancy should be studied and all outcomes assessed. Many analytical studies use the **cohort** approach, in which a specific adverse outcome is studied in women who were exposed to the same toxic agent. Sometimes, case-control studies within cohort groups of women are conducted. These lead to the identification of possible statistical associations between the exposure and outcome.

Prolonged use of certain medicines during pregnancy is likely to cause fetal harm. Women who have epilepsy, diabetes, or thyroid dysfunction often regularly use long-term medications, making pregnancy especially dangerous. Also, women with psychiatric illnesses may require fetotoxic medications on a long-term basis.

✱ Apply Your Knowledge 40.4 ▬▬▬▬▬

The following questions focus on what you have just learned about drug effects on fetuses.

CRITICAL THINKING

1. What is the reason that the placenta allows oral medications to pass to the fetus?
2. In which month of pregnancy does the liver of the fetus begin to activate or inactivate chemical substances by the process of oxidation?
3. What methods may be used to assess the risks of toxicity concerning embryos or fetuses?
4. What term is used to study a specific adverse outcome in women who were exposed to the same toxic agent?
5. What may be the long-term effects on the fetus of drugs used to treat psychiatric illnesses in the mother?

Drugs Used During Pregnancy

Nearly 80% of pregnant women use prescription or OTC drugs. Exposures to occupational and environmental agents while pregnant are also very common. It is best to avoid taking any medications unless absolutely necessary when pregnant. Illegal drugs, tobacco, and alcohol must be avoided. Classifications of drugs in relation to pregnancy are primarily based on human toxicity testing.

RISKS OF MEDICATIONS DURING PREGNANCY

Most pregnant women take between three and eight different medications during their pregnancies. The risks of each medication should be discussed between pregnant patients and their physicians before beginning use or before patients even become pregnant. If a patient has already taken any medication and is pregnant, the physician should continue to communicate with her about potential outcomes. This communication should include whether diagnostic procedures may be required to assess any fetal harm and consideration of termination of pregnancy if the harm is severe. It is not enough to rely on safety warnings printed on package inserts, reference books, and other sources to inform patients about the potential toxicities of medications.

TOXIC STATES

Reproductive toxicology is the study of the effects of toxic agents during the entire reproductive process. **Developmental toxicity** involves adverse effects that occur before adulthood. **Teratology** is the study of structural birth defects in general, although it also relates to certain functional defects. **Embryotoxicity** or **fetotoxicity** involves toxic effects resulting from prenatal exposure as well as structural or functional abnormalities of the

postnatal manifestations of these effects. **Teratogenicity** is defined as a manifestation of developmental toxicity by induction or an increase of frequency of structural disorders in the embryo or fetus.

Poor nutrition has been linked to many birth defects, as have such disease states as German measles (rubella) and toxoplasmosis. Perhaps the most famous case of severe birth defects occurred in the thalidomide disaster, wherein the mild sedative thalidomide taken by pregnant women caused fetal limb deformities. Although the prevalence of birth defects, which affect between 3 and 4% of babies, is not increasing, the potential for them as caused by the use of toxic agents is real. Another area of concern is exposure to environmental toxicity, often in the workplace.

The best prevention of toxic states on fetuses is achieved through public education. Curbing such habits as smoking and alcohol use is essential. Proper vaccination with all recommended vaccines is also critical. Drugs are classified into categories based on their potential to cause harm to developing fetuses, but these categories must be understood so they can be used properly. Also, when a metabolic disorder, such as **phenylketonuria**, is detected early enough, the diet may be adjusted so phenylalanine is present in only very low levels to prevent mental retardation. The removal of toxic agents from the market is the best way to avoid future harm.

In general, pregnant women must be educated so that no drugs of any kind are taken during pregnancy unless they are essential for proper health and development. When a drug is required, the potential risks must be discussed and understood. There are four established principles concerning a drug's potential to induce developmental disorders:

✱ **Principle 1:** Dose–effect relationship. The dose response is important in determining the level of toxicity. Most drugs have a threshold or "no effect" level. The daily dose is important to consider as well as the route of exposure.

✳ **Principle 2:** Species susceptibility. Not every drug has the same effects on humans as it does on other animals. Environmental factors may also be related.

✳ **Principle 3:** Period of development. Depending on the stage of development, drugs may have differing effects. This explains how during early development, **dysmorphology** (the study of birth defects, especially those that affect the anatomy) more likely occurs as a result of a specific drug that later in development causes functional disorders instead.

✳ **Principle 4:** Mode of action. To understand potential toxicity, a drug's molecular targets should be identified. The transport and metabolism of toxic agents play significant roles in this area.

✳ Apply Your Knowledge 40.5

The following questions focus on what you have just learned about drugs used during pregnancy.

CRITICAL THINKING

1. Why is the education of pregnant women important to inform them not to take any medications unless they are absolutely necessary?
2. What term is used to study the effects of toxic agents during the entire reproductive process?
3. What is the definition of *teratogenicity*?
4. What is phenylketonuria?
5. What is the definition of the term *dysmorphology*?
6. What was the result when pregnant women took the drug thalidomide?

Pharmacotherapy During Lactation

Breast milk receives secretions that carry a large number of drugs, although this has only been documented as causing a few infant injuries. Safer alternative drugs are usually available for use during lactation. Studies of drugs used during lactation must continue to fully understand their effects. Drugs that are highly lipid soluble are most likely to enter the breast milk. These include central nervous system medications. Usually, these agents exist in the breast milk at lower than clinically significant levels. Drugs that exist in the maternal plasma (such as warfarin) and are bound to albumin are not able to penetrate the mother's breast milk.

Drugs that should be avoided during breastfeeding are listed by the American Academy of Pediatrics' Committee on Drugs. Health care professionals working with pregnant and breastfeeding women should pay attention to drug guides and the information they contain about the risks of using specific drugs during these times. Table 40-2 ■ lists specific drugs associated with adverse effects during breastfeeding.

Table 40-2 ■ Specific Drugs Associated with Adverse Effects During Breastfeeding

GENERIC NAME	TRADE NAME	EFFECTS
acebutolol	Sectral	Bradycardia, hypotension, tachypnea
amiodarone	Cordarone	Hypothyroidism
atenolol	Tenormin	Bradycardia, cyanosis
bromocriptine	Parlodel	Suppression of lactation and potential hazards to the mother
ergotamine	Ergomar	Diarrhea, vomiting, and convulsions (when used in the recommended doses for migraine medications)
fluoxetine	Prozac	Colic, feeding and sleeping disorders, reduced weight gain

(continued)

Table 40-2 ■ **Specific Drugs Associated with Adverse Effects During Breastfeeding** (*continued*)

GENERIC NAME	TRADE NAME	EFFECTS
haloperidol	Haldol	Decline in developmental scores
lithium	Eskalith	One-third to one-half therapeutic blood concentration in infants
phenobarbital	Phenobarbital	Methemoglobinemia, sedation, infantile spasms after weaning from milk containing phenobarbital
primidone	Mysoline	Feeding problems, sedation
sulfasalazine	Azulfidine	Bloody diarrhea

Other drugs that may have adverse effects during breast-feeding include various amphetamines, which can cause irritability and poor sleeping patterns. Aspirin and other salicylates can cause metabolic acidosis. Cocaine can cause cocaine intoxication, diarrhea, irritability, tremulousness, seizures, and vomiting.

If possible, the use of a potentially risky drug during lactation should be postponed until the baby is weaned. Alternatively, a safer medicine should be used instead. If a drug must be used that has potentially risky effects, it should be administered immediately after breastfeeding so time will lapse between administration and the next breastfeeding. New mothers should be educated about the effects of alcohol, illicit drugs, and tobacco products during lactation.

Some drugs do not affect the nursing infant because they are destroyed in the infant's GI system or cannot be absorbed across the GI tract. Therefore, although a drug may be present in the breast milk, it is usually in such small amounts that no noticeable harm will be caused. However, premature, neonatal, and extremely ill infants may be at a greater risk for adverse drug effects because they lack drug-metabolizing enzymes. In general, drugs with shorter half-lives are preferable because those with longer half-lives (or active metabolites) can accumulate in the plasma of the infant. If possible, drugs with a high protein-binding ability should be selected because they are not secreted into the milk as readily. Because of a lack of testing, all OTC herbal products and dietary supplements should be avoided during lactation.

Recreational Drugs

Recreational drugs may also be harmful to developing embryos and fetuses and to nursing infants. They include alcohol, nicotine, opiates, caffeine, cannabis, cocaine, and other drugs.

ALCOHOL

Nursing infants receive about 10% of the alcohol consumed by their mothers. Alcohol can change the taste of breast milk and result in feeding problems. Milk levels of alcohol decrease along with plasma levels of alcohol. The faster alcohol is consumed, the faster its levels change in breast milk. Sipping an alcohol drink slowly does not cause levels of alcohol in breast milk to rise sufficiently because the body has time to metabolize it. Studies show that one to two servings of alcoholic beverages per week have no effect on nursing infants, but amounts higher than that have been shown to pose more significant risks to infant health. When an alcoholic beverage is consumed, the mother should avoid breastfeeding for 2 hours so the alcohol can be fully metabolized. If alcohol use is chronic or excessive, the baby should be weaned from breastfeeding and given baby formula instead.

NICOTINE

Smoking tobacco products has been linked to poor milk supply as well as poor nursing, restlessness, and vomiting by the infant. Secondhand smoke causes a higher rate of infant respiratory illnesses. Mothers who continue smoking tend to breastfeed their infants less than those who do not. It is important to realize that infants who are bottle-fed instead of breastfed also have nicotine in their urine. Secondhand smoke is dangerous for infants regardless of the manner of their feeding. Nicotine and its major metabolite—cotinine—pass into breast milk quickly. Levels increase with the number of cigarettes smoked. Many other chemicals are also present in the breast milk of smoking mothers.

OPIATES

All opiates penetrate breast milk, including heroin, morphine, methadone, and others. There have been documented cases of infant death caused by extremely high levels of opiates in breast milk. Infants may also become addicted to opiates if used in sufficient quantities. Methadone is safer than other opiates, but in general, all these agents should not be used by mothers when they are nursing their babies. Each case should be individually reviewed, and abrupt weaning should be avoided so withdrawal from opiates does not occur in the infant.

Focus Point

Codeine

Codeine is a morphine derivative with a more restricted analgesic and sedative effect during pregnancy than morphine.

CAFFEINE

Caffeine is quickly absorbed and readily enters breast milk. Because the livers of infants are immature, the elimination of caffeine takes much longer than in adults. Normal amounts of coffee are usually well tolerated by infants, but continued use of higher than normal amounts causes infants to become irritable, jittery, and not satisfied by breastfeeding. Often, it takes weeks for the infant to clear the caffeine level. Babies consuming caffeine often cannot sleep normally and may not be receiving normal amounts of iron from breast milk.

CANNABIS

Cannabis (marijuana or hashish) can be detected in breast milk and is stored in the brain and fat. The main effects of cannabis are related to the motor development of exposed infants, which is delayed. If cannabis is used regularly, the infant must be weaned from breast milk consumption.

COCAINE

Cocaine can be detected in breast milk but is cleared much more quickly than substances such as cannabis. However, the metabolites of cocaine are cleared much more slowly. Effects of cocaine on infants include hypertonia, tachycardia, excitation, and trembling. Habitual users of cocaine should avoid breastfeeding entirely.

Focus Point

Alcohols

Alcohols may be used topically as disinfectants during pregnancy. However, the consumption of alcohol during pregnancy causes a specific complex of congenital organic and functional developmental defects known as fetal alcohol syndrome.

The consumption of alcohol during pregnancy can cause fetal alcohol syndrome.

Diego Cervo/Shutterstock

❋ Apply Your Knowledge 40.6

The following questions focus on what you have just learned about recreational drugs.

CRITICAL THINKING

1. Why are fat-soluble drugs passed more quickly than other drugs to lactating infants?
2. What are the signs and symptoms of cocaine intoxication in lactating infants?
3. What are the adverse effects on infants whose mothers drink too much coffee?
4. If a mother consumes an alcoholic beverage, how long should she wait before breastfeeding her infant?
5. Why is smoking tobacco prohibited during lactation and breastfeeding?

Vaccinations During Pregnancy and Lactation

Protective and booster immunizations should be given before pregnancy for safety. Although no vaccines have proven embryotoxic or teratogenic effects, it is wise that excessive medication use be limited during the first trimester. Routine immunization should be avoided during pregnancy. However, when there is a high risk of infection because the mother has not received a common vaccine, she should be vaccinated regardless.

One of the concerns of vaccinations during pregnancy is that ethyl mercury is used as a preservative in vaccines, which may be a risk for fetuses' brains. Measles and mumps vaccines are contraindicated because fetuses may contract either disease. Most vaccines in general should be avoided during pregnancy unless there is an actual high risk of contracting a specific disease without the vaccination.

Most of the normally administered vaccinations are not contraindicated during lactation. However, the live oral polio vaccine should not be given to the mother until the infant has been immunized at 6 weeks or older. The killed-virus injectable form of the smallpox vaccine is recommended during lactation.

Focus Point

Tetanus Vaccine

There are no indications of embryotoxic properties in the tetanus vaccine and it is safe to administer to pregnant women.

PRACTICAL SCENARIO 1

A 32-year-old woman who is 7 months pregnant has consumed four to five glasses of wine per week and has been unable to quit smoking. She also consumes three to four cups of coffee per day. She is admitted to her local hospital and delivers her baby prematurely.

Wavebreakmedia/Shutterstock

Critical Thinking Questions

1. What would be the best way to prevent premature delivery of the baby in this scenario?
2. What are the effects of nicotine, alcohol, and caffeine on fetuses?
3. Which of these three substances is most dangerous to premature babies?

PRACTICAL SCENARIO 2

A 21-year-old woman went to the emergency room with a high fever, dyspnea, and chest pain. Her radiographs showed bilateral pneumonia, and her blood tests indicated a bacterial infection. She received antibiotics for 10 days (orally and intravenously). After discharge from the hospital, she took a pregnancy test and brought the results to her gynecologist, who determined she was 6 weeks pregnant.

Phovoir/Shutterstock

Critical Thinking Questions

1. What are the adverse effects of any medications during the early stages of pregnancy?
2. What is the possibility of adverse effects on her baby?

Chapter Capsule

This section repeats the objectives from the beginning of the chapter and then provides a summary of the most important concepts for that objective. Use this section as a quick review and to check your knowledge.

Objective 1: Describe various stages of reproduction that may potentially be affected by drug toxicity.

■ Drug toxicity may occur at different times and be highly unpredictable. Many structural malformations occur during organogenesis. They can also occur from 1 week before the missed menstrual period until the woman is 44 days past due. Because organ and system maturation occurs beyond organogenesis and the prenatal period, responses may occur over a much longer period of time.

Objective 2: Identify at least one example drug for each pregnancy risk category.

■ Category A—Folic acid, insulin, prenatal multivitamins, thyroxine

■ Category B—Acetaminophen, azithromycin, cephalosporins, penicillins, ibuprofen in first and second trimesters

■ Category C—Most prescription medications, most antihypertensives, antimicrobials (such as clarithromycin, cotrimoxazole, and fluoroquinolones), corticosteroids, SSRIs

■ Category D—ACE inhibitors and ARBs in second and third trimesters, alcohol, gentamicin, ibuprofen in third trimester, nicotine, conjugated estrogens, tetracyclines

■ Category X—Isotretinoin, misoprostol, thalidomide

Objective 3: Define the terms *reproductive toxicology*, *developmental toxicity*, and *embryotoxicity* and *fetotoxicity*.

■ Reproductive toxicology—the study of effects of toxic agents during the entire reproductive process

■ Developmental toxicity—adverse effects that occur before adulthood

■ Embryotoxicity and fetotoxicity—toxic effects resulting from prenatal exposure as well as structural or functional abnormalities of the postnatal manifestations of these effects

Objective 4: Explain the four principles concerning a drug's potential to induce developmental disorders.

- **Principle 1:** Dose–effect relationship. The dose response is important in determining the level of toxicity. Most drugs have a threshold or "no effect" level. The daily dose is important to consider as well as the route of exposure.

- **Principle 2:** Species susceptibility. Not every drug has the same effects on humans as it does on other animals. Environmental factors may also be related.

- **Principle 3:** Period of development. Depending on developmental stage, drugs may have differing effects. In early development, dysmorphology more likely occurs as a result of a specific drug that later in development causes functional disorders instead.

- **Principle 4:** Mode of action. To understand potential toxicity, a drug's molecular targets should be identified. Transport and metabolism of toxic agents plays a significant role.

Objective 5: Define *pharmacokinetics* in pregnant women.

- During pregnancy, metabolism and kinetics of drugs are more complicated; gastrointestinal motility and distribution to plasma proteins are decreased compared to other times during life; however, nearly all other resorptive, distributive, metabolic, and excretive processes are increased

- Pregnant women experience increased lung function, skin-blood circulation, distribution to plasma volume, distribution to body water, distribution to fat deposition, and the glomerular filtration rate

- Because total body water may be increased up to 81% during pregnancy, drugs can be distributed in a greatly increased volume

- Increased female hormones because of pregnancy may inactivate certain medications and environmental agents

Objective 6: Discuss the possible outcomes if toxic agents contact a developing embryo or fetus during embryogenesis or organogenesis.

- Embryogenesis: spontaneous abortion, birth defects, chromosomal defects, low birth weight, stillbirth

- Organogenesis: spontaneous abortion, birth defects, retarded development, functional disorders (such as autism), transplacental carcinogenesis

Objective 7: Describe which drugs used during lactation can cause disruption to the infant's normal sleeping patterns.

- Fluoxetine, various amphetamines, and caffeine

Objective 8: Define the term *teratology*.

- Teratology is the study of structural birth defects in general, although it also relates to certain functional defects

Objective 9: Discuss immunizations during pregnancy.

- Protective and booster immunizations should be given before pregnancy for safety. Although no vaccines have proven embryotoxic or teratogenic effects, excessive medication use should be limited during the first trimester. Routine immunization should be avoided during pregnancy. However, when there is a high risk of infection because the mother has not received a common vaccine, she should be vaccinated regardless. Because ethyl mercury is used as a preservative in vaccines, there may be a risk for fetal brain damage. Measles and mumps vaccines are contraindicated because fetuses may contract the disease. Most vaccines, in general, should be avoided during pregnancy unless there is an actual high risk of contracting a specific disease without the vaccination.

Objective 10: Identify which vaccine may be administered during pregnancy without any harm to the mother or baby.

- The tetanus vaccine is safe for pregnant women, with no indications of embryotoxic properties.

Internet Sites of Interest

- The stages of human reproduction are discussed at: **www.nature.com/scitable/ topicpage/meiosis-genetic-recombination-and-sexual-reproduction-210**
- For information about drugs during pregnancy, see: **www.cdc.gov/pregnancy/ meds/index.html**
- Drug use during pregnancy is discussed at: **www.merckmanuals.com/home/ women-s-health-issues/drug-use-during-pregnancy/drug-use-during-pregnancy**
- Developmental disorders are explained at: **www.firstsigns.org/delays_disorders/ other_disorders.htm**
- Information about a proper diet during pregnancy is listed at: **http://americanpregnancy.org/pregnancy-health/diet-during-pregnancy/**
- The Teratology Society's website is located at: **https://www.teratology.org**

Checkpoint Review 5

Select the best answer for the following questions.

1. Which of the following over-the-counter medications should be avoided by nursing mothers?

   a. Iodine
   b. Ascorbic acid
   c. Nicotinamide
   d. Cold remedies

2. Elderly patients appear to have reduced host defenses caused by alterations in the function of which of the following leukocytes?

   a. B-lymphocytes
   b. T-lymphocytes
   c. Macrophages
   d. Monocytes

3. Which of the following experiences the most age-related pharmacokinetic changes?

   a. Lean body mass
   b. Heart weight
   c. Kidney weight
   d. Body water

4. Which of the following age groups have higher percentages of water?

   a. Neonates
   b. Infants
   c. Teenagers
   d. Older adults

5. Prescribing multiple medications to a single patient simultaneously is called:

   a. Polydactylism
   b. Polypharmacy
   c. Pharmacology
   d. Polypharmacology

6. Pharmacokinetics deal with all the following except:

   a. Distribution
   b. Elimination
   c. Metabolism
   d. Mechanisms of action

7. Most of the common disorders seen in older adults concern which of the following systems?

   a. Respiratory
   b. Cardiovascular
   c. Urinary
   d. Integumentary

8. All elderly patients who receive antihypertensive drugs should be regularly monitored for:

   a. Orthostatic hypotension
   b. Hyperglycemia
   c. Hypouricemia
   d. Hypernatremia

9. Suicides are more than twice as common in which of the following age groups?

   a. Young children
   b. Teenagers
   c. Young adults
   d. Older adults

10. Which of the following is present in higher percentages in neonates compared with adults?

    a. Water
    b. Fat
    c. Plasma protein
    d. Lean mass

11. Which of the following drug forms is most popular for pediatric administration?

    a. Powders and pills
    b. Intramuscular injections
    c. Elixirs and suspensions
    d. Suppositories

12. Tetracyclines show up as about 70% of maternal serum concentrations, and breastfeeding may cause which of the following adverse effects in infants?

    a. Staining of incoming teeth
    b. Staining of urine and tears
    c. Staining of skin and hair
    d. Renal failure

13. Exposure to radioactivity during pregnancy may increase the risk of cancer in infants. Which of the following organs is at most risk?

    a. Pancreas
    b. Thyroid
    c. Spleen
    d. Liver

14. All the following drugs may produce pharmacologic effects in nursing infants except:

    a. Lithium and alcohol
    b. Antacids and vitamins
    c. Sedatives and hypnotics
    d. Heroin and antibiotics

For questions 15 to 19, match the lettered trade name to the numbered generic name.

GENERIC NAME	TRADE NAME
15. ____ fluoxetine	a. Tenormin
16. ____ lithium	b. Mebaral
17. ____ primidone	c. Mysoline
18. ____ mephobarbital	d. Eskalith
19. ____ atenolol	e. Prozac

Select terms from your reading to fill in the blanks.

20. In newborns, the glomerular filtration rate is much _____ than in older children or adults.

21. Creatinine clearance is an indicator of glomerular _____.

22. The administration of many drugs together is more common in the _____ because of the use of different physicians and specialties.

23. Pregnancy registries are maintained by special interest groups, governmental agencies, and _____ _____.

24. The pregnancy drug category that indicates a drug should never be used during pregnancy is drug category _____.

25. The study of birth defects is referred to as _____.

26. Precursor cells from which oocytes develop are called _____.

27. Agents that cause congenital malformations and developmental abnormalities are called _____.

28. Prenatal and postnatal drug exposure may be toxic during _____ _____ of development.

29. During pregnancy, cardiac output and regional blood flow may be increased, causing the dilution of drugs and _____ plasma protein concentration.

30. Many structural malformations occur during the period of _____.

31. Drugs can be distributed in a greatly increased volume because total _____ _____ may be increased up to 81% during pregnancy.

32. Drugs cross the placenta by _____ diffusion.

Appendix A

Top 200 Drugs by Prescription

Number	Generic Name	Trade Name
1	hydrocodone w/APAP	Hydrocodone w/APAP
2	atorvastatin	Lipitor
3	amoxicillin	Trimox
4	lisinopril	Prinivil, Zestril
5	hydrochlorothiazide	Diaqua, Esidrix
6	atenolol	Tenormin
7	azithromycin	Zithromax
8	furosemide	Lasix
9	alprazolam	Xanax
10	metoprolol	Toprol XL
11	albuterol	Proventil
12	amlodipine	Norvasc
13	levothyroxine	Synthroid
14	metformin	Glucophage, Glucophage XR
15	sertraline	Zoloft
16	escitalopram	Lexapro
17	ibuprofen	Motrin
18	cephalexin	Keflex
19	zolpidem	Ambien
20	prednisone	Deltasone
21	esomeprazole magnesium	Nexium
22	triamterene	Dyrenium
23	propoxyphene napsylate	Darvon-N
24	simvastatin	Zocor
25	montelukast	Singulair
26	lansoprazole	Prevacid
27	metoprolol tartrate	Lopressor
28	fluoxetine	Prozac
29	lorazepam	Ativan
30	clopidogrel	Plavix
31	oxycodone w/APAP	Oxycodone w/APAP
32	salmeterol	Serevent

Number	Generic Name	Trade Name
33	alendronate	Fosamax
34	venlafaxine	Effexor, Effexor XR
35	warfarin	Coumadin
36	paroxetine hydrochloride	Paxil
37	clonazepam	Klonopin
38	cetirizine	Zyrtec
39	pantoprazole	Protonix
40	potassium chloride	Potassium Chloride
41	acetaminophen/codeine	Tylenol-Codeine
42	trimethoprim/sulfamethoxazole	TMP-SMZ
43	gabapentin	Neurontin
44	conjugated estrogens	Premarin
45	fluticasone	Flonase
46	trazodone	Desyrel
47	cyclobenzaprine	Flexeril
48	amitriptyline	Elavil, Enovil
49	levofloxacin	Levaquin
50	tramadol	Ultram
51	ciprofloxacin	Cipro
52	amlodipine/benazepril	Lotrel
53	ranitidine	Zantac
54	fexofenadine	Allegra
55	levothyroxine	Levoxyl
56	valsartan	Diovan
57	enalapril	Vasotec
58	diazepam	Valium
59	naproxen	Anaprox, Naprosyn
60	fluconazole	Diflucan
61	lisinopril/HCTZ	Zestoretic
62	potassium chloride	Klor-Con
63	ramipril	Altace
64	bupropion	Wellbutrin, Wellbutrin XL
65	celecoxib	Celebrex
66	sildenafil citrate	Viagra
67	doxycycline hyclate	Vibra-Tabs
68	ezetimibe	Zetia

(continued)

Number	Generic Name	Trade Name
69	rosiglitazone maleate	Avandia
70	lovastatin	Mevacor
71	valsartan/hydrochlorothiazide	Diovan HCT
72	carisoprodol	Soma, Rela
73	drospirenone/ethinyl estradiol	Yasmin 28
74	allopurinol	Alloprin
75	clonidine	Catapres
76	methylprednisolone	Medrol
77	pioglitazone hydrochloride	Actos
78	pravastatin	Pravachol
79	risedronate sodium	Actonel
80	norelgestromin/ethinyl estradiol	Ortho Evra
81	citalopram hydrobromide	Celexa
82	verapamil	Calan
83	isosorbide mononitrate	Ismotic
84	penicillin V	Penicillin VK
85	glyburide	Micronase
86	amphetamine sulfate	Adderall
87	mometasone furoate	Nasonex
88	folic acid	Folacin
89	quetiapine fumarate	Seroquel
90	losartan potassium	Cozaar
91	fenofibrate	Tricor
92	carvedilol	Coreg
93	methylphenidate hydrochloride	Concerta
94	ezetimibe	Vytorin
95	insulin glargine	Lantus
96	promethazine hydrochloride	Phenergan
97	meloxicam	Mobic
98	tamsulosin hydrochloride	Flomax
99	rosuvastatin	Crestor
100	glipizide	Glucotrol XL
101	norgestimate/ethinyl estradiol	Ortho Tri-Cyclen Lo
102	temazepam	Restoril
103	omeprazole	Prilosec
104	cefdinir	Omnicef
105	albuterol	Ventolin

Number	Generic Name	Trade Name
106	risperidone	Risperdal
107	rabeprazole sodium	AcipHex
108	digoxin	Digitek
109	spironolactone	Aldactone
110	valacyclovir hydrochloride	Valtrex
111	latanoprost	Xalatan
112	metformin	Fortamet
113	losartan potassium/hydrochlorothiazide	Hyzaar
114	quinapril	Accupril
115	clindamycin	Cleocin
116	metronidazole	Flagyl
117	triamcinolone	Atolone
118	topiramate	Topamax
119	ipratropium bromide/albuterol sulfate	Combivent
120	benazepril	Lotensin
121	gemfibrozil	Lopid
122	irbesartan	Avapro
123	glimepiride	Amaryl
124	norgestimate/ethinyl estradiol	Trinessa
125	estradiol	Alora, Climara
126	hydroxyzine	Atarax
127	metoclopramide	Maxolon, Reglan
128	fexofenadine/pseudoephedrine	Allegra-D 12 Hour
129	doxazosin mesylate	Cardura
130	warfarin	Jantoven
131	glipizide	Glucotrol
132	diclofenac sodium	Voltaren
133	raloxifene hydrochloride	Evista
134	diltiazem	Cardizem, Tiazac
135	tolterodine tartrate	Detrol, Detrol LA
136	meclizine	Antivert, Bonamine
137	glyburide/metformin	Glucovance
138	atomoxetine	Strattera
139	duloxetine hydrochloride	Cymbalta
140	nitrofurantoin	Furadantin
141	promethazine/codeine	Phenergan with Codeine

(continued)

Number	Generic Name	Trade Name
142	olmesartan medoxomil	Benicar
143	mirtazapine	Remeron
144	bisoprolol/HCTZ	Ziac
145	desloratadine	Clarinex
146	oxycodone	OxyContin
147	minocycline	Arestin, Minocin
148	sumatriptan	Imitrex
149	nabumetone	Relafen
150	olanzapine	Zyprexa
151	lamotrigine	Lamictal
152	cetirizine/pseudoephedrine	Zyrtec-D
153	polyethylene glycol	Glycolax
154	acyclovir	Zovirax
155	propranolol	Inderal
156	triamcinolone acetonide	Nasacort AQ
157	donepezil hydrochloride	Aricept
158	butalbital/acetaminophen/caffeine	Fioricet
159	niacin	Niaspan
160	azithromycin	Zmax
161	divalproex sodium	Depakote
162	buspirone	Buspar
163	norgestimate/ethinyl estradiol	Tri-Sprintec
164	methotrexate	Amethopterin, MTX
165	oxycodone	Roxicodone
166	budesonide	Rhinocort Aqua
167	olmesartan medoxomil hydrochlorothiazide	Benicar HCT
168	terazosin	Hytrin
169	metaxalone	Skelaxin
170	clotrimazole/betamethasone	Lotrisone
171	tadalafil	Cialis
172	irbesartan/hydrochlorothiazide	Avalide
173	fexofenadine	Telfast
174	norgestimate/ethinyl estradiol	Ortho Tri-Cyclen
175	bupropion hydrochloride	Wellbutrin, Zyban
176	benzonatate	Tessalon
177	olopatadine hydrochloride	Patanol

Number	Generic Name	Trade Name
178	quinine	Quinamm, Quiphile
179	diltiazem hydrochloride	Cartia XT
180	insulin lispro, rDNA origin	Humalog
181	paroxetine	Paxil CR
182	levonorgestrel and ethinyl estradiol	Aviane
183	digoxin	Lanoxin
184	amphetamine	Adderall XR
185	famotidine	Pepcid, Pepcid AC
186	digoxin	Lanoxicaps
187	levothyroxine	Levothroid
188	nifedipine	Adalat, Procardia
189	nortriptyline	Aventyl
190	hydrocodone polistirex/ chlorpheniramine polistirex	Tussionex
191	nitroglycerin	NitroQuick
192	phenytoin	Dilantin
193	budesonide	Endocet
194	etodolac	Lodine, Lodine XL
195	atenolol/chlorthalidone	Tenoretic
196	phentermine	Fastin
197	tramadol/acetaminophen	Ultracet
198	tizanidine	Zanaflex
199	cetirizine hydrochloride/ pseudoephedrine	Virlix-D
200	divalproex sodium	Depakote ER

Appendix B

Poisons and Antidotes

Drug	Antidote
acetaminophen	acetylcysteine
anticholinesterases (cholinergics)	atropine, pralidoxime
antidepressants (monoamine oxidase inhibitors and tyramine-containing foods)	phentolamine
benzodiazepines	flumazenil
cyanide	amyl nitrite, sodium nitrite, sodium thiosulfate
digoxin (digitoxin)	digoxin immune Fab (Digibind)
fluorouracil (5-FU)	leucovorin calcium
heparin	protamine sulfate
ifosfamide	mesna
iron	deferoxamine
lead	edentate calcium disodium, dimercaprol, succimer
methotrexate	leucovorin calcium
opioid analgesics, heroin	nalmefene, naloxone
thrombolytic agents	aminocaproic acid (Amicar)
tricyclic antidepressants	physostigmine
warfarin (Coumadin)	phytonadione (vitamin K)

Appendix C

Common Sound-Alike Drug Names

The following is a list of common sound-alike drug names. Trade names are capitalized and generic names are in lowercase. In parentheses next to each drug name is the pharmacological classification/use of the drug. Source: *www.pharmacytimes.com*

Drug Name and Purpose	Looks Like/Sounds Like
Accupril (ACE inhibitor)	Accutane (antiacne drug)
acetazolamide (antiglaucoma drug)	acetohexamide (oral antidiabetic drug)
Aciphex (proton pump inhibitor)	Accupril (ACE inhibitor)
Aciphex (proton pump inhibitor)	Aricept (anti-Alzheimer's drug)
Actos (oral hypoglycemic)	Actonel (diphosphonate—bone-growth regulator)
Adriamycin (antineoplastic)	Aredia (bone-growth regulator)
albuterol (sympathomimetic)	atenolol (beta-blocker)
Aldomet (antihypertensive)	Aldoril (antihypertensive)
Alkeran (antineoplastic)	Leukeran (antineoplastic)
Alkeran (antineoplastic)	Myleran (antineoplastic)
allopurinol (antigout drug)	Apresoline (antihypertensive)
alprazolam (antianxiety agent)	lorazepam (antianxiety agent)
Amaryl (oral hypoglycemic)	Reminyl (anti-Alzheimer's drug)
Ambien (sedative-hypnotic)	Amen (progestin)
amiloride (diuretic)	amlodipine (calcium channel blocker)
amiodarone (antiarrhythmic)	amrinone (inotropic agent)
amitriptyline (antidepressant)	nortriptyline (antidepressant)
Apresazide (antihypertensive)	Apresoline (antihypertensive)
Aripiprazole (antipsychotic)	Lansoprazole (proton pump inhibitor)
Arlidin (peripheral vasodilator)	Aralen (antimalarial)
Artane (cholinergic blocking agent)	Altace (ACE inhibitor)
Asacol (anti-inflammatory drug)	Avelox (fluoroquinolone antibiotic)
asparaginase (antineoplastic agent)	pegaspargase (antineoplastic agent)
Atarax (antianxiety agent)	Ativan (antianxiety agent)
atenolol (beta-blocker)	timolol (beta-blocker)
Atrovent (cholinergic blocking agent)	Alupent (sympathomimetic)
Avandia (oral hypoglycemic)	Coumadin (anticoagulant)
Avandia (oral hypoglycemic)	Prandin (oral hypoglycemic)
Bacitracin (antibacterial)	Bactroban (anti-infective, topical)
Benylin (expectorant)	Ventolin (sympathomimetic)
Brevital (barbiturate)	Brevibloc (beta-adrenergic blocker)
Bumex (diuretic)	Buprenex (narcotic analgesic)

(continued)

Drug Name and Purpose	Looks Like/Sounds Like
bupropion (antidepressant; smoking deterrent)	buspirone (antianxiety agent)
Cafergot (analgesic)	Carafate (antiulcer drug)
calciferol (vitamin D)	calcitriol (vitamin D)
carboplatin (antineoplastic agent)	cisplatin (antineoplastic agent)
Cardene (calcium channel blocker)	Cardizem (calcium channel blocker)
Cardura (antihypertensive)	Ridaura (gold-containing anti-inflammatory)
Cataflam (NSAID)	Catapres (antihypertensive)
Catapres (antihypertensive)	Combipres (antihypertensive)
cefotaxime (cephalosporin)	cefoxitin (cephalosporin)
cefuroxime (cephalosporin)	deferoxamine (iron chelator)
Celebrex (NSAID)	Cerebyx (anticonvulsant)
Celebrex (NSAID)	Celera (antidepressant)
Cerebyx (anticonvulsant)	Celera (antidepressant)
chlorpromazine (antipsychotic)	chlorpropamide (oral antidiabetic)
chlorpromazine (antipsychotic)	prochlorperazine (antipsychotic)
chlorpromazine (antipsychotic)	promethazine (antihistamine)
Clinoril (NSAID)	Clozaril (antipsychotic)
clomipramine (antidepressant)	clomiphene (ovarian stimulant)
clonidine (antihypertensive)	Klonopin (anticonvulsant)
Combivir (AIDS drug combination)	Combivent (combination for COPD)
Cozaar (antihypertensive)	Zocor (antihyperlipidemic)
cyclobenzaprine (skeletal muscle relaxant)	cyproheptadine (antihistamine)
cyclophosphamide (antineoplastic)	cyclosporine (immunosuppressant)
cyclosporine (immunosuppressant)	cycloserine (antineoplastic)
Cytovene (antiviral drug)	Cytosar (antineoplastic)
Cytoxan (antineoplastic)	Cytotec (prostaglandin derivative)
Cytoxan (antineoplastic)	Cytosar (antineoplastic)
Dantrium (skeletal muscle relaxant)	danazol (gonadotropin inhibitor)
daunorubicin (antineoplastic)	doxorubicin (antineoplastic)
desipramine (antidepressant)	diphenhydramine (antihistamine)
dexamethasone (corticosteroid)	dextromethorphan (antitussive)
DiaBeta (oral hypoglycemic)	Zebeta (beta-adrenergic blocker)
digitoxin (cardiac glycoside)	digoxin (cardiac glycoside)
diphenhydramine (antihistamine)	dimenhydrinate (antihistamine)
dopamine (sympathomimetic)	dobutamine (sympathomimetic)
Doribax (antibiotic)	Zovirax (antiviral)
DTaP (diphtheria, tetanus toxoids, and acellular pertussis)	Tdap (tetanus toxoid, reduced diphtheria toxoid, and acellular pertussis)
Durasal (salicylate)	Durezol (corticosteroid)
Edecrin (diuretic)	Eulexin (antineoplastic)
enalapril (ACE inhibitor)	Anafranil (antidepressant)
enalapril (ACE inhibitor)	Eldepryl (anti-Parkinson agent)
Eryc (erythromycin base)	Ery-Tab (erythromycin base)

Drug Name and Purpose	Looks Like/Sounds Like
etidronate (bone-growth regulator)	etretinate (antipsoriatic)
etomidate (general anesthetic)	etidronate (bone-growth regulator)
E-Vista (antihistamine)	Evista (estrogen receptor modulator)
Femara (antineoplastic)	Femhrt (estrogen–progestin combination)
Fioricet (analgesic)	Fiorinal (analgesic)
Flomax (alpha-adrenergic blocker)	Volmax (sympathomimetic)
flurbiprofen (NSAID)	fenoprofen (NSAID)
folinic acid (leucovorin calcium)	folic acid (vitamin B complex)
Gantrisin (sulfonamide)	Gantanol (sulfonamide)
glipizide (oral hypoglycemic)	glyburide (oral hypoglycemic)
glyburide (oral hypoglycemic)	Glucotrol (oral hypoglycemic)
Hycodan (cough preparation)	Hycomine (cough preparation)
hydralazine (antihypertensive)	hydroxyzine (antianxiety agent)
hydrocodone (narcotic analgesic)	hydrocortisone (corticosteroid)
Hydrogesic (analgesic combination)	hydroxyzine (antihistamine)
hydromorphone (narcotic analgesic)	morphine (narcotic analgesic)
Hydropres (antihypertensive)	Diupres (antihypertensive)
Hytone (topical corticosteroid)	Vytone (topical corticosteroid)
imipramine (antidepressant)	Norpramin (antidepressant)
Inderal (beta-adrenergic blocker)	Inderide (antihypertensive)
Inderal (beta-adrenergic blocker)	Isordil (coronary vasodilator)
Indocin (NSAID)	Minocin (antibiotic)
K-Phos Neutral (phosphorus-potassium replenishment)	Neutra-Phos-K (phosphorus-potassium replenishment)
Lamictal (anticonvulsant)	Lamisil (antifungal)
Lamictal (anticonvulsant)	Ludiomil (alpha- and beta-adrenergic blocker)
Lamisil (antiviral)	Ludiomil (alpha- and beta-adrenergic blocker)
Lanoxin (cardiac glycoside)	Lasix (diuretic)
Lantus (insulin glargine)	Lente insulin (insulin zinc suspension)
Lioresal (muscle relaxant)	lisinopril (ACE inhibitor)
Lithostat (lithium carbonate)	Lithobid (lithium carbonate)
Lithotabs (lithium carbonate)	Lithobid (lithium carbonate)
Lodine (NSAID)	codeine (narcotic analgesic)
Lopid (antihyperlipidemic)	Lorabid (beta-lactam antibiotic)
lovastatin (antihyperlipidemic)	Lotensin (ACE inhibitor)
Ludiomil (alpha- and beta-adrenergic blocker)	Lomotil (antidiarrheal)
Medrol (corticosteroid)	Haldol (antipsychotic)
metolazone (thiazide diuretic)	methotrexate (antineoplastic)
metolazone (thiazide diuretic)	metoclopramide (GI stimulant)
metoprolol tartrate (beta-adrenergic blocker)	metoclopramide hydrochloride (GI stimulant)
metoprolol (beta-adrenergic blocker)	misoprostol (prostaglandin derivative)
Monopril (ACE inhibitor)	minoxidil (antihypertensive)

(continued)

Drug Name and Purpose	Looks Like/Sounds Like
morphine sulfate (analgesic)	morphine sulfate extended release (analgesic)
nelfinavir (antiviral)	nevirapine (antiviral)
nicardipine (calcium channel blocker)	nifedipine (calcium channel blocker)
Norlutate (progestin)	Norlutin (progestin)
Noroxin (fluoroquinolone antibiotic)	Neurontin (anticonvulsant)
Norvasc (calcium channel blocker)	Navane (antipsychotic)
Norvir (antiviral)	Retrovir (antiviral)
Ocufen (NSAID)	Ocuflox (fluoroquinolone antibiotic)
Orinase (oral hypoglycemic)	Ornade (upper respiratory product)
Percocet (narcotic analgesic)	Percodan (narcotic analgesic)
paroxetine (antidepressant)	paclitaxel (antineoplastic)
Paxil (antidepressant)	paclitaxel (antineoplastic)
Paxil (antidepressant)	Taxol (antineoplastic)
penicillamine (heavy metal antagonist)	penicillin (antibiotic)
pindolol (beta-adrenergic blocker)	Parlodel (inhibitor of prolactin secretion)
pitavastatin (anticholesterol agent)	pravastatin (anticholesterol agent)
Pitocin (neuromodulator that induces childbirth)	Pitressin (antidiuretic hormone)
Plaquenil (antimalarial drug)	Provigil (analeptic drug for sleep disorders)
Platinol (antineoplastic)	Paraplatin (antineoplastic)
Pletal (antiplatelet drug)	Plavix (antiplatelet drug)
Pravachol (antihyperlipidemic)	Prevacid (GI drug)
Pravachol (antihyperlipidemic)	propranolol (beta-adrenergic blocker)
prednisolone (corticosteroid)	prednisone (corticosteroid)
Prilosec (inhibitor of gastric acid secretion)	Prozac (antidepressant)
Prinivil (ACE inhibitor)	Prilosec (GI drug)
Prinivil (ACE inhibitor)	Proventil (sympathomimetic)
Procanbid (antiarrhythmic)	Procan SR (antiarrhythmic)
propranolol (beta-adrenergic blocker)	Propulsid (GI drug)
Provera (progestin)	Premarin (estrogen)
Prozac (antidepressant)	Proscar (androgen hormone inhibitor)
quinidine (antiarrhythmic)	clonidine (antihypertensive)
quinidine (antiarrhythmic)	Quinamm (antimalarial)
quinine (antimalarial)	quinidine (antiarrhythmic)
Regroton (antihypertensive)	Hygroton (diuretic)
risperidone (antipsychotic)	ropinirole (anti-Parkinsonism agent)
sulfadiazine (antibiotic)	sulfasalazine (anti-inflammatory agent)
tramadol (analgesic)	trazodone (antidepressant)
zolmitriptan (antimigraine serotonin agonist)	zolpidem (hypnotic)

ACE, angiotensin-converting enzyme; **GI**, gastrointestinal; **NSAID**, nonsteroidal anti-inflammatory drug.

Glossary

absence seizures Brief seizures characterized by the arrest of activity and occasional muscle contractions and relaxations

absorption The process of drug movement into the systemic circulation

abstinence syndrome The physiologic changes experienced when an individual abruptly stops taking a substance upon which he or she is physically dependent

abuse potential The potential for a drug to cause dependence, abuse, or both

accommodation Focusing of the lens of the eye

acetaminophen An analgesic used to relieve mild to moderate pain; it also has antipyretic properties

acids Substances that react with bases; aqueous acids have a pH of less than 7

acromegaly (ak-roh-MEG-uh-lee) A disorder in which the extremities, such as the hands, feet, and head, are greatly enlarged

active immunity (ih-MYOO-nih-tee) A form of acquired immunity that develops in an individual in response to an immunogen

acute (a) Characterized by sharpness or severity (acute pain; an acute infection); (b) having a sudden onset, sharp rise, and short course (an acute disease; an acute inflammation)

Addison's disease (ADD-iss-uns) Adrenocortical insufficiency caused by an autoimmune response to the adrenal gland

additive effect When two substances or actions used in combination produce a total effect the same as the sum of the individual effects

additives Chemicals that are added to foods to facilitate their processing and preservation, enhance their restorative or stimulating properties, and control natural contaminants

adenocarcinoma (ah-deh-no-kar-sih-NO-muh) A malignant tumor arising from a glandular origin

adenohypophysis (add-eh-no-hy-PO-fih-sis) Anterior lobe of the pituitary gland

adjuvant (AJ-eh-vant) Aiding or contributing to

adrenergic (add-ruh-NUR-jik) Referring to neurons that release norepinephrine, epinephrine, or dopamine

adverse effects The harmful effects of drugs or other substances

affinity Attractive force, such as when a drug is attracted to a target receptor

agonist (AH-go-nist) A drug that binds to a receptor and produces an appropriate physiologic response that is similar to what an endogenous substance would do

agonist-antagonist (AH-go-nist an-TAH-go-nist) Partial agonist, which produces weaker or less effective responses than an agonist

akathisia (ak-kuh-THIS-zee-uh) Difficulty in initiating muscle movement

alanine aminotransferase (ALT) (AL-uh-neen ah-mee-no-TRANS-feh-rays) An enzyme that is most commonly found in the liver, and catalyzes the alanine cycle; used to assess liver health

alimentary canal Part of digestive system that includes the mouth, pharynx, esophagus, stomach, small intestine, large intestine, rectum, and anus

alkalies Basic, ionic salts that dissolve in water; soluble bases have a pH of more than 7

alkaloids (AL-kuh-loyds) Organic nitrogen-containing compounds that are alkaline and usually bitter tasting; combine with acids to make a salt

alkylating agents (AL-kih-lay-ting) Agents that cause the replacement of hydrogen by an alkyl group, specifically one that inhibits cell division and growth

alopecia (al-o-PEE-shuh) Hair loss

alpha-adrenergic (AL-fuh add-ruh-NUR-jik) receptors Parts of cells that respond to adrenaline

alpha tocopherol (AL-fa toh-KAW-fer-rol) Vitamin E; a substance that protects fragile red blood cell walls (mainly in premature infants) from breaking down

aluminum hydroxide Base element used as an antacid

alveolar duct (al-vee-OH-lar dukt) End of each bronchiole

alveolar sacs Thin-walled air sacs in the bronchioles

alveoli (al-VEE-oh-lie) Microscopic air sacs in the capillary networks of bronchioles

Alzheimer's disease (AL-zhymerz) A disease characterized by progressive memory and cognitive function impairment, which may lead to a completely vegetative state and, ultimately, death

amebiasis (ah-mee-bee-AY-sis) A disease caused by the parasite *Entamoeba histolytica* that occurs most commonly in tropical areas with poor sanitary conditions; symptoms include diarrhea, stomach pain and cramping, and, if severe, bloody stools and fever

amylase (AM-mil-lace) Digestive enzyme

anabolic steroids (AN-uh-bol-lik STER-oidz) Hormonal substances related to estrogen, progestins, testosterone, and corticosteroids that promote muscle growth

analgesia (ah-nul-JEE-zee-ah) Insensibility to pain without loss of consciousness

analgesic (ah-nul-JEE-zik) Relating to, characterized by, or producing pain relief with or without antipyretic or anti-inflammatory action

anaphylactic shock (an-nuh-fih-LAK-tik) A sudden and severe allergic reaction that may be life-threatening

androgens Male sex hormones

anemia (uh-NEE-mee-uh) A deficiency of hemoglobin, red blood cell number, or red blood cell volume

anesthesia (an-ess-THEE-zee-ah) Loss of sensation or consciousness

anesthetics (an-ess-THET-iks) Substances that produce anesthesia

angina pectoris (an-JY-nuh pek-TOR-iss) A common form of ischemic heart disease that often precedes and accompanies myocardial infarction; described as chest pain and squeezing pressure that can radiate to the jaw and arm

angiogenesis (an-jee-oh-JEH-neh-sis) The physiological process in which new blood vessels form from preexisting vessels

anions (AN-eye-ons) Negatively charged ions

antagonist (an-TAH-go-nist) An agent that acts in physiologic opposition; in pharmacology, an agent that prevents an agonist from binding to a receptor, thereby blocking its effects

antibacterial spectrum (an-tie-BAK-tee-ree-ul SPEK-trum) The range of bacteria against which an agent is effective

antibiotics (an-tie-by-AW-tik) Substances produced by microorganisms that in low concentrations are able to inhibit or kill other microorganisms

antibodies (an-tih-BAH-deez) Special proteins manufactured by the lymphocytes when a foreign substance invades the body

anticholinergics (AN-tee-kol-in-UR-jiks) Drugs that inhibit the actions of acetylcholine by occupying the acetylcholine receptors

antidiuretic hormone (ADH) A hormone (also called *vasopressin*) that is released from the posterior lobe of the pituitary gland; exerts an antidiuretic effect; its absence can cause diabetes insipidus

antidote A drug or other substance that opposes the actions of another drug or substance

antigens (AN-tih-jenz) Specific chemical targets—usually pathogens or parts or products of pathogens—or other foreign compounds against which antibodies react

antihistamines Drugs that inhibit the action of histamine by blocking it from attaching to histamine receptors

antimetabolites (an-tee-meh-TAH-bo-lytz) Substances that prevent cancer cell growth by affecting DNA production; effective only against cells that are actively participating in cell metabolism

antimicrobial (an-tie-my-KRO-bee-ul) An agent that destroys or inhibits the growth of microorganisms, especially pathogenic microorganisms

antioxidant An agent that prevents cellular structure from being broken down by oxygen

antipsychotics Any of the powerful tranquilizers (e.g., phenothiazines or butyrophenones) used especially to treat psychosis and believed to act by blocking dopamine nervous receptors; also *neuroleptics*

antipyretics (an-tih-pye-REH-tiks) Drugs that reduce elevated body temperature (fever) to normal levels

antitumor antibiotics Agents made from natural products produced by species of the soil fungus *Streptomyces*; very effective in the treatment of certain tumors

antitussives (an-tee-TUSS-ivz) Agents that reduce coughing

anxiety A clinical state characterized by apprehension and dread.

apolipoprotein B-100 (ah-poh-ly-poh-PRO-teen) A form of low-density lipoprotein (LDL) that plays a role in cholesterol distribution throughout the body

apolipoprotein E A form of lipoprotein that is essential for normal catabolism of triglyceride-rich lipoprotein constituents

apoptosis (ah-pop-TOE-sis) Programmed cell death

apothecary system (ah-PAW-thuh-keh-ree) A very old English system of measurement that has been replaced by the metric system

aqueous humor (AY-kwee-us) Watery fluid that fills the space between the cornea and lens, helps nourish these parts, and aids in maintaining the shape of the front of the eye; secreted from the ciliary body

Arabic number A number commonly used in expressing quantity and value, such as 0, 1, 2, 3, 4, 5, 6, 7, 8, and 9

arsenic A trace element that is present in very small amounts in water, foods, supplements, and chemicals; however, in high amounts, it is poisonous and causes abdominal pain, hemolysis, shock, and death

ascites (eh-SY-teez) Accumulation of fluid in the peritoneal cavity that is usually linked to cirrhosis, severe liver disease, or metastatic cancer

ascorbic acid (as-SCOR-bik) Vitamin C; a substance required for building and maintaining strong tissues for wound healing, resistance to infection, and enhanced iron absorption

aseptic (ay-SEP-tik) Handwashing and other precautions to reduce the risk of infection

aspartate aminotransferase (AST) (ah-SPAR-tayt ah-mee-no-TRANS-feh-rays) An enzyme found throughout the body that is important in amino acid metabolism; used to assess liver health

aspergillosis (as-per-jul-LOH-sis) A fungal infection caused by *Aspergillus*, a common mold; people with weakened immune systems or lung diseases are at higher risk of developing related health problems, which include allergic reactions, lung infections, and other types of infections

asplenia (as-PLEN-ee-yuh) Loss of the spleen

asthma A chronic disease caused by increased reactivity of the tracheobronchial tree to various stimuli

ataxia An inability to coordinate muscle activity

atelectasis (at-tuh-LEK-tuh-sis) Absence of gas in the lungs, causing collapse

atrioventricular (AV) node (AY-tree-oh-ven-TRI-kyoo-ler) Node that provides the only normal conduction pathway between the atrial and ventricular syncytia; its fibers delay impulse transmission; located in the inferior portion of the septum, which separates the atria, and just beneath the endocardium

atrium (AY-tree-um) Smaller upper-receiving chamber of the heart

atropine An alkaloid extracted from various plants that has competitive antagonist actions for muscarinic acetylcholine receptors

attenuated (ah-TEN-yoo-ay-ted) Reduced severity of (a disease) or virulence or vitality of a pathogenic agent

aura A sensation a person feels before the onset of other symptoms.

autoimmunity The condition in which the immune system attacks its own cells; it may be triggered by certain drugs

automaticity (aw-toe-muh-TIH-sih-tee) The heart impulse's automatic, spontaneous initiation

bacteria Single-celled organisms with a cell wall and cellular organelles that allow them to live independently in the environment

bactericidal (bak-tee-ree-uh-SY-dul) Capable of killing microbes

bacteriostatic (bak-tee-ree-oh-STAH-tik) Capable of inhibiting microbial growth

basal ganglia A group of cell bodies in the medulla involved in the regulation of motor activity

benign (be-NYN) Of a mild type or character that does not threaten health or life; related to cancer; slow growing

benzene An organic chemical compound with carcinogenic properties that is used as an industrial solvent as well as an ingredient in many industrial chemicals

benzodiazepines Psychotropic agents used as antianxiety agents, muscle relaxants, sedatives, and hypnotics

beriberi (BEH-ree BEH-ree) A disease caused by a deficiency of thiamine and characterized by edema, cardiovascular abnormalities, and neurologic symptoms

beta-adrenergic receptors (BAY-tuh add-ruh-NUR-jik) Receptors that respond to norepinephrine or epinephrine

bevel The slanted part at a needle's tip

binary fission (BY-nah-ree) Asexual reproduction by a separation of an organism's body into two new bodies; DNA is duplicated then divided, and each new organism receives one copy of the DNA

bioavailability The degree and rate at which a substance (as a drug) is absorbed into a living system or is made available at the site of physiologic activity

biologics Medicinal preparations made from living organisms and their products, such as serums or vaccines

biotransformation The process of conversion of drugs within the body, also known as *metabolism*

black box warning A cautionary label for therapeutic agents or products that the FDA considers hazardous to health if correctly used

blastomycosis (blas-toh-my-KOH-sis) A fungal infection caused by *Blastomyces*, which causes fever, cough, night sweats, muscle aches or joint pain, weight loss, chest pain, and fatigue

blepharitis (blef-fah-RY-tis) Inflammation of one or both eyelids

blood–brain barrier The highly selective, semipermeable barrier separating the blood from the brain's extracellular fluid in the CNS; it prevents entry of many undesirable chemicals

blood pressure Commonly means *arterial pressure*; pressure created in the vessels by the pumping action of the heart; varies from one vessel to another within the systemic circuit

blood volume Total amount of blood in vascular system

booster A substance that increases the effectiveness of a medication

bradycardia (bray-dee-KAR-dee-uh) An abnormally slow heartbeat

bradykinesia (bray-dee-kuh-NEE-shuh) Extremely slow movement

bradykinin (brah-dee-KYE-nin) A polypeptide that mediates inflammation, increases vasodilation, and contracts smooth muscle

broad-spectrum Referring to agents that are effective against a wide range of organisms

bronchioles (BRONG-kee-ols) The portion of the bronchial tubes that are less than 1 mm in diameter and have abundant smooth muscle and elastic fibers

bronchitis Inflammation of the mucous membrane of the bronchial tubes

bronchodilators Agents that widen the diameter of the bronchial tubes

bronchospasm Contraction of smooth muscle in the walls of the bronchi and bronchioles

bundle of His A large group of fibers that enters the upper part of the intraventricular septum and are divided into right and left bundle branches lying just beneath the endocardium—between the atrioventricular node and the Purkinje fibers; also known as the *atrioventricular bundle*

calciferol (kal-SIH-fuh-rol) Vitamin D$_3$

calcitonin (kal-sih-TOE-nin) A thyroid hormone that lowers blood levels of calcium and phosphate and promotes bone formation

calcitriol (kal-SIH-tree-ol) The active vitamin D hormone

calibrated Marked with graduated measurements

Candida albicans **(KAN-dih-dah AL-bih-kans)** A fungus that causes opportunistic oral

and genital infections as well as candidal onychomycosis, an infection of the nail plates

candidemia (kan-dih-DEE-mee-ah) The presence of the fungus *Candida* in the blood

candidiasis (kan-dih-dy-AY-sis) An infection or disease caused by *Candida spp.*, especially *Candida albicans*, usually resulting from debilitation, physiologic change, prolonged administration of antibiotics, and barrier breakage

cannabinoids Organic substances, such as tetrahydrocannabinol (THC), found in cannabis

cannula (KAN-yoo-luh) The actual metal length that makes up the majority of the needle; attached to the hub

capsid The protein shell of a virus that encloses its genetic material

capsules Solid dosage forms featuring a drug contained inside an external shell

carbohydrates Any of a large group of compounds that contain carbon, hydrogen, and oxygen and can be broken down to release energy in the body

carbon monoxide (CO) A gas that is highly toxic in large quantities; it forms when there is not enough oxygen to produce carbon dioxide

carcinogenic (kars-ih-no-JEN-ik) Cancer causing

cardiac output Volume of blood pumped per minute

carotene (KAH-roh-teen) Substance found in dark green and yellow vegetables and fruits and converted to vitamin A in the human body

cataract A clouding of the lens of the eye or its surrounding transparent membrane that obstructs the passage of light

catecholamines (kah-teh-KOH-luh-meenz) Any of various amines (epinephrine, norepinephrine, and dopamine) that contain a dihydroxybenzene ring; are derived from tyrosine; and function as hormones, neurotransmitters, or both

cations (KAT-eye-ons) Positively charged ions

CD4 T-lymphocytes Also called *helper t-cells*; they act by triggering the body's response to infections

cell-mediated immunity Immunity obtained when cells attack the antigens directly rather than producing antibodies; lymphocytes are the primary cells that provide this immunity

central nervous system (CNS)   The brain and spinal cord

cerebrum (seh-REE-brum)   The largest part of the brain that includes nerve centers associated with sensory and motor functions and provides higher mental functions, including memory and reasoning

Chagas disease (SHAH-gus)   Also called *American trypanosomiasis*; a parasitic infection caused by *Trypanosoma cruzi*, transmitted by insects; primarily in Latin American countries

chelation therapy (kee-LAY-shun)   A chemical process in which a synthetic solution called *EDTA* (ethylenediaminetetraacetic acid) is injected into the bloodstream to remove heavy metals and minerals from the body

chemical name   The name describing the chemical makeup of a drug

cholecalciferol (koh-luh-kal-SIH-feh-rol)   Vitamin D_3; a substance that controls calcium metabolism in bone building

cholesterol (koh-LES-ter-rawl)   A natural lipid found in cell membranes, particularly in animal muscle and organ cells

cholesterol ester   A dietary lipid with lower solubility in water; hydrolyzed by pancreatic enzymes to produce cholesterol and free fatty acids

cholinergic (kol-i-NUR-jik)   Referring to neurons that release acetylcholine

cholinergic blockers   Drugs that inhibit the actions of acetylcholine by occupying the acetylcholine receptors

choroid layer (KO-royd)   The middle layer of the eye

chromomycosis (kro-mo-my-KOH-sis)   A localized chronic fungal infection of the skin, with rough, irregular lesions

chronic   Lasting a long time or marked by frequent recurrence

chylomicrons (ky-loh-MY-kronz)   Lipoprotein particles consisting of triglycerides, phospholipids, cholesterol, and proteins that transport dietary lipids from the intestines to other areas of the body

ciliary body (SIL-ee-ayr-ee)   The thickest part of the middle layer of the eye; extends forward from the choroid layer and forms an internal ring around the front of the eye

ciliary muscle   Muscle in the eye that enables the lens to adjust shape to facilitate focusing

cirrhosis (sih-ROH-sis)   A slowly progressing disease in which healthy liver tissue is replaced with scar tissue, eventually preventing normal function

coagulation (koh-ag-yew-LAY-shun)   Blood clotting

cobalamin (koh-BAL-luh-min)   Vitamin B_{12}; a substance that promotes the normal function of all cells, especially normal blood formation, and is necessary for proper nervous system function

coccidioidomycosis (kok-sid-dee-oy-doh-my-KOH-sis)   Also known as *valley fever*; a fungal infection caused by *Coccidioides*, primarily in the southwestern United States as well as Mexico, Central America, and South America; transmitted by breathing in fungal spores

cognitive   Relating to intellectual processes, such as thinking, reasoning, and remembering

cohort (KO-hort)   A group of people who share a common characteristic or experience within a defined period

common fraction   A fraction that represents equal parts of a whole; subclassified as proper, improper, mixed, and complex

comorbidities   Two or more coexisting medical conditions or disease processes

complementary and alternative medicine (CAM)   Various systems of diagnosis, treatment, and prevention that are not based on conventional Western medicine; examples include acupuncture, herbs, and homeopathy

congenital hypothyroidism   Deficiency of thyroid hormones (hypothyroidism) during infancy that results in dwarfism and severe mental retardation

congestive heart failure (CHF)   A condition in which the heart pumps blood at an insufficient rate, the kidneys retain salt and water, and fluid accumulates in interstitial spaces

connective tissue   Tissue that consists of fibroblasts, macrophages, and interlacing protein fibers (collagen) that supports, surrounds, and binds together other tissues and includes adipose tissue, tendons, ligaments, aponeuroses, cartilage, and bone

controlled substances   Drugs whose possession and use are controlled by the comprehensive Drug Abuse Prevention and Control Act

conversion   The changing of units

convulsion   An abnormal violent and involuntary contraction or series of contractions of the muscles; violent spasms

cornea The window of the eye that helps to focus entering light rays

creatinine (kree-AT-tih-neen) A chemical waste molecule produced in skeletal muscle tissue by the breakdown of creatine phosphate

creatinine clearance An indicator of the glomerular filtration rate; creatinine, a by-product of the muscle breakdown of stored proteins, is excreted by the kidneys

cryoanesthesia (KRY-o-an-ess-THEE-zee-ah) Reduction of nerve conduction by localized cooling

cryptococcosis (krip-toh-koh-KOH-sis) A fungal infection caused by various *Cryptococcus* species that usually affects immunocompromised patients; spread by inhalation of airborne fungi and causes a pneumonia-like illness

Cushing's disease (KUSH-ings) A disease in which Cushing's syndrome is caused by a tumor in the pituitary gland

Cushing's syndrome A condition that affects the trunk of the body in which a pad of fat develops between the shoulders, producing a buffalo hump, and the face becomes round and moon shaped

cutaneous flush (kew-TAY-nee-us) Skin reddening

cyanide A highly toxic chemical compound that is found in many plants; produced by certain bacteria, fungi, and algae

cyclic GMP The abbreviation for *cyclic guanosine monophosphate*, a nucleotide that acts as a "second messenger," activating protein kinases and producing various cell functions

cyclooxygenase (SYE-klo-OKS-ih-jeh-nase) The name for a group of enzymes required to produce prostaglandins from arachidonic acid

cystic fibrosis (SIS-tik fy-BRO-sis) A disorder marked by abnormal secretions of the exocrine glands, causing obstruction of bronchial pathways

cytochrome P450 (SY-toh-krohm) An enzyme, of which there are many different types, that functions in drug pharmacokinetics and responses; present in every type of cell except red blood cells and skeletal muscle cells

decimals Any real numbers expressed as a fraction of 10

decongestants A class of drugs that reverse excessive blood flow (congestion) into an area

dehydration (dee-hy-DRAY-shun) Excessive loss of body water

delirium tremens (DT) An acute, sometimes fatal episode usually caused by withdrawal or abstinence from alcohol after habitual excessive drinking; symptoms include sweating, trembling, anxiety, confusion, and hallucinations

denominator (dee-NAW-mih-nay-ter) The part of a fraction that is below the line and that functions as the divisor of the numerator (number above the line)

dermatitis (der-mah-TY-tis) Inflammation of the skin

dermatophyte (der-MAT-toh-fyt) One of three types of fungus that commonly cause infections of the skin, hair, and nails; examples of these infections include ringworm (tinea) and onychomycosis

designer drugs Drugs produced by a minor modification in the chemical structure of an existing drug, resulting in a new substance with similar pharmacologic effects

desired dose The amount of drug to be administered at one time (must be in the same unit of measurement as the dosage unit)

detergents Surfactants, or mixtures of surfactants, having cleaning properties in dilute solutions

detoxification The physiological or medicinal removal of toxic substances from a living organism, including the period of withdrawal

developmental toxicity (tok-SIH-sih-tee) Adverse effects induced during pregnancy or as a result of parental exposure that can be manifested at any point in the lifespan of the organism

diabetes insipidus (dy-uh-BEE-tees in-SIP-uh-dus) A disorder that is caused by the insufficient secretion of vasopressin by the pituitary gland or by a failure of the kidneys to respond to circulating vasopressin; characterized by intense thirst and the excretion of large amounts of urine

diabetes mellitus (dy-uh-BEE-tees MEL-uh-tiss) A serious endocrine disorder characterized by hyperglycemia (high blood glucose levels), resulting from deficient insulin secretion or decreased sensitivity of insulin receptors on target cells

diaphoresis (dy-uh-for-EE-sis) Also called *sweating*; excretion of fluid by the sweat glands of the skin

diastole Ventricles contract and eject blood

dietary supplements   Products containing vitamins, herbs, enzymes, amino acids or other ingredients, taken orally, to supplement the diet by providing missing nutrients

dilutions (dye-LOO-shuns)   Less concentrated mixtures

dissolution (dis-oh-LOO-shun)   The process of dissolving

distribution   The passage of an agent through blood or lymph to various body sites

diuretics (dy-yoo-REH-tiks)   Drugs that promote water loss from the body into the urine

dose   The amount of a drug that a patient takes for an intended therapeutic effect

dose–effect relationship   The relationship between the dose of a drug (or other agent) that produces harmful effects and the severity of the effects on the patient

drams   Fluidrams; apothecary unit of weight (equivalent to 1/8 oz)

drug   A therapeutic agent used in the prevention, diagnosis, alleviation, treatment, or cure of disease

drug targets   Biological components, usually proteins or nucleic acids, that experience modified effects due to specific drugs

dwarfism (DWARF-izm)   A condition in which the body is abnormally undersized

dyshidrotic eczema (dis-hy-DRAW-tik EK-zih-mah)   A type of dermatitis of unknown cause that is characterized by an itchy vesicular eruption on the fingers, palms, and soles

dysmorphology (dis-mor-FAH-lo-jee)   The study of human congenital malformations (birth defects), particularly those affecting the morphology (anatomy) of the individual

dysphagia (dis-FAY-jee-uh)   Difficulty swallowing

dysphasia (dis-FAY-zhuh)   A partial or complete impairment of the ability to communicate, resulting from brain injury

dysrhythmia (dis-RITH-mee-uh)   Disturbance of the heart rhythm; also called *arrhythmia*

echinocandin (ee-ky-no-KAN-din)   An antifungal drug that has actions that are similar to the way in which penicillins act against bacteria; it inhibits synthesis of components of fungal cell walls

eczema (EK-zih-mah)   The most common inflammatory skin condition, caused by endogenous and exogenous agents

edema (eh-DEE-muh)   An abnormal fluid accumulation in the body

efflux (EE-flucks)   The process of flowing out; something that is given off

electrocardiogram (ECG or EKG) (ee-lek-tro-KAR-dee-oh-gram)   A test that records the electrical activity of the heart; an electrograph is the tracing made on paper

elixirs (ee-LICKS-ers)   Alcoholic solutions that offer consistent dissolution and distribution of the drugs they contain; sweetened and contain alcohol and water

embolus (EM-bo-lus)   An abnormal particle circulating in blood, such as an air bubble or blood clot

embryo (EM-bree-oh)   A human between the stages of fertilization and the beginning of the third month of pregnancy; after this, the embryo is called a fetus

embryotoxicity (em-bree-oh-tok-SIH-sih-tee)   The degree to which a substance can damage an embryo or fetus

emollients (ee-MOLE-ee-ents)   Skin-softening agents

emphysema (em-fih-ZEE-muh)   Condition of the lung that is marked by distension and eventual rupture of the alveoli with progressive loss of pulmonary elasticity that is accompanied by shortness of breath with or without cough and that may lead to impaired heart action

endocardium (en-do-kar-dee-um)   The thin membrane lining the inside of the cardiac muscle

endogenous (en-DAH-jeh-nus)   Caused by factors within the body or mind or arising from internal structural or functional causes (*endogenous* malnutrition or *endogenous* psychic depression); relating to or produced by metabolic synthesis in the body

endogenous pathway   The connections between the liver, other tissues, intestines, and cells that act together to form very low-density lipoproteins (VLDLs), then LDLs, which are stored, converted to bile acids, or used in hormone production or cell membrane synthesis; excess LDL leads to formation of harmful plaque

endorphins (en-DOR-finz)   Any of a group of endogenous peptides (such as enkephalin and dynorphin) found especially in the brain that bind chiefly to opiate receptors and produce some of the same pharmacologic effects (such as pain relief) as do opiates

enkephalins (en-KEH-fuh-linz)   Peptides with opiate and analgesic activity that occur naturally in the brain and have a marked affinity for opiate receptors

enzyme induction (EN-zym in-DUK-shun) The process in which a drug changes the function of the hepatic microsomal enzymes and increases metabolic activity in the liver

epicardium (ep-ih-KAR-dee-um) Membrane lining the outside of the myocardium

epidemiological (ep-ih-dee-mee-oh-LAH-jih-kul) Related to epidemiology; the study of patterns of health and illness and associated factors at the population level

***Epidermophyton floccosum* (ep-ih-der-MOF-ih-ton flaw-KOH-sum)** A type of fungi that flourishes in human hosts and may cause *tinea pedis, tinea cruris, tinea corporis,* or *onychomycosis*

epidural anesthesia (ep-eh-DUR-al) Anesthesia produced by injection of a local anesthetic into the epidural (lumbar or caudal) space via a catheter that allows repeated infusions

epilepsy (EH-pih-lep-see) Various disorders marked by abnormal electrical discharges in the brain and typically manifested by sudden brief episodes of altered or diminished consciousness, involuntary movements, or convulsions

ergosterol (er-GAW-steh-rol) A sterol found in cell membranes of fungi and protozoa that is important for survival of these organisms

eructation (ee-ruk-TAY-shun) Burping or belching air from the stomach through the mouth

erythema (ear-ih-THEE-mah) Skin redness caused by capillary dilation

erythema multiforme (ear-ih-THEE-mah MUL-tee-form) A skin condition of unknown cause, usually following an infection or exposure to a drug; it causes raised, reddened lesions and has the potential to become life-threatening

esophagoscopy (eh-saw-fah-GA-sco-pee) A procedure in which a flexible endoscope is inserted through the mouth or nostrils into the esophagus, allowing magnified images to be displayed on a video screen

essential amino acids Components of proteins that cannot be synthesized by the body and must be provided by the diet; there are nine essential amino acids

estrogens One of two major groups of female sex hormones; stimulate enlargement of the vagina, uterus, uterine tubes, ovaries, and external reproductive structures

ethics Standards of behavior, including concepts of right and wrong, beyond what legal considerations are in any given situation

ethylene glycol A toxic organic compound used commercially in automotive antifreeze and as an ingredient in various plastics

euphoria A state of pleasure, well-being, happiness, and excitement

excretion The last stage of pharmacokinetics that removes drugs from the system via the kidneys

exogenous pathway (ek-ZAW-jeh-nus) The connections within the gastrointestinal tract in which triglycerides and cholesterol esters are digested and processed, eventually reaching the lacteals, lymphatic vessels, and bloodstream

expectorants Medications capable of dissolving or promoting liquefaction of mucus in the lungs

extremes The two outside terms in a proportion

fatty acids A group of acids that must be provided by the diet and can be either saturated or unsaturated

fermentation An anaerobic cellular process in which organic foods are converted into simpler compounds and chemical energy (ATP) is produced

fetal (FEE-tul) Related to a fetus, a developing mammal, or other vertebrate after the embryonic stage and before birth

fetotoxic (fee-toh-TOK-sik) Toxic to a fetus

fetotoxicity (fee-toh-tok-SIH-sih-tee) The state of being toxic to a fetus

fiber A type of complex carbohydrate that does not supply energy or heat to the body

fibrillation (fib-rih-LAY-shun) Very rapid, irregular contractions or twitching of the individual muscular fibers of the atria or ventricles

fight-or-flight response Reaction in the body when faced by a sudden threat or source of stress

first-pass effect Immediate exposure of orally administrated drugs to metabolism by liver enzymes before they reach the systemic circulation

flatulence (FLAT-yoo-lentz) The presence of excess gas in the stomach and intestines

fluorides Agents that are forms of fluorine, having beneficial properties in low quantities, but which may be highly toxic in larger quantities

flutter Rapid, regular atrial contractions that often produce sawtooth waves in an electrocardiogram (ECG); rapid ventricular tachycardia that appears as a regular, undulating pattern in an ECG without QRS and T waves, as would normally be found

formaldehyde An organic compound that is a precursor to many other chemical compounds; used in many industrial applications but has toxic, allergenic, and carcinogenic properties

formic acid A chemical commonly found in the bites and stings of insects that also has uses as a preservative or pesticide

fraction A number usually expressed in the form a/b; expresses one or more equal parts of a whole

frequency distribution curve A graphical representation used for a variety of reasons in medicine, such as to show the number of patients that respond to a drug's action at different doses

fulminant hepatitis (FUL-mih-nant heh-pa-TY-tis) A severe, rapidly progressive loss of hepatic function due to hepatitis B viral infection or inflammatory destruction of liver tissue

fungi (FUN-jeeor FUN-gee) Nonphotosynthetic, eukaryotic single or multicellular organisms that are found throughout the environment; fungi have a cell wall containing *sterol*

fungicidal (FUN-jih-sy-dul) Having a killing action on fungi

gastrostomy tube (gah-STRAWS-toh-mee) A surgically placed tube into the stomach that provides a route for feeding and administering medication

gastrotomy (gas-STRAW-toh-mee) Surgical incision into the stomach

gauge Diameter of the needle shaft that varies from #18 to #28; the larger the gauge, the smaller the shaft's diameter

generic name A drug's approved nonproprietary or official name

genome The genetic material of a human or other organism; it includes genes and noncoding sequences of sequences of DNA and RNA

genome medicine An emerging medical discipline involving use of genomic information as part of clinical care

gestation (jes-STAY-shun) The period of fetal development from conception until birth; about 40 weeks

gestational diabetes mellitus (jeh-STAY-shuh-nul) Disorder that may develop during pregnancy; symptoms may be similar to type 2 diabetes

gigantism (jy-GANT-izm) A condition in which the entire body or any of its parts is abnormally large

gingival hyperplasia (JIN-jih-vul hi-per-PLAY-zhuh) An increase in the number of cells in the gums of the mouth, causing them to have a swollen appearance

gingivostomatitis (jin-jih-voh-sto-mah-TY-tis) Sores in the mouth caused by a viral infection such as herpes simplex virus type 1 (HSV-1)

glaucoma (glauw-KO-muh) A disorder that damages the optic nerve and is often caused by elevated intraocular pressure

globulins (GLOB-yoo-linz) Proteins present in blood that contain antibodies

glomerular capsule (gloh-MAYR-yoo-lar KAP-sool) A thin-walled, sac-like structure of the renal corpuscle that surrounds the glomerulus

glomerular filtration Separation of wastes from body water to produce urine; occurs in the glomerulus

glomerulus (gloh-MAYR-yoo-lus) A filtering unit of the nephron composed of a cluster of blood capillaries

glucagon (GLOO-kuh-gon) Hormone secreted when blood glucose levels are low

glucuronidation (gloo-kyoor-on-ih-DAY-shun) The addition of glucuronic acid to a substrate, often involved in metabolism of drugs and other substances; also called *glucuronosylation*

glycerol (GLIH-ser-rawl) Also called *glycerine* or *glycerin*; a sugar alcohol compound used as a sweetener, moistening substance, or component of pharmaceutical formulations

glycoprotein A specific serum protein that binds to many basic drugs

glycoside (GLY-ko-side) An organic compound that yields sugar and non-sugar substances when hydrolyzed; an important cardiac glycoside is digoxin

goiter (GOY-ter) A swelling of the thyroid gland resulting from a shortage of iodine in the diet

grain Basic unit of weight of the apothecary system

gram The unit of weight of the metric system (equivalent to 15.432358 grains)

Gram-negative Refers to bacteria that cannot resist decolorization with alcohol after being treated with Gram's crystal violet; among these bacteria are *Escherichia coli*, *Salmonella spp.*, and other *Enterobacteriaceae*, *Pseudomonas*, *Moraxella*, *Helicobacter*, and *Legionella spp.*

Gram-positive Refers to bacteria that have the ability to resist decolorization with alcohol after being treated with Gram's crystal violet stain, imparting a violet color to the bacterium when viewed by a microscope; includes *Bacillus*, *Listeria*, *Staphylococcus*, *Streptococcus*, *Enterococcus*, and *Clostridium spp.*

Graves' disease   A disorder in which the thyroid gland is overactive; characterized by numerous eye problems

half-life (t1/2)   The time taken for the blood or plasma concentration of the drug to decrease from full to one-half

hallucinogens   Psychedelics, dissociatives, and deliriants—all of which are psychoactive drugs that can cause subjective changes in perception, thought, emotion, and consciousness

hapten   A small molecule that elicits an immune response only when attached to a protein or other large carrier

helper T-lymphocytes   T-cells that play an important role in the adaptive immune system; they release T-cell cytokines, which help the activities of other immune cells; essential in B-cell antibody class switching, actions of cytotoxic T-cells, and in maximizing bactericidal activity of phagocytes

hemostasis (hee-mo-STAY-sis)   A physiologic progression of several steps that stops bleeding

heparin (HEH-puh-rin)   An anticoagulant commonly administered subcutaneously

herpes keratitis (HER-pees keh-rah-TY-tis)   An HSV infection of the cornea of the eye, which may lead to scarring of the cornea or blindness

herpes labialis (HER-pees lay-bee-AL-lis)   Also called *cold sores*, a type of herpes simplex occurring on the lips or around the mouth; the lesions may recur, usually one to three times per year

histoplasmosis (his-toh-plaz-MOH-sis)   A fungal disease caused by *Histoplasma capsulatum*, found in soil or animal droppings, which primarily affects the lungs; common in AIDS patients

household system   System of measurement used in most American homes that is not precisely accurate

hub   Part of the needle that fits onto the syringe

humoral immunity (HYOO-moh-rul)   Immunity based on the antigen–antibody response; obtained when B cells produce circulating antibodies to act against an antigen

hybridomas (hy-brih-DO-muhz)   Fusion of a single immune cell to tumor cells that are grown in cultures

hydrophilic (hy-dro-FY-lik)   The state of being attracted to, absorbing, or dissolved by water

hypercholesterolemia (hy-per-koh-les-ter-raw-LEE-mee-uh)   Higher-than-normal levels of cholesterol in the blood

hyperglycemia   High blood sugar; a condition in which an excessive amount of glucose circulates in the blood plasma

hyperkalemia (hy-per-kah-LEE-mee-uh)   An abnormally high amount of potassium ions in blood

hyperplasia (hy-per-PLAY-shuh)   Abnormal cell growth

hypersensitivity   A set of undesirable reactions from the normal immune system, which includes allergies and autoimmunity; also called *intolerance* or *hypersensitivity reaction*

hypertension   Blood pressure that is elevated above the normal limits

hypertensive crisis   Severely elevated blood pressure

hyperthyroidism (hy-per-THY-royd-izm)   Overactivity of the thyroid gland

hyperuricemia (hy-per-yoo-rih-SEE-mee-uh)   Elevated blood level of uric acid

hypervitaminosis (hy-per-vy-tuh-mih-NOH-sis)   Excess intake of vitamins

hypodermic (hy-po-DER-mik)   Refers to the administration of drugs under the skin; of or relating to the needles used

hypoglycemia (hy-po-gly-SEE-mee-uh)   An abnormally low blood glucose level

hypokalemia (hy-po-kah-LEE-mee-uh)   An abnormally low concentration of potassium ions in blood

hyponatremia (hy-po-nuh-TREE-mee-uh)   An abnormally low concentration of sodium ions in blood

hypoparathyroidism (hy-po-par-uh-THY-royd-izm)   A rare disorder in which the body produces little or no parathyroid hormone, resulting in an abnormally low level of blood calcium (hypocalcemia)

hypopituitarism (hy-po-pih-TOO-ih-tayr-izm)   Underactivity of the pituitary gland

hypotension   An abnormal condition in which blood pressure is not adequate for full oxygenation of the tissues

hypothyroidism (hy-po-THY-royd-izm)   Underactivity of the thyroid gland

iatrogenic (eye-ah-troh-JEH-nik) Produced inadvertently by medication or other treatment

idiosyncratic (ih-dee-oh-sin-KRAT-ik) Occurring rarely and unpredictably

immune response A specific defense of the body in response to a foreign substance

immunity The ability to resist infection and disease through the activation of specific defenses

immunocompromised (im-myoo-no-KOM-pro-miezd) A weakened immune system

immunoglobulins (ih-myoon-o-GLOB-yoo-linz) Antibodies, derived from human plasma, formed by the body to specific antigens

impotence Also called *erectile dysfunction*; the inability to achieve or maintain an erection long enough to engage in sexual intercourse

improper fraction A fraction with a numerator that is greater than or the same as the denominator

infants Children who are between 29 days old and walking age (typically 1 year)

injectable Medication that can be administered by intradermal (within the skin), subcutaneous (into fatty tissue under the skin), intramuscular (IM; into the muscle), and intravenous (IV; into the vein) injection

insomnia (in-SOM-nee-uh) Inability to sleep normally

insulin (IN-suh-lin) A pancreatic hormone that stimulates glucose metabolism

international units Units standardized by an international agreement; used to show the amount of drug required to produce a certain effect

interstate commerce The commerce, traffic, transportation, and exchange among states of the United States

invasive Pertaining to a route of medication administration that requires insertion of an instrument or device through the skin or a body orifice

iodine A chemical element with nutritive properties; in excessive quantities, it can be cytotoxic

iris Thin diaphragm in the eye that is composed mostly of connective tissue and smooth muscle fibers; the colored portion of an eye

ischemia (is-KEE-mee-uh) Insufficient blood flow to the myocardium

islets of Langerhans (EYE-lits of LANG-ur-hans) Small clusters of cells within the pancreas

isopropyl alcohol A chemical compound commonly used for cleaning and disinfecting; highly toxic if ingested

isotypes (EYE-so-typz) Species of atoms of a chemical element with the same atomic number and position in the periodic table and nearly identical chemical behavior but with differing atomic mass or mass number and different physical properties

jaundice (JAWN-dis) Also called *icterus*; a yellowish pigmentation of the skin, sclera, and other mucous membranes due to high blood bilirubin levels; often seen in liver disease or biliary tract obstruction

keratinization (keh-rat-in-eh-ZAY-shun) Formation of keratin (a horny layer of skin)

keratinocytes (keh-RAH-tin-oh-syts) Epidermal cells that produce keratin

keratolytic (keh-rat-oh-LIH-tik) Referring to agents that separate or loosen the horny layer of the epidermis

kernicterus (ker-NIK-ter-rus) A serious form of jaundice in newborns

lavage (luh-VAAZH) Irrigation or washing-out of an organ or body cavity

lead An element that exists as a soft, malleable metal; used in many construction applications; if ingested, it is toxic to the nervous system

legend drugs Prescription drugs

lens Transparent part of an eye; adjusts to facilitate focusing

leukotriene inhibitors (loo-ko-TRY-een) Drugs that inhibit the production of leukotrienes, which are the cause of the inflammatory response in asthma

lipoatrophy (ly-poh-AT-troh-fee) Localized loss of fat tissue, or atrophy of subcutaneous fat

lipophilic (ly-poh-FIL-lik) Related to the ability to dissolve more easily in lipids than in water

lipoproteins (LY-poh-pro-teenz) Combinations of proteins and lipids, transported within a protein outer shell that allows fats to move through water outside of cells

liter (LEE-ter) The unit of volume of the metric system (equivalent to 1.056688 quarts)

lithium (LITH-ee-um) A drug that reduces the activity of certain neurotransmitters and is used in the treatment of bipolar disorder

loading dose A comparatively large dose given at the beginning of treatment to quickly obtain therapeutic effects

loop of Henle (HEN-lee) A long, U-shaped part of the renal tubule extending through the medulla from the end of the proximal convoluted tubule to the beginning of the distal convoluted tubule

lymph (limf) The fluid that flows through the lymphatic vessels

lymphatic vessels (lim-FAH-tik) Network of vessels of the lymphatic system that begins in peripheral tissues and ends at connections to the venous system

lymphocytes (LIM-foh-sites) White blood cells that manufacture antibodies to overcome infection and disease

lymphoid organs (LIM-foyd) Organs connected to the lymphatic vessels that contain large numbers of lymphocytes

lysosomes (LY-soh-sohmz) A membrane-bound cell organelle, spherical in shape, that contains enzymes able to break down most types of biomolecules

macrominerals (mak-ro-MIH-neh-ruls) Dietary minerals needed by the human body in high quantities

macrophages (MAK-ro-fah-jez) Immune cells derived from monocytes

magnesium carbonate Base element used as an antacid

magnesium sulfate A chemical compound containing magnesium, sulfur, and oxygen; its salt form is used for mineral baths

maintenance doses Doses that keep the plasma drug concentration of a drug continuously in the therapeutic range

major minerals Elements that occur in large amounts in the body (i.e., calcium) and have a daily requirement of more than 100 mg/d

Malassezia furfur **(mal-ah-SEH-zee-ah fur-fur)** A spherical, lipophilic yeast believed to be the causative agent of skin disorders such as *pityriasis versicolor*, *seborrheic dermatitis*, and *dandruff*

malignant (mah-LIG-nent) In terms of cells, rapidly proliferating with an atypical appearance

mast cells Large white blood cells found in connective tissue that contain a wide variety of biochemicals, including histamine; involved in inflammation secondary to injuries and infections and are sometimes implicated in allergic reactions

maximal efficacy The largest effect that a drug can produce

means The two inside terms in a proportion

median effective dose The amount of medication needed to produce a specific response in 50% of patients; abbreviated as ED_{50}

median lethal dose The dose of a medication that is lethal in 50% of a group of test animals; abbreviated as LD_{50}

median toxicity dose The dose of a medication that produces a given toxicity in 50% of patients; abbreviated as TD_{50}

medication A drug or other substance used to treat disease or injury

medication error The inappropriate or incorrect administration of a drug that should be preventable through effective system controls

medication reconciliation Keeping track of a patient's medications as they change health-care providers

melanosis Abnormal dark pigmentation

menorrhagia (men-no-RAH-jee-uh) Abnormally heavy or prolonged menstruation

mercury A chemical element that is a liquid metal at room temperature; it has many industrial applications but is highly toxic upon contact

metabolic acidosis A pH imbalance in which the body has accumulated too much acid and lacks sufficient bicarbonate to neutralize the resulting effects

metabolic alkalosis A pH imbalance in which the body has accumulated too much alkaline, such as bicarbonate, and lacks sufficient acid to neutralize the resulting effects

metabolic tolerance Drug tolerance that results from increased drug metabolism and results in dosages having to be increased to maintain therapeutic levels

metabolism The sum of chemical and physical changes in the tissues, consisting of anabolism and catabolism; also known as *biotransformation*

metabolites (meh-TAB-oh-lyts) Intermediates and products of metabolism

metastasis (meh-TAS-tuh-sis) The spreading of cancer cells from the primary site to secondary sites

meter A unit of length of the metric system (equivalent to 39.37007874 inches)

methyl alcohol Methanol; it has many applications in solvents and fuels but is highly toxic and can cause permanent blindness and death

metric system The most common, most accurate, and safest system of measurement; based on the decimal system

metrorrhagia (mee-tro-RAH-jee-uh) Uterine bleeding that occurs independent of the normal menstrual period

microglial cells (my-kro-GLEE-al) Cells derived from the bone marrow that are native to the central nervous system and retinas; part of the phagocytic system, activated by disease or injury

microminerals Minerals required for normal body functions, but only in trace amounts from the diet

microsomal enzymes Liver enzymes, such as *cytochrome P450*, that play major roles in drug metabolism

migraine A severe headache usually characterized by unilateral pain, with various focal disturbances of the nervous system

milliequivalents (mil-lee-ee-KWIH-vuh-lentz) Measurements used to indicate the strength of certain drugs; more specifically, an expression of the number of grams of equivalent weight of a drug contained in 1 mL of a normal solution

minims (MIH-numz) The basic units of volume of the apothecary system

minimum effective concentration The plasma drug level below which therapeutic effects do not occur

minuend (min-YOO-end) In subtraction, the number from which another number (subtrahend) is subtracted

miscible (MIS-sih-bul) Capable of mixing in any ratio without separation of two different phases

mitosis (my-TOH-sis) The splitting of one cell into two new cells

mixed fraction A fraction that has a whole number and a proper fraction combined and whose value is always greater than one

molds Minute fungi that may form on vegetable or animal matter, associated with decay or dampness; such a mold may also be referred to as *mildew*

monoclonal antibodies (maw-noh-KLO-nul) Types of human proteins that are produced by fusing a single immune cell to tumor cells that are grown in cultures

mucocutaneous (myoo-ko-kyoo-TAY-nee-us) Related to the mucous membranes and skin; especially where these meet, such as at the nasal, oral, vaginal, and anal orifices

mucolytics (myoo-ko-LIT-tiks) Medications capable of dissolving or promoting liquefaction of mucus in the lungs

multiplicand (mul-tih-plih-KAND) The number that is to be multiplied by another number

multiplier (MUL-tih-ply-er) The number that multiplies another number (multiplicand)

muscarinic (mus-kah-RIN-ik) receptors Receptors that innervate smooth muscle and slow the heart rate

Mycoplasma pneumoniae **(MY-koh-plaz-ma noo-MO-nee-yay)** An atypical bacterium that commonly causes respiratory infections, such as tracheobronchitis (chest cold), sore throat, or pneumonia

mycoses (my-KOH-seez) Fungal infections

myocardial infarction (my-oh-KAR-dee-ull in-FARK-shun) MI; heart attack; occurs when a portion of the heart is deprived of blood supply, causing cells to die

myocardium (my-oh-KAR-dee-um) The middle layer and most important structure of the heart; contains the heart muscles that regulate cardiac output

myxedema (mix-uh-DEE-muh) The most severe form of hypothyroidism; often develops in older children and adults and is characterized by swelling of the hands, feet, and face (especially around the eyes); can lead to coma and death

narcotic a medication that induces sleep or stupor and alters mood and behavior

nasogastric (NG) tube (nay-zo-GAS-trik) Tube that is inserted through the nose for feeding or removing gastric secretions

NDA review The process of approval of a new drug application, in which various clinical studies are analyzed for the drug's safety and effectiveness before it is approved

nebulizer (NEH-byoo-ly-zer) A device that disperses a fine-particle mist of medication into the deeper parts of the respiratory tract

necrosis (neh-KRO-sis) Death of cells and tissues, often in a localized area

neonates (NEE-oh-nayts) Newborns from birth to 28 days old

nephrons (NEH-fronz) The functional units of kidneys

nephrotic syndrome (neh-FROT-ik) A clinical state characterized by edema, various abnormal substances present in the urine, decreased plasma albumin, and increased blood cholesterol

neurohypophysis (noor-oh-hy-PO-fih-sis) Posterior lobe of the pituitary gland

neuroleptic Referring to psychotropic drugs used to treat psychosis

neurons Nerve cells

neurotransmitters (noo-roh-TRANZ-mih-ters) Certain chemical substances, concentrated in various parts of the central nervous system, that are released by neurons and allow communication from one nerve cell to another

nicotinic receptors (nik-oh-TIN-ik) Receptors that respond to acetylcholine and nicotine and affect skeletal muscles

nomogram (NAW-mo-gram) A numerical chart that shows relationships between two values

nonherbal supplements Specialty supplements obtained from various animal or plant sources, usually used only for very specific conditions; examples include chondroitin and glucosamine

nonproductive cough A sudden ejection of air from the lungs and through the mouth that does not expel (produce) mucus or fluid from the throat or lungs

nuclear pharmacy A specialty area of pharmacy practice dedicated to the compounding and dispensing of radioactive materials for use in nuclear medicine procedures

nucleoside (NOO-klee-oh-sied) Derived from a nucleic acid

nucleotides (NOO-klee-oh-tiedz) The basic structural subunits of DNA

numerator (NOO-meh-ray-ter) The top number in a fraction

nutrition The process of how the body takes in and uses food and other sources of nutrients for growth and repair of tissues

nystagmus (nis-TAG-mus) A constant, involuntary movement of the eye

oligospermia (ol-lih-go-SPER-mee-uh) A subnormal concentration of spermatozoa in ejaculate

oncogenes (ON-koh-jeenz) Cancer genes that develop from normal genes

oocytes (OO-oh-sites) Female sex cells

oogonia (ooh-ooh-GO-nee-uh) Immature reproductive cells of a female

opiates (OH-pee-uts) Drugs such as morphine, heroin, and codeine, containing or derived from opium and tending to induce sleep and to alleviate pain

opioids (OH-pee-oyds) Drugs that possess some properties characteristic of opiate narcotics, but are not derived from opium

optic nerve Nerve that runs through the back of the eye; transmits electrical pulses from the retina to the brain, providing vision

orphan drugs Drugs developed under the Orphan Drug Act, which provides federal financial incentives to nonprofit and commercial organizations for the development and marketing of drugs used to treat rare diseases (those that affect fewer than 200,000 people in the United States)

osmolality (oz-moh-LAL-ih-tee) The concentration of particles in plasma

osmosis (oz-MOH-sis) The process in which sodium and magnesium ions attract water into the bowel, causing a more liquid stool to be formed

osteopenia (os-tee-oh-PEE-nee-uh) Reduced bone mass

osteoporosis (os-tee-oh-por-OH-sis) Reduced bone mass that compromises normal function and often leads to fractures

ounces Household unit of measurement of weight equivalent to 480 grains or 31.10349 g

overdose A toxic dose of a drug or another substance

oxytocin (awk-see-TOH-sin) A hormone that stimulates powerful uterine contractions; aids labor in its later stages

P-glycoprotein Also known as *permeability glycoprotein*; an important cell membrane protein that pumps many foreign substances out of cells

palliative (PAH-lee-uh-tiv) Able to ease a disease's effects but not able to cure

parafollicular cells (par-uh-fo-LIK-u-lur) Cells in the thyroid gland that release calcitonin

paralytic ileus (par-uh-LIT-ik ILL-ee-us) Absence of peristaltic movements in the intestines

parasites (PAH-rah-syts) Protozoans, roundworms, flatworms, and arthropods

parasympathetic nervous system (pair-ah-sim-pah-THET-ik) The part of the nervous system that slows the heart rate, increases intestinal and glandular activity, and relaxes muscles

parasympatholytics (pair-ah-sim-pah-tho-LIH-tiks) Drugs that inhibit the actions of acetylcholine by occupying the acetylcholine receptors

parenteral (puh-REN-teh-rul) Introduction of a drug outside of the gastrointestinal tract; generally in injectable form

parkinsonism Any of several neurological conditions that resemble Parkinson's disease and that result from a deficiency or blockage of dopamine caused by degenerative disease, drugs, or toxins

partial response Relating to chemotherapy, a 50% or greater decrease in the tumor size or other objective disease markers and no evidence of any new disease for at least 1 month

passive immunity   The transfer of the effectors of immunity, which are called *immunoglobulins*, from an immune individual to another

pathogenic (pah-thoh-JEH-nik)   Disease causing

pathogens (PAH-tho-jenz)   Bacteria or viruses that invade the body

peak concentration   The highest level at which a drug is present in the body

pediculicides (puh-DIK-yoo-lih-sydz)   Pharmacologic agents that kill lice

pellagra (peh-LEH-gruh)   A condition caused by a deficiency of vitamin B₃ and marked by dementia, dermatitis, diarrhea, and death

peptidoglycan (pep-tih-doe-GLY-kan)   A polymer composed of polysaccharide and peptide chains, found especially in bacterial cell walls; also called a *mucopeptide* or *murein*

percent   A term meaning "hundredths" that can be expressed as a fraction, decimal, or ratio

perinatal (peh-ree-NAY-tul)   Related to the period around childbirth, especially 5 months before and 1 month after birth

peripheral blood circulation   Circulation in the body's extremities

peripheral nervous system (peh-RIF-er-al)   Part of the nervous system that is outside the brain and spinal cord

peripheral resistance   Friction in the arteries as blood flows through the vessels

peristalsis (payr-ih-STALL-sis)   The rhythmic movement of the intestine

petroleum distillates   Compounds extracted by distillation during the refining of crude oil; found in many products, including cosmetics, fertilizers, solvents, and fuels

pH partitioning   The tendency for acids to accumulate in basic fluid compartments and for bases to accumulate in acidic compartments, due to changes in electrical charges

pharmacodynamic tolerance   Drug tolerance that results from receptors adapting to a drug over time because of long-term administration; results in increased drug levels being needed to achieve desired effects

pharmacodynamics (far-muh-koh-dy-NAH-mix)   The biochemical and physiologic effects of drugs and mechanisms of drug action

pharmacogenomics (far-muh-koh-gee-NO-miks)   The use of an individual's genome to choose drugs and doses for treatment

pharmacognosy (far-muh-KOG-nuh-see)   The study of drugs derived from herbal and other natural sources

pharmacokinetics (far-muh-koh-kih-NEH-tix)   The study of the absorption, distribution, biotransformation, metabolism, and excretion of drugs

pharmacology   The study of drugs, including their actions and effects in living body systems

pharmacotherapeutics (far-muh-koh-thayr-ruh-PYOO-tix)   The study of how drugs may be best used in the treatment of illnesses and which drug is most or least appropriate to use for a specific disease

phenol   Carbolic acid; an organic compound produced as a precursor to many materials, primarily plastics and related materials

phenylketonuria   A genetic disorder in which the body lacks the enzyme necessary to metabolize phenylalanine to tyrosine

phospholipid (FOS-foh-lih-pid)   A type of lipid that is a major component of all cell membranes; an example is *lecithin*, found in egg yolks

phosphorus   A highly reactive chemical element used in many products, including explosives, pesticides, toothpaste, and detergents

photophobia   Also called *light sensitivity*; a common symptom of migraine headaches, but may also be related to encephalitis, meningitis, subarachnoid hemorrhage, corneal abrasion, scleritis, conjunctivitis, or dry eye syndrome

photoreceptors   Visual receptor cells of the eye

phylloquinone (fil-loh-KWIH-nohn)   Dietary form of vitamin K₁, which aids in blood clotting and bone development; treatment for warfarin (Coumadin) overdose

physiochemical   Pertaining to both physiology and chemistry

phytomedicine   Herbal-based traditional medical practice using various plant materials for prevention and therapy

placebo   A supposedly inert substance, such as a sugar pill, administered to cause an effect based on the recipient's belief of the substance's effectiveness

plant alkaloids   Physiologically active organic bases containing nitrogen (and usually oxygen) that are found in seed plants; prevent cell division (or meiosis); also called *mitotic inhibitors*

plasma albumin (PLAZ-ma al-BYOO-min)   The major plasma protein in the body, completely synthesized in the liver; it acts as a transport protein for free fatty acids, certain ions, bilirubin, and many drugs

Plasmodium (plaz-MO-dee-um)   A type of protozoa that includes the parasite that causes malaria

plateau (plah-TOH)   A steady level of a drug in the body, built up because of repeated dosages

platelet plug (PLATE-let)   Plug formed by platelets that become sticky and adhere to the inner lining of the injured vessel and to each other

platelets (PLATE-lets)   Megakaryocyte fragments important in the clotting of blood

poison   A substance with chemical actions that may injure, impair, or kill an organism

polar molecules (PO-lar MAW-leh-kyools)   Those in which the center point of the positive charges is different from the center point of the negative charges

polymorphisms (paw-lee-MOR-fiz-ums)   Changes in genomes; also, occurrences of two or more different forms, or *alternative phenotypes*, within the population of a species

polyneuropathy (paw-lee-noo-RAW-pah-thee)   A disease involving a number of peripheral nerves that affects distal fibers most severely; usually symmetrical

polypharmacy   The practice of simultaneously prescribing multiple medicines to a single patient

polysubstance abuse   The overusage of a minimum of three psychoactive substances within a 12-month period

porphyria (por-FEE-ree-uh)   A genetic disorder caused by a deficiency of enzymes of the heme biosynthetic pathway

preanesthetics (pree-an-ess-THEH-tiks)   Agents used to partially sedate patients before surgery

preeclampsia (pre-eh-KLAMP-see-ah)   A disorder of pregnancy characterized by high blood pressure and a large amount of protein in the urine; it usually occurs in the third trimester, worsening over time; it may result in seizures, at which point it is called *eclampsia*

prescription   Prescription is a written order for the preparation of medication

priapism (PRY-uh-pizm)   A painful and prolonged erection

primary hypertension   Hypertension that has no known cause; accounts for 90% of cases

productive cough   A cough that brings up fluid or mucus from the lungs

progesterones   One of the major groups of female sex hormones; promote changes in the uterus during the reproductive cycle

prophylactic dose   A dose that is given in order to prevent a disease

prophylaxis (pro-fih-LAK-sis)   Prevention, as in drug treatment or other therapy that is given to prevent a disease

prostaglandins (prah-stuh-GLAN-dinz)   Hormone-like substances that control blood pressure, contract smooth muscle, and modulate inflammation

protozoan (pro-toh-ZOH-un)   A single-celled, highly mobile microorganism

pruritus (proo-RY-tus)   Itching

psoriasis (soh-RY-uh-sis)   A chronic, relapsing inflammatory skin disorder

psychological treatment   Psychotherapy, involving an intentional, interpersonal relationship used by a trained psychotherapist to aid a client or patient in the problems of living

psychotropic (sy-koh-TRO-pik)   Affecting mental activity, behavior, or perception

ptosis (TOE-sis)   Drooping eyelid

puberty   The phase in development when an individual becomes reproductively functional

pupil   Circular opening in the iris of the eye

Purkinje fibers (pur-KIN-jee)   Specialized conductive fibers located within the walls of the ventricles that conduct an electrical stimulus or impulse that enables the heart to contract in a coordinated fashion

radical cure   A treatment that eliminates a microorganism from blood and tissue

ratio   A mathematical expression that compares the relationship of one number with another number or expresses a part of a whole number

receptor   A specific protein in cell membranes that specific drugs bind to, producing a pharmacologic effect

recommended dietary allowances (RDAs)   Guidelines released every 5 years by the Food and Nutrition Board that are computed to meet the needs of all healthy individuals

red man syndrome   An infusion reaction caused by certain drugs, such as vancomycin, administered too quickly; characterized by flushing and/or erythematous rash affecting the face, neck, and upper torso

refractory (ree-FRAK-toh-ree)   The period during repolarization when cells cannot respond normally to a second stimulus

regional anesthesia Affects a large but limited part of the body and is often used in obstetrics (labor and delivery)

reimportation Importation of a drug into the United States that was originally manufactured in the United States

renal corpuscle (REE-nul KOR-pus-sul) A filtering unit of the nephron composed of a cluster of blood capillaries called a *glomerulus*

renal tubule (REE-nul TOO-byool) The part of the nephron that leads away from the glomerular capsule and becomes highly coiled

renin (REE-nin) A hormone secreted by the kidneys that converts angiotensinogen to angiotensin I

reproductive toxicology Adverse effects on the reproductive system caused by exposure to a toxic chemical

respiratory acidosis An acid imbalance, in which there are excessive amounts of acid, caused by a problem related to breathing

respiratory alkalosis An alkaline imbalance, in which there are excessive amounts of alkaline, caused by a problem related to breathing

retina The inner layer of the eye that contains the visual receptor cells

retinal detachment Separation of the retina from the corneal layer of the eye

retinopathy (ret-tih-NOP-ah-thee) Degeneration of the blood vessels of the retina

reverse transcriptase (tran-SKRIP-tays) An enzyme used to generate complementary DNA from an RNA template in a process called *reverse transcription*; usually linked to a retrovirus such as the hepatitis B virus (HBV)

rickets A deficiency of calcitriol that is characterized by the malformation of skeletal tissue in growing children

risk management departments Divisions of organizations that focus on the identification and management of potential risks in order to minimize them

Roman numeral A number represented by a letter (e.g., I = 1, V = 5, X = 10)

root cause analysis (RNA) A method used in many health care facilities to identify causes of mistakes, reduce risks, and prevent future occurrences

salicylism Aspirin overdose; it can be acute or chronic, with symptoms including nausea and vomiting, abdominal pain, seizures, and cerebral edema

salpingitis (sal-pin-JY-tis) Inflammation or infection of a fallopian tube

sarcomas (sar-KO-muhs) Malignant growths of muscle or connective tissue

scabicides (SKAY-bih-sydz) Pharmacologic drugs that kill mites

scabies (SKAY-beez) A group of dermatologic conditions caused by mites that burrow into the skin, causing intense itching

sclera The outer layer of eye

scored Notched

seborrheic dermatitis (seb-oh-REE-ik der-mah-TY-tis) Also called *dandruff*; a recurring form of dermatitis affecting the scalp, face, and torso, causing the skin to appear flaky, itchy, reddened, and scaly; in infants, this condition is called *cradle cap*

second messenger An intracellular signaling molecule released by a cell to trigger physiological changes such as differentiation, proliferation, migration, survival, and apoptosis

sedatives Tranquilizers; substances that induce sedation by reducing irritability or excitement

seizures Abnormal electrical activity in the brain

sentinel events Unexpected occurrences involving death or serious physical or psychological injury or risk thereof

serotonin (sayr-uh-TOH-nin) A neurotransmitter that causes the blood vessel to go into spasms

serum sickness A reaction to a foreign serum

side effects Consequences other than a condition for which an agent is used; usually considered less severe than adverse effects

sinoatrial (SA) node (syn-oh-AY-tree-ull) The pacemaker; specialized cardiac muscle tissue that initiates one impulse after another; located just beneath the epicardium in the right atrium near the opening of the superior vena cava

soaps Salts of fatty acids, mainly used for washing, bathing, and cleaning and as components of lubricants

somnolence (SAHM-no-lents) A state of near sleep, a strong desire for sleep, or sleeping for unusually long periods

spasticity (spas-TIH-sih-tee) Inability of opposing muscle groups to move in a coordinated manner

sperm Male sex cells

spina bifida (SPY-nuh BIFF-ih-duh) A condition wherein the spinal column is imperfectly closed, resulting in the protrusion of the meninges or spinal cord

spinal anesthesia Injection of anesthetic agent into the subarachnoid space through a spinal needle

spirits Alcohol-containing liquids that may be used pharmaceutically as solvents; also known as *essences*

sporotrichosis (spor-oh-trik-KOH-sis) A fungal infection caused by *Sporothrix schenckii*, found in soil and vegetation; it usually affects the skin

stable disease In terms of cancer, a tumor that neither grows nor shrinks in size

stat (or STAT) Immediately

steatorrhea (stee-at-oh-REE-ah) Elimination of large amounts of fat in the stool

Stevens-Johnson syndrome A form of toxic epidermal necrolysis that is life-threatening, in which cell death causes the epidermis to separate from the dermis

stroke Cerebrovascular accident

stupor (STOO-por) Significant reduction of cognitive sensibility, which may be caused by a disease, narcotics, intoxicants, or other substances

subarachnoid (sub-uh-RAK-noyd) Area of spinal cord beneath the arachnoid membrane or between the arachnoid and pia mater and filled with cerebrospinal fluid

substance abuse Drug abuse; a maladaptive pattern of use of a substance that is not considered dependent but does not exclude dependency

substance-dependent The state of needing a drug or another substance regardless of problems that occur, which are related to the use of the substance

substantia nigra (sub-STAN-shee-uh NY-gra) A large cell mass involved in metabolic disturbances associated with Parkinson's disease

subtherapeutic doses Drug doses that are below the level used to treat diseases

subtrahend (SUB-truh-hend) In subtraction, the number that is to be deducted from another

suspensions Dosage forms that contain undissolved drug particles and must be shaken to evenly distribute them

sustained-release Tablets and capsules that are specially coated and contain several doses so they dissolve at specific times; also called *delayed release* or *timed release*

sympathetic (sim-puh-THEH-tik) Relating to the sympathetic part of the autonomic nervous system or the fight-or-flight response

sympathetic nervous system The part of the nervous system that accelerates heart rate, constricts blood vessels, and raises blood pressure

sympathomimetics (sim-pah-tho-mi-MEH-tiks) Adrenergic agonists

symptomatology The branch of medicine focused on symptoms of disease, their productions, and the indications they relate to

synapses (SIN-aps-eez) The point of contact between nerve cells and each other or other types of cells

syndrome (SIN-drohm) A collection of signs and symptoms that together signify a specific disease

syrups Aqueous solutions containing a high concentration of sugars; also known as *linctuses*

systole Ventricles relax and heart stops ejecting blood

tablet A solid dosage form that is made by compressing the powdered form of a drug and bulk filling material under high pressure

tachycardia (tak-ee-KAR-dee-uh) An abnormally fast heartbeat

tachyphylaxis (tak-ee-fih-LAK-sis) A reduction in response to a drug caused by repeated doses over a short period of time

tachypnea (tak-IP-nee-uh) Abnormally rapid breathing

tachyzoites (tah-kee-ZO-eyetz) Rapidly multiplying cells as part of certain coccidial infections such as toxoplasmosis

tardive dyskinesia (TAR-div dis-kih-NEE-zhah) Slowed ability to make voluntary movements

target molecules Specific molecules to which a hormone or other substance or agent is attracted; a target molecule has functional receptors for these substances or agents

teratogenic (teh-rah-toh-JEN-ik) Able to cause birth defects in fetuses

teratogenicity (teh-rat-oh-jeh-NIH-sih-tee) Related to the development of malformations of an embryo or fetus

teratogens (teh-RAT-oh-jens) Agents that can cause birth defects

teratology (the-rat-TAH-lo-jee) The study of birth defects

testosterone The most abundant androgen

tetrahydrocannabinol (THC) The main psychoactive substance found in the cannabis plant

therapeutic Meant to treat a disease or disorder

therapeutic index Information about a drug that is used to predict whether a certain dosage is safe for a specific patient

therapeutic range A level between the minimum effective concentration of a drug and its toxic concentration; drug dosing is based on keeping plasma drug levels within this range

thermodynamics A branch of physics concerned with heat and temperature and their relation to energy and work

thiazides The most commonly prescribed class of diuretics

thrombi (THROM-by) Blood clots that form within a blood vessel and attach to the site of formation

thromboembolism (throm-bo-EM-bo-lizm) The blocking of a blood vessel by a particle that has broken away from a blood clot at its site of formation

thrombophlebitis (throm-bo-fleh-BY-tis) Swelling (inflammation) of a vein caused by a blood clot

thrush A yeast infection in the mouth caused by *Candida albicans*, a normal resident of the gastrointestinal tract and vagina

thyrotoxicosis (thy-ro-toks-ih-KOH-sis) Graves' disease; a disorder in which the thyroid gland is overactive; characterized by numerous eye problems

tidal volume (TY-dul) The lung volume representing the normal volume of air displaced between normal inspiration and expiration when extra effort is not applied

tinea corporis (TIN-ee-ah KOR-poh-ris) A fungal infection of the skin, usually on the arms or legs

tinea cruris (TIN-ee-ah KROO-ris) Also called *jock itch*; a fungal infection of the groin region that mostly affects males

tinea pedis (TIN-ee-ah PEH-dis) Also called *athlete's foot*; a fungal infection of the feet, primarily between the toes

tinea versicolor (TIN-ee-ah VER-sih-kul-ler) A fungal infection of the trunk and proximal extremities

tobacco dependence The need for tobacco regardless of problems it may be causing to the health of the user

toddlers Children between approximately 1 and 3 years of age

tolerance The body's slow adaptation to a drug; increasingly higher doses are required to achieve the same effect; reduced responsiveness to a drug

toluene A clear, water-insoluble liquid that is an important organic solvent; if inhaled, it can cause severe neurological harm

tonic–clonic Contraction–relaxation

total body water Amount of water in the body

total parenteral nutrition (TPN) Intravenously administered fluids that supply all of a patient's daily nutritional requirements

toxic concentration The plasma level at which toxic effects of a drug begin to occur

toxic effects Outcomes produced by an intensification of drug effects that would normally produce a therapeutic response

toxic epidermal necrolysis (neh-KRAW-lih-sis) A potentially life-threatening dermatologic disorder characterized by widespread erythema, necrosis, and bullous detachment of the epidermis and mucous membranes; results in exfoliation and possible sepsis and/or death

toxicity (tok-SIH-sih-tee) The state of being noxious; refers to a drug's ability to poison the body

toxin (TOKS-in) A chemical produced by a microorganism that can be harmful

toxoids (TOKS-oyds) Protein toxins that have been modified to reduce their hazardous properties without significantly altering their antigenic properties

***Toxoplasma gondii* (tok-so-PLAZ-ma GON-dy)** A parasitic protozoan that causes the disease *toxoplasmosis*, which may be spread from cats to humans

trade name A drug's proprietary or brand name

transplacental (trans-plah-SEN-tul) Related to the ability of a toxin or pathogen to cross the physical and biological barriers of the placenta separating the mother and fetus, to whom such substances may be dangerous

***Trichophyton mentagrophytes* (trih-KAW-fih-ton men-tay-gro-FY-teez)** A fungus primarily spread from animals to humans that produces inflammatory skin or scalp lesions

***Trichophyton rubrum* (trih-KAW-fih-ton ROOB-rum)** A fungus that colonizes the upper layers of dead skin; the most common cause of athlete's foot, onychomycosis, jock itch, and ringworm

triglyceride (try-GLIH-ser-ryd) An ester derived from glycerol and three fatty acids that is the main constituent of body fat; in the blood, triglycerides enable transference of adipose fat and blood glucose from the liver

trough concentration The lowest level at which a drug is present in the body

***Trypanosoma cruzi* (trih-pan-oh-SO-ma KROO-zee)** A species of parasitic protozoan that may cause *trypanosomiasis* diseases such as *Chagas disease* or *sleeping sickness*; the protozoan is transmitted through insect bites

tubular reabsorption The method by which the kidneys selectively reclaim just the right amounts of substances that the body requires, such as water, electrolytes, and glucose

tubular secretion The method by which the cells of the tubules remove certain substances from the blood and deposit them into the fluid in the tubules

tumor suppressor genes A category of genes involved in carcinogenesis; they regulate and inhibit inappropriate cellular growth and proliferation

ulcers Breaks in skin or mucous membrane with loss of surface tissue, disintegration and necrosis of epithelial tissue, and often, pus

unit A standard of measure, weight, or any other similar quality

urea (yoo-REE-uh) The most abundant organic waste that results in the breakdown of amino acids

uric acid (YOO-rik) A type of waste molecule formed by the recycling of nitrogenous base from RNA molecules

vaccination (vak-sih-NAY-shun) Active immunization

vaccine (vak-SEEN) A preparation of killed microorganisms, living attenuated organisms, or living virulent organisms that are administered to produce or artificially increase immunity to a particular disease

vasodilation (vass-oh-dy-LAY-shun) Dilation of blood vessels; this action relaxes the smooth muscle of the peripheral arterioles

vasopressin (vaz-oh-PRESS-in) A peptide hormone of the posterior pituitary gland; also called *antidiuretic hormone (ADH)*

vasospasms (VAY-soh-spah-zims) Spasms of the blood vessels

ventricles (VEN-trih-kuls) The lower heart chambers that pump blood out of the heart

vertigo (VER-tih-go) A sensation of revolving—either of the patient themselves or of their environment

virions Complete viral particles that are extracellular, and can survive in crystalline forms to infect living cells

virulence (VEER-roo-lents) The degree to which a microorganism is able to produce disease

viruses Tiny genetic parasites that require the host cell to replicate and spread

vitreous humor (VIT-ree-us) Transparent, jelly-like fluid in the posterior cavity of the eye; supports the internal parts of the eye and helps maintain the eye's shape

volatile liquids Inhalation of anesthetic agents that are easily vaporized liquids

water deficit Low levels of body water; dehydration

water of metabolism The volume of body water that is a by-product of the oxidative metabolism of nutrients (about 10%)

wheal A slightly reddened, raised lesion

whooping cough Also known as *pertussis*; a bacterial infection of the nose and throat, with cold-like symptoms, that eventually develops coughing spells that have a "whooping" sound as the patient tries to breathe in air

withdrawal The effects felt by a person when discontinuing or reducing the use of a substance

xanthine derivatives (ZAN-theen) A group of drugs chemically related to caffeine that dilate bronchioles in the lungs

xenobiotics (zee-no-by-AW-tik) Chemical compounds, including drugs, that are foreign to an organism since they are not normally produced or expected to be present

yeasts Eukaryotic, single-celled fungi that reproduce by mitosis or budding; certain species, such as *Candida albicans*, are opportunistic pathogens that can cause various infections

Index